Drugs in Use

Clinical case studies for pharmacists

Fourth edition

Edited by

Linda J Dodds

London • Chicago Pharmaceutical Press

For Peter, Graham and Elizabeth
and my parents Alan and Jean Birdsell

Published by the Pharmaceutical Press
An imprint of RPS Publishing

1 Lambeth High Street, London SE1 7JN, UK
100 South Atkinson Road, Suite 200, Grayslake, IL 60030-7820, USA

First edition published 1991
Second edition published 1996
Third edition published 2004
Fourth edition published 2010

Typeset by Photoprint, Torquay, Devon, UK
Printed in Great Britain by TJ International, Padstow, Cornwall, UK

ISBN 978 0 85369 791 6

A catalogue record for this book is available from the British Library.

Front cover image: © Steve Percival/Science Photo Library

Contents

Preface

When I first conceived this book, back in the late 1980s, cutting-edge pharmaceutical practice was taking place primarily in hospitals, and 'clinical pharmacist' was a somewhat elitist term applied to the smallish number of hospital pharmacists who contributed to the direct care of patients on hospital wards but rarely got involved in actually writing the prescription or independently adjusting drug dosage.

Twenty years on, most practising pharmacists can justly be described as 'clinical' pharmacists. Pharmacists are independent prescribers in a wide range of clinical areas and working under patient group directions to supply and administer medicines without a prescription. In hospitals, consultant pharmacists have their own case load of patients and provide the highest levels of pharmaceutical care as well as contributing to research and development in their chosen specialty, whereas in the community, pharmacists with a special interest are being commissioned to provide high-level services that contribute to the overall care of patients in their specialty area. In hospitals most pharmacists spend a large part of their day working on the wards providing direct patient care, such as taking drug histories, advising on and monitoring therapy, and supporting discharge. In the community pharmacists are being commissioned to contribute to the management of patients with long-term as well as acute conditions, provide medicines use reviews to support adherence, and are seen as a key source of advice and support for preventative health measures, providing immunisations, helping patients to stop smoking and lose weight, and carrying out NHS health checks. The career opportunities for pharmacists in primary care have also expanded. Pharmacists can now be found working in GP surgeries, helping GPs to optimise their prescribing, and running medication review or specialist clinics, and pharmacists in NHS commissioning organisations are bringing their knowledge and skills to the commissioning and monitoring of NHS services involving medicines, as well as to the area of public health.

Each of these roles requires clinical knowledge and skills. This places new and exciting demands on individual pharmacists which need to be supported by undergraduate and postgraduate education, and followed up by appropriate – and now mandatory – continuing professional development.

Translating the knowledge acquired during undergraduate and postgraduate pharmacy courses into the clinical skills required to optimise the therapy of an individual patient and identify and meet all that patient's other pharmaceutical needs can seem a daunting task. Patients rarely have a single disease with a textbook presentation, and many factors can influence the choice of therapy, such as comorbidities and their treatments, previous medical and drug history, changes in clinical opinion on drug use etc. In addition, the patient's views on their treatments and the need for medicines must be taken into account in the care plan that is drawn up. Without an appreciation of all of these factors it can be difficult to understand the reason for a therapy decision that has already been taken, or to respond appropriately to questions regarding the choice of agent from a selection of similar products, or even to know when it is appropriate to offer drug-related information. If it is not clear why a particular product has been prescribed, it is also more difficult to monitor its usage appropriately and to counsel the patient.

One way of acquiring the extra knowledge and skills needed to contribute effectively to the care of individual patients is to work with, and to learn from, experienced clinical pharmacists. Unfortunately, such role models are not accessible to all. This book was therefore conceived as a method of helping pharmacists to 'bridge the gap' between the acquisition of theoretical knowledge about drugs and its practical application to individual patients.

Pharmacists with considerable experience of the clinical use of drugs have been asked to share their expertise by contributing a case study in an area of special interest to them. The topics chosen for inclusion in the book are ones which are either commonly encountered, associated with particular difficulties in dosage individualisation, or in which major advances in therapeutics have occurred in recent years. This fourth edition has been expanded to include new disease areas such as Crohn's disease, oncology, substance misuse, eczema and psoriasis, and many of the chapters featured in previous editions have had a major revision to reflect new evidence concerning optimal care, thereby reinforcing the importance of the need for all healthcare practitioners to keep abreast of medical advances and changes in practice. The chapters have been written by practitioners in primary and secondary care, and the cases cover patients who present and require pharmaceutical care in both sectors. Because patients move between care settings in the course of their disease and treatment, it is vital that pharmacists who care for them at any point along their path have the knowledge and skills to ensure their medicines management is optimal wherever they receive care.

I should like to take this opportunity to thank all the pharmacists who have contributed material for this fourth edition of *Drugs in Use*. Preparing case studies requires an enormous amount of time and effort, and everyone involved has given unstintingly of both. Once again the authors have had to adhere to a tight schedule to ensure the shortest possible time between the preparation of material and its publication. The reward for all this is largely the hope that the book will be of use to pharmacists who are committed to improving their clinical skills.

Linda J Dodds
May 2009

About the editor

Linda Dodds is currently Joint Acting Director of Clinical Pharmacy for East and South East England Specialist Pharmacy Services. This specialist pharmacy services team supports pharmacists working in all sectors across four Strategic Health Authorities which cover approximately 40% of the UK population, with the clinical pharmacy directorate having the responsibility to drive innovation and development in clinical pharmacy services. Linda is also a teacher practitioner at the Medway School of Pharmacy, where she has developed and delivers postgraduate programmes, including a Masters in Medicines Management, and the Diploma in General Pharmacy Practice for hospital and community pharmacists.

Prior to these roles Linda was a pharmaceutical adviser, first to a Health Authority and latterly to primary care organisations, but for a large part of her career she worked in hospitals, most recently as a Clinical Services Manager and Clinical Trainer. She has contributed as an author and editor to a variety of clinical pharmacy publications, and worked part-time as a community pharmacist. In 1992 and 1996 she was external examiner for the MSc in Clinical Pharmacy at the University of Otago, Dunedin, New Zealand.

Throughout her career Linda has undertaken and published pharmacy practice research on a variety of topics. Most recently she has been involved in projects to support the implementation of the NPSA/NICE safety solution on medicines reconciliation, and in supporting hospital clinical services redesign.

Contributors

Christopher Acomb, BPharm, MPharm, MRPharmS
Clinical Pharmacy Manager (Professional Development), Leeds Teaching Hospitals, Leeds UK

Caroline Ashley, BPharm, MSc, MRPharmS
Lead Pharmacist Renal Services, Royal Free Hampstead NHS Trust, London, UK

Rosemary Blackie, MPharm, MRPharmS, IPresc
Community Pharmacist

David Bryant, BSc, MSc (Clin Pharm), MRPharmS
Pharmaceutical Services Manager, Luto Research Limited, Leeds Innovation Centre, Leeds, UK

Toby G D Capstick, BSc, DipClinPharm, MRPharmS
Lead Respiratory Pharmacist, Leeds Teaching Hospitals NHS Trust, Leeds, UK

Gillian F Cavell, BPharm, MSc (Clin), MRPharmS, IPresc
Consultant Pharmacist in Medication Safety and Deputy Director of Pharmacy, Medication Safety, King's College Hospital, London, UK

Christine M Clark, BSc, MSc, PhD, FRPharmS, FCPP (Hon)
Freelance medical writer and independent pharmaceutical consultant and Chairman of the Skin Care Campaign

Andrew Clark, BSc, MSc (Clin), MRPharmS
Specialist Clinical Pharmacist Gastroenterology and Surgery, Guy's and St Thomas' NHS Foundation Trust, London UK

Anne Cole, BSc, MSc, MRPharmS
Specialist Clinical Pharmacist, Somerset Partnership NHS Foundation Trust, Taunton, UK

Aileen D Currie, BSc, MRPharmS,
Senior Pharmacist Renal Services, Crosshouse Hospital, Kilmarnock, UK

Elizabeth Davies, BSc, DipPharmPrac, MRPharmS, IPresc
Macmillan Specialist Pharmacist (Lead Pharmacist for Haematology and HIV Services), Central Manchester University Hospitals NHS Foundation Trust, Manchester, UK

Stan Dobrzanski, BPharm, PhD, MRPharmS
Pharmacy Clinical Services Manager, Bradford Teaching Hospitals NHS Foundation Trust, Bradford, UK

Benjamin J Dorward, BSc, DipClinPharm, MRPharmS
Lead Neurosciences Pharmacist, Sheffield Teaching Hospitals NHS Foundation Trust, Sheffield, UK

Tobias Dreischulte, MSc (Clin), MRPharmS
Research Pharmacist, NHS Tayside and Community Health Sciences Division, University of Dundee, Dundee, UK

Jacqueline Eastwood, BSc, MRPharmS
Pharmacy Manager, St Mark's Hospital, Harrow, London, UK and Chairman of the British Pharmaceutical Nutrition Group

Simon Gabe, MD, MSc, BSc, MBBS, FRCP
Consultant Gastroenterologist, St Mark's Hospital, Harrow, London UK and Co-chair Lennard-Jones Intestinal Failure Unit and Honorary Senior Lecturer

Stuart Gill-Banham, BSc, MRPharmS, MCMHP
Clinical Lecturer, Medway School of Pharmacy and Honorary Senior Clinical Pharmacist, Oxleas NHS Foundation Trust, Bexley, UK

Rachel Hall, BPharm, MRPharmS, PGCert, IPresc
Clinical Pharmacist at The Old School Surgery, Bristol, UK

Tina Hawkins, BSc, Clin Dip Pharm, MRPharmS, IPresc
Advanced Clinical Pharmacist – Rheumatology, Leeds Teaching Hospital NHS Trust, Leeds, UK

Colin Hardman, MPharm, MRPharmS, MCPP
Senior Pharmacist, United Lincolnshire Hospitals NHS Trust, Lincoln, UK

Stephen A Hudson, BPharm, MPharm, FRPharmS
Professor of Pharmaceutical Care, Strathclyde Institute of Pharmacy and Biomedical Sciences, University of Strathclyde, Glasgow, UK

Sarah Knighton, MPharm, DipClinPharm, MRPharmS, IPresc
Pharmacy Team Leader, Liver Services, King's College Hospital NHS Foundation Trust, London, UK

Kym Lowder, BPharm, MSc, MRPharmS
Independent Pharmaceutical Adviser and NPC Medicines Management Facilitator, Kent, UK

Jonathan Mason, BSc, MSc, DIC, MPhil, MRPharmS
Head of Prescribing and Pharmacy, NHS City and Hackney, London UK and National Clinical Director for Primary Care and Community Pharmacy, Department of Health

John J McAnaw, BSc, PhD, MRPharmS
Head of Pharmacy, NHS 24 and Honorary Lecturer in Clinical Practice, University of Strathclyde, Glasgow, UK

Duncan McRobbie, BPharm, MSc (Clin), MRPharmS
Associate Chief Pharmacist, Clinical Services, Guy's and St Thomas' NHS Foundation Trust, London UK and Visiting Professor, London School of Pharmacy.

Sharron Millen, BSc, Clin Dip, MRPharmS
Head of Clinical Pharmacy, Southampton General Hospital, Southampton, UK

Charles Morecroft, BSc(Pharm), BSc(Psychol), Msc, PhD, PGCert, FHEA, FRPharmS
Principal Lecturer, Pharmacy Practice and Programme Leader, Postgraduate Pharmacy, Liverpool John Moores University, Liverpool, UK

Anna C Murphy, BSc, MSc (Clin), MRPharmS
Consultant Respiratory Pharmacist, University Hospitals of Leicester NHS Trust, Leicester, UK

Carol Paton, BSc, DipClinPharm, MRPharmS
Chief Pharmacist, Oxleas NHS Foundation Trust, Bexley, Kent, UK

Stuart Richardson, BPharm, DipClinPharm, MRPharmS
Deputy Chief Pharmacist, Ealing Hospital, Ealing UK (and previously Lead Clinical Pharmacist, neurosciences, King's College Hospital, London)

John A Sexton, BPharm, MSc, PGCertEd (HE), MRPharmS, MCCP
Principal Pharmacist Lecturer-Practitioner, Royal Liverpool and Broadgreen University Hospitals NHS Trust and Liverpool John Moores University, Liverpool, UK

Nicola Stoner, BSc, PhD, MRPharmS, SPresc, IPresc, FCPP
Consultant Pharmacist – Cancer, Oxford Radcliffe Hospital and Honorary Principal Visiting Fellow, The School of Pharmacy, University of Reading, UK

Denise A Taylor, MSc, DipPharm(NZ), MRPharmS, FHEA
Senior Teaching Fellow in Clinical Pharmacy and Programme Lead for Pharmacist Prescribing, University of Bath, Bath, UK

Derek Taylor, BPharm, MSc (Clin), MCPP, MRPharmS
Deputy Chief Pharmacist (Medical Services), Liverpool Heart and Chest Hospital NHS Trust, UK & Chairman, UKCPA Care of the Elderly Group

Peter A Taylor, BPharm, MPharm, MRPharmS
Director of Pharmacy and Medicines Management, Airedale NHS Trust, Yorkshire, UK and Honorary Visiting Professor of Pharmacy Practice, University of Bradford.

Helen Thorp, BSc, DipClinPharm, MRPharmS
Medicines Finance and Commissioning Pharmacist, Leeds Teaching Hospitals NHS Trust, Leeds, UK

Stephen Tomlin, BPharm, MRPharmS, ACPP
Consultant Pharmacist – Children's Services, Guy's and St Thomas' NHS Foundation Trust, London UK and Chair of the Faculty of Neonatal & Paediatric Pharmacists Group (CPP)

Helen Williams, BPharm, PgDip Clin Cardiol, MRPharmS, IPresc
Consultant Pharmacist for Cardiovascular Disease, South East London and Lead Pharmacist for the South London Cardiac and Stroke Networks

Notes on the use of this book

This book has been written to help demonstrate how the specialised knowledge and skills possessed by pharmacists can be applied to the care of individual patients. It is a teaching aid and should not be regarded, or used, as a pharmacology textbook.

The case studies and questions have been kept separate from the answers in order to encourage readers to formulate their own answers before reading the author's. A short reading list can be found at the end of each case study. This should help to supplement the information supplied in the answers.

The background information provided on each patient has been kept to the level that should be easily accessible to the pharmacist, either by consulting the medical notes or through discussions with the patient's physician. Although many of the patients in this book are presented as hospital inpatients, the problems suffered by most of them, and the consequent need for pharmacist input, could just as easily occur if they were living in the community and receiving care from their GP.

The questions interspersing the case presentation aim to reflect those frequently asked by other healthcare professionals, plus those that should be considered by a pharmacist when the prescription is seen. In some cases questions have also been inserted to help ensure the reader appreciates the specialist techniques used to assess patients with the problems under discussion. In order to ensure that the overall pharmaceutical care of the patient is considered, as well as specific problems, at least one question for each patient relates to the construction of a pharmaceutical care plan.

The observant reader will notice that the reference ranges for some laboratory indices vary between case studies. This reflects the normal practice of an individual laboratory setting its own reference ranges.

The answer sections illustrate how the questions should be approached and what factors should be taken into consideration when resolving them. The answers are based on clinical opinion current at the time of writing, but to some degree they also represent the opinions of the authors themselves. It is thus highly likely that after studying the literature and taking into account new drugs and new information that may have become available since the case studies were prepared, some readers will disagree with decisions arrived at by the authors. This is entirely appropriate in a book endeavouring to teach decision-making skills in complex areas where there is rarely an absolutely right or wrong answer. Indeed, it is hoped that the questions raised in the case studies will generate discussion and argument between pharmacists, as it is through such debate that communication skills are developed. The ability to put forward and defend drug therapy decisions to other healthcare professionals is almost as important a skill to the pharmacist wishing to develop his or her clinical involvement as the ability to make such decisions.

Finally, as this book is intended for teaching purposes and not as a reference work, it has been indexed to disease states and approved drug names only.

Abbreviations

5-ASA	5-aminosalicylic acid
5-HT	5-hydroxytryptamine
6MP	6-mercaptopurine
8-MOP	8-methoxypsoralen
ABCD	disc-shaped cholesteryl sulphate–amphotericin B complexes
ACCP	American College of Chest Physicians
ACE	angiotensin-converting enzyme
ACEI	angiotensin-converting enzyme inhibitor
ACS	acute coronary syndrome
AD	Alzheimer's disease
ADAS-cog	Alzheimer's Disease Assessment Scale – cognitive subscale
ADL	activities of daily living
ADP	adenosine diphosphate
ADR	adverse drug reaction
AED	antiepileptic drug
AF	atrial fibrillation
AGE	advanced glycation end-product
AIDS	acquired immunodeficiency syndrome
ALD	alcoholic liver disease
ALG	anti-lymphocyte immunoglobulin
ALP	alkaline phosphatase
ALT	alanine aminotransferase
AMI	acute myocardial infarction
AMP	adenosine monophosphate
AMTS	Abbreviated Mental Test Score
ANA	antinuclear antibody
ANC	absolute neutrophil count
APD	automated peritoneal dialysis
APTT	activated partial thromboplastin time
ARB	angiotensin receptor blocker
ARCD	age-related cognitive decline
ARF	acute renal failure
ARR	absolute risk reduction
AST	aspartate aminotransferase
ATG	anti-thymocyte immunoglobulin
AUC	area under the curve
BAD	British Associaton of Dermatologists
BCG	Bacillus Calmette–Guérin
BCIS	British Cardiovascular Intervention Society
B-CLL	B-cell chronic lymphocytic leukaemia
BHIVA	British HIV Association
BHS	British Hypertension Society
BMD	bone mineral density
BMI	body mass index
BNF	*British National Formulary*

BP	blood pressure/*British Pharmacopoeia*
bpm	beats per minute
BPSD	behavioural and psychological symptoms in dementia
BSG	British Society of Gastroenterologists
BSR	British Society for Rheumatology
BTS	British Thoracic Society
CABG	coronary artery bypass grafting
CAN	chronic allograft neuropathy
CAPD	continuous ambulatory peritoneal dialysis
CAST	Chinese Acute Stroke Trial
CBT	cognitive behavioural therapy
CCB	calcium-channel blocker
CCF	congestive cardiac failure
CD	controlled drug/Crohn's disease
CDAI	Crohn's Disease Activity Index
CDS	continuous dopaminergic stimulation
CFC	chlorofluorocarbon
CHD	coronary heart disease
ChEI	cholinesterase inhibitor
CIBIC	Clinician's Interview-based Impression of Change
CIN	contrast-induced nephropathy
CISH	chromogenic *in situ* hybridisation
CK	creatine kinase
CKD	chronic kidney disease
CK-MB	creatine kinase isoenzyme specific for myocardium
CK-MB%	CK-MB expressed as a percentage of total CK
CMV	cytomegalovirus
CNI	calcineurin inhibitor
CNS	central nervous system
COMT	catechol-*O*-methyl-transferase
COPD	chronic obstructive pulmonary disease
COX	cyclo-oxygenase
CrCl	creatinine clearance
CRP	C-reactive protein
CSM	Committee on Safety of Medicines
CT	computed tomography
CV	cardiovascular
CVD	cardiovascular disease
CVP	central venous pressure
DAAT	Drug and Alcohol Team
DBP	diastolic blood pressure
DEXA	dual energy X-ray absorptiometry
DMARD	disease-modifying anti-rheumatic drug
DRESS	drug rash with eosinophilia systemic symptoms
DSM	*Diagnostic and Statistical Manual of Mental Disorders*
DVLA	Driver & Vehicle Licensing Authority
DVT	deep-vein thrombosis
DXA	dual X-ray absorptiometry
ECG	electrocardiograph/electrocardiogram
ECT	electroconvulsive therapy
EEG	electroencephalogram
EGFR	epidermal growth factor receptor
eGFR	estimated glomerular filtration rate
EMEA	European Agency for the Evaluation of Medicinal Products
EMS	eosinophilia myalgia syndrome
EPSE	extrapyramidal side-effect
ERF	established renal failure

ESA	erythropoietic stimulating agent
ESP	encapsulating sclerosing peritonitis
ESR	erythrocyte sedimentation rate
FBC	full blood count
FEV	forced expiratory volume
FEV_1	forced expiratory volume in 1 minute
FFP	fresh frozen plasma
FISH	fluorescence *in situ* hybridisation
FVC	forced vital capacity
GABA	gamma-aminobutyric acid
G-CSF	granulocyte colony-stimulating factor
GDH-PQQ	glucose dehydrogenase pyrroloquinolinequinone
GFR	glomerular filtration rate
GGT	gamma-glutamyltransferase
GI	gastrointestinal
GM-CSF	granulocyte–macrophage colony-stimulating factor
GMP	guanosine monophosphate
GP	general practitioner
GPwSI	general practitioner with a special interest
GTN	glyceryl trinitrate
GUM	genito-urinary medicine
HAART	highly active antiretroviral therapy
HAMD	Hamilton Depression (scale)
Hb	haemoglobin
HbA_{1c}	glycated haemoglobin
HCA	healthcare assistant
HDL	high-density lipoprotein
HIV	human immunodeficiency virus
HLA	human leukocyte-associated antigen
HMG	hydroxymethylglutaryl
HMG-CoA	hydroxymethylglutaryl coenzyme A
HOPE	Heart Outcomes Prevention Study
HPA	hypothalopituitary–adrenal/Health Protection Agency
HPLC	high-performance liquid chromatography
HR	heart rate
HRT	hormone replacement therapy
HSA	human serum albumin
IBD	inflammatory bowel disease
IBW	ideal body weight
ICS	inhaled corticosteroids
ICU	intensive care unit
IDU	intravenous drug user
IFX	infliximab
IHD	ischaemic heart disease
IL	interleukin
INR	international normalised ratio
IP	intraperitoneal
IPD	idiopathic Parkinson's disease
iPTH	intact parathyroid hormone
IRS	immune reconstitution disease/syndrome
IST	International Stroke Trial
IV	intravenous/intravenously
IVb	intravenous bolus
JME	juvenile myoclonic epilepsy
LABA	long-acting $beta_2$-agonist
LD	loading dose
LDH	lactate dehydrogenase

LDL	low-density lipoprotein
LFT	liver function test
LMWH	low-molecular-weight heparin
LTOT	long-term oxygen therapy
LVEF	left ventricular ejection fraction
LVSD	left ventricular systolic dysfunction
MAC	*Mycobacterium avium* complex
MAG3	^{99m}Tc mercapto acetyl triglycene
MAOBI	monoamine oxidase B inhibitor
MAOI	monoamine oxidase inhibitor
MAP	mean arterial pressure
MCH	mean cell haemoglobin
MCI	mild cognitive impairment
MCV	mean cell volume
MD	maintenance dose
MDI	metered-dose inhaler
MDS	monitored-dosage system
MED	minimal erythemogenic dose
MHRA	Medicines and Healthcare products Regulatory Agency
MI	myocardial infarction
MMF	mycophenolate mofetil
MMSE	Mini Mental State Examination
MPD	minimal phototoxic dose
MRC	Medical Research Council
MRI	magnetic resonance imaging
MRSA	meticillin-resistant *Staphylococcus aureus*
MSA	multiple system atrophy
MUR	medicines use review
NEAD	non-epileptic attack disorder
NFAT	nuclear factor of activated T cells
NHL	non-Hodgkin's lymphoma
NICE	National Institute for Clinical Excellence
NMDA	*N*-methyl-D-aspartate
NMS	non-motor symptoms
NNRTI	non-nucleoside reverse transcriptase inhibitor
NNT	numbers needed to treat
NPSA	National Patient Safety Agency
NRTI	nucleoside reverse transcriptase inhibitor
NSAID	non-steroidal anti-inflammatory drugs
NSF	National Service Framework
NSTEMI	non-ST-elevated myocardial infarction
NYHA	New York Heart Association
OA	osteoarthritis
OBRA	Omnibus Budget Reconciliation Act
OGD	oesophagogastroduodenoscopy
OTC	over-the-counter
PAMI	primary angioplasty
PASI	Psoriasis Area Severity Scale
PCA	patient-controlled analgesia
PCI	percutaneous coronary intervention
PCP	*Pneumocystis carinii* pneumonia
PCT	primary care trust
PCV	primary care visitor/packed cell volume
PD	peritoneal dialysis
PDS	Progressive Deterioration Score
PE	pulmonary embolism
PEF	peak expiratory flow

PI	protease inhibitor
PMR	polymyalgia rheumatica
PODs	patient's own drugs
PPI	proton pump inhibitor
PSP	progressive supranuclear palsy
PT	prothrombin time
PTCA	percutaneous transluminal coronary angioplasty
PTH	parathyroid hormone
PUD	peptic ulcer disease
PUFA	polyunsaturated fatty acids
PUVA	psoralen with ultraviolet A
PV	plasma viscosity
RA	rheumatoid arthritis
RBC	red blood cell
RCT	randomised controlled trial
RRT	renal replacement therapy
RT	rapid tranquillisation
rt-PA	alteplase or recombinant tissue-type plasminogen activator
SBP	systolic blood pressure/spontaneous bacterial peritonitis
SCDT	short-contact dithranol treatment
SD	standard deviation
SERM	selective oestrogen receptor modulator
SIGN	Scottish Intercollegiate Guidelines Network
SLE	systemic lupus erythematosus
SMBG	self-monitoring of blood glucose
SPC	Summary of Product Characteristics
SPECT	single photon emission computed tomography
SpO_2	oxygen saturation
SRH	stigmata of recent haemorrhage
SSRI	selective serotonin reuptake inhibitor
STEMI	ST-elevated myocardial infarction
STN	subthalamic nucleus
STN-DBS	subthalamic deep brain stimulation
SUDEP	sudden unexplained death in epilepsy
TB	tuberculosis
TC	total cholesterol
TCA	tricyclic antidepressant
Th	T-helper (cell)
TIA	transient ischaemic attack
TIPS	transjugular intrahepatic portosystemic shunt
TMPT	thiopurine methyl transferase
TNF	tumour necrosis factor
TNK-tPA	tenecteplase
tPA	tissue plasminogen activator
UA	unstable angina
U&E	urea and electrolytes
UVA	ultraviolet A
UVB	ultraviolet B
VTE	venous thromboembolism
WBC	white blood cell

1

Hypertension

Charles Morecroft and John Sexton

Case study and questions

Day 1 Mr FH, a 48-year-old van driver, was identified by his general practitioner (GP) as having a resting blood pressure of 162/92 mmHg. He was in reasonably good health and purchased over-the-counter (OTC) ibuprofen 400 mg, which he took up to three times daily for arthritis-type pain when necessary. He weighed 95 kg, was 5′7″ tall, and had a resting pulse rate of 82 beats per minute (bpm). He smoked 15 cigarettes per day and drank at least 6 units on 4 nights each week. His total cholesterol (TC) had been measured as 5.9 mmol/L and his high-density lipoprotein (HDL) as 1.5 mmol/L (TC:HDL ratio 4.5).

Q1 Why is it important to control blood pressure?
Q2 How would you assess Mr FH's cardiovascular disease (CVD) risk?
Q3 According to current guidelines, should Mr FH be treated for hypertension?
Q4 What non-drug approaches can Mr FH adopt to reduce his blood pressure and/or his cardiovascular (CV) risks, and why are these important?
Q5 What first-line treatments would be suitable for Mr FH's hypertension?

Month 3 Mr FH had had his blood pressure recorded twice more and the values had been recorded as 160/91 mmHg and 164/92 mmHg. His GP decided to start Mr FH on ramipril.

Q6 Suggest a suitable initial dose, titration regimen, and any monitoring required. What counselling would Mr FH require?
Q7 What other investigations, if any, might be appropriate for Mr FH as a patient newly diagnosed with hypertension?
Q8 What target blood pressure is appropriate for Mr FH?
Q9 How frequently would you monitor Mr FH's progress, in terms of blood pressure values, biochemical tests and possible side-effects?
Q10 Should Mr FH be started on aspirin and a statin?

Mr FH continued to visit his medical centre at 2-monthly intervals, but his blood pressure remained raised, despite the prescribed ramipril. Nine months later, Mr FH was admitted to the Acute Medical Assessment Unit of the local hospital, having collapsed at work with chest pains, which resolved rapidly after sublingual glyceryl trinitrate. He admitted that he had been getting chest pains on exertion for 'a couple of months'. His blood pressure was measured as 165/99 mmHg. His haematology and biochemistry results were as follows:

- Sodium 140 mmol/L (135–145)
- Potassium 4.9 mmol/L (3.5–5)
- Creatinine 130 micro mol/L (<110)
- Haemoglobin 11.2 g/dL (12–18)
- TC 7.1 mmol/L
- Blood glucose 4.1 mmol/L
- Glycated haemoglobin (HbA1c) 6.7%

His current therapy was:

- Ramipril 5 mg daily
- Simvastatin 10 mg daily
- Paracetamol 1 g four times daily when required
- Aspirin 75 mg daily

He admitted to continuing to buy OTC ibuprofen and not being terribly compliant with his statin therapy.

Q11 How can adherence be promoted and a concordant relationship with Mr FH developed?
Q12 What additional medication can be added to further control Mr FH's blood pressure?
Q13 Mr FH wishes to monitor his own blood pressure at home. What would be your recommendation?
Q14 Outline a pharmaceutical care plan for Mr FH.
Q15 What special considerations apply to the management of hypertension in the elderly?

Answers

Why is it important to control blood pressure?

A1 **There is a statistical association between elevated blood pressure values (hypertension) and the development of cardiovascular disease (CVD) and other organ damage, in particular to the eyes and kidneys.**

Large-scale epidemiological studies have shown that morbidity and mortality from ischaemic heart disease (IHD), congestive cardiac failure, cardiac hypertrophy, myocardial infarction (MI) and stroke all increase with rising blood pressure values.

The prevention and treatment of CVD has significantly improved since the introduction of the National Service Framework for Coronary Heart Disease in 2000. Hypertension is only one among many risk factors for developing CVD. Other risk factors include those that are modifiable, for example high cholesterol levels, smoking, impaired glucose metabolism and obesity, and those that are not modifiable, for example age, history of CVD events and gender. However, there is no 'normal' blood pressure, nor is it possible to predict precisely which individual patients are at risk of developing CVD.

Hypertension is a modifiable risk factor for CVD and meta-analysis from the Blood Pressure Lowering Treatment Triallists Collaboration indicates that reducing blood pressure with antihypertensive medication reduces cardiovascular (CV) risk in both young (<65 years of age) and older (≤65 years of age) people. The evidence to date indicates a potential 33% reduction in stroke mortality, 26% reduction in coronary mortality, and a 22% decrease in CV mortality between the treatment and control groups.

Patients who have already developed CVD, or who are considered at high risk (>20% over 10 years) of developing it, require more aggressive and earlier management of their hypertension; however, the management of hypertension should not be viewed in isolation, and other interventions, such as the prescribing of a statin and aspirin, should be considered, based on the assessment of the patient's CVD risk or history of CVD events.

How would you assess Mr FH's cardiovascular disease (CVD) risk?

A2 **In patients with no existing CVD such as Mr FH, a full assessment of risk should be carried out using a validated risk assessment tool, for example the Joint British Societies CV risk assessment charts published in the *British National Formulary* (BNF). This assessment should be used to inform the discussions and decisions regarding possible care options, such as how intensively to intervene, and whether to use pharmacological interventions for blood pressure and associated CV risk.**

Formal estimation of CVD risk should consider age, gender, systolic blood pressure, TC, HDL cholesterol, smoking status and the presence of left ventricular hypertrophy. Other factors should also be taken into account when managing a person's overall CVD risk. These include abdominal obesity, impaired glucose regulation, raised fasting triglyceride levels, and a family history of premature CVD. It is important to be aware that risk assessment tools can under- or overestimate the CVD risk of people from some ethnic groups. For example, the CVD risk for people originating from the Indian subcontinent can be 1.5 times higher than that predicted by an assessment tool.

Mr FH's CVD risk can be calculated using the Joint British Societies risk assessment tool to be about 18% in the next 10 years. Obviously, the clinician carrying out the assessment would also consider his weight, family history, race, and other factors when making a guess about how this crude estimate might apply to Mr FH. Interestingly, Mr FH might be shown how a similar non-smoker has a risk of only 10.9%, which might motivate him to attempt to stop smoking.

The threshold pressure for initiation of therapy is chosen to balance the probable clinical benefit (of avoiding CV events), potential harm (side-effects) and affordability. In the UK, a 'high-risk' patient is one in whom the CVD risk is greater or equal to a 20% risk of suffering CVD over 10 years. This level of risk determines the threshold for initiation of drug treatment for hypertension, and consideration of the use of aspirin and/or a statin. Assessing CVD risk is unnecessary in patients with existing CVD or those considered to be at high risk of CVD because of an existing medical condition, such as diabetes or a familial lipid disorder.

According to current guidelines, should Mr FH be treated for hypertension?

A3 **Not immediately. He is otherwise in good health, has several modifiable risk factors, and is only marginally over one of the two values normally considered as thresholds for drug treatment (160/100 mmHg in most guidelines). The decision to start an otherwise healthy patient on potentially lifelong drug therapy should not be taken lightly, and for patients with a lower CVD risk it might be possible to attempt lifestyle modifications before drug treatment is initiated, and to thus delay the initiation of therapy.**

Thresholds for the treatment of raised blood pressure should take account of the overall CVD risk as well as the blood pressure values. The greater the CVD risk, the greater the potential benefit from treatment. NICE Guidelines for the management of hypertension in primary care published in 2006, and the British Hypertension Society Guidelines, agree that for adults without CV complications and not at high risk (10-year risk ≥20%) of developing CVD, the threshold for treatment should be a sustained blood pressure of ≥160/100 mmHg. If only the diastolic or the systolic pressure is raised, treatment should still be initiated. If there is existing CVD or other organ damage, a 20% or greater chance of developing CVD (or in some guidelines, type 2 diabetes mellitus) then a blood pressure threshold of 140/90 mmHg applies.

Blood pressure is constantly changing, and any individual reading is influenced by a number of factors, such as posture, the time of the day, emotions and exercise. In addition, 'white-coat syndrome', in which the act of engaging in a medical consultation elevates blood pressure, is well recognised. As a result, the potential for misdiagnosis of raised blood pressure is high. To overcome this and to ensure the patient is as relaxed as possible, several readings need to be taken over a period of time before a diagnosis of hypertension is made. The recommended period of time and the number of readings vary according to the severity of the raised blood pressure. The average of the recorded blood pressure values should be used in the risk assessment.

What non-drug approaches can Mr FH adopt to reduce his blood pressure and/or his cardiovascular (CV) risks, and why are these important?

A4 **Non-drug approaches that could be used to reduce Mr FH's blood pressure include losing weight, stopping smoking, reducing his alcohol intake, taking more exercise, amending his intake of salt and caffeine, and avoiding certain over-the-counter (OTC) drugs.**

The use of non-drug approaches may avoid the necessity for drug therapy, or reduce the number of therapies and their doses required to control his blood pressure. In addition, some non-drug therapies that do not in themselves affect blood pressure may radically improve his CV risk, to which blood pressure is only one contributor.

To improve blood pressure values and overall CVD risk patients like Mr FH should:

(a) Adjust their body weight to that approaching an ideal body weight through reduced fat and total calorie intake. Mr FH has a BMI (body mass index) of 32.9 kg/m^2 and is probably obese, though this would require observation as he might just be very muscular. There is an association between overweight and hypertension for patients of all ages, although it is reduced in elderly patients. A reduction in weight usually brings about a corresponding – albeit small – reduction in blood pressure. However, compliance with weight-reducing diets is a problem and not easily maintained. The usual aim is to change specific areas of food intake, particularly the amount of fat consumed. Any changes to a person's diet should incorporate the adoption of a balanced diet and an increase in the consumption of a variety of fruit and vegetables. Mr FH should be encouraged to take responsibility for his weight reduction and should be referred to a dietitian for advice on a suitable diet.

(b) Limit alcohol consumption to 21 units weekly for men or 14 units for women. Mr FH is currently over this limit. It is also important that alcohol consumption, to the recommended value, is spread evenly across the week.

(c) Avoid salty foods and reduce dietary sodium intake to less than 2.4 g/day – the equivalent of 6 g of salt. This is recommended for all patients regardless of whether or not they are receiving active pharmacological treatment. There is some evidence that sodium restriction will result in a small reduction in systolic blood pressure. Although a very significant reduction is difficult, a high sodium intake can negate the effectiveness of antihypertensives and diuretics. Mr FH should receive advice about using salt substitutes (for example Lo-salt), not using salt in cooking, and reducing his intake of high-sodium foods. Increasing the amount of potassium in his diet (for example eating bananas) could also forestall any possible hypokalaemic adverse drug reactions (ADRs) due to diuretics, and is in itself hypotensive.

(d) Take regular physical exercise, especially dynamic rather than isometric exercise. Mr FH has a sedentary job as a van driver. Walking or swimming (for 30–45 minutes three or four times a week) can bring about a modest reduction in blood pressure. It is important that the exercise is regularly maintained, as any benefit is lost 14 days after the exercise ceases.

(e) Stop smoking. Mr FH smokes. Stopping smoking has benefits with respect to his overall CVD risk, although guidelines disagree about whether stopping smoking leads to a direct reduction in blood pressure values. Mr FH should be given advice about smoking cessation programmes and support groups. Drug therapy for smoking cessation should be checked to ensure there are no cautions or contraindications to the use of particular products.

(f) Avoid excessive consumption of coffee (>5 cups) and other caffeine-rich products as these can raise blood pressure.

(g) Some groups of OTC medications may cause problems for hypertensive patients, and all patients should be advised to consult their community pharmacist before purchasing any such medications. For example, antacids can reduce the adsorption of angiotensin-converting enzyme inhibitors (ACEIs), and oral sympathomimetic decongestants can cause an increase in blood pressure. Mr FH should also be advised to be cautious of medications, both prescribed and OTC, that have a high sodium content, e.g. Gaviscon or medications presented in an effervescent formulation. Mr FH is purchasing an OTC-available non-steroidal anti-inflammatory drug NSAID (ibuprofen) for his arthritic-type pain. This class of drug can cause fluid retention and a subsequent increase in blood pressure, and should thus be avoided.

Combinations of the above lifestyle modifications may achieve significant reductions in blood pressure. Approximately 25% of patients undertaking multiple lifestyle modifications achieve an estimated 10 mmHg or more reduction in their blood pressure values in the first year. However, lifestyle alterations can be difficult to achieve. Patients need to be highly motivated, and require regular follow-up and considerable support over a long period of time.

What first-line treatments would be suitable for Mr FH's hypertension?

A5 **The choice of first-line treatment for Mr FH should be influenced by his age, ethnicity and comorbidities. Obviously, some patients will have compelling reasons owing to their comorbidities to use or not use certain therapies, but otherwise the 'ACD' rule can be used as outlined below. This evidence-based guidance looks at the place of three groups of antihypertensives: A(CEIs), C(alcium-channel blockers) and D(iuretics), and guides drug choice based on ethnicity and age.**

Comorbidities. It is important first to consider whether Mr FH has any compelling or relative indications or contraindications to any of the main classes of medication with a substantial evidence base that might be recommended. For example, heart failure would indicate ACEI therapy (or angiotensin receptor blocker therapy if cough is a problem) even in groups for whom they might not otherwise be the preferred initial choice.

Age. Meta-analysis undertaken by NICE recommends that Mr FH (as he is aged <55 years) should be prescribed an ACEI unless he is black. Had Mr FH been 55 or older, a calcium-channel blocker (CCB) or diuretic would have been a more appropriate initial choice.

Ethnicity. If Mr FH was black (of African or Caribbean descent, but not mixed race, Asian or Chinese) guidelines advise that a thiazide diuretic or CCBs (rate-limiting or dihydropyridine) would have been appropriate, regardless of his age.

Given the situation in which the prescriber has a choice of first-line treatments, the actual choice should be made in conjunction with the patient and take account of clinical judgement, risk of adverse effects and patient preferences.

Beta-blockers are no longer considered appropriate for the initial treatment of hypertension unless there are compelling reasons, for example IHD. Beta-blockers have been shown to be less effective than other classes of drug in reducing major CV events, especially stroke, and less effective than ACEIs or CCBs in reducing the risk of diabetes, especially when co-prescribed with a thiazide diuretic.

Suggest a suitable initial dose, titration regimen, and any monitoring required. What counselling would Mr FH require?

A6 The licensed initial dose of ramipril in hypertension is 1.25 mg, increasing every 1–2 weeks to a maximum of 10 mg. Mr FH's renal function and potassium levels should be monitored as well as his blood pressure. Counselling should cover the reasons why his blood pressure is being controlled and what lifestyle issues should be addressed, as well as specific information about ramipril.

The renin–angiotensin–aldosterone system plays a central role in hypertension, producing the potent vasoconstrictor angiotensin II and releasing aldosterone. ACEIs competitively block the enzyme responsible for the conversion of angiotensin I to the active angiotensin II. They promote sodium excretion, both by reducing aldosterone levels and by causing renal vasodilation. They reduce the breakdown of the vasodilatory bradykinins and inhibit local formation of angiotensin II in the tissues. In elderly patients low renin levels are common, but ACEIs still seem effective in reducing blood pressure. They can also be helpful for patients with claudication because of their vasodilatory effects.

Mr FH's baseline serum electrolytes and creatinine levels should be measured. After initiating ramipril Mr FH should have his blood pressure monitored, but also his serum potassium (hyperkalaemia is possible) and his serum creatinine should be rechecked, ideally after a week. ACEIs can cause abrupt renal dysfunction, especially in the presence of renal artery stenosis. Renal artery stenosis, or narrowing, leads to reduced glomerular filtration pressure. Angiotensin II constricts the efferent glomerular arteriole and helps to increase the pressure gradient across the glomerulus. This necessary effect is antagonised by ACEIs and renal hypoperfusion results. Although there is no evidence that Mr FH has renal stenosis, the risk of silent renal artery stenosis is increased if peripheral vascular disease is present.

Mr FH should be given verbal advice and information on why he is taking this medication and what may happen if he does not. Any advice given should be supported with leaflets and a selection of suitable website addresses, as appropriate. As an additional source of information, he should be directed to the patient information leaflets provided with his prescribed antihypertensive medications.

Mr FH should also be told that the first doses of ramipril might be better taken at bedtime, in case a dip in blood pressure leads to dizziness, and that if he develops a dry cough or any perceived adverse event he should report this to his prescriber or pharmacist. In addition, as with any initiation of an antihypertensive treatment, he needs to appreciate that:

(a) He should adhere to the prescribed dose to ensure that he maximises the reduction in blood pressure values for the minimum level of drug therapy.
(b) It may take several changes of dose and drug before his ideal blood pressure is achieved.
(c) He should discuss or report any possible adverse events to his prescriber or pharmacist.
(d) The lifestyle modifications described earlier need to be implemented as they are an adjuvant to reducing blood pressure.
(e) Hypertension is symptomless and he will not feel better in himself (he may feel worse); failure to understand this leads to poor adherence.
(f) OTC NSAIDs (ibuprofen and naproxen) can potentially increase his blood pressure and he should no longer purchase them.

What other investigations, if any, might be appropriate for Mr FH as a patient newly diagnosed with hypertension?

A7 **A number of additional routine biochemical tests are appropriate for newly diagnosed hypertensive patients to aid the accurate profiling of CVD risk, to help detect diabetes or damage to the heart and kidneys caused by raised blood pressure, and to look for possible causes of secondary hypertension such as kidney damage.**

Urine strip test for protein and blood. The presence of protein or blood (proteinuria) in the urine can help to identify patients with kidney damage but cannot distinguish those who have renal disease and secondary hypertension from those whose kidneys have been damaged by the raised blood pressure.

Blood electrolytes and creatinine. Sodium and potassium levels should be checked to exclude hypertension resulting from adrenal disease. Similarly, serum urea and creatinine levels reflect kidney function and are used to exclude kidney disease as a cause of secondary hypertension.

Blood glucose and glycated haemoglobin (HbA_{1c}). These are required to determine whether or not the patient has diabetes.

Serum total and HDL cholesterol. These are required to determine the patient's cholesterol profile.

Currently there is little evidence to support the use of electrocardiograms (ECGs) as a routine investigation to determine the patient's heart rate, rhythm, conduction abnormalities, left ventricular size and damage to heart muscle. However, an ECG might be used to confirm or refute the presence of left ventricular hypertrophy, a variable in the CVD risk assessment.

What target blood pressure is appropriate for Mr FH?

A8 **NICE advises a target blood pressure of <140/90 mmHg.**

This target is supported by the British Hypertension Society (BHS) for uncomplicated patients; however, the BHS Guidelines and the BNF advise a tighter target for high-risk patients (identified as those with CVD, 10-year risk >20%, organ damage, type 2 diabetes mellitus) of 130/80 mmHg, and thus there is some confusion in practice. In renal patients or those with proteinuria even lower targets may be advised.

Of course, some patients never achieve these targets even if motivated and with good professional support, because adverse effects limit what is practicable. For people with hypertension any reduction in blood pressure values is beneficial. Decisions regarding the intensity of treatment and treatment goals should be reached in discussion with the patient.

How frequently would you monitor Mr FH's progress, in terms of blood pressure values, biochemical tests and possible side-effects?

A9 **Blood pressure should be monitored routinely until stable and at the desired level. The Summary of Product Characteristics (SPC) for ramipril suggests increasing the dose every 1–2 weeks, but clearly this depends on the effect it is having, the development of ADRs, and the urgency of the need to reduce blood pressure. Patient adherence to therapy is crucial, so it is essential that they reach an agreement with the prescriber as to the need for treatment. Some guidelines suggest assessing blood pressure after 4 weeks of unchanged therapy before considering the effect of a particular drug dose. After titration is complete, rechecking depends on the patient's condition. Initially the prescriber or the practice nurse might wish to recheck Mr FH's blood pressure monthly, but this could drop to as little as annually in some cases. At each visit, Mr FH can be asked about side-effects. His renal**

function should be monitored a week or so after each increase in ACEI dose, and then annually thereafter.

ACEIs are associated with few serious side-effects. Renal dysfunction may occur, so monitoring of renal function (urea and creatinine) is required. As noted earlier, the deterioration in renal function can be dramatic, and serum urea and creatinine must be checked prior to treatment and shortly after starting an ACEI. Potassium levels may increase because of the inhibition of aldosterone, and should be monitored. For this reason ACEIs should not be co-prescribed with potassium-sparing diuretics.

A dry, irritating cough occurs in up to 15% of patients and should be actively enquired about. It is thought to be mediated by an increase in bradykinin levels.

In addition, each interaction with the patient gives the healthcare professional an opportunity to continue the development of a concordant relationship by identifying and responding to the patient's concerns and anxieties, reaffirming the need for lifestyle modifications, and ascertaining the patient's degree of adherence to the treatment regimen.

Should Mr FH be prescribed aspirin and a statin?

A10 Probably not, unless other risk factors are identified.

Most sources agree that aspirin is reserved for patients over 50 who have either diabetes, a 20% risk over 10 years of developing CVD, or CVD or other organ damage. In addition, blood pressure should be controlled before initiating aspirin. The HOT trial suggests that for well-controlled hypertensive patients over 50 years, aspirin 75 mg daily can reduce CV events by 15% and MI by 36%. However, the risk of non-cerebral bleeding does increase, and this would have to be balanced against the benefits of reducing the risk of coronary heart disease for individual patients.

Similarly, in an otherwise healthy, low-risk patient statins are not currently promoted in the UK, but it would be important for the prescriber to consider Mr FH's family history, CV risk prediction and serum cholesterol level. If the latter was raised, statin therapy might well be indicated for dyslipidaemia.

How can adherence be promoted and a concordant relationship with Mr FH developed?

A11 A more engaged, non-judgemental, and structured approach is indicated.

Mr FH needs to understand the dangers of seemingly benign hypertension. In addition, now that he has developed signs of CVD, tight blood pressure control is even more important. Showing a patient the coloured tables at the back of the BNF often highlights the benefits to be had from smoking cessation. Perhaps the prescriber could try alternative analgesia to avoid Mr FH buying NSAIDs. Is the statin causing muscle pains? Mr FH needs to understand the need for, and benefits of, BP control and risk factor management. As a pharmacist, you need to identify any problems that pharmaceutical intervention could ameliorate.

It is important to ensure that Mr FH understands how to take his medication, and it should be checked that he can, for example, open child-resistant tops and read the container labels.

As with any patient with an increasingly complex drug regimen, tactful enquiries should be made as to how well he manages to take his treatment as prescribed. He should be given further advice on when and how to take his medication. Counselling about drug treatment should be ongoing: a single session is unlikely to have a lasting impact.

Despite the benefits of antihypertensive medication, population studies have demonstrated that hypertensive patients continue to have a substantially higher risk of coronary heart disease and stroke than non-hypertensive individuals, even after several years of treatment.

What additional medication can be added to further control Mr FH's blood pressure?

A12 **A stepped approach to antihypertensive treatment is recommended to achieve target blood pressure values, with the addition of other drugs as necessary. Second-line therapy for Mr FH would be a CCB or diuretic (following the ACD rule); however, as he now has a diagnosis of IHD, his second-line therapy needs to be reconsidered.**

The HOT study suggested that 70% of patients achieve their target blood pressure with more than one antihypertensive, and 24% of patients require three (Mr FH's target would be considered by some doctors to have tightened to <130/80 mmHg because he has developed IHD, although NICE 2006 does not specify this).

When the first-line antihypertensive does not adequately control blood pressure additional drugs should be added in a sequential manner, ideally according to the A(B)/CD rule. As beta-blockers are no longer included in the rule, at least for initial choices of therapy, for the reasons mentioned previously, the rule has become ACD. This means that someone like Mr FH who was started on an ACEI should have a CCB or diuretic added to their regimen at Step 2 (i.e. A + C or D). Step 3 is then to move to A+C+D. If this fails to control blood pressure, fourth-line agents may be required. Using this stepwise approach helps achieve one of the aims of hypertension therapy, which is to obtain maximum control of the blood pressure with minimal therapy, thereby reducing possible side-effects and increasing the chance of adherence.

If it can be ascertained that Mr FH has been taking his ramipril at a dose of 5 mg, then consideration could first be given to increasing this dose to the recommended maximum of 10 mg daily. Alternatively, the application of the ACD rule would suggest that either a CCB or a thiazide diuretic would be appropriate additional therapy to control his blood pressure; however, as Mr FH has developed IHD it could be argued there is a compelling reason to consider starting either a beta-blocker, or if this were not possible, a rate-limiting CCB. In this kind of situation the ACD rule does not apply again until this therapy has been initiated, titrated up, adherence ensured, and blood pressure and any adverse events rechecked. Other groups of antihypertensives outside the ACD rule have a lower evidence base in terms of outcomes and are best reserved for when first- and second-line therapies have either failed or were not tolerated. In addition, the BHS Guidelines advise that submaximal combinations of more than one drug may be more effective and better tolerated (fewer side-effects) than pushing a drug to its maximum dose.

In practice, CCBs are categorised into two classes: rate limiting (verapamil and diltiazem) and non-rate limiting (e.g. nifedipine, amlodipine, nicardipine), which are quite similar in their efficacy as antihypertensive agents. They act at different sites to slow calcium influx into vascular smooth muscle cells, causing vasodilation and hence reduced blood pressure. They have varying degrees of negative inotropic effects, with verapamil having the greatest effect and nicardipine the least. Negatively inotropic CCBs are therefore cautioned against or contraindicated in heart failure

Alpha-blocking agents such as prazosin, doxazosin and terazosin act as vasodilators upon both arterioles and veins. They have the advantages of not reducing cardiac output, and of having a positive effect on cholesterol and triglyceride levels. They do not exacerbate peripheral vascular disease; however, there is a risk of first-dose and postural hypotension, particularly with prazosin. The newer agents can be prescribed as single daily doses. If Mr FH proves unable to tolerate a CCB, or if CCB therapy proves ineffective, one of these agents would be the logical next step. However, these fourth-line alternatives have a weak evidence base and the ALLHAT study indicated higher mortality with doxazosin.

It is important that Mr FH receives further counselling about his medication, owing to the increasing complexity of his drug regimen. An opportunity should also be taken to enquire how he has been able to reduce his other risk factors. Once the correct dose of each respective agent has been established, there may be a case for using a combined preparation, if one exists, to simplify his regimen.

Mr FH wishes to monitor his own blood pressure at home. What would be your recommendation?

A13 **Home monitoring or self-measurement of blood pressure is popular with patients. There are a number of automated, small and lightweight home blood pressure monitors available. All are oscillometric and measure the blood pressure on the upper arm, wrist or finger. However, due to possible peripheral vasoconstriction, sensitivity to posture and the distal location of finger devices, home monitoring may lead to inaccurate measurements.**

Home monitoring can offer some advantages over traditional clinical measurement. They include more reliable measurements, as frequent measurement produces average values that are more reliable than a one-off clinic measurement, and the removal of a number of biases (for example white-coat hypertension). Home monitoring allows a patient to assess their own response to treatment, and may increase their adherence to their prescribed regimen.

There are, however, a number of disadvantages, which should be taken into account when advising patients. First, some research studies have indicated that home monitoring can cause anxiety and obsessive self-interest in some patients. The main potential disadvantages are: the need for appropriate training to use the device effectively; using an inappropriately fitted cuff; and measuring blood pressure after or during exercise. One study has indicated that only 30% of patients using a manual home monitoring device adhered correctly to the recommended protocol. Another difficulty is that there is no consensus regarding the frequency, timing or number of measurements to determine a mean blood pressure value. For these reasons home monitoring of blood pressure is not currently recommended in the UK as its value has not been adequately established.

Outline a pharmaceutical care plan for Mr FH.

A14 **The pharmaceutical care plan should consider each of the problems identified on his admission with chest pain: hypertension; IHD; anaemia; raised creatinine and cholesterol levels. His continued smoking also needs to be addressed.**

Mr FH now has a number of problems which need to be addressed in the pharmaceutical care plan.

Hypertension. Appropriate management is discussed in **A12.**

Ischaemic heart disease IHD. There is now a clinical indication to start sublingual glyceryl trinitrate therapy on an as-required basis, and to continue his therapy with aspirin 75 mg daily. A statin is also indicated for both his hyperlipidaemia and his raised CV risk (reasons for the initiation of both aspirin and statin therapy earlier were weak, but guidelines support their use now). The reason for non-compliance with the simvastatin needs to be investigated and the dose increased to the licensed CVD dose (40 mg daily). If his cholesterol level does not reduce to <4 mmol/L (as per NICE guidelines, May 2008), the dose could be further increased or a more potent statin tried. Beta-blocker therapy should also be considered, as it will improve his anginal symptoms and also his blood pressure; beta-blockers improve CV outcomes in patients with IHD.

Anaemia. The lower haemoglobin level recorded during his admission will both increase the demands on his heart output to supply oxygen and reduce the oxygen reaching the heart. Anginal symptoms are thus more likely. It is worth investigating whether Mr FH has had a minor gastrointestinal bleed secondary to NSAIDs, and stopping the ibuprofen and starting a proton pump inhibitor may enable the aspirin therapy to be continued. Ferrous sulphate therapy may also be required temporarily.

Smoking. Because smoking reduces blood oxygen levels, it has the same effect as anaemia on worsening anginal symptoms. In addition, it is a major contributor to the chances of Mr FH's angina progressing to MI, and he needs to understand this.

Raised creatinine. Mr FH's raised creatinine level needs investigating if it proves to be sustained. Hypertension is a risk factor for renal disease, and even though Mr FH does not have diabetes mellitus, it may be an early warning of hypertensive nephropathy. If sustained, referral to a nephrologist is warranted to delay the progression of renal impairment towards end-stage renal disease. The pharmaceutical care plan would thus include the following:

(a) Ensure adequate and appropriate relief is provided for chest and arthritic pains.
(b) Ensure he is treated optimally for IHD (aspirin, statin, beta-blocker).
(c) Ensure he receives appropriate antihypertensive therapy and help him to reduce his risk factors for hypertension and CVD (smoking, obesity, high salt intake).
(d) Ensure he has an adequate understanding of his medication regimen, in order to maximise his adherence.
(e) Advise on future OTC therapy (no NSAIDs etc.).
(f) Monitoring: all his therapies should be monitored for efficacy and side-effects. Specifically: aspirin, check for side-effects; pain relief,

enquire about efficacy; antihypertensive therapy, monitor blood pressure, sodium, potassium, urea and creatinine levels; statin therapy, regular monitoring of TC, HDL and triglyceride levels plus LFTs (liver function tests). Ask about muscle pain.

What special considerations apply to the management of hypertension in the elderly?

A15 **The elderly have been shown to gain benefit from blood pressure management where it may contribute to the development of vascular dementia and heart failure. Treatment can be initiated up to the age of 80, and continued beyond this. The BHS Guidelines advise that the patient's biological age be considered, not the date on their birth certificate.**

A meta-analysis of the data from a number of studies has indicated that treatment of patients aged 80 years and older prevented 34% of strokes and reduced the rates of major CV events by 22% and heart failure by 39%; however, there was no effect on CV mortality.

The elderly benefit particularly from the use of thiazides and dihydropyridine CCBs. It must be remembered, however, that the elderly have pharmacokinetic and pharmacodynamic changes that may mean they are more susceptible to adverse events, especially if doses are not reduced initially. In particular, vasodilating drugs that impair the orthostatic response and drugs that limit cardiac output may contribute to postural hypotension, dizziness, confusion and falls, and generally make life very difficult for the patient.

Further reading

Blood Pressure Lowering Treatment Triallists' Collaboration. Effects of different blood-pressure-lowering regimens on major cardiovascular events: results of prospectively-designed overviews of randomised trials. *Lancet* 2003; **362**: 1527–1535.

Joint British Societies (JBS 2). Joint British Societies' guidelines on prevention of cardiovascular disease in clinical practice. *Heart* 2005: **91**(Suppl 5), v1–v52.

Kjeldensen SE, Hedener T, Jamerson K *et al*. Hypertension optimal treatment (HOT) study: home blood pressure in treated hypertensive subjects. *Hypertension* 1998; **31**: 1014–1020.

National Collaborating Centre for Chronic Conditions. *Hypertension. Management of Hypertension in Adults in Primary Care: Pharmacological Update (full NICE guideline)*. Clinical guideline 18 (update). Royal College of Physicians and British Hypertension Society, London, 2006.

National Institute of Health and Clinical Excellence. CG34. *Hypertension: Management of Hypertension in Adults in Primary Care*. NICE, London, June 2006.

National Institute of Health and Clinical Excellence. CG67. *Lipid Modification. Cardiovascular Risk Assessment and the Modification of Blood Lipids for the Primary and Secondary Prevention of Cardiovascular Disease*. NICE London, May 2008.

Padwal R, Straus SE, McAlister FA. Evidence based management of hypertension: cardiovascular risk factors and their effects on the decision to treat hypertension: evidence based review. *Br Med J* 2001; **322**: 977–980.

West R, McNeill A, Raw A. Smoking cessation guidelines for health care professionals: an update. *Thorax* 2000; **55**: 987–999.

Williams B, Poulter NR, Brown MJ *et al*. Guidelines for management of hypertension: report of the fourth working party of the British Hypertension Society, 2004-BHS IV. *J Hum Hypertens* 2004; **18**: 139–185.

Useful addresses

National Service Framework for Older People and the National Service Framework for Coronary Heart Disease. Department of Health, London.

Examples of patients' experiences of hypertension and links to other patient-related medical sites can be found on www.healthtalkonline.org

2

Ischaemic heart disease

Duncan McRobbie

Case study and questions

Day 1 Mr CW, a 62-year-old businessman, presented to A&E complaining of central chest pain which was only partly relieved by the glyceryl trinitrate (GTN) spray he carried with him. On examination he was tachycardic, with a blood pressure of 156/90 mmHg.

He had a previous medical history of angina. His attacks had become more frequent over the last few weeks, but this was the first one that had not been completely relieved by his GTN spray. He was a diet-controlled type 2 diabetic and his random blood sugar was 11 mmol/L and his glycated haemoglobin (HbA_{1c}) was 7.2% at admission.

He had a history of hypercholesterolaemia and had been started on simvastatin by his (general practitioner (GP). His last recorded fasting cholesterol was 7.2 mmol/L. He had never been hospitalised for his heart condition.

His father had died of a heart attack at age 68. His mother and his sister were still living. He was married with three adult sons, none of whom had any cardiac complaints. He smoked 30 cigarettes a day and his job required him to entertain regularly, resulting in his drinking 20–30 units of alcohol a week. He weighed 95 kg, with a body mass index (BMI) of 31.

His regular medicine consisted of:

- Aspirin 75 mg enteric-coated tablet, one daily
- Omeprazole 20 mg every morning
- Nicorandil 10 mg orally twice a day
- Isosorbide mononitrate sustained-release 60 mg orally every morning
- Atenolol 100 mg orally daily
- Simvastatin 20 mg orally in the evening
- GTN spray sublingually when required

Q1 Discuss Mr CW's risk factors for coronary heart disease (CHD).
Q2 What are the aims of treatment in angina?

Q3 Before this admission, Mr CW had been treated for stable angina. Comment on the appropriateness of each of Mr CW's medicines on admission. Are any changes to these therapies appropriate?

Q4 What other medications could have been added to this therapy regimen?

After initial assessment he was referred to the cardiology team who documented that he had no obvious symptoms of jaundice, anaemia, cyanosis, clubbing or oedema. His abdominal and respiratory examinations revealed nothing of note. His 12-lead electrocardiogram (ECG) showed transient ST segment changes (>0.05 mV) that developed during symptomatic episodes, but resolved when asymptomatic. No Q waves were observed. His urea and electrolytes were within the normal reference ranges and his full blood count revealed nothing remarkable. His creatine kinase isoenzyme specific for myocardium (CK-MB) fraction was less than 4%. An initial troponin-T test was negative and a subsequent test was ordered for 12 hours after the initial onset of his chest pain.

Q5 What is the reason for performing a CK-MB fraction and troponin-T test?

An acute myocardial infarction (AMI) was excluded and the cardiologist's impression was that he was suffering from non-ST segment elevation myocardial infarction (NSTEMI).

Q6 What is NSTEMI, and what are the implications for Mr CW?

Q7 Identify Mr CW's pharmaceutical care needs during the acute phase of his hospitalisation.

Mr CW continued to suffer intermittent chest pain and was admitted to the coronary care unit for medical management. He was prescribed:

- Aspirin 75 mg orally once daily
- Clopidogrel 600 mg orally for one dose, then 75 mg orally daily
- Enoxaparin 95 mg twice a day subcutaneously
- Eptifibatide 17 mg immediately by intravenous (IV) bolus, then 11.4 mg/h by IV infusion
- GTN IV infusion 50 mg in 50 mL at a rate of 1–5 mg/h titrated to response
- Actrapid insulin IV sliding scale to keep blood sugars between 4 and 8 mmol/L
- Atenolol 100 mg orally daily
- Atorvastatin 80 mg orally daily

His pain settled on this medication regimen.

Q8 Comment on the rationale for the combination of antiplatelet therapy prescribed.

Q9 What risks are associated with the use of combination antiplatelet therapy?

Q10 How should Mr CW be monitored?

Q11 How should Mr CW's GTN infusion be 'titrated to response'?

After 12 hours of treatment his troponin-T result was positive. He was consented for angiography/angioplasty with or without coronary artery stent insertion or coronary artery bypass grafting (CABG) for the following morning.

Q12 Discuss the implications of interventional cardiology.

Day 2 The angiogram revealed 90% occlusion of the left anterior descending coronary artery. An angioplasty was performed and a coronary artery stent was successfully inserted. He was pain free after the procedure and returned to the cardiology ward. His medication immediately after the procedure was:

- Aspirin 75 mg orally daily
- Clopidogrel 75 mg orally daily
- Actrapid insulin sliding scale to keep blood sugars between 4 and 8 mmol/L
- Atenolol 100 mg orally daily
- Atorvastatin 80 mg orally daily
- GTN spray two puffs sublingually when required

Q13 What is the place of drug-eluting stents? Would one have benefited Mr CW?
Q14 Was it appropriate to discontinue his enoxaparin?
Q15 Why has his nicorandil and isosorbide mononitrate therapy not been restarted?

Mr CW's femoral sheaths were removed 4 hours after the procedure.

Day 3 Mr CW's CK-MB was not elevated on the day following the procedure, indicating that no further myocardial damage had occurred during the procedure. Ramipril 2.5 mg orally once daily was initiated. Mr CW remained pain free and his discharge was planned for the following day, with a referral to the cardiac rehabilitation team and a cardiology outpatient appointment made for 6 weeks later. His blood pressure and renal function remained stable. Metformin 850 mg orally twice a day was initiated.

Q16 Why was metformin initiated?

Day 4 Mr CW remained pain free. His blood pressure remained stable at 150/85 mmHg.

His discharge medication was:

- Aspirin 75 mg daily
- Clopidogrel 75 mg orally daily
- Atenolol 100 mg orally daily
- Metformin 850 mg orally twice a day
- Atorvastatin 80 mg orally daily

- Ramipril 2.5 mg orally daily
- GTN spray two sprays sublingually when required

Q17 How long should Mr CW remain on his antiplatelet therapy?
Q18 What information should be communicated to the GP?
Q19 What points would you wish to discuss with Mr CW prior to discharge?
Q20 Should Mr CW be offered nicotine replacement therapy?

Answers

Discuss Mr CW's risk factors for coronary heart disease (CHD).

A1 **Mr CW presents with many factors that increase his risk of CHD, which is one of a spectrum of cardiovascular diseases (CVDs). Fixed factors include: his age; being male; and having a previous history of ischaemic heart disease (IHD) and a family history of IHD. Modifiable factors include: hypertension, diabetes, hypercholesterolaemia, cigarette smoking and obesity.**

People who have multiple risk factors for heart disease are typically three to five times more likely to die, or to suffer a heart attack or other major cardiovascular event than people without such conditions or risk factors. People who have already had a heart attack, have angina, or who have undergone coronary revascularisation are at particularly high risk. Identifying and treating those at greatest risk is one of the highest priorities of the National Services Framework for Coronary Heart Disease.

Various tools are available that allow clinicians to calculate quickly and easily an individual's cardiovascular risk (e.g. Joint British Societies Coronary Risk Prediction Chart, Sheffield Risk Table). These permit the calculation of risk status in patients without a confirmed diagnosis of IHD; however, as Mr CW has already been diagnosed and treatment begun, his risk cannot now be calculated using these tools.

The Interheart study published in the *Lancet* in 2004 identified nine modifiable risk factors which together predict 90% of the risk for heart attacks. These are high cholesterol, hypertension, diabetes, abdominal obesity, smoking, psychological factors such as stress and depression, diet, exercise and excess alcohol intake. As well as having pre-existing CHD, Mr CW has a number of modifiable risk factors for CHD.

(a) **Hypertension.** Hypertension is defined as systolic blood pressure (SBP) of ≥140 mmHg, diastolic blood pressure (DBP) of ≥85 mmHg, or the use of antihypertensive drugs. The Framingham Heart Study demonstrated that hypertensive patients have an excess risk of

CHD, stroke, peripheral artery disease and heart failure compared to patients with normal blood pressure. Hypertensive individuals with one or more major CHD risk factors make up the bulk of the hypertensive population, and more aggressive blood pressure targets are set for these people. As Mr CW has diabetes, the NICE Guideline recommends a target blood pressure of 140/80 mmHg or lower. More stringent targets are identified for patients with retinopathy, cerebrovascular disease or microalbuminuria.

(b) **Diabetes.** The mortality rates from CHD are up to five times higher for people with diabetes, and the risk of stroke is up to three times higher. Mr CW has both elevated random blood sugars and an elevated HbA_{1c}. Lifestyle modifications to reduce blood sugar levels should be continued, but as they appear unsuccessful at reducing his HbA_{1c} to <6.5%, oral hypoglycaemic agents should be considered.

(c) **Smoking.** The risk of CVD is two to four times higher in heavy smokers (those who smoke at least 20 cigarettes per day) than in those who do not smoke. Other reports estimate the age-adjusted risk for smokers of more than 25 cigarettes per day is five to 21 times that of non-smokers.

(d) **High cholesterol levels.** Studies have repeatedly demonstrated the benefit of reducing cholesterol, especially low-density lipoprotein (LDL) cholesterol, in patients with CHD. Earlier studies focused on patients with 'elevated' cholesterol, but the Heart Protection Study demonstrated that all patients with coronary risk factors will benefit from reduction of their serum cholesterol level. In 2008 NICE recommended that in addition to offering lifestyle advice to patients, statins should be prescribed for primary prevention of CVD in adults with a > 20% 10-year risk of developing CVD, and to all patients with established CVD.

(e) **Obesity.** Obese patients are at an increased risk for developing many medical problems, including insulin resistance and type 2 diabetes, hypertension, dyslipidaemia, CVD, stroke and sleep apnoea. Excess body weight is also associated with substantial increases in mortality from all causes, in particular CVD. A study in US nurses estimated this increase in risk to be two to three times that of lean persons. Mr CW has a BMI of 31, which makes him 'obese' according to the World Health Organization classification.

What are the aims of treatment in angina?

A2 The National Service Framework for Coronary Heart Disease states that the aims of treatment for stable angina are:

(a) To relieve symptoms.
(b) To prolong life and minimise cardiac risk.

Treatment to relieve symptoms should include the use of sublingual nitrates for immediate symptom control plus beta blockers and/or nitrates and/or calcium antagonists for long-term symptom control.

In order to minimise his cardiovascular risk, Mr CW should receive advice and treatment about how to adjust his modifiable risk factors.

(a) Stop smoking.
(b) Increase physical activity.
(c) Reduce alcohol consumption.
(d) Manage his diabetes.
(e) Advice and treatment to maintain his blood pressure below 140/80 mmHg.
(f) Continue low-dose aspirin therapy to reduce the chance of future cardiac events.
(g) Continue statin therapy, plus adhere to dietary advice to lower serum cholesterol concentration. It is now recommended that for secondary prevention a total cholesterol level of <4 mmol/L and an LDL cholesterol of <2 mmol/L should be aimed for.
(h) Education about the symptoms of heart attack and, should they develop, instruction to seek help rapidly by calling '999'.

Before this admission, Mr CW had been treated for stable angina. Comment on the appropriateness of each of Mr CW's medicines on admission. Are any changes to these therapies appropriate?

A3 The choice of agents for stable angina is appropriate. Aspirin and statin therapy reduces the risk of further cardiovascular events. Nitrates and nicorandil therapy reduce the frequency and severity of anginal symptoms, and beta blockers are the mainstay of anti-anginal therapy as they reduce both symptoms and risks. However, a number of adjustments to his current therapy should be considered.

(a) **Aspirin.** People at increased risk of heart disease, including men older than 40 years of age, post-menopausal women and younger persons with heart disease risk factors (smoking, diabetes or hypertension) will benefit from low-dose (75–150 mg/day) aspirin. Regular aspirin use in these groups has been linked to a 28% reduction in cardiac events.

For 1000 patients with a 5% risk of cardiac events in the next 5 years, aspirin would prevent six to 20 myocardial infarctions (MIs). At the same time, aspirin would cause zero to two haemorrhagic strokes and two to four major gastrointestinal bleeding episodes. If the 5-year risk was 1%, only one to four infarctions would be prevented, but just as many bleeding events would occur.

In an extensive review of the literature, the Antiplatelet Triallists Collaboration demonstrated an absolute risk reduction of 2% per year in patients with established CHD.

As Mr CW is known to have CHD he would benefit from remaining on his aspirin; however, there is no evidence that enteric-coated aspirin products reduce gastrointestinal bleeding episodes, so a switch to dispersible aspirin should be considered and he should be encouraged to take the dose after a meal.

(b) **Omeprazole.** Gastrointestinal bleeding and dyspepsia are more frequent with aspirin than with placebo. However, the absolute risk of these occurring is small, and patients should not be automatically started on acid-suppression medication. In addition, the combination of enteric-coated preparations, which are specifically designed to dissolve in the higher pH of the duodenum, with a proton pump inhibitor (PPI) which reduces acid secretion in the stomach, is not logical.

If Mr CW has a previous history of gastrointestinal bleeding or dyspepsia, a low dose of a PPI has been shown to be superior to H_2 antagonists at reducing the risk of gastrointestinal bleeding in patients on aspirin. If he has no previous history, acid suppression is probably not required.

(c) **Statins.** Numerous trials have demonstrated the benefit of statins with respect to lowering serum cholesterol. Primary prevention studies, including WOSCOPS and the Heart Protection Study, have consistently demonstrated the benefit of lowering total and LDL cholesterol.

Substantially more benefit is gained in patients with established CHD. It is now recommended that for secondary prevention a total cholesterol level of <4 mmol/L and an LDL cholesterol of <2 mmol/L should be aimed for.

Mr CW's cholesterol is currently considerably above 4 mmol/L and, provided he is compliant with his current therapy, his dose should be increased to 40 mg simvastatin.

(d) **Beta-blockers.** Various studies have demonstrated the beneficial effect of beta-blockers in angina, and they are now considered first-line therapy in national and international guidelines. Beta-blockers achieve a reduction in myocardial oxygen demand by blocking beta-adrenergic receptors, thereby reducing heart rate and the force of left ventricular contraction. Beta-blockers are particularly useful in exertional angina. Patients treated optimally should have a resting heart rate of around 60 beats per minute (bpm).

The Atenolol Silent Ischaemia Study showed a trend for atenolol to be superior to placebo in reducing anginal attacks and cardiac complications. The results demonstrated that seven patients need to be treated to prevent one primary end-point (death, resuscitation from ventricular tachycardia, non-fatal MI, unstable or worsening angina, or revascularisation), but 55 need to be treated to prevent one death.

Beta-blockers should be used with caution in patients with diabetes, as the production of insulin is under adrenergic system control and thus their concomitant use may worsen glucose control. Beta-blockers can also mask the symptoms of hypoglycaemia, and patients in whom the combination is considered of value should be warned of this; however, most clinicians now believe that the benefits of taking beta-blockers, even in diabetics, outweigh the risks and they are frequently prescribed.

Mr CW's pulse should be monitored to ensure his dose is appropriately titrated, and his adherence with the medication assured.

(e) **Nitrates.** Reduced myocardial oxygen consumption can be achieved by reducing the vasomotor tone of the blood vessels. Various vasoactive substances, most notably endothelium-derived relaxing factor and nitric oxide, have been identified. Nitrates, which release nitric oxide when metabolised, have an established role in the treatment and prevention of angina.

The problem of tolerance with nitrates (where increased doses are required to achieve the same effect) means that short-acting preparations need to have their timings staggered to achieve an 8-hour nitrate-free period every day; however, this can be overcome with the use of a modified-release preparation. Although modified-release nitrate formulations provide a nitrate-free period, they also confer a treatment-free period, usually just before waking. This is of concern, as it is the period of greatest risk for an acute coronary event. For this reason nitrates are not optimal first-line monotherapy. In addition, trials have so far not established any mortality gain from the use of oral nitrate preparations, although their role in providing symptom relief is well established.

GTN spray is an important diagnostic tool in establishing the severity of anginal pain. Its rapid onset of action results in relief of pain, whereas failure to relieve this pain through the use of repeated (up to six) sprays indicates progression of stable angina to a more acute condition (unstable angina (UA) or myocardial infarction (MI)). The spray formulation has largely replaced sublingual GTN tablets as it does not oxidise on contact with air and therefore retains its effectiveness for up to 3 years.

Mr CW should be regularly questioned as to his usage of GTN spray and its effectiveness.

(f) **Nicorandil.** Nicorandil combines the properties of an organic nitrate with a potassium channel activator. It causes dilation of coronary arteries and arterioles and reduces systemic vasculature resistance. In small studies monotherapy appears to be as effective as other anti-anginal medications. The IONA trial demonstrated a positive effect on mortality, and may raise nicorandil above nitrates in the anti-anginal prescribing hierarchy. Mr CW is on a small dose of nicorandil and this could have been increased if his anginal symptoms were not being controlled.

What other medications could have been added to this therapy regimen?

A4 **Calcium-channel blockers (CCBs) are effective at reducing anginal symptoms and angiotensin-converting enzyme inhibitors (ACEIs) have an emerging role in reducing the development of coronary events in patients with IHD. Ivabradine or CCBs may be used to control heart rate when beta-blockers are contraindicated.**

(a) **CCBs.** Although short-acting CCBs have been implicated in the exacerbation of angina owing to the phenomenon of 'coronary steal', longer-acting preparations of dihydropyridines, e.g. amlodipine and nifedipine LA, have demonstrated symptom-relieving potential similar to beta-blockers.

CCBs with myocardial rate control as well as vasodilatory properties (e.g. diltiazem) and those with predominantly rate-controlling effects (e.g. verapamil) have also been shown to improve symptom control, reduce the frequency of anginal attacks and increase exercise tolerance. They should be avoided in patients with compromised left ventricular function and conduction abnormalities. They should also be used with caution in patients already receiving beta-blockers, as bradycardia and heart block have been reported with this combination.

(b) **ACEIs.** Although they are well-established treatments for heart failure, the vasoactive properties of ACEIs are still to be fully understood.

The Heart Outcomes Prevention Study (HOPE) provided compelling evidence that ramipril will reduce cardiovascular death, non-fatal MI, stroke, heart failure and the need for revascularisation in patients with angina but without heart failure. The HOPE investigators randomised over 9500 patients with IHD to receive either ramipril (titrated to 10 mg/day) or placebo as well as conventional anti-anginal therapy. At the end of 4 years the ramipril group had a 3% absolute risk reduction of MI, stroke or cardiovascular death compared to the placebo group. A significant number of patients achieved, and were maintained on, the 10 mg dose and the dropout rate in both groups was the same. There was a small reduction in blood pressure in the ramipril group (136/76 mmHg compared to 139/77 mmHg), which may have contributed to some, but not all, of the effect.

Further evidence for the benefit of ACEIs with respect to reducing cerebrovascular events has been provided by the PROGRESS study.

(c) **Ivabradine.** Heart rate control is an essential modification in patients with angina. This is traditionally achieved with beta-blockers; however, a number of patients are unable to take beta-blockers because of contraindications or side-effects. In clinical studies ivabradine, a novel I_f current inhibitor, reduced heart rate as effectively as beta-blockers. At the time of writing ivabradine is licensed in the UK as an alternative rate control agent when beta-blockers are contraindicated or not tolerated. In practice, many clinicians would choose a rate-limiting CCB as the second-line rate control agent.

What is the reason for performing a CK-MB fraction and troponin-T test?

A5 CK-MB and troponin T are tests used to identify whether myocardial damage has occurred. The tests are used to help differentiate between different types of myocardial chest pain.

The term acute coronary syndrome (ACS) covers a group of conditions with a common theme of myocardial ischaemia. There is considerable emphasis on accurate diagnosis of these conditions, as their drug management differs considerably. Traditionally, four factors contribute to the diagnosis of ACS: history, examination, ECG and cardiac markers.

The ideal cardiac marker should be present in the myocardial tissue only, released into the systemic circulation in a direct proportion to the amount of myocardial injury, then remain in the circulation long enough to provide a therapeutic window. Finally, it should be assessed by a cheap, easy to perform and readily available assay. Currently no such marker exists.

CK is a muscle-bound protein that is released into the systemic circulation after muscle damage. CK-MB is still an acceptable diagnostic test. Rapid, cheap and accurate assays are available; however, it loses specificity in the setting of skeletal muscle injury or surgery. It has low sensitivity during the early (first 6 hours after the onset of symptom) and late (over 36 hours after onset of symptoms) phases. Combined with a positive history and sustained ECG changes, a CK-MB > 4% indicates that an MI has occurred.

Cardiac troponins are more sensitive and specific markers of myocardial necrosis. Their ability to detect minor myocardial damage enhances their prognostic value beyond CK-MB levels. Troponin T is a protein that binds strongly to tropomycin on the filaments of myocardial tissue and is released into the blood system when the myocardium is damaged. 'Troponin-positive' patients with normal CK-MB values at presentation have an increased risk of death and cardiac complications compared to those who are 'troponin negative'. There is also an excellent linear correlation between increasing troponin levels and worsening outcome. Troponins T and I are the preferred markers, as the isoform C shows significant similarity with smooth and skeletal muscle.

Troponin T has low sensitivity in the early stages of symptoms and tests should be carried out 8–12 hours after the onset of chest pain. Its long half-life (up to 2 weeks) means that it has limited ability to detect reinfarction.

The recent ACC/AHA guidelines consider UA and non-ST segment elevation myocardial infarction (NSTEMI) to be closely related conditions whose pathogenesis and clinical presentations are similar but of differing severity. Myocardial damage severe enough to release detectable amounts of troponin is considered to be NSTEMI, whereas if no troponin is detected the patient is considered to have UA.

The combination of Mr CW's history (previous diagnosis of and worsening of angina, plus chest pain at rest), transient ECG changes, normal CK-MB with a raised troponin T, led the cardiologist to a diagnosis of NSTEMI.

What is NSTEMI, and what are the implications for Mr CW?

A6 **NSTEMI can be defined as new-onset angina at rest or prior existing angina which is increasing in severity, duration or frequency. Both UA and NSTEMI result from the rupture of atheromatous**

plaques in the coronary vasculature, which initiates the formation of platelet plugs. This is a dynamic process with endogenous antiplatelet factors in competition with platelet-activating factors. Without aggressive management a significant number of patients will develop a thrombus, which may completely occlude a coronary blood vessel, resulting in an MI.

The conditions grouped as acute coronary syndrome (ACS) often present with similar symptoms of chest pain which is not – or only partially – relieved by GTN. These conditions include acute myocardial infarction (AMI), unstable angina (UA) and non-ST-elevated MI (NSTEMI). AMI with persistent ST segment elevation on the ECG usually develops Q waves indicating transmural infarction (see Chapter 3). UA and NSTEMI present without persistent ST segment elevation and are managed differently, although a similar early diagnostic and therapeutic approach is employed.

UA is defined as angina that occurs at rest or with minimal exertion, or new (within 1 month) onset of severe angina or worsening of previously stable angina. Modern approaches consider NSTEMI (or non-Q wave MI) to be a more severe state of the same clinical syndrome.

In England and Wales about 115 000 new patients are diagnosed with UA or NSTEMI each year. Despite the use of standard therapy the rate of adverse outcomes (such as death, non-fatal MI or refractory angina requiring revascularisation) remains at 5–7% at 7 days and about 15–30% at 30 days; 5–14% of patients with UA or NSTEMI die within the first year of diagnosis.

Patients presenting with UA/NSTEMI can be classified into three categories depending on their risk of death or developing an AMI. High-risk patients (those with ST segment changes during chest pain, chest pain within 48 hours, troponin T-positive patients, and those who are already on intensive anti-anginal therapy) can be effectively managed with aggressive medical and interventional therapy. This results in lower event rates (development of AMI) and costs. Mr CW is classified as a high-risk patient and would be suitable for interventional therapy.

Identify Mr CW's pharmaceutical care needs during the acute phase of his hospitalisation.

A7 **The pharmaceutical care needs of Mr CW can be viewed in the context of his key therapeutic aims, which are to:**

(a) Reduce his chance of death or MI.
(b) Control his symptoms of chest pain.
(c) Reduce his long-term cardiovascular risk.

Each of these three priorities should be evaluated in order to ensure that:

(a) Mr CW is prescribed all necessary drug therapies at an optimal dose.
(b) The drug therapy is safe.
(c) The drug therapy is effective.
(d) He can comply with the drug therapy.

Comment on the rationale for the combination of antiplatelet therapy prescribed.

A8 Aspirin, clopidogrel and low-molecular-weight heparins each inhibit different platelet activation pathways. This combination has been shown to be superior to the use of individual antiplatelet agents in reducing the risk of AMI in NSTEMI. Eptifibatide inhibits the binding of fibrinogen to receptors on platelets and prevents platelet adhesion. This drug is especially beneficial in patients with UA who are going to undergo percutaneous coronary intervention (PCI).

Ischaemia develops as a result of decreased myocardial perfusion caused by platelet aggregation following the disruption of an atherosclerotic plaque. After vessel wall injury platelets initially adhere to the site of the injury, with von Willebrand factor acting as a binding ligand. This process initiates a cascade of platelet activation which is stimulated via numerous mechanisms, of which collagen, thrombin, thromboxane A_2, serotonin, and adenosine diphosphate (ADP) are the most significant. These stimulants cause a change in platelet conformation and the activation of glycoprotein IIb/IIIa receptors on the surface of the platelet. Platelet aggregation (plugging) results from the binding of these receptors with fibrinogen and the eventual development of a thrombus, which may partially or completely occlude the coronary artery. The development of these platelet plugs is a dynamic process, with endogenous antiplatelet factors attempting to effect clot dissolution. Pharmaceutical intervention is aimed at reducing platelet activation and aggregation.

The combination of aspirin (150 mg) and enoxaparin (1 mg/kg twice a day) is now recognised to be superior to aspirin and unfractionated heparin (5000 units stat, then 30 000 units/24 hours with the aim of keeping the activated partial thromboplastin time (APTT) 1.5–2.5 times that of the control). The combination of these agents has a pharmacological logic, as they act on different platelet activation pathways, and their use results in a reduction in the incidence of MI and death. The addition of the ADP inhibitor clopidogrel (300 mg initially, then 75 mg daily) confers significant additional benefit to the combination of thromboxane A_2 inhibitor and antithrombin agent, especially in the acute phase.

Prasugrel, a new ADP receptor antagonist, has recently been licensed in the UK to be used in combination with aspirin in patients with ACS undergoing PCI. This drug was shown to be significantly superior to clopidogrel in reducing major cardiac events in the TRITON TIMI-38 study published in 2008. However, this study also demonstrated an increase in bleeding events in the prasugrel arm, especially in patients with previous transient ischaemic attacks or stroke, in the elderly and in those under 60 kg, making its place in therapy unclear at the present time.

A recent study (OASIS 5) indicated that fondaparinux, a synthetic factor Xa inhibitor, at a dose of 2.5 mg subcutaneously once a day was at least as effective as enoxaparin in preventing the combined endpoint of death, MI or refractory ischaemia. Patients in the fondaparinux arm suffered significantly fewer bleeds; however, trends towards an increase in periprocedural events, especially catheter-related thrombi, have limited its use in patients undergoing early intervention.

Although reducing platelet activation via these mechanisms is important, over 90 other factors that activate platelets have been identified, and the prevention of platelet aggregation via inhibition of the glycoprotein IIb/IIIa receptor has attracted particular attention in recent years. There is a financial implication to using these products, as well as an increased risk of bleeding; however, these drugs have demonstrated a significant reduction in death and MI in high-risk patients, with the maximum benefit seen in those high-risk patients who go on to percutaneous transluminal coronary angioplasty (PTCA), as PTCA disrupts atheromatous plaques and initiates the platelet activation cascade. As a result, the use of glycoprotein IIb/IIIa inhibitors is recommended by NICE as an adjunct to PCI for all patients with diabetes undergoing elective PCI, and for those patients undergoing complex procedures. The glycoprotein IIb/IIIa receptor inhibitors eptifibatide or tirofiban should thus be considered for Mr CW, especially as he has a raised troponin level. It should be initiated before the start of the procedure and continued for 12 hours after it ends.

The results of trials involving thrombolytic therapy, either alone or in combination with a glycoprotein IIb/IIIa receptor antagonist in NSTEMI, have so far not shown any benefit, but have resulted in a significant increase in the risk of bleeding complications.

What risks are associated with the use of combination antiplatelet therapy?

A9 **The main risks associated with combination antiplatelet therapy are an increase in bleeding events and an increase in thrombocytopenia.**

The combination of antiplatelet agents has the benefit of reducing platelet adherence, but at the risk of increased bleeding. Bleeding events are usually defined as fatal, major bleeds or minor bleeds. The definitions of the latter two are not necessarily consistent between trials, making interpretation of data difficult.

Using aspirin alone is not without risk. Although there is no increase in the number of fatal bleeds that occur, there is a 2% absolute increase in major and minor bleeds.

Adding heparin (either unfractionated or low molecular weight) increases the absolute risk of major and minor bleeds to about 7%. Again, no increase in fatal bleeds has been noted.

Better awareness of the bleeding risks associated with the combination of glycoprotein IIb/IIIa inhibitors and heparin has resulted in a dramatic reduction in reported bleeding rates. A meta-analysis of glycoprotein IIb/IIIa trials indicated the risk of major bleeds to be 1.4% on heparin alone and 2.5% on a glycoprotein IIb/IIIa inhibitor plus heparin. Minor bleeds were not reported, and there was no increase in intracranial haemorrhage.

The ESPRIT study pre-treated patients undergoing stent procedures with aspirin and clopidogrel (or ticlopidine, another thienopyridine), dose-adjusted heparin and either eptifibatide or placebo. The rate for both major and minor bleeds increased in the eptifibatide group (1% versus 0.4% and 2.8% versus 1.7%, respectively).

The CURE study demonstrated a significant increase in overall bleeding from 5% to 8.5% in patients taking clopidogrel and aspirin compared to those taking aspirin only (minor bleeding: 5.1% versus 2.4%; major bleeding: 3.7% versus 2.7%).

Although laboratory testing has been traditionally used to titrate the dose of unfractionated heparin, there is no routine assay for monitoring either low-molecular-weight heparin or glycoprotein IIb/IIIa receptor antagonist therapy. One advantage of low-molecular-weight heparin is that its anti-Factor Xa activity is predictable, obviating the need to monitor anticoagulant activity in the majority of cases.

Unfractionated heparin, low-molecular-weight heparin and the glycoprotein IIb/IIIa receptor inhibitors have all been associated with thrombocytopenia. Thrombocytopenia can be defined as a fall in platelet count to below 100 000 cells/micro L, but again this definition is not consistent across all trials.

The ESSENCE trial compared enoxaparin and dose-adjusted heparin in UA and reported a thrombocytopenia rate (defined as a drop in platelet count of >50% from baseline) of 2.5% in the enoxaparin group and 3.7% in the unfractionated heparin group.

Abciximab, the first glycoprotein IIb/IIIa inhibitor to be marketed, appears to be the one most prone to cause thrombocytopenia. A review of three abciximab studies demonstrates a significant increase in thrombocytopenia from 2% to 3.7%. All patients also received unfractionated heparin. Only two patients in the ESPRIT study developed thrombocytopenia, both in the eptifibatide arm.

There was no increase in the incidence of thrombocytopenia between the clopidogrel and the placebo arm in the CURE study.

How should Mr CW be monitored?

A10 Mr CW should be monitored for symptoms of ischaemic chest pain and for side-effects of medicines.

Monitoring for ischaemic chest pain should include ECG and evaluation of his cardiac markers after the angioplasty, to ensure no periprocedural ischaemic event occurs.

Antiplatelet agents should be monitored by observing for signs of bleeding and thrombocytopenia. Dyspepsia should also be monitored, and a PPI may be required. Mr CW's blood sugars should be controlled to 4–8 mmol/L, and his pulse and blood pressure should be monitored to ensure the effectiveness of the β-blocker. His renal function should be monitored every few days to ensure there is no reduction in creatinine clearance after the initiation of the ACEI.

In ACSs NICE recommends a high-intensity statin and suggest that treatment should not be delayed if cholesterol levels are not available. Recent concerns regarding an increased risk of myalgia with high-dose simvastatin resulting in many interventional centres recommending atorvastatin 80 mg in line with the data published in the PROVE-IT study. It is recommended that liver function be evaluated on admission to give a base line and fasting cholesterol and liver function tests should be measured at 3 months.

How should Mr CW's GTN infusion be 'titrated to response'?

A11 IV nitrates reduce myocardial oxygen demand by reducing the workload of the heart. Traditionally, IV nitrates are made up to a strength of 1 mg/mL by diluting 50 mg GTN in 50 mL of sodium chloride 0.9% and running the infusion into a peripheral venous line via a syringe driver. The drug should be initiated at a dose of 5 micrograms/kg/min and the dose increased until the patient is pain free, or until headaches become intolerable or hypotension (SBP <100 mmHg) necessitates dose reduction.

Discuss the implications of interventional cardiology.

A12 **Interventional cardiology encompasses various invasive procedures that aim to improve myocardial blood delivery, either by opening up the blood vessels or by replacing them. Percutaneous coronary interventions (PCIs) open stenosed coronary vessels and are less invasive than coronary bypass surgery, where the coronary vessels are replaced.**

A percutaneous (through the skin) transluminal (through the lumina of the blood vessels) coronary (into the heart) angioplasty (surgery or repair of the blood vessels) (PTCA) was first carried out on a conscious patient by Andeas Gruentzig in Zurich in 1977. Now over 2 million people a year undergo PCIs. The procedure is less invasive than CABG surgery, although the overall effectiveness and cost-effectiveness are still contested.

PCI involves the passing of a catheter via the femoral artery and aorta into the coronary vasculature under radiocontrast guidance. Inflation of a balloon at the end of the catheter in the area of the atheromatous plaques opens the lumen of the artery.

For patients undergoing PCI there is a risk of death, MI and long-term re-stenosis. This is reduced by the insertion of a coronary artery stent. Over the last 10 years the proportion of patients undergoing PCTA in which a stent is implanted has increased markedly. In 2005 the British Cardiovascular Intervention Society (BCIS) reported that stents were used in 94% of all PCI procedures.

After stent insertion there is a short-term risk of thrombus formation until the endothelial lining of the blood vessel has been re-established. Traditional anticoagulation with warfarin required patients to be heparinised and therefore hospitalised, until a therapeutic international normalised ratio (INR) was achieved. This option was replaced by the combination of the ADP receptor antagonist ticlopidine and aspirin, which, albeit effective, had a high incidence of neutropenia. The combination of the newer antiplatelet agent clopidogrel (300 mg initiated before the procedure and 75 mg daily thereafter) and aspirin has been shown to be safer and equally as effective, and to reduce the duration of hospital stay.

What is the place of drug-eluting stents? Would one have benefited Mr CW?

A13 **Diabetic patients face a greater risk of complications and events following coronary intervention, and there is some evidence that drug-eluting stents may be more effective at reducing the risk of re-stenosis in this population.**

Re-stenosis occurs after PCI due to hyperplasia of the new intimal lining of the blood vessels. Re-stenosis rates following PTCA were originally as high as 40%; however, stent implantation reduced this to <30% and intracoronary brachytherapy (irradiation of the blood vessel) to <10%. Drug-eluting stents appear to reduce re-stenosis rates to 0–5%.

Drug-eluting stents are balloon-expandable stents which have been impregnated with a variety of agents to prevent re-stenosis. Immunosuppressants (e.g. sirolimus (RAVEL and SIRIUS studies) and more recently everolimus) and antineoplastic agents (e.g. paclitaxel (TAXUS-I and ELUTES studies)) have both so far shown dramatic reductions in re-stenosis rates at 1 year. Dexamethasone-coated stents are no longer available in the European Union. At the time of writing, trials are ongoing or planned with migration inhibitors such as batimastat and halofunginone, and with enhanced healing agents including vascular endothelial growth factor, 17-β-oestradiol and hydroxymethylglutaryl coenzyme A (HMG-CoA) reductase inhibitors.

It appears that there are some groups of patients whose vessels are more likely to re-stenose. The absolute rate of revascularisation has been shown to be greater in patients with small vessels (<3 mm in calibre) or long lesions (>15 mm). This means that these groups of patients are most likely to benefit from drug-eluting stents, and NICE now recommends such stents in these patients only. Although there is considerable clinical opinion that diabetes is also associated with an increase in re-stenosis risk, NICE has not supported this usage at the time of writing.

BCIS reported that by 2006 drug-eluting stents made up 62% of all stents used in the UK. Concerns relating to late complications have led to the US FDA and BCIS to issue recommendations with regard to the duration of dual antiplatelet therapy, increasing this to 12 months after drug-eluting stent insertion. The decision to use a drug-eluting stent thus also needs to be carefully considered in light of the need for extended dual antiplatelet therapy, as this limits the opportunity for surgery, either cardiac or other surgery, as there may be a need to stop clopidogrel to reduce the risk of bleeding.

Was it appropriate to discontinue his enoxaparin?

A14 **Yes. It is important to discontinue heparin at the end of the procedure and at least 4 hours before the femoral sheaths are removed, to prevent haematomas and oozing at the incision site.**

In trials comparing low-molecular-weight with unfractionated heparin, where patients went on to revascularisation (ESSENCE and TIMI 11B), the low-molecular-weight heparin was discontinued before the procedure and substituted with unfractionated heparin. The unfractionated heparin was discontinued at the end of the procedure. A consensus document was produced as a result of a review of the available literature, and this suggested that low-molecular-weight heparin can be used as a safe alternative to unfractionated heparin in combination with a glycoprotein IIb/IIIa receptor inhibitor.

Why has his nicorandil and isosorbide mononitrate therapy not been restarted?

A15 PCI procedures restore the coronary blood flow and result in less anginal pain, and this opportunity should be taken to reduce Mr CW's tablet load.

Discontinuation of anti-anginal drugs, particularly those for symptom relief, would be beneficial at this time. These drugs can be restarted should symptoms recur; however, drugs prescribed to reduce his long-term cardiovascular risk should be continued.

Why was metformin initiated?

A16 To provide better control of his diabetes.

CVD remains the major cause of morbidity and mortality in the diabetic population, who continue to have a three- to fivefold greater risk of developing CVD than do non-diabetics. Prospective data have linked elevated HbA_{1c} with increased cardiovascular morbidity and mortality, and in both the Diabetes Control and Complications Trial and the United Kingdom Prospective Diabetes Study reduction in HbA_{1c} resulted in a reduced incidence of CVD.

Metformin can be used as monotherapy as an adjunct to diet. It has an approximately equal effect as sulphonylureas on fasting blood glucose and HbA_{1c}, but should be considered first-line in obese patients such as Mr CW, as body weight is significantly lower after long-term metformin than after sulphonylurea treatment. A sulphonylurea can be added to the metformin therapy if appropriate blood sugars are not achieved.

How long should Mr CW remain on his oral antiplatelet therapy?

A17 Clopidogrel (with aspirin) has demonstrated superiority over aspirin alone in patients suffering from NSTEMI. National guidelines now suggest that the duration of dual therapy for this group of patients should be 12 months. Aspirin should be continued indefinitely.

In order to prevent intrastent thrombus formation in planned bare metal stent procedures, the combination of aspirin and clopidogrel should be continued for a month; however, in patients with high-risk ACS (such as Mr CW) the recommended duration of dual antiplatelet therapy is a year. Drug-eluting stent insertion also requires longer dual therapy because of the inhibition of re-epithelialisation. Aspirin should be continued indefinitely.

Early discontinuation of dual antiplatelet therapy, in particular in patients with drug-eluting stents, has been associated with an increase in acute MI and death.

The combination of aspirin and clopidogrel is associated with an increased bleeding risk. The discontinuation of clopidogrel (and/or aspirin) in patients showing symptoms of bleeding needs to be carefully weighed against the risk of an increase in cardiovascular events.

What information should be communicated to the GP?

A18 **Apart from the traditional information provided (drug name, dose and frequency), GPs find guidance on duration of treatment, monitoring, new patient allergies and any changes in therapy particularly important.**

The summary information for Mr CW would comprise:

(a) Drugs started

(i) Clopidogrel 75 mg for 1 year in accordance with NICE guidance. A full blood count should be performed after 1 week (if not done in hospital) to check for thrombocytopenia.

(ii) Ramipril 2.5 mg initiated. Increase the dose by 2.5 mg increments until the target dose of 10 mg daily is achieved or side-effects occur (drop in blood pressure, reduced renal function or intolerable cough). Continue treatment long term.

(iii) Metformin initiated to control blood sugars. Review renal function annually and stop if renal function decreases. Review blood sugars regularly and add other oral hypoglycaemic agents as required.

(iv) Atorvastatin. Statin switched and dose increased to 80 mg daily (see also Chapter 3, **A22**). Cholesterol levels should be checked in 6 weeks, together with liver function tests. Continue therapy indefinitely. Target total cholesterol levels of <4 mmol/L should be achieved. If Mr CW experiences side-effects from the high dose of statin, this could be reduced or an alternative statin considered.

(b) Dose changed

(i) Enteric-coated aspirin changed to 75 mg dispersible form, as no benefit from use of enteric-coated form. Continue long term. Review for dyspepsia.

(c) Drugs stopped

(i) Omeprazole, as no clear indication for use and data are emerging about an increase in cardiac events in post-ACS patients on aspirin and clopidogrel who are also prescribed a PPI. Current recommendations from the licensing authorities ate that PPIs should be avoided unless considered essential in these patients.

(ii) Nicorandil. Successful PCI should reduce chest pain. Restart only if chest pain recurs.

(iii) Isosorbide mononitrate, as nicorandil.

(d) Drug therapies unchanged

(i) Atenolol and GTN spray.

What points would you wish to discuss with Mr CW prior to discharge?

A19 **Patient adherence to their medication regimen is associated with how satisfied they are with the quality of information they have received about their medicines, and not necessarily the *quantity* of that information. It is therefore important to establish Mr CW's need for information, and to provide this as far as possible.**

Patient beliefs about medicines are influenced by many factors. These can be divided largely into beliefs about the importance of the medicine and concerns about its harmful effects. In order to ensure compliance with medication regimens it is necessary to address each individual patient's beliefs and concerns.

One approach to counselling Mr CW may be to divide the medications prescribed into those used to reduce the risk of heart attacks and death, and those for symptom control. Key points to be discussed include side-effects and what to do if they occur, the need to continue medication until told otherwise, and to ensure he does not run out of medication.

In relation to each prescribed medicine, specific information might include:

(a) **Aspirin** is used long term to reduce the chance of a heart attack by reducing the formation of clots in the blood system, in particular the blood vessels that feed the heart muscle. The dose should be taken after food (not on an empty stomach), as aspirin can cause indigestion. If indigestion is a problem, this should be reported to the patient's GP, who may prescribe a drug to counter this effect.

(b) **Clopidogrel** is used to enhance the effect of aspirin while the stent settles. Evidence from the CURE study shows that this should be continued for up to 12 months in patients with NSTEMI. If a blood test has not been done in hospital (to check platelets), it should be done after a week. The patient's GP can do this. Both the patient and the GP need to be given clear information regarding the duration of treatment. Many units now provide the patient with a 'Clopidogrel Card' which augments verbal information.

(c) **Atorvastatin.** There are primarily two types of fat that circulate in the blood: low-density lipoproteins (LDLs), which cling to the blood vessel wall, resulting in narrowing of blood vessels, and high-density lipoproteins (HDLs) which do not narrow blood vessels. The target for cholesterol lowering is to reduce the total amount of cholesterol in the blood, but also to shift the balance of fats by reducing LDL and increasing HDL. Cholesterol-lowering drugs work best in conjunction with a low-fat diet. It is therefore important to reduce intake of animal fats, including cheese and dairy products, which contain the LDLs. Fish and olive oil contain the 'good' HDLs. Antioxidants are thought to be beneficial, and are found in fresh fruit and salads. These are normally obtained as part of a fully balanced diet, and there is little evidence that taking additional vitamin supplements makes any difference. The target for total cholesterol should be a level <4 mmol/L. The GP should do a blood test in 12 weeks' time to see how much reduction has occurred, and to check for side-effects of the medicine. It may be necessary to modify the therapy if the target has not been achieved. Appointments to take blood should be booked with the surgery. Blood should normally be taken in the morning, and ideally the patient should not have eaten beforehand. Any muscle aches and pains should be reported immediately to the patient's GP.

(d) **Atenolol.** Chest pain (angina) occurs when the heart muscle requires more oxygen than the blood vessels can deliver (because they are narrowed with cholesterol). Often angina occurs when the heart beats faster or harder than normal. Atenolol (a beta-blocker) reduces the workload of the heart, thereby reducing its need for oxygen. This therefore reduces angina. Atenolol will reduce the heart rate increase that normally occurs during exercise or emotion. Patients often feel tired when first starting on atenolol, but will usually adjust to this. Other common side-effects include cold hands and feet, and impotence in men. Any of these should be discussed with the patient's GP, who may initially try other medicines from the same class. Patients with angina usually need to take a beta-blocker for a prolonged period.

(e) **Ramipril** has been shown to reduce further damage to the heart. The ideal dose is 10 mg daily and the GP will try to increase the dose to this target; however, not all patients can tolerate this dose. Ramipril (as well as atenolol) can reduce blood pressure. This has positive effects, provided the blood pressure does not decrease too much. The GP will monitor this. Ramipril can sometimes cause cough, which may occur at night. If this becomes troublesome it should be reported to the GP, who may change the medicine. Ramipril may also be required long term.

(f) GTN spray is used when symptoms of chest pain occur. Simply resting (sitting down and taking deep breaths) may sometimes alleviate chest pain, but if this has not occurred after 5 minutes, the spray should be used. Two puffs should be sprayed onto the tongue or the inside of the cheek. Symptoms of flushing or headache mean that the drug is working and will go away relatively quickly. If the chest pain is not relieved after 5 minutes then another two sprays should be used. Should this be unsuccessful, then urgent medical attention should be sought (usually by going to A&E or dialling 999), as a clot may be forming in the arteries that feed the heart. It is important to carry the spray at all times, and it is often easier to have two or three sprays (at work, in the car, etc.). If the patient notices that they need to use the spray more frequently, they should tell their GP who may adjust their regular medicines.

Should Mr CW be offered nicotine replacement therapy?

A20 Yes: any and every opportunity should be taken to encourage him to stop smoking.

High-quality research has demonstrated that simple treatments and important lifestyle changes can substantially reduce cardiovascular risk, and can slow and perhaps even reverse the progression of established coronary disease. When used appropriately, these interventions can be more cost-effective than many other treatments currently provided by the NHS.

Within a matter of months after smoking cessation, CHD risk begins to decline. Within 2–3 years of smoking cessation, the risk decreases to approximately the level found in people who have never smoked, regardless of the amount smoked, the duration of the habit and the age at cessation.

A meta-analysis of structured cessation programmes has indicated that nicotine replacement therapy almost doubles smokers' chances of successfully stopping smoking (18% versus 11%). Mr CW should be offered advice on stopping smoking and encouraged to attend specialist smokers' clinics to further improve his chances of quitting.

Further reading

Anderson JL, Adams CD, Antman EM *et al.* ACC/AHA 2007 guidelines for the management of patients with unstable angina/non–ST-elevation myocardial infarction: a report of the American College of Cardiology/American Heart Association Task Force on Practice Guidelines (Writing Committee to Revise the 2002 Guidelines for the Management of Patients With Unstable Angina/Non–ST-Elevation Myocardial Infarction): developed in collaboration with the American College of Emergency Physicians, American College of Physicians, Society for Academic Emergency Medicine, Society for Cardiovascular Angiography and Interventions, and Society of Thoracic Surgeons. *J Am Coll Cardiol* 2007; **50**: e1–157.

Antiplatelet Trialists' Collaboration. Collaborative overview of randomised trials of antiplatelet therapy I: prevention of death, myocardial infarction and stroke by prolonged antiplatelet therapy in various categories of patients. *Br Med J* 1994; **308**: 81–106.

Boersma E, Harrington RA, Moliterno DJ *et al.* Platelet glycoprotein IIb/IIIa inhibitors in acute coronary syndromes: a meta-analysis of all major randomised clinical trials. *Lancet* 2002; **359**: 189–198.

CURE. Effects of clopidogrel in addition to aspirin in patients with acute coronary syndromes without ST segment elevation. *N Engl J Med* 2001; **345**: 494–502.

De Lorgeril M, Salen P, Martin J-L *et al.* Mediterranean diet, traditional risk factors, and the rate of cardiovascular complications after myocardial infarction. Final report of the Lyon Diet Heart Study. *Circulation* 1999; **99**: 779–785.

Department of Health. *National Service Framework for Coronary Heart Disease.* Department of Health, London, 2001.

Department of Health Coronary Heart Disease Policy Team. *Shaping the Future Progress Report 2006.* The Coronary Heart Disease National Service Framework January 2007.

Heart Protection Study Collaborative Group. MRC/BHF Heart Protection Study of cholesterol lowering with simvastatin in 20,536 high risk individuals: a randomised placebo-controlled trial. *Lancet* 2002; **360**: 7–22.

Heart Outcomes Prevention Evaluation Study Investigators. Effects of an angiotensin-converting-enzyme inhibitor, ramipril, on cardiovascular events in high-risk patients. *N Engl J Med* 2000; **342**: 145–153.

Hill RA, Boland A, Dickson R *et al.* Drug-eluting stents: a systematic review and economic evaluation. *Health Technol Assess* 2007; **11**(46): iii, xi–221.

Kereiakes DJ, Montalescot G, Antman EM *et al.* Low-molecular-weight heparin therapy for non-ST-elevation acute coronary syndromes and during percutaneous coronary intervention: an expert consensus. *Am Heart J* 2002; **144**: 615–624.

National Collaborating Centre for Chronic Conditions. *Type 2 Diabetes: National Clinical Guideline for Management in Primary and Secondary Care (Update)*. Royal College of Physicians, London, 2008.

National Institute of Health and Clinical Excellence TA47. *Glycoprotein iib/iiia Inhibitors in the Treatment of Acute Coronary Syndromes*. NICE, London, 2002.

National Institute of Health and Clinical Excellence CG34. *Hypertension: Management of Hypertension in Adults in Primary Care*. (Partial update of NICE Clinical Guideline 18). NICE, London, 2006.

National Institute of Health and Clinical Excellence CG67. *Lipid Modification: Cardiovascular Risk Assessment and the Modification of Blood Lipids for the Primary and Secondary Prevention of Cardiovascular Disease*. NICE, London, 2008.

National Institute of Health and Clinical Excellence TA80. *Clopidogrel in the Treatment of Non-ST-Segment-Elevation Acute Coronary Syndrome*. NICE, London, 2004.

National Institute of Health and Clinical Excellence TA152. *Drug-Eluting Stents for the Treatment of Coronary Artery Disease*. (Part review of NICE technology appraisal guidance 71). NICE, London, 2008.

Pi-Sunyer FX. Medical hazards of obesity. *Ann Intern Med* 1993; **119**: 655–660.

Raw M, McNeill A, West R. Smoking cessation guidelines for health professionals. A guide to effective smoking cessation interventions for the health care system. *Thorax* 1998; **53**[suppl. 5(1)]: S1–38.

Scottish Intercollegiate Guidelines Network. *Management of Stable Angina*. February 2007.

Task Force on the Management of Stable Angina Pectoris of the European Society of Cardiology. Guidelines on the management of stable angina pectoris. *Eur Heart J* 2006; **27**(21): 2606.

Yusuf S, Hawken S, Ôunpuu T *et al*. Effect of potentially modifiable risk factors associated with myocardial infarction in 52 countries (the INTERHEART study): case–control study. *Lancet* 2004; **364**: 937–952S.

3

Myocardial infarction

Helen Williams

Case study and questions

Day 1 Mr BY, a 52-year-old sales representative, presented to A&E via ambulance following the onset of chest pain approximately 2 hours earlier while he was replacing some guttering on his house. He had tried several doses of sublingual glyceryl trinitrate (GTN), but his pain had not resolved. He had become increasingly breathless and clammy, with a tight crushing pain across his chest and left shoulder. His past medical history was documented as 'angina'. He was noted to be obese (estimated body weight >100 kg). His drug history on admission was recorded as nifedipine and isosorbide mononitrate (doses were not stated). On examination his blood pressure (BP) was found to be 150/110 mmHg with a heart rate (HR) of 112 beats per minute (bpm).

Q1 What routine tests should be carried out to confirm a diagnosis of acute myocardial infarction (AMI)?

Mr BY was initially prescribed one dose of each of the following drugs:

- Morphine 5 mg intravenously (IV)
- Metoclopramide 10 mg IV
- Aspirin 300 mg orally
- Clopidogrel 300 mg orally

Q2 What actions of morphine are particularly useful in the acute phase of an AMI?
Q3 Why is metoclopramide necessary? What alternative antiemetics could be considered?
Q4 Why should intramuscular injections generally be avoided in patients suffering with AMI?
Q5 What is the rationale for aspirin and clopidogrel administration during an AMI?
Q6 What other drug therapies should be considered at this stage?

The electrocardiogram (ECG) showed 2–3 mm ST elevation in leads V2–V4 with some evidence of ischaemia in the lateral leads, indicating that Mr BY had suffered an anterior myocardial infarction (MI). Laboratory results were as follows:

- Qualitative troponin (bedside) negative
- Sodium 138 mmol/L (reference range 135–145)
- Potassium 3.8 mmol/L (3.5–5.0)
- Creatinine 104 micromol/L (45–120)
- Urea 6 mmol/L (3.3–6.7)
- Glucose 18 mmol/L (3–7.8 fasting)
- Haemoglobin 14.2 g (14–18)
- Red blood cells (RBC) 6.4×10^{12}/L (4.5–6.5)
- White blood cells (WBC) 6.1×10^{9}/L (4–11)
- Platelets 167×10^{9}/L (150–400)

Following analysis of the ECG a decision was taken to thrombolyse him. In accordance with local protocol a bolus dose of tenecteplase 50 mg was administered. IV heparin and a sliding-scale insulin infusion were also initiated.

Q7 What is the rationale for thrombolysis in the management of AMI?
Q8 When should thrombolysis be administered to gain maximal benefit?
Q9 What are the contraindications to thrombolysis?
Q10 What pharmaceutical issues should be considered when choosing a thrombolytic?
Q11 What monitoring should be undertaken for patients prescribed and administered thrombolytic therapy?
Q12 What alternative strategies to thrombolysis could be employed?
Q13 Is IV heparin indicated for Mr BY?
Q14 What other therapies might be considered at this stage?

Mr BY was successfully thrombolysed and transferred to the Coronary Care Unit for further care. On arrival he was found still to be breathless, although his chest pain had resolved. A repeat ECG at 90 minutes post thrombolysis showed resolution of the ST segments, indicating successful thrombolysis. He had coarse crackles at the left lung base, and a chest X-ray showed some pulmonary oedema. His blood gases showed reduced oxygen saturations on room air, so oxygen therapy was continued. IV furosemide was prescribed at a dose of 80 mg over 20 minutes.

- BP 105/65 mmHg
- HR 103 bpm

He was prescribed:

- Morphine 2.5–5 mg IV when required
- Metoclopramide 10 mg three times daily orally or IV, as required
- Humidified oxygen at 4 L/min
- Human Actrapid insulin 50 units in 500 mL to run over 24 hours according to a sliding-scale regimen

- GTN 400 micrograms sublingually when required
- Aspirin 75 mg orally daily
- Clopidogrel 75 mg orally daily

Day 2 Following three IV doses of furosemide, Mr BY's symptoms had settled with no further episodes of chest pain and improved oxygen saturations. A repeat chest X-ray showed a good response to diuretic therapy, with resolution of pulmonary oedema. On the ward round a cardiac echo was requested by the registrar, alongside repeat blood tests.

- BP 94/63 mmHg
- HR 88 bpm

His biochemistry results were:

- Sodium 143 mmol/L (135–145)
- Potassium 3.1 mmol/L (3.5–5.0)
- Glucose 4.8 mmol/L (3–7.8)
- Urea 5 mmol/L (3.3–6.7)
- Creatinine 110 micromol/L (45–120)
- Haemoglobin 13.2 g/dL (14–18)
- RBC 5.2×10^{12}/L (4.5–6.5)
- WBC 6.0×10^{9}/L (4–11)
- Platelets 172×10^{9}/L (150–400)

From admission bloods:

- Total cholesterol 5.6 mmol/L (<5.0)
- Triglycerides 4.2 mmol/L (<1.8)

Q15 Outline a pharmaceutical care plan for Mr BY.
Q16 Why are his potassium levels a cause for concern? What other electrolytes should be monitored closely?
Q17 Comment on the drugs Mr BY was taking prior to admission.

Day 2 (pm) Mr BY continued to respond well to treatment and was beginning to mobilise. He was haemodynamically stable (BP 92/50 mmHg; HR 72 bpm). The echo report highlighted marked hypokinesia of the anteroseptal region of the left ventricle and an ejection fraction of 30–35%, indicating compromised ventricular function. Mr BY was started on ramipril 1.25 mg initially, then 2.5 mg twice daily thereafter, plus atorvastatin 80 mg daily.

Q18 What is the rationale for angiotensin-converting enzyme inhibitors (ACEIs) following MI? How should ACEI therapy be initiated?
Q19 Should beta-blocker therapy be considered at this stage?
Q20 What advice would you give about the initiation of a beta-blocker?
Q21 Should eplerenone be prescribed for Mr BY?
Q22 Comment on Mr BY's cholesterol level. How should this be managed?
Q23 How should Mr BY's blood sugar levels be controlled over the longer term?

Day 5 Mr BY had made good progress over the past 3 days, although he was complaining of a dry cough.

- BP 92/56 mmHg
- HR 58 bpm
- Sodium 141 mmol/L (135–145)
- Potassium 4.2 mmol/L (3.5–5.0)
- Glucose 5.1 mmol/L (3–7.8)
- Urea 5.3 mmol/L (3.3–6.7)
- Creatinine 121 micromol/L (45–120)

He was stabilised on the following regimen for discharge:

- Aspirin tablet 75 mg orally daily
- Clopidogrel 75 mg once daily for 1 month, then stop
- Ramipril 2.5 mg orally twice daily
- Carvedilol 3.125 mg orally twice daily
- Eplerenone 25 mg once daily
- Atorvastatin 80 mg orally daily
- Human Actrapid insulin 8 units subcutaneously three times daily
- Human Insulatard 10 units subcutaneously at night
- GTN spray 400 micrograms sublingually as required

Q24 What lifestyle issues should be discussed with Mr BY?

Q25 What issues should be highlighted during discharge counselling for this patient?

Answers

What routine tests should be carried out to confirm a diagnosis of AMI?

A1 **A 12-lead electrocardiogram (ECG) should be performed and a blood sample taken for measurement of troponin levels.**

A 12-lead ECG is the key diagnostic tool used to distinguish ST-elevated MI (STEMI – classic myocardial infarction) from other acute coronary syndromes, including non-ST-elevated MI and unstable angina. Key ECG features of STEMI include ST elevation of more than 1 mm in two adjacent limb leads, or more than 2 mm in two adjacent chest leads, or the presence of new left bundle branch block.

Cardiac enzyme measurements are used to determine the presence or absence of myocardial necrosis. In the past, creatine kinase (CK) and CK isoenzyme specific for myocardium (CK-MB) have been used routinely in the diagnosis of AMI. Other cardiac markers include myoglobin and lactic dehydrogenase. All of these markers have limitations in clinical practice. For example, CK only becomes raised a number of hours after the onset of MI, and as a result the usefulness of the test in the early phase of treatment to guide thrombolytic therapy is limited. In addition, CK and CK-MB levels only increase after significant degrees of infarct damage have occurred, and therefore cannot detect smaller areas of ischaemic damage. In view of the limitations of standard biochemical markers of cardiac damage, new diagnostic tests with greater sensitivity and specificity have been identified. Troponins are cardiac contractile proteins which, if raised, indicate thrombotic activity and recent myocardial damage. Troponin levels become raised within 3–12 hours after the onset of pain, even after minor damage to the cardiac muscle, and are more sensitive and specific for myocardial damage than CK or CK-MB. A troponin is considered raised where it exceeds the 99th percentile of the normal reference range; however, this will vary by laboratory depending on the assay used for measurement. As troponin levels only become raised a few hours after the onset of chest pain, their utility in the acute treatment phase is limited. Serial negative tests are required over a 12–24-hour period after pain onset to exclude myocardial damage and allow safe discharge from hospital in patients complaining of chest pain.

Any increase in the levels of these biochemical markers indicates some degree of myocardial damage, but only in the presence of characteristic ECG changes can the diagnosis of STEMI be confirmed. Additional care must be taken as troponin levels may also be increased in the presence of other acute or chronic conditions, such as myocarditis, heart failure, hypertensive crisis, septicaemia or renal dysfunction.

Mr BY presented early after the onset of his symptoms and the cardiac enzymes might not yet have become raised. This emphasises the importance of the ECG in making an accurate and timely diagnosis to maximise the benefits of treatment. Troponin levels may be re-measured to confirm the working diagnosis of AMI and assess the extent of myocardial damage.

What actions of morphine are particularly useful in the acute phase of an AMI?

A2 Morphine has analgesic, anxiolytic and vasodilating effects.

All of these effects are beneficial in AMI. Analgesia is required to provide immediate relief from chest pain; vasodilatation improves blood supply to the myocardium and may contribute to the anti-ischaemic effects. As the symptoms of MI frequently cause patients to panic and further exacerbate the situation, the anxiolytic effect of morphine can calm the patient rapidly and facilitate the administration of further therapy. These effects are not unique to morphine and other opiates may be considered, although pethidine is generally avoided because of its short duration of action and propensity to increase BP.

Why is metoclopramide necessary? What alternative antiemetics could be considered?

A3 During the acute phase of MI the majority of patients suffer from significant nausea and vomiting, which may be further

exacerbated by administration of an IV opiate. Metoclopramide is a suitable agent for use in this setting as it can be administered IV for a rapid onset of action.

IV cyclizine 50 mg up to three times daily would be a suitable alternative, although occasionally this agent may cause a significant reduction in BP and, in the presence of heart failure, may reduce cardiac output.

Why should intramuscular injections generally be avoided in patients suffering with AMI?

A4 The administration of drugs by the IV route allows a rapid and predictable onset of action.

Patients experiencing an AMI, are likely to suffer some degree of shock, with a resultant reduction in muscle perfusion, which could in turn affect the distribution of medicines administered via the intramuscular route.

What is the rationale for aspirin and clopidogrel administration during an AMI?

A5 In the acute phase, the administration of aspirin has been shown to reduce mortality at 5 weeks by approximately 23%, and recent data have confirmed a small additional benefit from the co-administration of clopidogrel

ISIS-2 demonstrated that the administration of aspirin reduces the mortality and morbidity associated with AMI. A dose of 300 mg should be given immediately, regardless of prior aspirin use. Patients should be advised to chew the tablet before swallowing to aid early absorption. Aspirin therapy has also been shown to reduce the rates of reocclusion and reinfarction. A meta-analysis of antithrombotic interventions in high-risk patients has concluded that, when used chronically, aspirin reduces the risk of MI by approximately 25%. Aspirin should therefore be continued indefinitely post MI at a dose of 75 mg daily.

More recently, two studies (COMMIT and CLARITY) have looked at the use of aspirin and clopidogrel dual therapy following STEMI. A recent meta-analysis based on these two studies concluded that the addition of clopidogrel to aspirin slightly reduces all-cause and cardiovascular mortality in patients with STEMI, but also increases the risk of bleeding. The studies in question continued clopidogrel for a maximum of 4 weeks after the event. For this reason the NICE guidance for secondary prevention post STEMI recommends that clopidogrel should be stopped after 4 weeks, unless there is an indication for a longer duration, such as the insertion of a drug-eluting stent.

What other drug therapies should be considered at this stage?

A6 At this stage the diagnosis is unclear. A number of potential drug therapies should therefore be under consideration.

Heparin, glycoprotein IIb/IIIa receptor antagonists, or thrombolysis with or without IV beta-blockers may be indicated pending test results. Patients with ongoing pain or evidence of left ventricular dysfunction may benefit from IV GTN. Oxygen should be administered early to improve myocardial oxygen supply and limit the extent of ischaemia.

What is the rationale for thrombolysis in the management of AMI?

A7 Thrombolytic therapy has been shown to reduce 5-week mortality in AMI patients by 18%, with benefits being maintained for up to 10 years.

The majority of AMIs are caused by obstruction of blood flow in one or more coronary arteries by the formation of a blood clot. Thrombolytic therapy is targeted at breaking down the occluding thrombus through the process of fibrinolysis. Myocardial tissue does not die immediately, and early reperfusion following clot dissolution may salvage areas of heart muscle where blood flow has been compromised. As a result, thrombolytic therapy may limit infarct size, preserve left ventricular function and reduce deaths. A number of clinical trials have confirmed the benefits of thrombolysis in patients with acute STEMI, most notably ISIS-2, GISSI and GUSTO. ISIS-2 demonstrated a 25% reduction in 35-day mortality through the administration of streptokinase alone in AMI, and highlighted the benefits of combining aspirin and thrombolytic therapy, when a 42% mortality reduction was seen.

When should thrombolysis be administered to obtain maximal benefit?

A8 Thrombolytic therapy should be administered as early as possible after symptom onset to gain the maximum benefit from treatment.

The UK National Service Framework (NSF) for Coronary Heart Disease 'door-to-needle' target for the administration of thrombolytics is currently 30 minutes. Early treatment has been shown to improve survival from AMI. One study investigating the use of pre-hospital thrombolysis demonstrated a mortality of 1.2% in patients treated within 70 minutes of symptom onset, compared to 8.7% in the remainder who received therapy at 70 minutes or later. It has been calculated that for every hour earlier thrombolytic therapy is administered, an additional 1.6 lives per 1000 patients treated could be saved. Thrombolytic therapy offers significant benefits when administered up to 12 hours after symptom onset, although greater benefits are seen within the first 6 hours. At 12 hours and beyond, patients derive little benefit from the administration of thrombolytic therapy and other strategies should be considered.

What are the contraindications to thrombolysis?

A9 **Contraindications to thrombolytic therapy can be divided into those that are absolute (i.e. therapy must not be administered) and those that are relative (i.e. the benefits and risks of therapy must be considered for the individual patient requiring treatment).**

The absolute contraindications to thrombolytic therapy are previous haemorrhagic stroke, any cerebrovascular event within the previous year, active internal bleeding and suspected aortic dissection. Relative contraindications include uncontrolled hypertension (systolic blood pressure >180 mmHg), anticoagulant therapy or bleeding disorder, recent trauma or major surgery (within the previous 4 weeks), prolonged cardiopulmonary resuscitation and pregnancy. The decision to administer thrombolytic therapy to a patient with relative contraindications should be made following careful consideration of the risks and potential benefits on an individual basis.

What pharmaceutical issues should be considered when choosing a thrombolytic?

A10 **A number of issues should be considered, including comparative efficacy, dose, method of administration and adverse effects.**

Alteplase, reteplase, streptokinase and tenecteplase are the thrombolytics licensed at the time of writing for the treatment of AMI in the UK. They are all effective, but can be distinguished from one another in terms of their pharmacokinetic and pharmacodynamic profiles.

Streptokinase is supported by strong clinical trial data demonstrating mortality and morbidity benefits up to 10 years after administration, and is the cheapest thrombolytic agent available. However, it does have disadvantages, particularly the potential for allergic reactions and the development of neutralising antibodies within a few days that make re-administration inappropriate. Alteplase is also supported by strong clinical trial data, particularly when administered in a 'front-loaded' regimen. Earlier vessel patency rates have been demonstrated in clinical trials, but an increased incidence of intracranial haemorrhage has also been noted. Unfortunately, the early reperfusion achieved with alteplase has not been shown to improve survival significantly in comparison to streptokinase. Alteplase is not subject to the allergies and antibody responses that limit the usefulness of streptokinase, but it is significantly more expensive. Both of these drugs are administered by infusion, and alteplase is given by a complex 'front-loaded' regimen, in which 65% of the total dose is given during the first 30 minutes of the 90-minute infusion.

The ideal thrombolytic would be effective, easy to administer (ideally by bolus dosing), have a low rate of complications and be at least as effective as the 'gold standards' of streptokinase and alteplase. Reteplase (a double-bolus agent) and tenecteplase (a single-bolus agent) were licensed in the late 1990s. They are marginally more expensive than alteplase, with equivalent outcome data, but are much easier to administer. Many centres have changed to these therapies in an attempt to improve door-to-needle times so as to reach NSF targets, although there remains concern over the potential for these agents to precipitate intracranial bleeding, particularly in elderly patients.

What monitoring should be undertaken for patients prescribed and administered thrombolytic therapy?

A11 **Patients should be monitored closely throughout thrombolytic therapy as they are at risk of haemodynamic instability, reperfusion arrhythmias or other complications. The clinical efficacy of the thrombolysis should be assessed at 90 minutes with a repeat 12-lead ECG.**

Standard observations should be undertaken, including monitoring of BP (hypotension can occur), HR and rhythm. A repeat 12-lead ECG at 90 minutes should confirm resolution of the ST segment, thereby indicating successful thrombolysis.

Complications of thrombolytic therapy include haemorrhagic stroke, which occurs in approximately 1.2% of patients overall, but higher frequencies have been noted in hypertensive patients and the elderly. Other adverse effects include allergy (particularly to streptokinase), other haemorrhage (patients should be monitored for signs of bleeding, such as haematuria, epistaxis (nose bleeds) and haematemesis (coffee-ground vomit)) and systemic emboli. A full blood count should be checked prior to and after treatment to ensure there is no significant drop in haemoglobin, which may indicate haemorrhage. Patients are at risk of bleeding for up to 4 days following the administration of thrombolytic therapy.

What alternative strategies to thrombolysis could be employed?

A12 **The most effective strategy for managing AMI is primary angioplasty (direct angioplasty to the affected coronary artery, which may be combined with intracoronary stent placement), often**

referred to as PAMI. This has been shown to be superior to thrombolytic therapy in the majority of comparative studies, provided it can be undertaken within 90 minutes of symptom onset.

Nationally, there is a move towards treating AMI by primary angioplasty in place of thrombolysis, although this requires a full systems redesign with an integrated approach between ambulance centres, interventional centres and district general hospitals to ensure that patients are transported to a primary angioplasty centre as soon as possible for early intervention. Developing PAMI services in some areas of the country presents significant challenges, particularly where large geographical areas are involved. If transfer to an interventional centre for PAMI would mean a delay of more than 90 minutes, then thrombolytic therapy should instead be administered as early as possible at the presenting site. At the time of writing, approximately 75% of patients within London presenting with ST-elevation MI undergo PAMI.

In patients presenting late (48 hours or more after the acute event), myocardial damage is likely to be irreversible. Standard therapies such as heparin, aspirin and IV GTN may be considered if there is ongoing pain, with referral for early angiography. The early use of IV beta-blockers (with or without thrombolytic therapy) is recommended in most AMI guidelines, primarily to reduce the occurrence of ischaemia-related tachyarrhythmias and sudden cardiac death.

Is intravenous heparin indicated in this patient?

A13 **Yes. IV heparin should be administered at the same time as tenecteplase (TNK-tPA) and be continued for a minimum of 48 hours. The use of concomitant heparin therapy during thrombolysis is agent dependent.**

Heparin is indicated for use in combination with alteplase, reteplase and tenecteplase. The adjunctive use of heparin therapy is necessary to protect against reocclusion. By comparison, streptokinase should not be co-prescribed with heparin because of the increased risk of cerebral bleeds and a greater need for transfusions. Doses of IV heparin should be weight-adjusted to reduce bleeding complications, and should be initiated with a bolus dose followed by a continuous infusion. The activated partial thromboplastin time (APTT/APTTr) should be carefully monitored, particularly at initiation and after any dosage changes. In general, the aim is to achieve an APTT/APTTr twice that of the control. Alternatively, a low-molecular-weight heparin may be considered, although these remain unlicensed for use in combination with thrombolytic agents. Data from the ASSENT-3 study has demonstrated that a combination of enoxaparin and tenecteplase is both safe and effective in AMI.

What other therapies might be considered at this stage?

A14 In view of Mr BY's raised blood glucose on admission, an intensive insulin regimen should be initiated to ensure tight control of his blood sugars in order to improve survival.

Evidence from the DIGAMI study, published in 1997, has established the importance of aggressive blood sugar management in AMI. Sliding-scale insulin therapy is recommended for the first 24 hours in all patients with a raised blood sugar (>11 mmol/L) on admission, or any history of diet- or tablet-controlled diabetes mellitus. DIGAMI reported an absolute reduction in mortality of 11% at 1 year when an aggressive insulin/glucose/potassium infusion was prescribed for the first 24 hours, followed by a minimum of 3 months' subcutaneous insulin therapy. The majority of this benefit was established in younger patients, who had no previous diagnosis of diabetes. No outcome data exist to support the use of diet or oral medication to control blood glucose in post-MI patients.

Outline a pharmaceutical care plan for Mr BY.

A15 The pharmaceutical care plan for Mr BY should include the following:

(a) Ensure that evidence-based strategies are introduced in a timely manner.
(b) Ensure that all drugs are initiated at an appropriate dose and that dose titration is undertaken.
(c) Monitor for efficacy and adverse effects, notify relevant staff and advise on alternatives if necessary.
(d) Ensure that nursing staff are administering IV therapy correctly.
(e) Ensure that secondary prevention strategies are initiated.
(f) Ensure that adequate lifestyle advice has been given, and that the patient is being followed up by the appropriate specialist teams.
(g) Ensure that appropriate information on aims of therapy, dose titrations post discharge, duration of treatment and monitoring are provided to the general practitioner (GP).
(h) Counsel Mr BY on his discharge medication, including the rationale for therapy, appropriate monitoring, possible side-effects and how to deal with them, and how therapies should be continued in future.
(i) Reinforce patient counselling with written information on drug therapy and the provision of appropriate aids, such as a medication record card.

Why are his potassium levels a cause for concern? What other electrolytes should be monitored closely?

A16 **A reduction in serum potassium may predispose Mr BY to post-infarction arrhythmias. Serum magnesium and calcium should also be monitored, and corrected if necessary to further protect against arrhythmias. Serum sodium, creatinine and urea should be monitored throughout his diuretic therapy.**

A significant fall in serum potassium might be expected in this patient secondary to excess catecholamine release in response to the pain and anxiety caused by his AMI. In addition, the intensive insulin/glucose infusion prescribed and the use of repeated bolus doses of a loop diuretic will further reduce his serum potassium levels.

Oral potassium supplements could be started at this point, unless there are signs of impending arrhythmias, such as frequent ventricular ectopic beats or runs of ventricular tachycardia. In this situation, IV supplementation may be more appropriate.

Comment on the drugs Mr BY was taking prior to admission.

A17 **Mr BY's drug therapy on admission of nifedipine and isosorbide mononitrate should be reviewed.**

The SPRINT-2 study indicated that nifedipine may increase early mortality after MI and is not associated with a reduction in cardiac events in the long term. Therefore, his nifedipine therapy should be discontinued. Although isosorbide mononitrate is an effective anti-anginal agent, it has not been shown to improve outcomes in patients with coronary heart disease (CHD), and more suitable alternatives with secondary prevention benefits should be considered first. Mr BY has a number of comorbidities (hypertension, angina and raised blood glucose) which should all be considered when making decisions on drug therapy. His drug regimen on discharge should be designed to optimise cardiovascular outcomes in the long term.

What is the rationale for angiotensin-converting enzyme inhibitors (ACEIs) following MI? How should ACEI therapy be initiated?

A18 **A number of studies (SAVE, AIRE, GISSI-3, ISIS-4 and TRACE) have demonstrated the benefits of ACEIs following MI, with an overall reduction in 30-day mortality of 7%.**

ACEIs should be started in all patients post MI (in the absence of contraindications). The greatest benefits from therapy are seen in high-risk patients, such as those with a reduced left ventricular ejection fraction or overt clinical signs of heart failure (as in the case of Mr BY), diabetes, anterior infarcts or tachycardia. The longer-term benefits with respect to reduced morbidity and mortality in patients with cardiovascular disease were established in the HOPE study (which included post-MI patients) and, specifically following MI, in the AIREX study (an extension of the AIRE study).

Following publication of the GISSI-3 and ISIS-4 studies, early initiation of therapy (within 24 hours) is recommended. Where there is concern over haemodynamic instability (systolic blood pressure <90 mmHg) ACEIs may be temporarily delayed, but this should be reviewed on a daily basis. ACEIs should be started at low doses to avoid the problem of first-dose hypotension, and dose titration should then be undertaken to achieve the optimal doses used in clinical trials. Persistent hypotension may limit the extent to which dose titration can be undertaken during the acute hospital admission. Mr BY's BP and HR should be monitored closely throughout the initiation phase. His renal function should be checked prior to and within 48 hours of starting ACEI therapy, and should be rechecked within a few days of each dose increment. Renal dysfunction (except bilateral renal artery stenosis) is not a contraindication to ACEI therapy. It is recommended that ACEIs be continued indefinitely in the absence of any clear reason to stop therapy.

Angiotensin receptor blockers may be considered as an alternative in patients unable to tolerate ACEIs, but the evidence base to support this drug class for this indication is less robust.

Should beta-blocker therapy be considered at this stage?

A19 **Beta-blocker therapy has been shown to reduce mortality and morbidity post MI, and should therefore be considered for Mr BY. Consideration should be taken of his concurrent heart failure and reduced left ventricular ejection fraction, which may make early initiation of beta-blocker therapy inappropriate, and will also influence the choice of agent and dose regimen.**

Early IV beta-blocker therapy is recommended in the majority of guidelines to reduce the risk of post-infarct arrhythmias. Acute IV therapy would have been inappropriate for Mr BY because of the clinical signs of heart failure in the early phases of his illness. Long-term oral beta-blocker therapy post MI has been studied in a number of clinical trials and an overall 20% reduction in mortality has been established through meta-analysis. The majority of benefit is attributed to a reduction in sudden cardiac deaths.

In this case there are additional considerations. Mr BY has clinically evident left ventricular dysfunction, an indication for beta-blocker therapy in its own right, and there is evidence that beta-blockers can be initiated safely and effectively in patients with left ventricular dysfunction post MI. The CAPRICORN study, in which patients were randomised to carvedilol or placebo at 3–21 days post MI, demonstrated a 23% reduction in mortality over approximately 1 year. Beta-blocker therapy should therefore be considered for initiation over the next few days, provided Mr BY remains clinically stable, particularly with respect to his symptoms of heart failure.

The use of both ACEI and beta-blocker therapy following MI is recommended by NICE. It might be considered that ACEI therapy should be optimised before the addition of a beta-blocker; however, it should be remembered that although there are established benefits of ACEI dose titration, these are primarily morbidity benefits (reduced hospitalisations seen in the ATLAS study). In contrast, ACEIs and beta-blockers have both been shown to reduce mortality independently. Early initiation of agents from the two different drug classes may therefore be justified, but dose titration of each should be continued over the next few weeks to reach the maximal tolerated doses. For Mr BY, the key limitation of combined ACEI and beta-blocker therapy in the early phases will be his persistent low BP following his acute event.

What advice would you give about the initiation of a beta-blocker?

A20 **The beta-blocker therapy should be introduced cautiously, starting at a low dose and with careful monitoring of HR, BP, blood gases and symptoms of heart failure. The dose should be titrated to the maximum tolerated by doubling at 2-weekly intervals, unless cardiac symptoms prohibit this. Mr BY's symptoms may be exacerbated during the titration phase. If this happens, additional diuretic therapy may be required or the interval between titrations may need to be extended. Occasionally, a step down in dose may be required. Close follow-up should be arranged prior to discharge to ensure ongoing monitoring and dose titration.**

Should eplerenone be prescribed for Mr BY?

A21 **Yes. In line with NICE guidance, an aldosterone antagonist licensed for use post MI (eplerenone) should be prescribed within 3–14 days, preferably after ACEI therapy, for patients with symptoms and/or signs of heart failure and left ventricular systolic dysfunction (LVSD) and an ejection fraction ≤40%.**

In the EPHESUS trial, eplerenone therapy led to a 13% reduction in cardiovascular mortality or hospitalisation for cardiovascular causes over the 12 months of follow-up. The reduction in cardiovascular mortality was mainly due to a 21% reduction in sudden cardiac death.

Eplerenone should be started after the ACE inhibitor, with careful monitoring of renal function and potassium levels. Hyperkalaemia is often an issue during treatment and may require withdrawal of the drug in some cases, but a low-potassium diet should be instituted in the first instance.

Comment on Mr BY's cholesterol level. How should this be managed?

A22 **Mr BY has a raised cholesterol level which will increase his risk of further cardiovascular events. Lipid-lowering therapy should be initiated, as reducing serum cholesterol has been shown to reduce the risk of death, reinfarction or other cardiovascular events in this patient group. Mr BY should be given dietary advice in combination with the initiation of a high-dose statin.**

Cholesterol levels should be measured within 24 hours of symptom onset in patients with AMI, as after 24 hours cholesterol levels have been shown to fall and remain low for approximately 3 months. As the cholesterol level was measured on admission in this case, it is unreasonable to expect it to be a fasting sample and therefore only the measured total cholesterol levels can be considered reliable.

Patients should be encouraged to reduce their total fat intake, particularly of saturated fat, and to increase their intake of vegetables and fibre. A number of booklets on healthy eating for patients with CHD are available, e.g. *Cut the Saturated Fat from Your Diet* from the British Heart Foundation. Most patients find it difficult to achieve large reductions in total cholesterol using diet alone, with average reductions in the order of 5%.

Statins reduce total cholesterol by an average of 25–35%, with greater reductions in low-density lipoprotein (LDL), the cholesterol subtype that correlates most closely with cardiovascular risk. Reducing cholesterol with statins has been shown to reduce the risk of death, reinfarction and other cardiovascular events in this patient group.

High-intensity statins for patients following acute coronary syndromes were endorsed in the NICE Lipid Modification guideline (CG 67), which recommended the use of an agent which produced a greater lipid-lowering effect than simvastatin 40 mg, such as simvastatin 80 mg daily. This recommendation is based mainly on the results of the PROVE-IT study (atorvastatin 80 mg vs pravastatin 40 mg), which demonstrated a statistically significant reduction in the composite of cardiovascular mortality and morbidity in the atorvastatin-treated arm. A to Z (simvastatin 40 mg then 80 mg vs placebo then 20 mg) only demonstrated a trend in favour of higher-dose statin therapy. Since the publication of the NICE lipid guidance in 2008 there has been much controversy over the efficacy and the safety of simvastatin 80 mg daily, and, as a result, many clinicians are using atorvastatin 80 mg for this indication. In order to maximise the potential early benefits of statin therapy, treatment should be started as early as possible post AMI, even in the absence of baseline cholesterol levels, and should be aimed at reducing total cholesterol to <4 mmol/L and LDL cholesterol to <2 mmol/L in this high-risk group.

Mr BY's cholesterol should be rechecked in 3 months and therapy should be reviewed if levels remain high. Liver function tests should be performed throughout the first year of statin therapy. Routine monitoring of creatine kinase (CK) is not recommended, although patients should be advised to report any unusual muscle pain or weakness. If this occurs, CK levels should be checked to aid clinical decision making.

How should Mr BY's blood sugar levels be controlled over the longer term?

A23 **A subcutaneous insulin regimen should be initiated on cessation of his sliding-scale IV insulin.**

The preferred insulin regimen for Mr BY is the combination of a long-acting (basal) insulin with short-acting soluble insulin at mealtimes to mimic physiologic insulin patterns. Patient assessment, careful selection of insulin dose and administration device, and the provision of adequate education and support is essential to ensure successful management of blood sugar levels. All patients should be referred to a diabetic clinic to ensure appropriate follow-up. In the DIGAMI study, insulin therapy was maintained for a minimum of 3 months post infarction, but the optimal duration has not been clearly established. Long-term control of blood sugar is important following MI to reduce the risk of cardiac and non-cardiac complications of diabetes.

What lifestyle issues should be discussed with Mr BY?

A24 **Lifestyle advice should include the importance of diet, exercise and weight loss. Stopping smoking, modifying his diet and increasing exercise are all effective in reducing his risk of further coronary events. Mr BY should be encouraged to participate in a cardiac rehabilitation programme, where these issues will be addressed in greater depth.**

Within 1 year of smoking cessation the risk of cardiac events is halved, and after 2–3 years it has returned to that of a non-smoker. Interventions to improve cessation rates include counselling, the use of nicotine replacement therapies, and the prescription of bupropion or varenicline. Mr BY should be strongly encouraged to stop smoking at this point and appropriate cessation aids should be offered.

The adoption of a healthy balanced diet, low in saturated fats and high in vegetables and fibre, should be encouraged for Mr BY. Diets low in saturated fats and supplemented with polyunsaturated fatty acids (PUFAs) have been shown to improve survival in patients with CHD, who should be advised to eat two to four portions of oily fish each week to increase their intake of PUFAs. If they are unable or unwilling to do this, then prescription of an omega-3 fatty acid supplement should be considered. A reduction in calorie intake is appropriate in view of Mr BY's obesity, and a reduced saturated fat intake will contribute to cholesterol lowering. Weight loss will also improve his sensitivity to insulin and may reduce the need for long-term insulin therapy.

Exercise is also important and has been shown to reduce cardiac mortality. Mr BY should be advised on increasing his physical activity safely and encouraged to attend a cardiac rehabilitation programme, where he can begin to do this under supervision. Such a programme will support Mr BY in making the lifestyle changes necessary to reduce his cardiovascular risk.

What issues should be highlighted during discharge counselling for this patient?

A25 **Key areas for counselling include an explanation of the indication for and aim of each medicine, instruction on how each should be taken, information on appropriate follow-up, long-term monitoring, and dealing with potential adverse effects. The benefits of long-term cardiovascular risk reduction should be emphasised to encourage adherence to prescribed medications.**

It is essential to convey the importance of long-term drug treatment in patients with CHD. If the difference between risk reduction and symptom management is not clearly explained, patients may fail to adhere to therapy, particularly if they are asymptomatic. Mr BY should be advised that some of his drug doses may need to be increased over the next few weeks to achieve the optimal dose. Follow-up by a diabetic clinic and a heart failure clinic will be necessary to ensure appropriate long-term management. Clopidogrel therapy should be discontinued at 4 weeks, and the patient should be issued with a clopidogrel card as a reminder of this.

All of these points should be reinforced with written information and, ideally, an individual medication record card as an *aide-mémoire*. Additional information for patients, in the form of booklets such as *Medicines for the Heart*, is available from the British Heart Foundation. Mr BY should again be encouraged to attend a cardiac rehabilitation programme, which has been shown to improve outcome post MI.

Further reading

ACE-Inhibitor Myocardial Infarction Collaborative Group. Indications for ACE-inhibitors in the early treatment of acute myocardial infarction: systematic overview of individual data from 100 000 patients in randomised trials. *Circulation* 1998; **97**: 2202–2212.

AIRE Extension (AIREX) Study. Follow-up study of patients randomly allocated ramipril or placebo for heart failure after acute myocardial infarction. *Lancet* 1997; **349**: 1493–1497.

Anon. Lifestyle measures to reduce cardiovascular risk. *MeReC Brief* 2002; **19**.

Antithrombotic Triallists' Collaboration. Collaborative meta-analysis of randomised trials of antiplatelet therapy for prevention of death, myocardial infarction, and stroke in high risk patients. *Br Med J* 2002; **324**: 71–86.

Assessment of the Safety and Efficacy of a New Thrombolytic (ASSENT-2) Investigators. Single-bolus tenecteplase compared with front-loaded alteplase in acute myocardial infarction. The ASSENT-2 randomised double-blind trial. *Lancet* 1999; **354**: 716–722.

Assessment of the Safety and Efficacy of a New Thrombolytic Regimen (ASSENT-3) Investigators. Efficacy and safety of tenecteplase in combination with enoxaparin, abciximab, or unfractionated heparin. The ASSENT-3 randomised trial in acute myocardial infarction. *Lancet* 2001; **358**: 605–613.

Cannon CP, Braunwald E, McCabe CH *et al.* Intensive versus moderate lipid lowering with statins after acute coronary syndromes. *N Engl J Med* 2004; **350**: 1495–1504.

Dargie HJ (for the CAPRICORN Investigators). Effect of carvedilol on outcome after myocardial infarction in patients with left-ventricular dysfunction; the CAPRICORN randomised trial. *Lancet* 2001; **357**: 1385–1390.

CLARITY–TIMI 28 Investigators. Addition of clopidogrel to aspirin and fibrinolytic therapy for myocardial infarction with ST-segment-elevation. The CLARITY-TIMI 28 trial. *N Engl J Med* 2005; **352**: 1179–1189.

COMMIT Collaborative Group. Addition of clopidogrel to aspirin in 45 852 patients with acute myocardial infarction: randomised placebo-controlled trial. *Lancet* 2005; **366**: 1607–1621.

Dalby M, Bouzamondo A, Lechat P, Montalescot G. Transfer for primary angioplasty versus immediate thrombolysis in acute myocardial infarction: a meta-analysis. *Circulation* 2003; **108**(15): 1809–1814.

de Lemos JA, Blazing MA, Wiviott SD *et al.* Early intensive vs a delayed conservative simvastatin strategy in patients with acute coronary syndromes: phase Z of the A to Z trial. *J Am Med Assoc* 2004; **292**: 1307–1316.

Fibrinolytic Therapy Trialists' (FTT) Collaborative Group. Indications for fibrinolytic therapy in suspected acute myocardial infarction: collaborative overview of early mortality and major morbidity results from all randomised trials of more than 1000 patients. *Lancet* 1994; **343**: 311–322.

Freemantle N, Cleland J, Young P *et al.* Beta-blockade after myocardial infarction. Systematic review and meta-regression analysis. *Br Med J* 1999; **318**: 1730–1737.

Heart Outcomes Prevention Evaluation Study Investigators. Effects of an angiotensin-converting-enzyme inhibitor, ramipril, on cardiovascular events in high-risk patients. *N Engl J Med* 2000; **342**: 145–153.

Heart Protection Study Collaborative Group. MRC/*BHF* heart protection study of cholesterol lowering with simvastatin in 20 536 individuals: a randomised placebo-controlled trial. *Lancet* 2002; **360**: 7–22.

Helton TJ, Barry AA, Kumbhani DJ *et al.* Incremental effect of clopidogrel on important outcomes in patients with cardiovascular disease: a meta-analysis of randomized trials. *Am J Cardiovasc Drugs* 2007; **7**: 289–297.

Joint British Societies 2. Joint British Societies' guidelines on prevention of cardiovascular disease in clinical practice. *Heart* 2005; **91**(Suppl V): 1–52.

Joint ESC/ACCF/AHA/WHF Task Force for the Redefinition of Myocardial Infarction. Universal definition of myocardial infarction. *Eur Heart J* 2007; **28**: 2525–2538.

LaRosa JC, He J, Vupputuri S. Effect of statins on risk of coronary disease: a meta-analysis of randomized controlled trials. *J Am Med Assoc* 1999; **282**: 2340–2346.

Malmberg K, Norhammer A, Wedel H *et al.* Glycometabolic state at admission: important risk marker in conventionally treated patients with diabetes mellitus and acute myocardial infarction: long-term results from the Diabetes and Insulin-Glucose Infusion in Acute Myocardial Infarction (DIGAMI) study. *Circulation* 1999; **99**: 2626–232.

National Institute for Health and Clinical Excellence. CG48. *MI: Secondary Prevention. Secondary Prevention in Primary and Secondary Care for Patients Following a Myocardial Infarction.* NICE, London, 2007.

National Institute for Health and Clinical Excellence. CG67. *Lipid Modification.* NICE, London, 2008.

National Institute for Clinical Excellence. TA52. *Guidance on the Use of Drugs for Early Thrombolysis in the Treatment of Acute Myocardial Infarction.* NICE, London, 2002.

Pitt B, Remme W, Zannad F *et al.* Eplerenone, a selective aldosterone blocker, in patients with left ventricular dysfunction after myocardial infarction. *N Engl J Med* 2003; **348**: 1309–1321.

Task Force for Diagnosis and Treatment of Acute and Chronic Heart Failure 2008 of European Society of Cardiology. ESC Guidelines for the diagnosis and treatment of acute and chronic heart failure 2008. *Eur Heart J* 2008; **29**(19): 2388–2442. Epub 2008 Sep 17.

Van de Werf F, Ardissino D, Betriu A *et al*. Task Force on the Management of Acute Myocardial Infarction of the European Society of Cardiology. Management of acute myocardial infarction in patients presenting with ST-segment elevation. *Eur Heart J* 2003; **24**(1): 28–66.

4

Cardiac failure

Stephen Hudson, John McAnaw and Tobias Dreischulte

Case study and questions

Day 1 Mrs HMcC, a 71-year-old woman weighing 53 kg, was admitted to hospital. She had been treated for chronic heart failure for 3 years and had a history of atrial fibrillation (AF) and hypertension. She had now been referred to hospital by her general practitioner (GP) with a suspected deterioration in her condition. Over the past 3 months she had started complaining of increased tiredness and shortness of breath, which limited her walking. She also had some difficulty sleeping, which was notably affected by shortness of breath at night. Mrs HMcC reported episodes of discomfort in the chest, which she described as 'palpitations' rather than tightness or pain. Her medication on admission was:

- Bendroflumethiazide 2.5 mg daily
- Furosemide 40 mg daily
- Enalapril 10 mg daily
- Digoxin 125 micrograms daily
- Simvastatin 40 mg at night
- Warfarin 3 mg daily
- Co-codamol 8/500 tablets, two when required

On examination she was pale and her temperature was 37.3°C, pulse 130 beats per minute (bpm) and irregular, and her blood pressure (lying) was 155/89 mmHg. Her jugular venous pulse was elevated 3 cm and pitting oedema was present in both feet and ankles. The apex of the beat was difficult to locate, and crepitations were present in the right and left lung fields. There was slight enlargement of the liver beyond the costal margin, but no tenderness. The results of plasma biochemistry and haematology investigations on admission were:

- Sodium 137 mmol/L (reference range 135–145)
- Potassium 3.7 mmol/L (3.5–5.0)
- Urea 12.4 mmol/L (2.6–6.6)
- Creatinine 140 micromol/L (80–120)
- Haemoglobin 10.1 g/dL (12–16)
- Mean cell volume 71 fL (77–91)
- Mean cell haemoglobin concentration 0.30 g/dL (0.32–0.36)
- Digoxin 1.0 micrograms/L (0.8–2)
- Total cholesterol 3.8 mmol/L

An electrocardiogram (ECG) demonstrated rapid AF without ischaemic changes or signs of infarction. An echocardiogram confirmed left ventricular systolic dysfunction and marked left ventricular hypertrophy. The ejection fraction was 35%.

A diagnosis was made of cardiac failure, complicated by the presence of AF and anaemia associated with iron deficiency.

Q1 How can AF and anaemia exacerbate cardiac failure in a patient such as Mrs HMcC?
Q2 What symptoms of cardiac failure does Mrs HMcC exhibit?
Q3 What are the immediate therapeutic aims for Mrs HMcC?
Q4 Which evidence-based treatments may be of benefit to Mrs HMcC to slow disease progression and minimise the risk of further heart failure exacerbations? How do these treatments work, and which would you recommend for Mrs HMcC at this point in her illness?
Q5 Can a knowledge of digoxin pharmacokinetics guide digoxin dose optimisation? What dose would you recommend for Mrs HMcC?

Day 5 Mrs HMcC was discharged home with a New York Heart Association (NYHA) functional assessment of II/III and on the following medications:

- Digoxin 187.5 micrograms once daily
- Furosemide 40 mg each morning
- Enalapril 10 mg twice daily
- Ferrous sulphate 200 mg three times daily after food
- Warfarin 3 mg daily
- Simvastatin 40 mg at night
- Bisoprolol 1.25 mg daily

A 2-week follow-up appointment was arranged.

Q6 Outline your pharmaceutical care plan for Mrs HMcC.

Day 20 Mrs HMcC was seen in the outpatient heart failure clinic. She still seemed to be symptomatic at home and had some difficulty climbing stairs. Oedema was still present in both ankles and her pulse was 108 bpm.

Q7 Which medical conditions and drug treatments are known to exacerbate cardiac failure?
Q8 What is the likely explanation for Mrs HMcC's persisting cardiac failure?

Mrs HMcC's digoxin dose was increased to 250 micrograms daily, and her diuretic requirements were increased to furosemide 40 mg each morning and 20 mg at lunchtime. She was asked to return to clinic in 2 weeks.

Day 35 Mrs HMcC was visited at home by her GP after a week-long deterioration in her condition. She felt unwell, tired but restless, and nauseated. She had been unsociable and had not been out of the house for 3 days. She was readmitted to hospital with suspected digoxin toxicity.

Q9 What symptoms might lead you to suspect digoxin toxicity?
Q10 What is the role of plasma digoxin assay and when should blood samples be drawn?
Q11 What clinical factors predispose patients to digoxin toxicity, and why do you think Mrs HMcC might be demonstrating these symptoms?

On examination in hospital Mrs HMcC's pulse was found to be 52 bpm and regular. She was still nauseated, withdrawn and a little confused. An ECG demonstrated sinus rhythm with no abnormalities. Blood was sampled for urea, electrolytes, international normalised ratio (INR) and plasma digoxin. Her plasma potassium was 3.7 mmol/L (3.5–5.0) and her plasma digoxin concentration was 2.7 micrograms/L (1.0–2.0).

Q12 What are the cardiac effects of digoxin toxicity?
Q13 Apart from stopping the drug, how can digoxin toxicity be managed?

Because Mrs HMcC was demonstrating signs and symptoms of digoxin toxicity at the plasma digoxin concentration required to control her AF, digoxin was discontinued and amiodarone commenced. She improved mentally within 24 hours and became mobile over the following 2 days. She was discharged after 5 days on the following therapy:

- Furosemide 40 mg each morning, and 20 mg at lunchtime
- Enalapril 10 mg twice daily
- Amiodarone 200 mg three times a day
- Ferrous sulphate 200 mg three times daily after food
- Warfarin 3 mg daily
- Simvastatin 40 mg at night
- Bisoprolol 5 mg daily

Q14 Do you agree with the choice of amiodarone to control Mrs HMcC's AF? What issues would you now add to or change in the pharmaceutical care plan originally developed for Mrs HMcC and described in **A6**?

Day 70 Mrs HMcC was complaining of increasing shortness of breath and further ankle swelling.

Q15 What treatment options might you consider next to manage Mrs HMcC's cardiac failure?

Answers

How can AF and anaemia exacerbate cardiac failure in a patient such as Mrs HMcC?

A1 The heart fails when its output falls short of the perfusion needs of the tissues. Heart failure is most commonly due to sudden or insidious deterioration of cardiac function. Mrs HMcC's declining cardiac function is probably due to loss of cardiac contractility, but is also complicated by a persistent arrhythmia which may be contributing to the signs of left ventricular failure. Her iron-deficiency anaemia may be further complicating her inability to match her cardiac output to the perfusion demands of her muscles, as iron deficiency increases those perfusion demands.

When the heart pump is compromised by ventricular damage (e.g. ischaemia or infarction), persistent arrhythmia, valve disorder or outflow obstruction there is a resulting reduction in the rate of oxygen and nutrient delivery to the tissues.

In AF, the contractions of the atria are disorganised and frequent electrical impulses (>600 per minute) pass down the conducting fibres. The ventricles cannot contract at this rate, owing to the refractoriness of the conducting system (the atrioventricular node). Instead they contract irregularly, at a rate usually between 100 and 200 bpm. Cardiac output is lowered as a result of reduced ventricular filling arising from the loss of normal atrial contraction plus the short diastole (caused by the high ventricular rate). The poor control of Mrs HMcC's AF is thus likely to be exacerbating her cardiac failure. This may be reversed by an improvement in the control of her AF.

Anaemia can be a cause of what may be termed 'high-output' heart failure. The link between anaemia and heart failure is the reduced capacity of the blood to transport oxygen to the tissues owing to the low haemoglobin content of the red cells. In response to severe depletion of oxygen the normal heart can increase cardiac output in an effort to increase the blood supply to the tissues and therefore compensate for the reduced rate of oxygen delivery; however, the resulting increased demands placed on a failing heart can exacerbate symptoms of cardiac failure in a patient such as Mrs HMcC.

What symptoms of cardiac failure does Mrs HMcC exhibit?

A2 Dyspnoea, oedema and raised jugular venous pulse, pallor and tiredness.

In a patient with stable heart failure, presenting symptoms are often described using the New York Heart Association (NYHA) classification of

Table 4.1 NYHA classification of functional status of the patient with heart failure

I	No symptoms with ordinary physical activity (such as walking or climbing stairs)
II	Slight limitation with dyspnoea on moderate to severe exertion (climbing stairs or walking uphill)
III	Marked limitation of activity: less than ordinary activity causes dyspnoea (restricting walking distance and limiting climbing to one flight of stairs)
IV	Severe disability, dyspnoea at rest (unable to carry on physical activity without discomfort)

functional status outlined in Table 4.1. This system allows the grading of heart failure symptoms experienced by the patient according to severity; however, it is not consistently used in routine practice and so a patient's NYHA status may not be explicitly recorded in the case notes. It is nevertheless a well-understood categorisation system and is frequently used to describe populations of heart failure patients studied in clinical trials.

Mrs HMcC has been complaining of shortness of breath when walking and at night. This is typical. Dyspnoea occurs on exertion and on lying down (orthopnoea). Orthopnoea may progress to attacks of gasping at night, termed paroxysmal nocturnal dyspnoea, which are relieved by sitting or standing up. These symptoms arise from a reduced output from the left ventricle, which in turn results in an impaired blood supply to the tissues and organs where the function of muscle, kidney and nervous systems are particularly affected. Mrs HMcC could be described as NYHA stage II worsening to stage III.

In cardiac failure, retention of sodium and fluid leads to oedema in the lungs, ankles, wrists and abdomen. When the patient is lying down oedema is redistributed, and in the lungs this produces cough or breathlessness.

Congestion of blood in the lungs also produces increased pulmonary capillary pressure, which leads to pulmonary oedema and shortness of breath. Owing to the reduced compliance of the congested lungs, more effort is required to expand them. Failure of the right ventricle leads to congestion and oedema in the peripheral tissues. Venous congestion may be demonstrated in the reclining patient by visible elevation of the jugular venous pulse in the neck. This is seen in Mrs HMcC.

Muscle fatigue resulting from the reduced blood supply further diminishes tolerance to exercise. Symptoms are often insidious in onset, especially in the elderly, as patients may adjust their lifestyle to accommodate a loss of tolerance to exercise. Other symptoms resulting from a reduced blood supply to the tissues of the brain, kidneys, liver and gut are confusion, renal failure, enlargement of the liver (hepatomegaly) and abdominal distension, anorexia, nausea, and abdominal pain. The patient's complexion may be pale, and the hands cold and sweaty, due to stimulation of the sympathetic nervous system in response to reduced cardiac output. These are symptoms recorded for Mrs HMcC.

What are the immediate therapeutic aims for Mrs HMcC?

A3 (a) Treat her AF to control the ventricular rate.

In the management of AF either a rhythm-control or a rate-control strategy can be employed. In the former case restoration of sinus rhythm would be attempted via pharmacological or electrical cardioversion. However, in patients with marked left ventricular enlargement (ventricular wall diameter >5 cm) the chances of successful cardioversion and long-term maintenance of sinus rhythm are slim. It had therefore been decided to pursue a rate-control strategy for Mrs HMcC. Beta-blockers, digoxin and amiodarone are recommended for rate control in patients with heart failure and concurrent AF. Beta-blockers and digoxin exert their beneficial effects in AF mainly by slowing conduction down the atrioventricular node, whereas amiodarone acts primarily by increasing the refractory period. Both mechanisms control the ventricular rate and improve cardiac output. Although beta-blockers have been shown to reduce mortality and morbidity in heart failure patients in the longer term (see below), they may initially cause a deterioration of heart failure symptoms by reducing the contractile force of the myocardium, which is mediated by sympathetic activity. This is particularly true at higher doses, which are normally required for control of AF. Amiodarone has a neutral effect on myocardial contractility but has numerous extracardiac side-effects (see below). In contrast, digoxin has a positive inotropic effect on the myocardium, which is caused by an increase in myocardial intracellular ionic calcium that occurs secondary to the inhibition of sodium extrusion from the myocardial cell. The positive inotropic effect secures the contractile force of the myocardium, making it the preferred choice of initial drug therapy in Mrs HMcC's case. However, this effect of digoxin may not be sustained long term, and clear beneficial effects of digoxin on life expectancy have not been shown in outcome studies of patients in sinus rhythm (that is, in the absence of AF).

(b) Investigate and treat her suspected iron-deficiency anaemia.

A dietary and drug history is required, together with any history of blood loss from the body (e.g. gastrointestinal, postmenopausal, urinary). Laboratory tests should include serum iron, total iron-binding capacity and serum ferritin levels, to confirm or refute true iron deficiency. Mrs HMcC will require ferrous sulphate tablets 200 mg three times daily. In order to ensure that body iron stores are replenished, treatment must be continued beyond the restoration of haemoglobin concentration to within normal limits: a course of iron therapy may thus last up to 6 months.

(c) Control her oedema and symptoms of cardiac failure.

Diuretic therapy is normally prescribed for the control of sodium and water retention, although Mrs HMcC's oedema may reduce once her AF and the associated cardiac failure are successfully controlled.

There are two main classes of diuretic available for the treatment of cardiac failure: thiazides and loop diuretics. Thiazides are not often used as sole diuretic therapy, being reserved for cases of mild cardiac failure and where renal function is not compromised. Most patients with symptoms of cardiac failure require a more potent loop diuretic, usually bumetanide or furosemide. Torasemide is a newer loop diuretic with limited evidence of clinically relevant advantages over the other agents in this group.

Loop diuretics produce a more vigorous diuresis than thiazides, and thus carry a greater risk of causing hypovolaemia in the short term. A too-rapid and profound diuresis can exacerbate cardiac failure by reducing the circulating blood volume, and can also increase the patient's uraemia (pre-renal azotaemia). In practice, furosemide 40 mg is considered equipotent to bumetanide 1 mg. Clinical trials indicate that 5–10 mg torasemide is equivalent to 40 mg furosemide. Thiazides, on the other hand, produce a less profound diuresis, but pose the greater long-term risk of hypokalaemia and hyponatraemia, particularly in elderly patients. The thiazides have a longer duration of action (average 12–24 hours) than the loop diuretics (average 4–6 hours) but have a low ceiling effect. Bendroflumethiazide produces a maximum effect at 5 mg: any further increase in dose provides no added benefit, but increases the chance of adverse effects such as hyperglycaemia and hyperuricaemia.

Thiazide diuretics also lose effectiveness when renal function is markedly impaired, particularly when the patient's creatinine clearance is <25 mL/min. However, when used as an add-on to a loop diuretic, thiazides may produce a synergistic diuretic effect by reducing the compensatory rebound in sodium retention provoked by loop diuretics (sequential nephron blockade). Metolazone in particular is reserved for synergistic use with a loop diuretic and can produce profound diuresis, with potentially dramatic effects on electrolyte balance.

Mrs HMcC is exhibiting signs and symptoms of acute congestive cardiac failure (CCF) while being prescribed furosemide 40 mg, therefore an increase in dose is warranted during her hospital stay to control these symptoms. Because of this increase in her diuretic dose Mrs HMcC's potassium level must be monitored closely, as hypokalaemia increases the risk of digoxin toxicity. If required, potassium-sparing diuretics or adequate potassium supplements (e.g. 40–80 mmol/day) should be co-prescribed. Combination diuretic plus potassium products such as Burinex K (bumetanide 0.5 mg plus potassium 7.7 mmol) are not suitable as their potassium content is too low.

(d) Ensure effective antithrombotic prophylaxis.

AF predisposes to stroke, particularly in patients with rheumatic heart disease, congestive heart failure, arterial hypertension, diabetes mellitus or uncontrolled thyrotoxicosis. Randomised controlled trials have investigated the use of warfarin and aspirin for the prevention of first stroke (primary prevention) or further stroke (secondary prevention) in patients with AF. These trials have shown that anticoagulation reduces the risk of thromboembolic stroke by two-thirds in men and women with persistent or paroxysmal non-rheumatic AF. Anticoagulation mainly has a role in primary prevention of stroke in AF, with some benefit also shown in the prevention of a further stroke for those with a history of stroke. Warfarin should therefore be a therapeutic option for those patients over 65 years of age with non-valvular AF and at least one other risk factor for stroke. In the case of Mrs HMcC, three risk factors are present: age >65, a history of hypertension and the presence of heart failure. Therefore, warfarin is the best treatment option for her. However, the benefits and risks of warfarin therapy should be considered very carefully in patients over 75 years. Only where warfarin is refused by the patient or contraindicated should the use of aspirin 75–300 mg daily be considered. Although aspirin is considered to be a safer option, and a simpler and cheaper alternative to warfarin in the prevention of stroke in patients with AF over the age of 75, it is less effective than warfarin. In patients with AF under 65 years with no risk factors for stroke, such as diabetes mellitus or hypertension, the benefits of anticoagulant therapy are marginal (<2% reduction of risk).

(e) Control her blood pressure.

Control of underlying hypertension is important in order to reduce her risk of haemorrhagic stroke and other cardiovascular problems, such as coronary heart disease, myocardial infarction (MI) and organ damage. According to NICE guidance, the optimum blood pressure to be achieved in Mrs HMcC is <140/90 mmHg, therefore her current blood pressure of 155/89 mmHg demonstrates suboptimal control. Mrs HMcC is currently prescribed two antihypertensive agents (bendroflumethiazide 2.5 mg daily, and enalapril 10 mg daily), but there is scope to reduce her blood pressure by further optimising the angiotensin-converting enzyme inhibitor (ACEI) dose (also see **A4**).

Which evidence-based treatments may be of benefit to Mrs HMcC to slow disease progression and minimise the risk of further heart failure exacerbations? How do these treatments work, and which would you recommend for Mrs HMcC at this point in her illness?

A4 **Mrs HMcC currently receives diuretic treatment, enalapril and digoxin for treatment of heart failure. At this point she should have her ACEI therapy increased to the maximum tolerated dose and a low-dose beta-blocker such as bisoprolol introduced and titrated up to the maximum tolerated dose. Her digoxin and diuretic therapy should also be optimised.**

Although diuretics and digoxin have traditionally been used for symptomatic relief of heart failure symptoms, evidence of any long-term effects on mortality is scarce. In contrast, a number of clinical trials support the use of ACEIs, beta-blockers, low-dose aldosterone antagonists, angiotensin receptor blockers (ARBs) and hydralazine/nitrate combinations because of demonstrated benefits in morbidity and mortality for patients with left ventricular systolic dysfunction. Nevertheless, diuretics are required in the majority of patients to control oedema and dyspnoea, and digoxin remains important in heart failure patients such as Mrs HMcC, who has coexisting AF.

Specific recommendations are as follows:

(a) **ACEIs.** Large studies (CONSENSUS, SOLVD-T, SOLVD-P and V-HeFT II), have shown that ACEIs in combination with diuretics (with or without digoxin) can improve symptoms and prolong life in all grades of heart failure, as well as improving exercise tolerance. In patients who have suffered MI, similar improvements in outcomes have also been demonstrated (SAVE, AIREX and TRACE). ACEIs are thus regarded as a cornerstone in the management of heart failure. Progression of heart failure from mild to severe is reduced, as is hospitalisation, and survival is improved in all grades of heart failure. Some conditions, such as renovascular stenosis, aortic stenosis or outflow tract obstruction, are relative contraindications to ACEIs, but they tend to be well tolerated by most patients.

ACEIs act upon the renin–angiotensin–aldosterone system, and produce vasodilation by blocking the sequence of events leading to the production of the circulating vasoconstrictor angiotensin II and subsequent effects mediated by aldosterone. Through impairment of aldosterone formation, ACEIs also benefit heart failure by reducing sodium and water retention, thereby reducing venous congestion. This reduction contributes to an improved cardiac output, which in turn improves renal perfusion, leading to a reduction in oedema. ACEIs are therefore able to interrupt the cycle of secondary physiological events that occur in response to cardiac failure.

The major problems with all ACEIs are first-dose hypotension (worsened by an upright posture), skin rashes and renal toxicity signified by proteinuria. First-dose hypotension is particularly marked in patients who have recently received high doses of diuretics. The sensitivity of blood pressure to the introduction of an ACEI results from the high circulating angiotensin levels that maintain the blood pressure in circumstances of reduced blood volume secondary to diuresis. To minimise acute hypotension, high diuretic doses should therefore be curtailed, if possible for a few days prior to starting treatment with the ACEI, and a small first dose of the drug should be administered at bedtime. In patients at risk of hypotension, captopril is most commonly used. Even though captopril has the disadvantage of a faster onset of effect, it has the advantage of a shorter duration of action in the event of an exaggerated response. Other patients at particular risk of this first-dose effect include those who have activation of the renin–angiotensin system and secondary hyperaldosteronism (such as patients with liver disease).

Higher doses of ACEIs have been demonstrated to reduce hospitalisation rates compared to lower doses (ATLAS). After the initiation of an ACEI, the dose is therefore titrated towards that used in clinical trials associated with improvements in morbidity and mortality, e.g. enalapril 10–20 mg twice daily. Where a target dose is not achievable because of poor patient tolerance, the maximum tolerable dose is an acceptable alternative. As ACEIs can have a pronounced effect on blood pressure, it is important that titration towards a target dose is accompanied by blood pressure measurements after each increase.

All the ACEIs apart from captopril and lisinopril are prodrugs. The use of prodrugs means that there may be patient variability in response, affected by the bioavailability and the varying ability of patients to convert the prodrug into the active form. All ACEIs licensed for CCF at the time of writing are eliminated mainly by the kidney and require dosage adjustment in renal failure (creatinine clearance <60 mL/min). ACEIs can also impair renal function, although this is most likely to occur in a patient with pre-existing renal impairment or renal artery stenosis. This effect can occur with any ACEI, and therefore renal function should be carefully monitored when initiating therapy and after any subsequent increase in dose.

The risk of hyperkalaemia precludes the use of potassium upplements or potassium-sparing diuretics with ACEIs, unless potassium levels are carefully monitored.

Unwanted immunological effects on the skin and proteinuria occur more often with captopril than with the other agents, and are thought to be due to its sulphydryl group; however, these are rare side-effects in the usual therapeutic dose range, unless the patient has a connective tissue disorder such as rheumatoid arthritis. Alteration or loss of taste, cough and mouth ulcers are also recognised side-effects of ACEIs, but are not specific to any one agent.

(b) **Beta-blockers.** Beta-blockers were previously considered to be contraindicated in patients with heart failure; however, clinical trials involving carvedilol, bisoprolol, metoprolol SR and nebivolol (US Carvedilol, CIBIS II, MERIT-HF, COPERNICUS and SENIORS) have shown that they have a beneficial effect on morbidity and mortality in all grades of heart failure as an adjunct to ACEIs and diuretic therapy. In the UK at the time of writing only carvedilol, bisoprolol and nebivolol are licensed for the treatment of patients with chronic heart failure.

Beta-blockers counteract the chronic sympathetic overactivity that occurs when the heart fails to maintain sufficient cardiac output. They inhibit arterial constriction and the direct effects of noradrenaline (norepinephrine) and circulating catecholamines on the heart. These effects reduce the demands placed on the heart, thereby lessening the structural and physiological changes that occur with chronic heart failure. Clinical trial evidence has shown that initiation at a low dose and careful upward titration of dose are necessary to institute beta-blocker therapy safely. Titration is usually carried out over a period of weeks or months, during which time patients are likely to suffer from an initial worsening of symptoms with each dose increment. The goal is to titrate the dose towards those used in clinical trials that led to morbidity and mortality benefits, e.g. bisoprolol 5–10 mg daily. However, it is accepted that not all patients will be able to tolerate such doses, and therefore the maximum tolerated dose would be an acceptable alternative.

Close monitoring is needed during the initiation and titration of beta-blocker therapy in order to identify excessive bradycardia or marked deterioration of symptoms. The occurrence of these symptoms may limit the use of beta-blocker therapy in certain patients. Other limiting side-effects related to beta-blocker therapy may include fatigue and loss of libido.

(c) **ARBs.** ARBs can reduce sodium and water retention by preventing the release of aldosterone (reduction in venous congestion), and angiotensin II-mediated arterial vasoconstriction (reduction in afterload). They mimic the effect of ACEIs in that these effects combine to improve cardiac output and renal perfusion, thereby leading to an improvement in symptoms and a reduction in oedema. The main advantage over ACEIs is that ARBs rarely produce cough, and they should therefore be considered where ACEI-induced cough is persistent and troublesome to the patient. In studies of patients who were unable to tolerate an ACEI, ARBs have been demonstrated to be comparable to ACEIs in reducing cardiovascular mortality and rate of hospitalisation, and in the control of heart failure symptoms (CHARM Alternative, Val-HeFT). The use of ARBs as an adjunct to ACEI and beta-blocker therapy has been associated with significant reductions in cardiovascular events and hospitalisation rates (ValHeFT, CHARM Added). Although this finding is encouraging, the impact on mortality alone has so far been inconsistent, and there is no clear consensus on when to use an ARB as adjunctive therapy. As with the use of ACEIs, monitoring of renal function and plasma potassium concentration is important on initiation of therapy or after any increase in dose. This is particularly important in more elderly patients or those who have compromised renal function.

(d) **Hydralazine/nitrate combination.** Directly acting agents such as hydralazine and organic nitrates exert selective action on arteries and veins respectively. Although less effective than ACEIs and ARBs in reducing mortality, the combination of hydralazine in doses of 300 mg/day with isosorbide dinitrate at 160 mg/day has been associated with significant improvement in morbidity and mortality (VHeFT and VHeFT II). The nitrate component leads to vasodilation on the venous side, which reduces the rate of return of blood to the heart and the tendency of the ventricles to overfill. This in turn results in a reduction in pulmonary congestion and a reduction in symptoms. In order to achieve a balanced effect on the heart nitrates are mostly used in combination with an arterial vasodilator such as hydralazine, which reduces the arterial pressure against which the heart must work. The net effect is an improvement in cardiac output and a reduction in symptoms.

The combination of hydralazine plus nitrate has mainly been reserved as an alternative for patients who show intolerance to an ACEI and ARB (e.g. ACEI- or ARB-induced renal dysfunction) or a contraindication to ACEI and ARB use (bilateral renal artery stenosis, aortic stenosis, hypersensitivity). However, recent evidence suggests that the combination of hydralazine and isosorbide dinitrate in addition to ACEI and beta-blocker therapy may provide added benefits to African-American patients (A-HeFT).

In practice, it is more common to see isosorbide mononitrate being used in conjunction with hydralazine rather than isosorbide dinitrate. This is because the isosorbide 5-mononitrate metabolite derived from isosorbide dinitrate is responsible for producing venodilation. To reduce the risk of nitrate tolerance developing, it is important that an asymmetric dosing regimen is used to ensure a nitrate-free period.

There is a need to monitor the compliance of patients prescribed an asymmetric dosing regimen, and to monitor for side-effects such as postural hypotension, headache or dizziness. As there is a risk of hydralazine-induced systemic lupus erythematosus, it is also important to monitor patients for the appearance of a rash on the face (shaped like a butterfly) or neck.

(e) **Digoxin.** Digoxin has been shown to have a neutral effect on mortality, but is associated with a reduction in hospital readmission rate and an improvement in symptoms of patients who remain symptomatic despite adequate doses of an ACEI and diuretics (DIG). Digoxin is recommended for use in NYHA III–IV heart failure as an adjunct to ACEI and diuretic therapy. Other studies have shown that when digoxin is discontinued in patients in sinus rhythm there is a worsening of symptoms (RADIANCE and PROVED), therefore only a trial of digoxin discontinuation can demonstrate whether a patient in sinus rhythm is continuing to benefit from the drug.

Digoxin increases the force of contraction of the heart through direct stimulation of the heart muscle, thereby improving cardiac output. It also improves cardiac output in patients with atrial fibrillation through suppression of the atrioventricular node and control of ventricular rate. There is also some evidence to show that digoxin is linked to a reduction in sympathetic nerve activity as well as increased vagal stimulation. Both of these actions may be involved in the beneficial effects seen with digoxin.

Although the use of digoxin is associated with the treatment of AF, its use for patients with heart failure in sinus rhythm can lead to improved symptom control with much lower doses than those used to treat AF. There are no target plasma drug concentrations for the use of digoxin in sinus rhythm, therefore the dose is titrated against the symptoms. Owing to the long half-life associated with digoxin and the fact that it has a narrow therapeutic range, initiation of treatment involves the calculation of a suitable loading dose and subsequent maintenance dose to give to the patient. This will ensure that the plasma drug concentration is within the accepted range. Although drugs such as digoxin with a low therapeutic index require close patient monitoring for signs and symptoms of toxicity or lack of effect, routine plasma drug concentration monitoring is not recommended. Therapeutic drug monitoring is usually reserved for the confirmation or exclusion of toxicity, assessment of compliance, or confirmation of the plasma drug concentration following an increase in dose. Thus, most of the monitoring of digoxin therapy involves clinical assessment to identify poor control of symptoms, or to detect potential toxicity evidenced by symptoms such as nausea, vomiting, depressed appetite, visual disturbances or diarrhoea.

(f) **Aldosterone antagonists.** The use of an aldosterone antagonist as an adjunct to standard treatment has been shown to have a beneficial effect on morbidity and mortality in patients with heart failure. Aldosterone antagonists prevent aldosterone-mediated sodium and water retention, sympathetic activation and parasympathetic inhibition, all of which have a detrimental effect on the failing heart. They also help provide a more complete blockade of the renin–angiotensin–aldosterone system, which is activated in the presence of heart failure.

Spironolactone has been proved to significantly reduce mortality in patients with NYHA III–IV grades of heart failure (RALES). The use of eplerenone has also been shown to be associated with similar benefits in post-MI patients with symptomatic heart failure or post-MI diabetic patients with asymptomatic heart failure. Eplerenone has an advantage over spironolactone in that it does not cause gynaecomastia, and may therefore be considered as an alternative in male patients who are suffering from this side-effect.

Although aldosterone antagonists are potassium sparing, doses of up to 50 mg are considered to be safe when used in combination with potassium-conserving ACEIs or ARBs. Nevertheless, it is still important that plasma potassium be carefully monitored, and practitioners must be vigilant for any signs and symptoms of hyperkalaemia developing.

Table 4.2 (overleaf) summarises evidence-based standards for drug treatment of chronic heart failure. An assessment of drug regimens against these standards may facilitate a systematic identification of potential drug therapy problems regarding the implementation of clinical evidence in patients with chronic heart failure.

It is important to point out that although most of the above combinations have been shown to improve symptoms, the safety and efficacy of combining an ACEI, an ARB and aldosterone antagonist is uncertain, and it has been recommended to avoid the use of these three drugs together.

(g) **Aspirin.** Mrs HMcC's age and medical history (hypertension, AF, heart failure) put her at an increased risk of cardiovascular events. Aspirin would be indicated in addition to simvastatin for secondary prevention of cardiac events; however, aspirin and warfarin should normally not be co-prescribed (except in special circumstances, such as recurrent thromboembolism) because of an excessive risk of bleeding. As warfarin is the more effective agent for stroke prevention and equally effective as aspirin in preventing MI, it is appropriate that she is prescribed warfarin.

In summary, of the options available the first steps should be to optimise her ACEI therapy so as to realise the maximum benefits, and also to introduce a low-dose beta-blocker, which can be titrated up to the maximum tolerated dose. At the same time, her digoxin dose should be optimised in an attempt to control her AF, and her diuretic therapy should be adjusted to improve her symptoms of breathlessness and oedema.

Can a knowledge of digoxin pharmacokinetics guide optimisation of the digoxin dose? What dose would you recommend for Mrs HMcC?

A5 **Yes. Digoxin pharmacokinetics are relevant to the selection of a dosage regimen both when the drug is being initiated and when it is adjusted, as in Mrs HMcC's case. Mrs HMcC should have her dose increased to 187.5 micrograms daily. In order to achieve steady-state plasma levels rapidly she should first receive a loading dose of 500 micrograms (given as 250 micrograms twice daily for 1 day only).**

Table 4.2 Medication assessment tool for identification of potential drug therapy problems related to the implementation of guideline standards. Note: The specific circumstances of individual patients may justify deviation from these standards.

		Standards	*Standard met?*
	Patient with chronic heart failure . . .		
1	. . . and symptoms of heart failure	is prescribed diuretic treatment	☐
2	. . . and without contraindication or intolerance to an ACEI	is prescribed an ACEI or ARB	☐
3	. . . and not prescribed an ACEI or ARB	is prescribed a combination of hydralazine and oral nitrate	☐
4	. . . and without contraindication or intolerance to a beta-blocker (BB)	is prescribed a beta-blocker (except metoprolol tartrate)	☐
5	. . . and prescribed one of the following ACEIs: captopril (C), enalapril (E), lisinopril (L), perindopril (P), ramipril, (R) or trandolapril (T)	is prescribed target dose (C 50 mg tds, E 10–20 mg bd, L 20 mg od, R 10 mg od, P 8 mg od or T 4 mg od) or a documented maximum tolerated dose	☐
6	. . . and prescribed losartan (L), candesartan (C) or valsartan (V)	is prescribed target dose (L 50 mg od, C 32 mg od, V 160 mg bd) or a documented maximum tolerated dose	☐
7	. . . on carvedilol (C), bisoprolol (B) or nebivolol (N)	is prescribed target dose (C 25–50 mg bd, B or N 10 mg od) or a documented maximum tolerated dose	☐

8	. . . in NYHA II-III despite target or maximum tolerable doses (if less) of an ACEI and BB	is prescribed candesartan	□
9	. . . in NYHA III-IV despite target or maximum tolerable doses (if less) of an ACEI and BB	is prescribed spironolactone	□
10	. . . in NYHA III-IV despite target or maximum tolerable doses (if less) of an ACEI and BB and has developed gynaecomastia	is prescribed eplerenone	□
11	. . . and on spironolactone (S) or eplerenone (E)	is prescribed a target dose (S 25–50 mg od, E 50 mg od) or a documented maximum tolerated dose (if less)	□
12	. . . without AF and with current symptoms of heart failure despite optimal therapy	is prescribed digoxin	□
13	. . .	has received an annual influenza vaccination	□
14	. . .	has received a once-only pneumococcal vaccination	□
	Patient with chronic heart failure and AF . . .		
15	. . . and at least one additional risk factor for thromboembolism (aged >75 years, or >60 years with other risk factors such as hypertension, diabetes mellitus, or left ventricular dysfunction)	is prescribed warfarin	□
16	. . . and at least one additional risk factor for thromboembolism (aged >75 years, or >60 years with other risk factors such as hypertension, diabetes mellitus, or left ventricular dysfunction) and NOT prescribed warfarin	is prescribed antiplatelet therapy	□

Therapeutic plasma concentrations of digoxin (1–2 micrograms/L) will not be achieved until concentrations in the body compartments are equilibrated. Digoxin is absorbed slowly and bioavailability is incomplete. Digoxin is only 25% bound to plasma proteins and the drug distributes slowly into a large apparent volume of distribution (approximately 7 L/kg body weight). Therefore, to ensure a rapid onset of the therapeutic effects when therapy is initiated, most patients are given a loading dose of digoxin. As 99% of digoxin in the body is tissue bound, primarily to skeletal and cardiac muscle and minimally within body fat, a suitable oral loading dose can be calculated from the patient's lean body weight on the basis of 12–15 micrograms/kg. As Mrs HMcC is a thin woman, her actual body weight should have been used to calculate the dose, so a suitable loading dose at the start of digoxin therapy would have been approximately 795 micrograms orally, that is 750 micrograms given as three doses of 250 micrograms at 6-hourly intervals to reduce side-effects of nausea and vomiting.

If Mrs HMcC had been in urgent need of digitalisation at the time of digoxin initiation, e.g. if she had been suffering from acute dyspnoea as a result of her cardiac failure, intravenous (IV) digoxin therapy might have been more appropriate to control her tachycardia. An IV dosage regimen must, however, take into account the increased bioavailability of the drug by this route: the dose should be 70% of that calculated for oral administration, and the total dose should, whenever possible, be divided into aliquots, with an interval of 1–2 hours between injections to allow proper clinical evaluation. However, digitalisation in hospital often requires only the use of oral digoxin administered at suitable intervals over 6–24 hours.

If a loading dose is not given at the start of therapy, then the maximum clinical effect of a maintenance dose (MD) would only be seen after the plasma digoxin level is at steady state (i.e. when digoxin excretion equals daily digoxin intake), which is usually after four or five half-lives. In Mrs HMcC's case, this would have been 17–21 days.

When calculating an appropriate MD of digoxin for Mrs HMcC, several factors need to be considered. The first is her renal function. The half-life of digoxin is normally 36–40 hours. As the drug is excreted approximately 70% unchanged in the urine, any impairment of renal function will extend the half-life and must therefore be taken into account. Mrs HMcC's plasma creatinine level can be used to estimate her creatinine clearance (CrCl). When the equation of Cockcroft and Gault is used, it can be calculated that Mrs HMcC has a CrCl of 27 mL/min, which indicates that caution must be taken in choosing an MD. The extension of digoxin half-life can be calculated from:

$$\text{Extension in half-life} = \frac{1}{(1 - Fe) + (Rf \times Fe)}$$

where Fe = fraction of drug excreted unchanged in urine (for digoxin, 0.7) and Rf = fraction of normal renal function (patient's CrCl/100, for Mrs HMcC = 0.27).

For Mrs HMcC, the calculated extension in half-life is 2, i.e. her predicted digoxin half-life is double that of a person with normal renal function. Thus, as a guide, her renal impairment should be compensated for by a 50% reduction in MD.

The choice of MD can also be guided by estimating the proportion of the loading dose that will be excreted each day, and which must therefore be replaced, using the formula:

% loading dose excreted each day = (14% + patient's CrCl/5)

For Mrs HMcC, this gives a figure of 19% of the loading dose being excreted each day. If the loading dose were 750 micrograms, then the MD should be 142 micrograms.

A third method of calculating an appropriate MD is to use population values from reference texts. To do this the patient's renal function, expressed as CrCl, is first estimated using the Cockcroft and Gault equation. The estimated CrCl can then be used to predict the digoxin clearance for the patient. If the patient is more than 15% overweight, their ideal body weight rather than their true body weight should be used in these calculations.

Digoxin clearance (mL/min/kg) = 0.88 CrCl (mL/min/kg) + 0.33

where 0.88 is a coefficient which allows for a degree of heart failure (if no heart failure, then coefficient = 1). It is then necessary to convert digoxin clearance in mL/min/kg into L/h for the next stage:

$$\text{Average steady-state level of digoxin } (C_{ss}) = \frac{F \times S \times D}{CL \times T}$$

where F = bioavailability (0.6 for tablets), S = salt factor = 1, D = dose (in micrograms), CL = digoxin clearance (in L/h) and T = dosing interval (in hours). If it is necessary to convert the plasma concentration from micrograms/L to nanomol/L, then the C_{ss} value must be multiplied by 1.28.

Using this method, doses of 125, 187.5 and 250 micrograms would predict levels of approximately 1.3, 1.9 and 2.5 micrograms/L, respectively, for Mrs HMcC. This method can also be used in reverse after a plasma concentration has been measured, in order to calculate a patient's true digoxin clearance. This individualised clearance estimate can then be used when calculating the effects of altering dosages; however, as linear kinetics apply and plasma concentrations vary in proportion to dose, if the dosing interval remains constant such calculations are often unnecessary. This approach to dosage individualisation only applies if the dosage history is accurate, the sample is taken at the correct time, and the patient's medical condition is stable.

However, these dosing recommendations can only be a guide to Mrs HMcC's requirements, as interindividual variations in clinical response limit the usefulness of pharmacokinetic methods. In particular, doses needed to control AF may produce plasma concentrations that would be judged excessive (e.g. 2.5–3.5 micrograms/L) compared to the usually quoted reference range of 1–2 micrograms/L that is relevant to cardiac failure in general. Although in Mrs HMcC the MD needs to be reduced because of her renal function, her dose requirement may increase as her renal function improves following the control of her cardiac failure.

Mrs HMcC is already on digoxin and her plasma digoxin concentration estimate indicates a need to increase the dose. The required interim loading dose (LD) to increase her plasma digoxin from the present 1.0 micrograms/L to a new target of, say, 1.8 micrograms/L (an increase of 0.8 micrograms/L) can be estimated as:

LD = Target increase (micrograms/L) × volume of distribution of digoxin (L)

Using 7 L/kg as the volume of distribution of digoxin, and knowing Mrs HMcC's body weight to be 52 kg:

$$LD = 0.8 \times 7 \times 52 = 291 \text{ micrograms}$$

This is equivalent to 291/0.6 or 485 micrograms after oral bioavailability (0.6) has been taken into account.

In summary, an MD of 187.5 micrograms/day would be more appropriate for Mrs HMcC, as it is estimated this will produce a plasma digoxin concentration of approximately 1.9 micrograms/L. The new steady state will take several days to achieve if the MD is merely increased from 125 to 187.5 micrograms, but the required serum concentration can be achieved within 24 hours by prescribing an oral loading dose of approximately 500 micrograms (prescribed as 250 micrograms twice daily).

Outline your pharmaceutical care plan for Mrs HMcC.

A6 **The main points to be considered for her pharmaceutical care plan are as follows:**

(a) **Atrial fibrillation**

(i) Ensure appropriate drug therapy is prescribed to control her AF.

(ii) Ensure an appropriate digoxin maintenance regimen is prescribed.
(iii) Monitor urea and electrolyte levels regularly, particularly plasma creatinine and potassium.
(iv) Counsel the patient and advise other healthcare professionals to monitor for signs and symptoms of digoxin toxicity.

(b) **Iron-deficiency anaemia**

(i) Ensure an appropriate form and dose of oral iron supplement is prescribed.
(ii) Counsel the patient on the potential side-effects of oral iron therapy.
(iii) Monitor relevant haematological markers, e.g. haemoglobin, mean cell haemoglobin concentration.

(c) **Cardiac failure**

(i) Ensure appropriate diuretic therapy is prescribed.
(ii) Monitor the patient for improvement in signs and symptoms of CCF, e.g. reduced shortness of breath, reduced peripheral oedema, etc.
(iii) Monitor for side-effects/adverse events associated with increased ACEI dosage.
(iv) Monitor daily weight as a measure of fluid loss or retention to assess the appropriateness of diuretic therapy.
(v) Monitor patient tolerance of bisoprolol therapy during titration towards target dose.
(vi) Monitor all prescribed and over-the-counter medication use to ensure that medications known to exacerbate cardiac failure are avoided whenever possible, or caution exercised where such a medication is deemed appropriate, e.g. a non-steroidal anti-inflammatory drug (NSAID), corticosteroids, antidepressants, antihistamines.

(d) **Antithrombotic therapy**

(i) Ensure future changes to concomitant therapy take into account potential interactions with warfarin.
(ii) Counsel the patient on the purpose and potential side-effects of warfarin therapy.
(iii) Monitor the patient's international normalised ratio (INR) routinely.

(e) **Control of blood pressure**

(i) Ensure that control of blood pressure improves in response to changes in Mrs HMcC's therapeutic plan.
(ii) Monitor blood pressure routinely.

Which medical conditions and drug treatments are known to exacerbate cardiac failure?

A7 **Medical conditions include iron-deficiency anaemia, thyrotoxicosis, mitral valve disease and AF. A large number of drug treatments may exacerbate cardiac failure through a variety of mechanisms.**

Drug treatments that can exacerbate cardiac failure include:

(a) NSAIDs, corticosteroids, carbenoxolone, liquorice, lithium and products containing high sodium levels (effervescent formulations, some antacid preparations). These can all cause sodium and/or water retention.
(b) Tricyclic antidepressants may depress heart function and may also predispose the patient to cardiac arrhythmias.
(c) Beta-blockers in high doses produce negative inotropic and chronotropic effects.
(d) Class I and class III anti-arrhythmic agents (except amiodarone) cause negative inotropic effects and may lead to arrhythmias.
(e) Calcium-channel blockers (diltiazem, verapamil, first-generation dihydropyridines) all produce negative inotropic and neuroendocrine effects.
(f) Antihistamines, erythromycin and antifungal agents prolong the QT interval and may lead to arrhythmias.

What is the likely explanation for Mrs HMcC's persisting cardiac failure?

A8 **Non-adherence to the digoxin therapy, digoxin toxicity, or lack of response to digoxin therapy.**

Mrs HMcC's pulse rate suggests continuing poor control of her AF.

Loss of control of cardiac failure and AF may accompany digoxin toxicity, and this possibility needs to be excluded by inquiring about other symptoms of digoxin toxicity. Alternatively, Mrs HMcC may be non-compliant with the current digoxin regimen and this might explain the lack of control.

In her case, compliance was assured and toxicity ruled out, therefore the dose of digoxin prescribed was judged to be still suboptimal for the control of her AF.

What symptoms might lead you to suspect digoxin toxicity?

A9 **The loss of control of her cardiac failure, nausea, fatigue and her complaint of restlessness.**

Digoxin toxicity may easily go unrecognised, but is commonly signalled by gastrointestinal and/or central nervous system symptoms. These symptoms may be vague and insidious in onset, such as fatigue, apathy or restlessness, insomnia, confusion, abdominal discomfort or a change in bowel habits (especially diarrhoea). More overt signs are anorexia, nausea, vomiting, lethargy and psychosis. Visual disturbances (blurring, haloed or yellow vision, red–green colour blindness) are well documented, but are not often among the first symptoms volunteered by the patient.

What is the role of plasma digoxin assay and when should blood samples be drawn?

A10 **Although digoxin has a low therapeutic index there is little evidence to support the routine assessment of plasma digoxin concentration in patients prescribed this medication. Overuse of the digoxin plasma assay is both common and wasteful, and plasma drug concentration measurement should be reserved for the initiation of treatment, confirmation or exclusion of digoxin toxicity, or to confirm patient adherence to therapy. If an assay is appropriate, blood should be sampled for digoxin between 6 and 24 hours after a dose is administered.**

The slow distribution of the drug confers two-compartment pharmacokinetic characteristics. The equilibration between drug in the plasma and that in the myocardium (and other tissues) continues for up to 6 hours after a dose is taken. Up to this time the plasma digoxin concentration reflects drug distribution and is unrelated to the amount of digoxin in the tissues, and hence its effect on the myocardium. In addition, assay results cannot be interpreted if the sampling times are unrecorded or inappropriate.

What clinical factors predispose patients to digoxin toxicity, and why do you think Mrs HMcC has experienced symptoms of toxicity?

A11 **Hypokalaemia, hypomagnesaemia, hypercalcaemia, alkalosis, hypoxia and hypothyroidism can all predispose to digoxin toxicity; however, the development of digoxin toxicity in Mrs HMcC probably occurred as a result of the high plasma digoxin concentration that appears necessary to control her AF.**

Hypokalaemia, hypercalcaemia and hypomagnesaemia all lead to an increase in responsiveness of tissues to digoxin's cardiac effects and to toxic symptoms in general. The most common contributor to digoxin toxicity is hypokalaemia, and plasma digoxin concentrations can only be interpreted in conjunction with a plasma potassium measurement.

Alkalosis and hypoxia also potentiate digoxin toxicity, whereas hypothyroidism increases responsiveness to digoxin and elevates plasma concentrations by reducing the drug's clearance and apparent volume of distribution.

What are the cardiac effects of digoxin toxicity?

A12 Arrhythmias and loss of control of cardiac failure.

Digoxin increases the automaticity and slows conduction in all cardiac cells. Cardiotoxicity may occur without other warning symptoms, and the cells of the atrioventricular and sinoatrial nodes are particularly affected. Common arrhythmias include atrioventricular block with supraventricular tachycardias, junctional or escape rhythms, ventricular ectopic beats and ventricular tachycardia. Sinus bradycardia and sino-atrial arrest may occur. Loss of control of cardiac failure may also be a feature of digoxin toxicity.

Apart from stopping the drug, how can digoxin toxicity be managed?

A13 By correcting any underlying factors contributing to digoxin toxicity and, if clinically necessary, by using resins or digoxin-specific antibody fragments to increase digoxin elimination.

If present, hypokalaemia should be corrected, unless the presence of atrioventricular block contraindicates potassium use. When heart block persists, lidocaine and similar anti-arrhythmic agents (such as propranolol and phenytoin) are recommended, and cardiac pacing is indicated.

Attempts to reduce digoxin concentrations by dialysis are ineffective, as 99% of drug in the body is tissue bound and not in the plasma. The use of oral resins such as colestyramine and colestipol (bile acid-chelating agents which also bind digoxin) can increase elimination by interrupting enterohepatic circulation of the drug; however, severe toxicity requires the use of the digoxin-specific antibody fragment preparation Digibind by the IV route.

Digoxin has a much higher affinity for the digoxin-specific antibody fragment than for its receptor (Na, K-dependent ATPase) and hence is attracted away from its receptors in the heart tissue. The inactive complex that is formed is readily excreted by the kidney. The dosage of digoxin-specific antibody fragment depends on the amount of digoxin to be neutralised. There are various methods for calculating the digoxin-specific antibody fragment required, depending on how the toxicity occurred, the age of the patient, and whether or not a measured plasma digoxin concentration is available.

The digoxin level in Mrs HMcC's case probably does not warrant the use of digoxin-specific antibody fragment. However, if she showed life-threatening signs of cardiac toxicity after digoxin withdrawal and the correction of any electrolyte imbalances, then digoxin-specific antibody fragment would be an option. Under those circumstances, the formula below should be used to calculate the amount of Digibind required (rounding up to the nearest number of whole vials):

Dose (no. of vials) = (serum digoxin conc. (micrograms/L) × weight (kg)) /100

For Mrs HMcC:

Dose = (3.4 × 53)/ 100 = 2 vials

The contents of each vial would need to be dissolved in sterile Water for Injection by gentle mixing. This solution may then be diluted further to any convenient volume using sterile saline suitable for infusion. The final solution should be infused over a 30-minute period through a 0.22-μm membrane filter to remove any incompletely dissolved aggregates of Digibind.

Under circumstances in which cardiac arrest is imminent, then Digibind can be given as a bolus IV injection. ECG and electrolyte monitoring is required for at least 24 hours following Digibind administration.

Do you agree with the choice of amiodarone to control Mrs HMcC's AF? What issues would you now add to or change in the pharmaceutical care plan originally developed for Mrs HMcC and described in A6?

A14 **Yes, amiodarone was the best choice of agent for Mrs HMcC. As a result of this change in therapy, pharmaceutical care activity related to the treatment of her iron-deficiency anaemia and cardiac failure, the provision of thromboprophylaxis and the control of her blood pressure would remain unchanged, but the plans related to the management of her AF must be changed. In addition, the interaction of amiodarone and warfarin, which is due to inhibition of warfarin metabolism, leads to an increased anticoagulant effect, and would prompt more frequent monitoring of the INR and adjustment of her warfarin dose during the amiodarone titration period.**

In considering which agent to prescribe as a replacement for digoxin, rate-limiting calcium-channel blockers (verapamil, diltiazem) and class I antiarrhythmic agents are best avoided, as they would aggravate Mrs HMcC's heart failure. Increasing the dose of beta-blocker might have been attempted as long as Mrs HMcC was able to tolerate the higher dose, as this group of agents, albeit proven to be beneficial with regard to morbidity and mortality, can still aggravate heart failure symptoms. The prescription of amiodarone was therefore the most appropriate choice of alternative antiarrhythmic agent.

The care plan changes include removal of issues related to the prescription and use of digoxin, with the following additions relating to the introduction of amiodarone:

(i) Ensure that the reduction in the daily dose of amiodarone occurs over an acceptable period to an appropriate maintenance dose.
(ii) Ensure that appropriate control of AF is achieved with amiodarone.
(iii) Monitor thyroid function every 6 months.
(iv) Monitor liver function.
(v) Counsel the patient and advise other healthcare professionals on the signs and symptoms of adverse effects of amiodarone therapy.

The dose of amiodarone on initiation of therapy is usually 200 mg three times daily, reducing by 200 mg each week until a maintenance dose of 200 mg daily is achieved (or the lowest dose required to control the arrhythmia). Amiodarone has an unusual pharmacokinetic profile with high protein binding, a very high volume of distribution due to extensive deposition in tissues, and a long half-life (1–2 months). Amiodarone can cause hypo- or hyperthyroidism, and so baseline and then regular thyroid function tests are essential. It also produces corneal microdeposits in the eye: vision is usually unaffected, although some patients might be dazzled by car headlights at night; this should therefore be discussed with those still intending to drive. Phototoxic skin reactions can also occur and sunscreen protection is often required. Pulmonary and hepatic toxicity is also a risk for patients taking amiodarone, and where signs or symptoms develop therapy must be stopped immediately.

What treatment options might you consider next to manage Mrs HMcC's cardiac failure?

A15 **A number of options can be considered: optimise her diuretic therapy, add candesartan, consider the reintroduction of digoxin, or start treatment with spironolactone.**

Where symptoms of sodium and water retention continue there is further scope to increase the dose of furosemide. In cases where oedema is resistant, the addition of metolazone is often necessary. However, any increase in diuretic therapy will require careful monitoring of Mrs HMcC's renal function and plasma concentrations of potassium and other electrolytes.

Although spironolactone may increase plasma potassium levels it can usually be safely prescribed alongside an ACEI without causing hyperkalaemia; however, a dose of 25–50 mg daily should not be exceeded.

When co-prescribed, a more complete block of the renin–angiotensin–aldosterone system is achieved, accounting for the additional morbidity and mortality benefits observed in clinical trials. However, there have been cases where hyperkalaemia has developed, and so monitoring of renal function and plasma electrolytes is mandatory for patients prescribed this combination therapy.

The combination of all three drug groups (ACEI, ARB and aldosterone antagonist) is not recommended as evidence of safety and efficacy is lacking, and therefore a single agent to be co-prescribed with enalapril must be selected. The preferred choice of agent as an adjunct to optimised therapy with ACEIs and beta-blockers remains controversial. However, clinical trials support the addition of candesartan in patients with mild (NYHA II–III) – and spironolactone as the preferred option in patients with more severe symptoms of cardiac failure (NYHA III–IV).

Digoxin has been shown to have a neutral effect on survival but to improve symptoms of cardiac failure and reduce the rate of rehospitalisation. The doses required are much lower than those needed to control AF, therefore Mrs HMcC might still benefit from a reintroduction of this agent. Care must be taken if this option is followed, as the plasma concentration of digoxin is increased by amiodarone, and therefore the clinical and laboratory monitoring for signs and symptoms of digoxin toxicity discussed earlier must be reintroduced.

Further reading

CIBIS-II Investigators and Committees. The Cardiac Insufficiency Bisoprolol Study II (CIBIS-II): a randomised trial. *Lancet* 1999; **353**: 9–13.

Cohn JN, Tognoni G. A randomized trial of the angiotensin-receptor blocker valsartan in chronic heart failure. *N Engl J Med* 2001; **345**: 1667–1675.

Granger CB, McCMurray JJ, Yusuf S *et al.* Effects of candesartan in patients with chronic heart failure and reduced left-ventricular systolic function intolerant to angiotensin-converting-enzyme inhibitors: the CHARM-Alternative trial. *Lancet* 2003; **362**: 772–776.

Hall AS, Murray GD, Ball SG. Follow-up study of patients randomly allocated ramipril or placebo for heart failure after acute myocardial infarction: AIRE Extension (AIREX) Study. Acute Infarction Ramipril Efficacy. *Lancet* 1997; **349**: 1493–1497.

Krum H, Roecker EB, Mohacsi P *et al.* Effects of initiating carvedilol in patients with severe chronic heart failure: results from the COPERNICUS Study. *J Am Med Assoc* 2003; **289**: 712–718.

Lonn E, McKelvie R. Drug treatment in heart failure. *Br Med J* 2000; **320**: 1188–1192.

McMurray J, Cohen-Solal A, Dietz R *et al*. Practical recommendations for the use of ACE inhibitors, beta-blockers, aldosterone antagonists and angiotensin receptor blockers in heart failure: putting guidelines into practice. *Eur J Heart Fail* 2005; **7**: 710–721.

McMurray JJ, Ostergren J, Swedberg K *et al*. Effects of candesartan in patients with chronic heart failure and reduced left-ventricular systolic function taking angiotensin-converting-enzyme inhibitors: the CHARM-Added trial. *Lancet* 2003; **362**: 767–771.

MERIT-HF Study Group. Effect of metoprolol CR/XL in chronic heart failure: Metoprolol CR/XL Randomised Intervention Trial in Congestive Heart Failure (MERIT-HF). *Lancet* 1999; **353**: 2001–2007.

National Institute for Health and Clinical Excellence. CG05. *The Management of Congestive Heart Failure in Adults in Primary and Secondary Care*. NICE, London, 2003.

Packer M, Coats AS, Fowler MB *et al*. Effect of carvedilol on survival in severe chronic heart failure. *N Engl J Med* 2001; **344**: 1651–1658.

Packer M, Gheorgiade M, Young JB *et al*. Withdrawal of digoxin from patients with chronic heart failure treated with angiotensin-converting-enzyme inhibitors. RADIANCE Study. *N Engl J Med* 1993; **329**: 1–7.

Peterson RC, Dunlap ME. Angiotensin II receptor blockers in the treatment of heart failure. *Congest Heart Fail* 2002; **8**: 246–250, 256.

Pitt B, Zannad F, Remme WJ *et al*. The effect of spironolactone on morbidity and mortality in patients with severe heart failure. Randomized Aldactone Evaluation Study Investigators. *N Engl J Med* 1999; **341**: 709–717.

Pitt B, Remme W, Zannad F *et al*. Eplerenone, a selective aldosterone blocker, in patients with left ventricular dysfunction after myocardial infarction. *N Engl J Med* 2003; **348**: 1309–1321.

Scottish Intercollegiate Guidelines Network. *Management of Chronic Heart Failure. A National Clinical Guideline*. February 2007.

Scottish Intercollegiate Guidelines Network. *Cardiac Arrhythmias in Coronary Heart Disease. A National Clinical Guideline*. February 2007.

Yusuf S, Pfeffer MA, Swedberg K *et al*. Effects of candesartan in patients with chronic heart failure and preserved left-ventricular ejection fraction: the CHARM-Preserved Trial. *Lancet* 2003; **362**: 777–781.

5

Stroke

Derek Taylor

Case study and questions

Day 1 Mr DF, a 62-year-old-man, was admitted to hospital after collapsing and experiencing a brief loss of consciousness 3 hours earlier. On admission he was fully conscious and apyrexial. He had lost voluntary movement in both his left arm and leg. His blood pressure was 160/100 mmHg.

His previous medical history included hypertension, for which he had been prescribed bendroflumethiazide 2.5 mg daily for 6 years. He had also been on carbamazepine 400 mg twice a day for 10 years for epilepsy. He lived at home with his wife, and smoked 15 cigarettes per day and occasionally drank alcohol.

His serum biochemistry results were:

- Sodium 137 mmol/L (reference range 135–145)
- Potassium 4.9 mmol/L (3.5–5.0)
- Urea 4.7 mmol/L (2.5–7.0)
- Creatinine 95 micromol/L (50–130)

A diagnosis of ischaemic stroke was made. Mr DF was prescribed aspirin 300 mg orally and transferred to the Acute Stroke Unit. A computed tomography (CT) scan was ordered.

Q1 What risk factors did Mr DF have for developing a stroke?
Q2 What is the rationale for ordering a CT scan?
Q3 When should aspirin be administered if benefit is to be obtained, and what dose should be given?
Q4 Should Mr DF be prescribed prophylaxis against peptic ulceration?
Q5 What other agents, apart from aspirin, have been shown to be of benefit in the treatment of ischaemic stroke?
Q6 Would Mr DF be a suitable candidate for a thrombolytic agent?
Q7 What metabolic parameters should be monitored closely?
Q8 What supportive treatment does Mr DF require?

Q9 Should the carbamazepine therapy be discontinued?
Q10 How should Mr DF's hypertension be managed?

Day 3 Mr DF was still experiencing loss of movement and hemiplegic pain in his left arm and leg. He also had difficulty swallowing, and was therefore referred to the physiotherapist, speech and language therapist and dietitian. A nasogastric tube was inserted.

Q11 Outline a pharmaceutical care plan for Mr DF.
Q12 How would you recommend his pain be managed?
Q13 What other complications associated with his stroke might Mr DF experience?
Q14 What problems might occur when administering Mr DF's medication via the nasogastric tube?
Q15 What advice would you give to the nursing staff to overcome these problems?

Day 9 Mr DF was transferred to a rehabilitation ward. His blood pressure was 150/100 mmHg and he was therefore prescribed perindopril 2 mg daily. His serum cholesterol level was 5.2 mmol/L.

Q16 Should Mr DF be started on warfarin?
Q17 What are the alternative antiplatelet agents to aspirin?
Q18 What is the rationale for the initiation of an angiotensin-converting enzyme inhibitor (ACEI)?
Q19 Should a statin be prescribed for Mr DF?

Day 23 Mr DF's swallow reflex had partially returned. Therefore, he was started on a puréed diet during the day and given fluids overnight via the nasogastric tube.

Day 44 Mr DF had regained most of his limb function and his swallow reflex had almost fully returned. His nasogastric tube was therefore removed and he was discharged home on a soft diet. His medication on discharge was:

- Aspirin 75 mg orally daily
- Dipyridamole Retard 200 mg twice a day
- Bendroflumethiazide 2.5 mg orally daily
- Carbamazepine suspension 400 mg twice a day
- Amitriptyline 50 mg tablet at night
- Perindopril tablets 4 mg daily
- Simvastatin 40 mg at night

Q20 What lifestyle changes would you recommend?
Q21 How could the pharmacist contribute to Mr DF's discharge?

Answers

What risk factors did Mr DF have for developing a stroke?

A1 Hypertension, smoking and gender.

Hypertension is the major risk factor for stroke. Current trial data suggest that lowering blood pressure by 5–6 mmHg diastolic and 10–12 mmHg systolic for 2–3 years may reduce the annual risk of stroke from 7% to 4.8%. Smoking increases the risk of stroke by around 50%, and men are 25–30% more likely to have a stroke than women.

Other risk factors, which are not present in Mr DF, include alcohol abuse, drug abuse, cardiovascular disease (especially atrial fibrillation), diabetes mellitus, migraine headaches and previous transient ischaemic attacks.

What is the rationale for ordering a CT scan?

A2 To differentiate between an ischaemic stroke and a haemorrhagic stroke.

Approximately 85% of strokes are the result of an infarct in the brain (ischaemic), the remaining 15% being due to intracerebral or subarachnoid haemorrhage. A haemorrhagic stroke must be excluded by brain imaging before the prescribing of thrombolytics or anticoagulants can be considered.

When should aspirin be administered if benefit is to be obtained and what dose should be given?

A3 Aspirin 150–300 mg orally should be given within 48 hours.

The rationale for aspirin treatment in the acute phase of ischaemic stroke is to prevent further occlusion of blood supply to surrounding areas of brain tissue. A dose of 150–300 mg of aspirin should be administered as soon as possible after the onset of stroke symptoms if a diagnosis of haemorrhage is considered unlikely. The initial diagnosis of an ischaemic stroke is a clinical decision, and studies have shown that aspirin may be administered before a brain scan has been undertaken; however, a brain scan must always be undertaken before commencing anticoagulation or thrombolysis, owing to the significantly increased risk of intracerebral haemorrhage with these therapies.

This use of aspirin is supported by two large studies of the treatment of acute ischaemic stroke: the International Stroke Trial (IST) and the

Chinese Acute Stroke Trial (CAST). In the IST, those patients treated with aspirin 300 mg daily for 14 days had significantly fewer recurrent ischaemic strokes (2.8 vs 3.9%, $2P < 0.001$) and no significant excess of haemorrhagic strokes (0.9 vs 0.8%) within 14 days, compared with placebo. However, the reductions in deaths within 14 days (9.0 vs 9.4%) and the numbers of patients dead or dependent after 6 months (62.2 vs 63.5%, $2P = 0.07$) were not significant. In the CAST, those patients treated with aspirin 160 mg/day for up to 4 weeks (started within 48 hours of stroke onset) showed a small but significant reduction in recurrent ischaemic stroke rate (1.6 vs 2.1%, $2P = 0.01$) and a non-significant increase in haemorrhagic strokes (1.1 vs 0.9%, $2P > 0.1$) after 4 weeks, compared with placebo. In the CAST, overall mortality after 4 weeks was shown to fall from 3.9 to 3.3% ($2P = 0.04$).

The authors concluded that when the results of these two studies are combined, aspirin started early in hospital produces a small but definite net benefit, with about nine fewer deaths or non-fatal strokes per 1000 patients in the first few weeks ($2P = 0.001$) and about 13 fewer dead or dependent per 1000 patients at 6 months ($2P < 0.01$).

In line with the evidence from these trials, aspirin should be administered at a dose of 150–300 mg daily for at least the first 14 days after an ischaemic stroke. After this period the dose may be reduced to 75 mg daily for secondary prevention of further thromboembolic events.

Should Mr DF be prescribed prophylaxis against peptic ulceration?

A4 No.

Mr DF does not have a history of peptic ulcer disease. The incidence of major gastrointestinal bleeds with aspirin, at the doses used for cardiovascular protection, is 2–3%. There is still some debate over the relative risk–benefit ratio (for gastrointestinal bleeds) between using higher doses (>300 mg) and lower doses (<150 mg) of aspirin.

If prophylaxis is required, a maintenance dose of a proton pump inhibitor (PPI) may be prescribed, e.g. lansoprazole 15 mg daily. The current NICE guidelines recommend the use of low-dose PPI therapy for patients with a history of ulcers but not for those with a history of dyspepsia.

What other agents, apart from aspirin, have been shown to be of benefit in the treatment of ischaemic stroke?

A5 Thrombolytic agents.

The rationale behind the use of thrombolytics in the acute phase of an ischaemic stroke is to accelerate reperfusion of the affected area in the brain. A number of multicentre clinical trials in recent years (e.g. NINDS, ECASS-I, ECASS-II, Atlantis-A and B, CASES and SITS-MOST) have shown significant benefit from alteplase, especially when administered within 3 hours of onset of stroke symptoms. However, the use of thrombolysis in the treatment of acute ischaemic stroke is dependent on patients reaching hospital as soon as possible, and the availability of out-of-hours CT scanning to confirm the diagnosis.

In the National Institute of Neurological Disorders and Stroke rt-PA Stroke Study Group Trial, patients who received alteplase (0.9 mg/kg to a maximum of 90 mg) within 3 hours of ischaemic stroke onset were shown to have a significantly better outcome (no or minimum disability) at 3 months than those who received placebo. Unfortunately, there was no significant reduction in mortality at 3 months (17% in the alteplase group and 21% in the placebo group; $P = 0.30$). Trials with streptokinase have been stopped early owing to an increased incidence of early death, usually due to cerebral haemorrhage.

The IST indicated that the use of heparin did not confer any benefit in the treatment of acute ischaemic stroke. In this trial, subcutaneous heparin 5000 IU twice daily and 12 500 IU twice daily were compared with placebo. Heparin therapy produced a non-significant reduction in mortality within 14 days (9.0 vs 9.3%) compared with placebo. Patients receiving heparin had significantly fewer recurrent ischaemic strokes within 14 days (2.9 vs 3.8%, $2P = 0.005$) but this was offset by a similarly sized increase in haemorrhagic strokes (1.2 vs 0.4%, $2P < 0.00001$). When compared with the low-dose heparin regimen, heparin 12 500 IU twice daily was associated with significantly more transfused or fatal extracranial bleeds, more haemorrhagic strokes, and more deaths or non-fatal strokes within 14 days (12.6 vs 10.8%, $2P = 0.007$). Perhaps as a result of this, at 6 months the number of patients dead or dependent was identical to that with placebo after 6 months (62.9%).

Would Mr DF be a suitable candidate for a thrombolytic agent?

A6 **No.**

Mr DF did not present to hospital until 3 hours after the onset of his symptoms. The Royal College of Physician's National Clinical Guidelines for Stroke state that thrombolytic treatment with a tissue plasminogen activator (tPA) should only be given if the following criteria are met: tPA is administered within 3 hours of onset of stroke symptoms; haemorrhage has definitely been excluded (by CT scan); and the patient is in a specialist centre with appropriate experience and expertise in thrombolytic use. Because of the difficulties in meeting these rapid diagnostic deadlines, two ongoing clinical trials, ECASS-III and IST-3, have been set up to investigate the effectiveness of alteplase given to patients with acute ischaemic stroke within 3–4.5 hours and within 6 hours of symptom onset, respectively. The results from the ECASS–III trial, published late in 2008, supported the fact that alteplase does have some benefit within the 3–4.5-hour post-stroke window (although less benefit than within the 0–3-hour window); however, its use more than 3 hours after a stroke is outside the current product licence and at the time of writing the national guidance above still stands.

What metabolic parameters should be monitored closely?

A7 Mr DF's state of hydration, blood glucose level, temperature, oxygenation and blood pressure.

(a) **Hydration.** His fluid balance, urea, creatinine and sodium levels should be monitored closely. Excessive hydration can result in hyponatraemia, which can force fluid into neurons and hence exacerbate damage from ischaemia. Hyponatraemia can also lead to seizures, which may further affect the damaged neurons.

(b) **Blood glucose level.** Hypoglycaemia may lead to significantly worse clinical outcomes. It is therefore important that Mr DF's blood glucose levels are kept within the normal range.

(c) **Temperature.** Any pyrexia, such as that linked with infection, should be controlled with paracetamol, a fan, and treatment of the underlying cause.

(d) **Oxygenation.** The routine use of supplemental oxygenation is not recommended, and Mr DF should only receive supplemental oxygen if his oxygen saturation falls below 95%.

What supportive treatment does Mr DF require?

A8 He requires assessment of his level of consciousness, swallow reflex, pressure sore and venous thromboembolism risk, nutritional status, cognitive impairment, moving and handling needs, and bladder and bowel management needs.

These parameters should be assessed by suitably trained staff as part of the formal admission procedure. Those patients with identified swallowing needs should then have a specialist assessment of swallowing, ideally within 24 hours, but no more than 72 hours after admission. If Mr DF is unable to take adequate nutrition orally he should receive early tube feeding with a nasogastric tube, ideally within 24 hours of admission.

Dysphagia is common and occurs in about 45% of all stroke patients admitted to hospital. It is associated with more severe strokes and worse outcomes. The presence of aspiration may be associated with an increased risk of developing pneumonia after stroke. Malnutrition is also common and is found in about 15% of all patients admitted to hospital, increasing to about 30% a week after admission.

Venous thromboembolism often occurs in the first week of a stroke, most often in immobile patients with paralysis of the leg, but its impact after stroke is still unclear. Studies have shown that deep-vein thrombosis (DVT) occurs in up to 50% of patients with hemiplegia, but clinically apparent DVT probably occurs in fewer than 5%. Similarly, although autopsy has identified pulmonary embolism (PE) in a large percentage of patients who die, clinically evident PE occurs in only 1–2% of patients. To minimise the risk of venous thromboembolism patients should be adequately hydrated and mobilised as soon as possible following an appropriate assessment (e.g. sitting balance and falls risk). The effectiveness of compression stockings in the acute post-stroke phase is still being assessed in clinical trials. Prophylactic anticoagulation should not be routinely used in either the acute or the rehabilitation phases, as it increases the risk of cerebral haemorrhage; however, if a venous thromboembolism has been diagnosed clinically, anticoagulant treatment should be started.

Most patients presenting with moderate to severe stroke are incontinent at presentation and may still be incontinent on discharge. This is a major burden on carers and may impede rehabilitation. Management of both bladder and bowel problems must therefore be seen as an essential part of the rehabilitation process.

Should the carbamazepine therapy be discontinued?

A9 **No.**

Seizures may occur in up to 20% of stroke patients, and with his history of epilepsy and the dangers of fitting in the acute post-stroke phase, Mr DF should be continued on his carbamazepine therapy. He should remain on the same dose, but it should be administered using the suspension formulation.

How should Mr DF's hypertension be managed?

A10 **Mr DF should be maintained on his bendroflumethiazide. There should be no further attempts to reduce his blood pressure in the acute phase of his stroke, unless it continues to increase.**

Caution should be exercised in controlling Mr DF's blood pressure acutely, because reducing blood pressure too rapidly will compromise cerebral blood flow and expand the region of ischaemia and infarction, whereas hypertension will place him at greater risk for cerebral haemorrhage, especially if a thrombolytic agent is used. Therefore, blood pressure manipulation is only recommended in acute stroke where there is a hypertensive emergency or the patient has a serious concomitant medical condition, such as hypertensive encephalopathy, aortic dissection, hypertensive nephropathy, pre-eclampsia, hypertensive cardiac failure, or intracerebral haemorrhage with systolic blood pressure >200 mmHg.

Outline a pharmaceutical care plan for Mr DF.

A11 **The pharmaceutical care plan for Mr DF should include the following:**

(a) **Antiplatelet therapy**

- (i) Ensure antiplatelet agent is continued daily at the current dose.
- (ii) Monitor for signs of gastric irritation.

(b) **Dysphagia**

- (i) Determine his swallow reflex after liaison with the speech and language therapist.
- (ii) Assess suitable alternative formulations if an enteral feeding tube is in place.
- (iii) Check timing of medication doses if on an enteral feed.

(c) **Hypertension**

- (i) Regular monitoring of blood pressure.
- (ii) The optimal target blood pressure (in the rehabilitation phase) for patients with established cardiovascular disease is 130/80 mmHg, with a maximum of 140/90 mmHg.
- (iii) Do not increase doses or prescribe new doses of antihypertensives until at least 7 days after the initial stroke.

(d) **Aggravating drug therapy.** Centrally acting drugs should be avoided if possible, as they may compromise memory and cognition.

(e) **Monitor other parameters**

- (i) Urea and electrolytes.
- (ii) Blood glucose.
- (iii) Temperature.

How would you recommend his pain be managed?

A12 If the pain is genuinely hemiplegic, a low dose of amitriptyline should be prescribed.

It is very important that the correct cause of the pain is diagnosed. Other possible causes of post-stroke limb problems may be muscular, spasticity or joint related. These types of pain may respond to careful manipulation and physiotherapy. Appropriate medication, such as paracetamol, baclofen or intra-articular injections, may also be prescribed for each of these problems, respectively.

If the pain is central in origin, a low dose of amitriptyline, e.g. 25 mg at night, may be prescribed. This should be titrated at 25 mg intervals every week, according to response. The patient should be monitored closely for any signs of central nervous system (CNS) suppression, and therapy should not be commenced until the patient is medically stable. Alternative options include carbamazepine (which Mr DF is already on) and gabapentin.

What other complications associated with his stroke might Mr DF experience?

A13 Agitation, delerium, stupor, coma, cerebral oedema, pneumonia, pulmonary oedema, DVT, arrhythmias and depression.

Pneumonia, pulmonary oedema, DVT and arrhythmias after an ischaemic stroke may be related to further infarction, haemorrhage or cerebral oedema. Pneumonia and DVT are further exacerbated by inactivity, hence the need to mobilise Mr DF as soon as possible.

Stroke patients often experience psychological reactions. The most common is depression, which occurs in 40–50% of patients. If this interferes with recovery and rehabilitation, a selective serotonin reuptake inhibitor may be prescribed.

What problems might occur when administering Mr DF's medication via the nasogastric tube?

A14 Carbamazepine may bind to the feeding tube and interact with the enteral feed.

The first option when selecting alternative formulations for administration is to use a commercially available oral solution or dispersible tablet. If this is not an option, the next step is to crush and fully disperse the contents of the tablet or capsule. This should not be done with enteric-coated or modified-release preparations, as it may result in changes in bioavailability, with dangerous peaks or troughs, or blockage of the tube.

Carbamazepine suspension may bind to the material of the enteral tubing or interact with the feed itself. Both of these effects may alter the bioavailability and clinical effectiveness of the medication.

What advice would you give to the nursing staff to overcome these problems?

A15 **The feed should be stopped at least 1 hour before the dose. The carbamazepine suspension should be diluted with at least 30–60 mL of water and the tube flushed with at least an equal volume after the dose. The enteral feed should not be restarted until 2 hours after the dose.**

Should Mr DF be started on warfarin?

A16 **No.**

Anticoagulation should only be considered for patients in valvular or non-valvular atrial fibrillation. It should not be started until intracerebral haemorrhage has been excluded by brain imaging, and usually only after 14 days have elapsed. Meta-analysis of several trials into the use of warfarin has suggested a relative risk of stroke in patients receiving warfarin of 0.33 compared with placebo. This means that only one-third as many strokes occurred in patients receiving warfarin compared with those receiving placebo. There also appears to be a relative risk for deaths from causes other than stroke of 0.57 in patients receiving warfarin compared with placebo.

What are the alternative antiplatelet agents to aspirin?

A17 **Dipyridamole and clopidogrel.**

The European Stroke Prevention Study 2 compared the efficacy of low-dose aspirin, modified-release dipyridamole and the two agents combined for the prevention of ischaemic stroke in patients with prior stroke or transient ischaemic attacks. Risk of stroke (after 24 months) was reduced by 18% with aspirin (25 mg twice daily) alone ($P = 0.013$), 16% with modified-release dipyridamole (200 mg twice daily) alone ($P = 0.039$) and 37% with the combination ($P < 0.001$). The authors therefore concluded that when aspirin and dipyridamole are co-prescribed the protective effects against stroke appear to be additive and significantly greater than for either agent alone. Current NICE guidelines recommend that aspirin and modified-release dipyridamole should be prescribed as secondary prevention for all first-time ischaemic stroke patients. Therefore, Mr DF had dipyridamole Retard 200 mg twice a day added to his medication regimen once the acute phase of his stroke was over (i.e. after the first 14 days).

An alternative to this regimen, particularly in those patients who are aspirin intolerant, is the use of clopidogrel. This antiplatelet drug is a thienopyridine derivative which appears to be modestly superior to aspirin in reducing the incidence of thromboembolic events. In the CAPRIE trial, clopidogrel 75 mg daily showed a relative risk reduction of 8.7% (P = 0.043) versus aspirin 325 mg daily. Aspirin intolerance is defined as allergy to aspirin or a history of peptic ulcer disease. A history of simple dyspepsia, caused by taking aspirin on an empty stomach, is not a contraindication to low-dose aspirin therapy.

There is currently no evidence to support the combination of aspirin and clopidogrel for routine secondary prevention after an ischaemic stroke. The MATCH study demonstrated that a combination of aspirin and clopidogrel did not produce a significantly greater reduction in the risk of secondary stroke events than either agent used as monotherapy; however, the combination did produce a significantly greater risk of life-threatening bleeding than either agent used as monotherapy.

What is the rationale for the initiation of an angiotensin-converting enzyme inhibitor (ACEI)?

A18 To reduce the risk of Mr DF suffering a further stroke.

The management of Mr DF's hypertension should now be a priority, with a target blood pressure of 130/80 mmHg; however, his blood pressure should only be reduced gradually, and additional antihypertensives are not normally prescribed until at least 7 days after a stroke, as a sudden drop in blood pressure could impair cerebral perfusion, which may impair consciousness or result in further infarction.

In the PROGRESS study the combination of an ACEI (perindopril) and a thiazide diuretic (indapamide) produced a stroke risk reduction of 43% compared to placebo in both hypertensive and non-hypertensive patients. As Mr DF is already on bendroflumethiazide and was still hypertensive on day 9, it was decided to add in perindopril 2 mg daily and titrate the dose slowly upwards as needed.

There is still debate as to whether the reduction in stroke risk observed in the trial is a class effect, an effect unique to perindopril, or just the result of aggressive lowering of blood pressure. In the HOPE study, ramipril reduced the risk of stroke by 33% in high-risk patients with vascular disease or diabetes and one other risk factor. The resultant cardiovascular benefit was greater than that attributable to a reduction in blood pressure; however, HOPE was not specifically designed to examine the prevention of further strokes.

Should a statin be prescribed for Mr DF?

A19 **Yes.**

The Royal College of Physicians Stroke Guidelines state that a statin should be considered for all patients with a total serum cholesterol >3.5 mmol/L following stroke. This statement is supported by the results of the Heart Protection Study, in which simvastatin 40 mg daily led to a relative risk reduction of about one-quarter in all groups of patients, irrespective of their baseline serum cholesterol level.

What lifestyle changes would you recommend?

A20 **Smoking cessation, reduction of alcohol intake, weight reduction and moderate regular exercise.**

Mr DF should be advised about the availability and use of nicotine replacement therapy. A reduction in alcohol intake, regular, moderate exercise and dietary advice may also reduce his cardiovascular risk.

How could the pharmacist contribute to Mr DF's discharge?

A21 **The pharmacist can contribute to the discharge by providing pharmaceutical advice and support to the patient and his carers. There should also be effective liaison with his general practitioner (GP) and community pharmacist.**

The pharmacist can contribute to Mr DF's discharge in the following ways:

(a) **Counselling.** Mr DF should be given both written (patient information leaflets and a reminder chart) and verbal information regarding the purpose and use of his medicines. The importance of long-term antiplatelet therapy and good control of his blood pressure and cholesterol level should be stressed.

Early treatment of acute stroke appears to be the most important factor in determining outcome, therefore Mr DF and his carers should be carefully instructed to seek urgent medical attention if he experiences any weakness or paralysis, speech impairment, numbness, blurred or sudden loss of vision, or altered level of consciousness.

(b) **Compliance assessment.** This must be assessed in the light of any existing impairment of his manual dexterity or cognitive function as a result of the stroke. Mr DF still has some restriction in arm movement, which may impair the opening of his medication containers. The use of any compliance aids must be with the consent of Mr DF and his carers.

(c) **Liaison with his GP and community pharmacist.** Information regarding medication changes (i.e. the prescribing of aspirin, dipyridamole, perindopril, simvastatin and amitriptyline), alternative formulations of medicines (i.e. the carbamazepine suspension), nutritional products and compliance aids should be communicated to the patient's GP and community pharmacist.

(d) **Liaison with patient support groups.** Mr DF should be given contact information for organisations that provide support and information to both patients and carers, e.g. The Stroke Association, Different Strokes and The National Stroke Association.

Further reading

Bhatt DL, Hirsch AT, Ringleb PA. Reduction in the need for hospitalisation for recurrent ischaemic events and bleeding with clopidogrel instead of aspirin. CAPRIE investigators. *Am Heart J* 2000; **140**: 67–73.

CAST (Chinese Acute Stroke Trial) Collaborative Group. CAST: randomised placebo-controlled trial of early aspirin use in 20 000 patients with ischaemic stroke. *Lancet* 1997; **349**; 1641–1649.

Clark WM, Wissman S, Albers GW *et al.* Recombinant tissue-type plasminogen activator (alteplase) for ischaemic stroke 3 to 5 hours after symptom onset. The ALTANTIS Study: a randomised controlled trial. Alteplase Thrombolysis for Acute Noninterventional Therapy in Ischemic Stroke. *J Am Med Assoc* 1999; **282**: 2019–2026.

Diener HC, Cunha L, Forbes C *et al.* European Stroke Prevention Study 2. Dipyridamole and acetylsalicylic acid in the secondary prevention of stroke. *J Neurol Sci* 1996; **143**: 1–13.

Diener HC, Bogousslavsky J, Brass LM *et al.* Aspirin and clopidogrel compared with clopidogrel alone after recent ischaemic stroke or transient ischaemic attack in high-risk patients (MATCH): randomised, double-blind, placebo-controlled trial. *Lancet* 2004; **364**: 331–337.

Hacke W, Kaste M, Fieschi C *et al.* Intravenous thrombolysis with recombinant tissue plasminogen activator for acute hemispheric stroke. The European Cooperative Acute Stroke Study (ECASS). *J Am Med Assoc* 1995; **274**: 1017–1025.

Hacke W, Kaste M, Fieschi C *et al.* Randomised double-blind placebo-controlled trial of thrombolytic therapy with acute ischaemic stroke (ECASS-II). Second European–Australian Acute Stroke Study Investigators. *Lancet* 1998; **352**: 1245–1251.

Hacke W, Kaste M, Blumki E *et al*. Thrombolysis with alteplase 3 to 4.5 hours after acute ischaemic stroke. *N Engl J Med* 2008: **359**: 1317–1329.

Heart Outcomes Prevention Evaluation Study Investigators. Effects of an angiotensin-converting-enzyme inhibitor, ramipril on cardiovascular events in high-risk patients. *N Engl J Med* 2000; **342**: 145–153.

Hill MD, Buchan AM and Canadian Alteplase for Stroke Effectiveness Study (CASES) Investigators. Thrombolysis for acute ischaemic stroke; results of the Canadian Alteplase for Stroke Effectiveness Study. *Can Med Assoc J* 2005; **172**: 1307–1312.

Intercollegiate Working Party for Stroke. *National Clinical Guidelines for Stroke*, 3rd edn. Royal College of Physicians, London, 2008.

International Stroke Collaborative Group. The International Stroke Trial (IST): a randomised trial of aspirin, subcutaneous heparin, both, or neither among 19 435 patients with acute ischaemic stroke. *Lancet* 1997; **349**: 1569–1581.

MRC/BHF Heart Protection Study of cholesterol lowering with simvastatin in 20 536 high-risk individuals; a randomised placebo-controlled trial. *Lancet* 2002; **306**: 7–22.

PROGRESS Collaborative Group. Randomised trial of a perindopril-based blood-pressure lowering regimen among 6105 individuals with previous stroke or transient ischaemic attack. *Lancet* 2001; **358**: 1033–1041.

Wahlgren N, Ahmed N, Davolos A *et al*. Thrombolysis with alteplase for acute ischaemic stroke in Safe Implementation of Thrombolysis in Stroke Monitoring Study (SITS-MOST): an observational study. *Lancet* 2007; **369**: 275–282.

6

Type 1 diabetes in childhood

Stephen Tomlin

Case study and questions

Day 1 Vicky, a 6-year-old girl who lived with her mother and two younger sisters, was brought into A&E by her mother. She weighed 22 kg and had always been a healthy, active child. The whole family had had colds and fevers over the last few weeks, but Vicky was still suffering from flu-like symptoms as well as having some nausea, vomiting and a recurrent stomach ache. Her mother was concerned because her symptoms were not improving and she appeared to have lost weight over the last few weeks.

On questioning, it became apparent that Vicky had been drinking large quantities of water and juice over the last couple of months. She had also wet the bed on a number of occasions, which her mother had put down to her not getting on well at school.

Laboratory values for blood taken in A&E were:

- Glucose 22 mmol/L (reference range 3.5–10)
- Bicarbonate 11 mmol/L (22–29)
- Blood pH 6.7 (7.35–7.45)
- Ketones 5.5 mmol/L

Her urine also tested positive for ketones (normally 0).

A diagnosis of mild ketosis was made presenting secondary to newly diagnosed type 1 diabetes.

Q1 Describe the presenting symptoms that lead to a diagnosis of type 1 diabetes.
Q2 How do these symptoms compare to a classic presentation of the disease? Could there have been a misdiagnosis?
Q3 What are the aims of treatment for Vicky?
Q4 What initial treatment would you recommend for Vicky?
Q5 What long-term therapy would you recommend and why?

Vicky was managed as an inpatient over the next few days and was then started on Humulin M3 insulin (7 units in the morning and 4 units before her evening meal). She was carefully monitored and given a lot of information from members of the multidisciplinary team. After 5 days she was discharged home, but had daily visits from the diabetic nurse for the following 4 days.

Q6 Outline a pharmaceutical care plan for Vicky.
Q7 How should Vicky's therapy be monitored at home after discharge?

Week 5 Vicky was taken to a general practitioner (GP) during the family holiday complaining of headaches and nightmares. Her mother admitted that since they had been on holiday they had not been checking her blood sugars as often as they were recommended to, and that they had also missed the last hospital appointment. On top of this, Vicky had probably been running around more than usual on the beach. Her insulin regimen had not altered much over the first few weeks and from her last consultation was still 7 units of Humulin M3 in the morning and 4 units in the evening. Her mother was also concerned that Vicky's eating habits had become more erratic, even before the holiday, and was not sure of the consequences of this.

Q8 What do the presenting symptoms tell us about Vicky's condition?
Q9 Why is it so important to keep a close eye on blood sugar levels in the first few months after starting treatment?
Q10 What treatment changes would you recommend for Vicky?
Q11 What are the possible options for treating type 1 diabetes in children with erratic eating habits?

Vicky was discharged after another long consultation with the paediatrician and diabetic nurse. Her insulin type had not been changed, but the dose had been reduced to 4 units in the morning and 3 at night.

Over the next few months Vicky was not a regular clinic attender and her blood sugar diary was not well filled in; however, she did remain fairly well.

Month 6, day 1 Vicky was once again brought back to A&E by her mother. She was looking very pale and lethargic. She had been unwell for a few days with diarrhoea and vomiting following a friend's birthday party. Her mother said they had omitted the last couple of doses of insulin as Vicky had not been eating, but that she had carried on going downhill.

On examination Vicky was very lethargic, but just about responding. Her eyes looked sunken and her mouth was very dry. There was a distinctive fruity odour on her breath. Her abdomen was very tender and her pulse rate high, at 125 beats per minute (bpm). She was breathing deeply.

Laboratory results were:

- Blood glucose 25 mmol/L (3.5–10)
- Sodium 150 mmol/L (135–147)
- Potassium 5.6 mmol/L (3.5–5.0)
- Chloride 110 mmol/L (95–105)
- Bicarbonate 5 mmol/L (22–29)
- Creatinine 180 micromol/L (80–120)
- Urine 2% glucose and ketones (normal for both is 0)
- Weight 21.2 kg (last recorded weight was 23 kg a month ago)

Vicky's therapy had not varied greatly over the last few months, and her last regimen had still been using Humulin M3 at a dose of 4 units in the morning and 3 units at night.

Q12 What is the clinical diagnosis for Vicky?
Q13 Why might this have occurred?
Q14 What are the aims of treatment now?
Q15 What treatment would you recommend for Vicky?

Day 2 After 36 hours Vicky was able to tolerate oral feeds.

Day 3 Her fluid balance and electrolytes were finally completely corrected. She was given the first dose of her usual subcutaneous insulin an hour before her insulin infusion was turned off.

Because of the recent problems and a real loss of confidence in the treatment regimen on the part of Vicky and her mother, a thorough review was conducted by the consultant and specialist nurse. The options were discussed with Vicky and her mother, and included the use of insulin glargine, lispro and insulin pumps; however, it was decided that she would be better off at this time carrying on with the twice-daily biphasic insulin with regular support from the diabetic nurse.

Q16 Discuss the advantages and disadvantages associated with alternative methods and types of insulin. Why is it likely that the current regimen was finally decided on?
Q17 How should Vicky's mother be advised to manage minor illness in the future?
Q18 How should Vicky's specialist consultant and GP monitor her long-term therapy?

Answers

Describe the presenting symptoms that lead to a diagnosis of Type 1 diabetes.

A1 **Abdominal pain, weight loss, enuresis, thirst, elevated blood glucose, and ketones and glucose in the urine.**

The onset of type 1 diabetes is often preceded by an acute viral illness which can cause an autoimmune destructive response in the pancreas, leading to impaired insulin production.

Abdominal symptoms are often seen as the presenting symptoms of diabetic ketoacidosis, which is still fairly mild in Vicky's case. The keto-acidosis is due to an excessive mobilisation of free fatty acids to the liver, where they are metabolised to ketones. This process is activated by low insulin levels.

The weight loss will be the product of several of the presenting symptoms. When glucose levels reach the renal threshold, glucose spills into the urine, taking water with it by the process of osmotic diuresis. The loss of calories in water in this way leads to polyuria, enuresis, thirst, weight loss and fatigue. In addition, there will also be weight loss due to the ongoing viral illness reducing Vicky's desire to eat.

How do these symptoms compare to a classic presentation of the disease? Could there have been a misdiagnosis?

A2 **Vicky's symptoms are classic, but in children such symptoms may initially be associated with urinary tract infection, failure to thrive, gastroenteritis or psychological problems.**

Vicky's symptoms are typical of type 1 diabetes, with a relatively acute onset of symptoms at a young age following a traumatic life event (e.g. a viral illness). Unlike type 2 diabetes, there is rarely an association with a family history of diabetes and the patient is rarely obese.

It is uncommon for infants (under 1 year of age) to develop diabetes, but the incidence increases with age, with particular peaks between 4 and 6 years, and the largest peak in early adolescence.

Polyuria and bed-wetting in children are often linked to urinary tract infection, and this diagnosis is further supported by the presence of abdominal pain. Because of the gastrointestinal upset caused by the presenting ketoacidosis there is often weight loss due to lack of eating, vomiting, and the higher urine output. This in turn leads to fatigue and irritability. Consequently there are often problems at school, which may be picked up by the parents or teachers; however, these problems are then often blamed for the bed-wetting and emotional instability, thereby leading to an initial misdiagnosis.

Vicky's height and weight have been normal for her age, and the sequence of events alongside the laboratory results have led to the correct diagnosis.

What are the aims of treatment for Vicky?

A3 To obtain optimal glucose control, prevent diabetic complications (chronic and acute), and achieve normal growth and development.

Vicky had normal growth velocity before the onset of illness; however, any acute or chronic illness in a child can have a dramatic long-term influence on height and weight. They can thus be used as markers for Vicky's overall wellbeing as she grows up. The weight loss Vicky has already experienced should be corrected easily and quickly now that the diagnosis has been made. Her height and weight should be plotted at regular clinic appointments on a standard growth chart, so that progress can be monitored.

The Diabetes Control and Complications Trial Group demonstrated that tight blood glucose control reduced the incidence of complications, in terms of both microvascular (retinopathy and renal failure) and macrovascular (stroke, angina, myocardial infarction) complications. In older children and adults it is recommended that intensive control of blood sugar is adhered to, in order to reduce the long-term sequelae of diabetes. The same principle applies to younger children, but greater care must be taken in the implementation of this. Over-zealous control could lead to hypoglycaemias, and these must be avoided in children under the age of 8 as brain development may be impaired.

Glucose control can be assessed by measuring glycated haemoglobin. The HbA_{1c} fraction is commonly measured. It comprises the majority of glycated haemoglobin and is the least affected by recent fluctuations in sugar levels. It measures the percentage of haemoglobin A that has been irreversibly glycated, and its value is determined by the plasma glucose levels and the lifespan of a red blood cell (about 120 days). It can thus be said that HbA_{1c} is an indicator of glycaemic control over the preceding 2–3 months.

Glycated haemoglobin is thus normally monitored on a 3-monthly basis to give a longer-term view of blood sugar control. It is carried out on a finger-prick of blood. It has been shown that lowering HbA_{1c} can delay or stop the development of long-term complications. A normal HbA_{1c} is 4–6.5%; levels > 8.5% are seriously elevated. The target HbA_{1c} for a child such as Vicky would be 4–7.5% (making the target too tight can be discouraging to children, and so a real balance has to be achieved) but children will often have an HbA_{1c} of 8–10%. Children's blood sugars are notoriously hard to control owing to their varied lifestyles and lack of adherence to therapy and a set dietary regimen. It is important to encourage tight glucose control and praise when progress is being made, rather than condemn for being outside a specified range.

What initial treatment would you recommend for Vicky?

A4 **As Vicky has significant signs of ketoacidosis she should probably be started on a sliding-scale insulin regimen for about 24 hours, in order to bring her condition under control.**

The sliding-scale insulin method is probably still the most common initial treatment for newly diagnosed patients. The amount of insulin given over the first 24 hours is no longer used as a predictor of the patient's insulin requirement, but it is a safe way to gain initial control of hyperglycaemic symptoms.

A sliding scale works as follows. An intravenous (IV) infusion is set up of soluble insulin (Human Actrapid) 50 units made up to 50 mL with sodium chloride 0.9% in a syringe pump (i.e. 1 mL = 1 unit insulin). The giving set is flushed with insulin solution before it is connected to the child, in order to saturate the plastic's absorption of insulin.

The blood glucose level should be measured as soon as the insulin is started and the infusion rate adjusted according to the table below, in order to keep the blood glucose between 4 and 11 mmol/L. Blood glucose levels should be measured every hour for the first 4 hours, and then reduced to every 2 hours until stable. Once Vicky is stable, her ongoing insulin needs must be met.

Table 6.1 Insulin dosing using a sliding scale

Blood glucose (mmol/L)	*Insulin infusion (units/kg/h)*
0–5	0
6–10	0.05
11–15	0.1
16–20	0.15
>20	0.2

What long-term therapy would you recommend and why?

A5 **She could start on a twice-daily subcutaneous insulin regimen using a biphasic insulin mix via a preloaded pen. The dose should**

be based on 0.5 units/kg/day, with two-thirds given in the morning before breakfast and one-third given before the evening meal.

Severe insulin deficiency combined with the physical and psychological changes that accompany normal development through childhood make the management of type 1 diabetes particularly difficult. NICE do not specify a specific regimen for preschool and primary school children, and just recommend that it be appropriate and individualised to optimise glycaemic control.

As it is more important to prevent hypoglycaemia (which is potentially life-threatening) than hyperglycaemia, initial treatment should be cautious.

Initial insulin dosing in this age group will usually start at 0.25 units/kg/day, but will be higher if there are signs that ketoacidosis has been present for a while. Dosing of > 0.9 units/kg of insulin per day are rarely required in prepubertal children, but may increase up to 1.8 units/kg/day during puberty owing to the increased release of growth hormone at this time leading to reduced insulin sensitivity.

As Vicky has shown signs of ketosis for some days she should be started on a dose of 0.5 units/kg/day, with two-thirds being given in the morning before breakfast and one-third before the evening meal. A variety of insulins are available for long-term treatment, each with a different time to onset and peak of action, as well as duration of action.

The mixed preparations of insulin (biphasic) give a high initial peak and then a sustained level throughout the day when used twice daily. This is a good combination for children of school age, as they have limited support during lunchtime. These combinations have the advantage of providing peaks of insulin around main meal times (breakfast and evening), as well as continual lower levels throughout the day without the user having to draw up two different insulins. It is normal to start with a 70:30 ratio, e.g. Mixtard 30 (70% isophane and 30% regular) and to make any necessary changes thereafter.

Vicky could start by using a pen device giving 7 units in the morning and 4 units each evening (0.5 units/kg/day). These mixes may cause hypoglycaemic episodes in young children owing to the short-acting insulin peaks. It is thus essential that as well as eating three main meals, Vicky is encouraged to have three snacks during the day. Another solution may be for one or both of the doses to be swapped for an intermediate-acting insulin on its own, or to a different ratio of biphasic insulin. If Vicky shows signs of hypoglycaemia after a meal, the proportion of short-acting insulin is obviously too large and a different ratio biphasic could be tried.

Once children have lost their baby fat, subcutaneous injections are not as easy to give and care must be taken when choosing an injection site. During this period the abdomen may be a difficult site to use, so injections should be rotated between the thighs and the upper buttock area. Insulin pens have differently sized needles, so that the insulin is delivered directly into the subcutaneous tissue. The specialist nurse will assess a patient for the correct needle size.

Outline a pharmaceutical care plan for Vicky.

A6 **The pharmacist should contribute to Vicky's overall care and management by providing her and her family with information specifically about storage, administration and monitoring of insulin therapy. It is also essential that the pharmacist reinforce information on all relevant aspects of diabetic care given by other healthcare professionals.**

The care plan for an individual with type 1 diabetes must be individualised, as the treatment will affect their whole life. NICE recommends that children be offered an ongoing integrated package of care by a multidisciplinary paediatric diabetic care team, and should have 24-hour access to that team for advice. The key players in this team are: the consultant, who will perform the formal clinical assessments of the child, initially on a monthly basis; the specialist nurse, who will have regular contact with the family; and the dietitian, who will be involved initially to advise on diet and then intermittently, depending on Vicky's progress.

The key information Vicky and her carers need includes:

(a) Education on how to use an insulin pen device (the easiest initial method of administration). This includes checking the insulin expiry date; using a different needle each time; how to insert, hold and then remove the needle. It is also important that the family know how to use a syringe in case the pen is lost or damaged.

(b) The need to rotate injection sites, as injecting into the same site can cause lumps to form which will affect insulin uptake in the long term. Rotation guides are available if these are deemed necessary.

Patients are normally advised to inject insulin into the subcutaneous tissue of the abdomen, thighs and buttocks in rotation; however, younger children are often reluctant to inject into their abdomen. It is important that no one site is overused, as this may lead to lipohypertrophy and poor insulin absorption, resulting in erratic blood glucose concentrations.

The site of injection also influences the speed of absorption, with the abdomen and arms providing quickest absorption and the thighs and buttocks the slowest. More rapid absorption will be caused by exercise or heat, for example from a bath following the injection.

Practical instructions for the patient/carer could be as follows:

> Insulin should be given by subcutaneous injection, i.e. into the fat beneath the skin, not into the muscle. To avoid injecting into the muscle, it is important to lift a skin fold with the thumb and index finger ('two-finger pinch-up') and insert the needle at a 45° angle. Lifting a skin fold is important, even if you are using an 8 mm (1/3 inch) needle. With 5–6 mm needles, injections can be given without lifting a skin fold if there is enough subcutaneous fat (at least 8 mm, as skin layers may be compressed when injecting perpendicularly). Lean boys, however, usually have less fat, especially on the thigh.
>
> Wiggle the needle slightly before injecting. If the tip feels 'stuck' you have probably reached the muscle. If this is the case, withdraw the needle a little before injecting. You can also inject insulin into the buttocks, where there is usually a layer of subcutaneous fat thick enough to insert the needle perpendicularly without lifting a skin fold.

(c) How to dispose of needles safely.

(d) The need to keep spare insulin cartridges in the fridge. Opened insulin can be stored for 1 month out of the fridge.

(e) How to take blood glucose levels and, hopefully, keep them at 4–8 mmol/L. A single drop of blood from the side of a finger (not thumb) is usually put onto a test strip. It is important that blood level diaries are kept so that trends can be seen.

(f) How to assess for hyper- and hypoglycaemia and how to treat them. It is essential that this aspect of care is understood by all the child's carers, e.g. teachers. If a child has symptoms of hypoglycaemia they should take some sugar or a sugary drink straightaway, followed by a sandwich or biscuit. If they are unable to swallow, Glucogel (a sugary gel that can be rubbed into the lips or gums) can be used. If these measures do not work, glucagon injections may be given by the carer if they are deemed to have a good level of understanding of their use. Otherwise the patient and carer should be advised to go to a doctor. It is important that Vicky and her family always carry sugar or sweet food with them.

(g) Normal dietary advice includes:

  (i) avoiding fatty foods;
  (ii) eating mainly vegetables, fruit, cereal, rice and pasta;

(iii) eating only small amounts of refined sugar (jam, sweets etc.);
(iv) eating at regular intervals;
(v) carrying glucose tablets or sweets in case of hypoglycaemia.

(h) Information on what to do when the child is ill.
(i) Useful contact numbers.

How should Vicky's therapy be monitored at home after discharge?

A7 Initially blood glucose should be monitored before each meal and at bedtime. This level of monitoring can usually be reduced over time.

Immediately following diagnosis, monitoring is essential before each meal along with a final daily check before bedtime. Once glycaemic control is stable and appropriate, then monitoring can drop to two to three times a week, with three or four tests on each of those days prior to meals, or to twice daily each day to help adherence to blood testing. Monitoring should be increased during acute illness and at times of changed lifestyle.

Blood samples are usually taken from finger-pricks, although in younger children the heels and the earlobes may provide an alternative site.

Blood glucose monitoring must be tailored to an individual's life circumstances, and this is particularly important with children going to school. Enforcing a regimen that is not what the child wants when they are at school (this will vary with age) is likely to lead to a child who carries out no monitoring at all. Ideally, blood glucose levels should be maintained at 4–8 mmol/L apart from at bedtime, when 7–10 mmol/L would be ideal.

Parents should be taught to monitor as often as possible and to respond to altering glucose concentrations. If glucose levels are high, they may be taught to give additional insulin on top of the normal requirements. This will normally involve doses of short-acting insulin in doses of about 0.1 units/kg. These doses should not be given more frequently than 4-hourly to avoid hypoglycaemia. If this additional requirement is recurrent, then changes in dose will be recommended. In reality most additional insulin dose adjustments are made by the diabetic nurse and not taken on fully by the carer. Adjustments of the biphasic insulin dose, whether up or down, are usually made in increments of 10–20% of the original.

Children are usually monitored, either in the clinic or at home through visits by a specialist diabetic nurse on a regular basis. Initially home visits may be daily, reducing to weekly over time. The child and their carers will be given dietary advice on avoiding high glucose-containing foods and drinks. They will also be encouraged to fill in glucose diaries so that trends in blood glucose patterns can be seen.

What do the presenting symptoms tell us about Vicky's condition?

A8 **That Vicky is being overtreated with insulin and is suffering from hypoglycaemia.**

Nightmares, as in Vicky's case, poor sleep and crying are all potential signs of hypoglycaemia. Hypoglycaemia is a very serious and life-threatening consequence of diabetic treatment. It is particularly hard to spot in children and is more likely to occur as a result of their very varied activity levels throughout a day. Nocturnal hypoglycaemia has also been observed more frequently in children than in adults and, perhaps more worryingly, it is often asymptomatic.

Why is it so important to keep a close eye on blood sugar levels in the first few months after starting treatment?

A9 **A lot of patients have a 'honeymoon' period for the first few months after starting treatment, with their insulin requirements dropping off dramatically.**

Apart from the lack of sugar monitoring that Vicky has been receiving and the increased exercise burning off more sugar, she is at increased risk in the first few months after diagnosis of having lower insulin requirements.

Around a quarter of all patients who develop type 1 diabetes have what is known as a 'honeymoon' period within days or weeks of the onset of treatment. It is as if the patient has gone into remission, and it can be confusing for the patient/carer as it would appear that the condition has corrected itself. Some patients actually require no insulin during this phase, and this may last for weeks or months. It is usually best to keep treating with insulin, even if the requirements are negligible, to avoid possible insulin allergy upon re-exposure, and also to maintain a treatment regimen and not give false hope to the patient.

What treatment changes would you recommend for Vicky?

A10 **Vicky now needs increased monitoring and probably a reduction in her insulin dose, especially in the evening.**

The nightmares indicate that the hypoglycaemia is occurring at night, but increased daily monitoring should be encouraged to rule out an overall 'honeymoon' period. Both bedtime and early morning blood glucose monitoring should be carried out. It is important to have a good picture of what is happening to ensure the best changes to treatment. If a biphasic insulin is being given before the evening meal the overall dose may be too large, or perhaps the soluble insulin component needs altering. The most common treatment change to avoid nocturnal hypoglycaemia is to use a different ratio of biphasic insulin, such as 75:25 (e.g. Insuman Comb 25), thereby reducing the amount of fast-acting insulin. The use of biphasic insulin containing a very fast-acting phase, such as Humalog Mix25, could also be considered, as the action of the lispro insulin is short-lived. Alternatively, control may be almost correct and the only intervention needed is to give a small snack just before going to bed to keep the blood sugar up.

What are the possible options for treating type 1 diabetes in children with erratic eating habits?

A11 The answer to this is very patient specific, but may involve giving short-acting insulin more frequently (three times daily) and an intermediate-acting insulin before bed.

Set-regimen and combination (biphasic) insulins are the most convenient form to administer, provided the person's lifestyle and eating habits do not fluctuate greatly. Children are renowned for eating erratically, and for the quantity and content of what they eat having little to do with their daily routine (or lack of it).

Using the same total daily insulin dose, the soluble insulin may be given before the three main meals of the day (breakfast, lunch and dinner); a fourth dose of intermediate insulin is then given prior to going to bed.

Another option could be to use insulin lispro as the short-acting insulin in the above regimen. It is fast-acting (onset in about 15 minutes, peaking at 1 hour) with a short duration (about 5 hours), and can solve some of these problems as it can be used when necessary and will even be effective if given directly after a meal, instead of before.

In reality, erratic eating habits often go hand in hand with poor adherence, and education is the main support of treatment (see **A15**).

What is the clinical diagnosis for Vicky?

A12 Vicky has acute, life-threatening diabetic ketoacidosis.

As in the initial diagnosis, Vicky has signs of ketoacidosis; however, this time the signs and symptoms, as well as the laboratory results, show that it is serious and potentially life threatening.

Vicky has presented with a high blood glucose level, which in turn has led to an increase in plasma osmolarity. Osmotic diuresis has then set in, with loss of fluid and electrolytes. Dehydration can be rapid, causing changes in skin texture, sunken eyeballs, and eventually loss of consciousness. Excessive ketone production causes a distinctive fruity odour on the breath. High levels of ketones also cause a fall in pH, as they are organic acids. Hypercapnia then results, owing to the respiratory rate increasing to try to compensate for the metabolic acidosis.

Why might this have occurred?

A13 **Misinterpretation of her symptoms, leading to non-administration of insulin.**

Vicky was vomiting after the party. It could be assumed that she had gastroenteritis and thus was not eating, and therefore would not be needing any insulin. In reality, the nausea and vomiting were probably the first signs of ketoacidosis due to a large glucose intake at the party. Non-administration of the insulin has only made the situation worse, and has caused a critical ketoacidosis to develop.

What are the aims of treatment now?

A14 **The main aims of treatment for Vicky are to correct her dehydration and the hyperglycaemia.**

What treatment would you recommend for Vicky?

A15 **Fluid correction is vital and must be initiated immediately. This must be done cautiously, while bringing the blood sugars back under control.**

Children who are more than 5% dehydrated and/or drowsy will almost certainly require urgent IV fluids with electrolyte correction; however, this must be done with caution to avoid cerebral oedema and hypokalaemia, which are the leading causes of death in such cases.

Vicky is 1.8 kg lighter than she was a month ago and has therefore lost about 8% of her body weight through dehydration (weight loss should be based, as near as possible, on her current weight against her weight before dehydration started). This is severe dehydration, with 1 kg weight loss equating to 1 L of fluid loss. Treatment will be as if the dehydration were 8%, as using figures higher than this can lead to more complications and assessment can never be regarded as totally accurate. In cases of > 5% dehydration with shock, or in the young, it would be normal practice to treat the patient on a paediatric intensive care unit.

Children who are in shock due to the severity of the ketoacidosis (tachycardia, poor capillary refill time and hypotension) should initially be given 10 mL/kg of sodium chloride 0.9%. Vicky has some of these symptoms, and this should be the first treatment that she receives.

After this initial fluid a continuous rehydration infusion should be set up alongside an insulin infusion.

The rehydration regimen should be calculated so that fluid correction takes place over 48 hours as follows:

- 24 h correction = maintenance fluid + 0.5 × deficit + any continuing losses (vomiting)
- Maintenance = 0–2 years: 80 mL/kg/24 h
  3–5 years: 70 mL/kg/24 h
  6–9 years: 60 mL/kg/24 h
  10–14 years: 50 mL/kg/24 h
  >15 years: 35 mL/kg/24 h
- Deficit (mL) = % dehydration × body weight (kg) × 1000

For Vicky:

- Maintenance = 60 mL × 23 kg = 1380 mL/24 h
- Deficit = 8/100 × 23 × 1000 = 1840 mL

Thus, 24-hour correction for Vicky = maintenance + 0.5 × deficit = 1380 mL + 920 mL = 2300 mL, i.e. 4.6 L needs to be run in over the next 48 hours. Provided she is not anuric (which she is not), this fluid should be sodium chloride 0.9% with 20 mmol of potassium in each 500 mL bag.

An electrocardiogram monitor should be set up and her potassium levels should be checked every 2–4 hours throughout the first 24 hours. Levels should be corrected to keep them between 4 and 5 mmol/L.

The insulin regimen should be as follows. A continuous infusion of soluble insulin (Actrapid) should be set up. The insulin should be diluted to 1 unit/mL in a syringe using sodium chloride 0.9%. The infusion should be started at 0.1 units/kg/h. If the rate of fall of glucose is > 5 mmol/h, add glucose to the IV fluids, then the rate of the infusion should be halved. Rates of fall > 5 mmol/h can lead to large osmolarity changes, and this can in turn lead to cerebral oedema. When the blood glucose is 14–17 mmol/L the insulin infusion should be reduced and the fluid changed to glucose 5% + sodium chloride 0.9% with or without potassium, still running at the same rate.

Blood glucose levels should be held between 10 and 11 mmol/L. If levels start to dip below 7 mmol/L the glucose input should be increased. The insulin should not be stopped, as insulin is required to switch off ketone production.

Acidosis is usually self-limiting; however, profound acidosis with a pH <7 with shock and circulatory failure will require sodium bicarbonate infusion to reverse the acidosis slowly. This should be a very rare requirement if rehydration has been managed appropriately.

Discuss the advantages and disadvantages associated with alternative methods and types of insulin. Why is it likely that the current regimen was finally decided on?

A16 **Alternative methods do have their advantages, but they are generally felt to be best suited to patients with a thorough understanding of their disease state and a high level of motivation. This is not the case with Vicky and her family, so continuing with the current regimen is the best option here.**

Insulin glargine and detemir are long-acting insulin analogues. They are designed to have a flat release profile to mimic natural insulin release and have a longer duration of action than isophane insulin. A lower incidence of nocturnal hypoglycaemia has been demonstrated in some trials, although early morning hypoglycaemia may occur. Short-acting insulins still need to be administered before meals, and thus the number of injections daily is likely to be four or five, making it less convenient for patients with poor adherence.

Insulin pumps are available and being reviewed for their place in therapy as they provide an alternative to multiple injections. The insulin pump is a battery-operated pump with a computer that programs the delivery of predetermined amounts of soluble insulin from a chamber into a subcutaneously implanted catheter. The pump can deliver a constant flow as well as be activated for boluses by the operator 30 minutes before meals. Lispro insulin is also now being combined with the pumps so that shots of insulin can be given whenever a meal is eaten, rather than the user having to pre-plan and inject 30 minutes before meals. This type of device is likely to increase in use, as it can mimic normal insulin flow reasonably well; however, users must be highly motivated to use the device efficiently, and not all children take kindly to having a pump attached to them. This may well be a suitable device in the future for Vicky.

Vicky and her family are typical in terms of compliance with the treatment of type 1 diabetes. The best way to improve treatment is to continuously encourage adherence and to reach agreement about treatment which takes into account the social issues.

How should Vicky's mother be advised to manage minor illness in the future?

A17 **Vicky's mother should be advised never to stop giving insulin to her daughter even if she is unwell and not eating.**

Even when she is unwell and not eating, Vicky's body is still producing glucose from its stores. If the insulin is stopped, then Vicky could become hyperglycaemic and seriously ill. The dose of insulin may need to be adjusted during periods of illness, and thus careful monitoring of the patient is essential. Blood sugars usually rise during illness, especially if fever is involved, and thus increases in insulin may be necessary. This increase in requirements is usually short-lived and reductions will need to be made as soon as levels start dropping again. Increased requirements are usually only in the region of 10–20% of the original dose.

Hyperglycaemia is more common if dehydration occurs, and this is common during episodes of fever. Therefore, good fluid intake should be encouraged throughout the day.

If solid foods are not being taken then alternatives such as milk, fruit juice, soup, ice cream and fizzy drinks will help maintain the carbohydrate allowance, thereby avoiding hypoglycaemia.

During illness the urine should be monitored for sugar and ketones. The presence of both of these substances will indicate a lack of insulin. If there is no sugar and only ketones, this is an indication of lack of food intake, especially carbohydrates.

Vicky's mother should be advised to contact the healthcare team for advice during periods of illness.

How should Vicky's specialist consultant and GP monitor her long-term therapy?

A18 Alongside the blood glucose and HbA_{1c} monitoring there are a number of other parameters that should be monitored regularly. These include growth and development, injection-site checks and retinal field checks.

At this age growth and development must be plotted regularly on a standard growth chart.

It is important that the injection sites are checked to ensure that they are being rotated. If sites are used over and over again they may become red and lumpy, a condition called lipodystrophy. Insulin injected into these sites may not work properly, owing to poor absorption.

Because of the long-term risk of retinal damage, eye checks should be performed not only at initial diagnosis, but also on a yearly basis thereafter. This practice usually only starts once the child is 12 years old, but many clinicians will do random eye checks before this time, especially if diagnosis is at a very early age.

Further reading

Anon. When and how should patients with diabetes test blood glucose? *MeReC Bull* 2002; **13**(1).

Devendra D, Liu E, Eisenbarth GS. Type 1 diabetes: recent developments. *Br Med J* 2004; **328**: 750–754.

Diabetes Control and Complications Trial Research Group. The effect of intensive diabetes treatment on the development and progression of long-term complications in adolescents with insulin-dependent diabetes mellitus. *J Pediatr* 1994; **125**: 177–188.

Koda-Kimble MA, Young LY, Kradjan WA *et al.*, eds. *Applied Therapeutics: The Clinical Use of Drugs*, 7th edn. Lippincott Williams & Wilkins, Philadelphia, 2001.

National Institute of Clinical Excellence. *Type 1 diabetes in children, young people and adults*. NICE, London, 2004.

Rudolph CD, Rudolph AM, eds. *Rudolph's Pediatrics*, 21st edn. McGraw-Hill, New York, 2001.

Schober E, Schoente E, Van Dyk J *et al.* Comparative trial between insulin glargine and NPH insulin in children and adolescents with type 1 diabetes mellitus. *Pediatr Endocrinol Metab* 2002; **15**: 369–376.

Scottish Study Group for the Care of the Young Diabetic. Factors influencing glycaemic control in young people with Type 1 diabetes in Scotland. *Diabetes Care* 2001; **24**: 239–244.

Silverstein J *et al.* Care of children and adolescents with type 1 diabetes. *Diabetic Care* 2005; **28**(1): 186–212.

Sperling MA. Continuous subcutaneous insulin infusion and continuous subcutaneous glucose monitoring in children with Type 1 diabetes mellitus: boon or bane? *Paediatr Diabetes* 2001; **2**: 49–50.

Tamborlane WV, Bonfig W, Bowland E. Recent advances in treatment of youth with Type 1 diabetes: better care through technology. *Diabetic Med* 2001; **18**: 864–870.

Thompson R, Hindmarsh P. Management of Type 1 diabetes in children. *Prescriber* 2002; **19 April**: 77–85.

Tupola S, Komulainen J, Jääskeläinen J *et al.* Post-prandial insulin vs. human regular insulin in prepubertal children with Type 1 diabetes mellitus. *Diabetic Med* 2001; **18**: 654–658.

7

Type 2 diabetes mellitus

Rachel A Hall

Case study and questions

Day 1 Mr KB, a 61-year-old builder, made an appointment with his general practitioner (GP) because he had felt increasingly tired over the last few weeks and it was starting to affect his work. He also complained of feeling thirsty and of going to the toilet frequently to urinate, especially during the night, which was unusual for him. His late mother had a history of type 2 diabetes.

The GP dipped his urine, which was positive for glucose but not ketones and a trace of protein. His random blood sugar was 11.5 mmol/L and his blood pressure (BP) 156/90 mmHg. He rarely came to see the GP. His previous medical history was osteoarthritis of the knee, for which he was taking the following medications:

- Diclofenac 50 mg orally three times daily after food
- Omeprazole 20 mg orally daily for gastroprotection.

The GP asked Mr KB to come back for a fasting blood glucose test the next morning.

Day 4 His fasting blood glucose was reported as 8.1 mmol/L (reference range 6.0–7.0). An appointment was made for Mr KB to see the clinical pharmacist (a non-medical prescriber) to discuss the result.

Day 7 The clinical pharmacist explained to Mr KB that his reported symptoms plus one fasting plasma glucose ≥ 7 mmol/L confirmed a diagnosis of type 2 diabetes (as per World Health Organization criteria).

A thorough explanation of the cause of diabetes and how it can be managed was given. Mr KB was shocked and upset by the diagnosis, but was keen to understand what he could do to help himself feel better.

The clinical pharmacist discussed his diet and lifestyle and what impact this would have on his condition. Mr KB admitted to smoking

20–30 cigarettes per day, drinking 40 units of alcohol a week, eating lots of sugary and fatty foods and doing little physical activity. He was obese, with a weight of 105 kg (body mass index (BMI) 32) and a waist circumference of 124 cm. His BP was 152/96 mmHg.

Mr KB was advised to start modifying his diet and to increase his physical activity, building up to at least 30 minutes five times per week. He was also given a file of written information and leaflets about type 2 diabetes, diet, exercise and diabetes-related complications to reinforce the discussions. He consented to being referred to the primary care dietitian, for which he was asked to complete a food diary. He was also referred to the Structured Education Programme and for retinopathy screening, as well as being advised to make an appointment with an optician for a visual acuity test, and to notify his car insurance company of the diagnosis. A follow-up appointment was arranged for 1 month later.

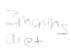

Q1 What risk factors does Mr KB have for the development of type 2 diabetes?
Q2 What are the management priorities for Mr KB?
Q3 Outline a pharmaceutical care plan for the initial management of Mr KB.
Q4 What dietary advice would you give to Mr KB?
Q5 Would it be appropriate to prescribe Mr KB an anti-obesity drug?
Q6 What information would you give Mr KB about alcohol consumption now that he has type 2 diabetes?
Q7 How would you explain to Mr KB why giving up smoking is so important, and how could you help him to achieve this?
Q8 How long should Mr KB be given to improve his glycaemic control through lifestyle measures before starting an oral hypoglycaemic agent?

Month 2 Mr KB returned to the clinical pharmacist, having seen the dietitian 2 weeks earlier. At that appointment he had been given detailed healthy eating advice after assessment of his food diary, and had also been advised to reduce his portion sizes and alcohol intake. He had been unaware that he was consuming excess calories and said he would try to cut down, although he knew this would not be easy. He was still feeling tired and urinating frequently, but preferred to continue diet control rather than start oral hypoglycaemic agents.

Mr KB's foot assessment was unremarkable and general foot care advice was given. He denied any erectile dysfunction.

His BP at this visit was 158/96 mmHg and his weight was 103 kg. A random blood sugar level was 12.7 mmol/L.

His serum biochemistry and haematology results were:

- Glycated haemoglobin (HbA_{1c}) 8.6% (reference range 6.5–7.5%)
- Thyroid-stimulating hormone 3.9 mU/L (0.35–5.0)

- Sodium 138 mmol/L (133–145)
- Potassium 4.1 mmol/L (3.5–5.2)
- Creatinine 78.0 μmol/L (50–95)
- Estimated glomerular filtration rate (eGFR) 71 mL/min/1.73 m^2 (chronic kidney disease stage 2 if there is evidence of existing renal disease)
- Alinine aminotransferase (ALT) level 46 IU/L (5–40)
- Alkaline phosphatase 37 IU/L (5–40)
- Albumin 39 g/dL (35–50)
- Total cholesterol 6.1 mmol/L (<4)
- High-density lipoprotein (HDL) cholesterol 0.9 mmol/L (>1.2)
- Low-density lipoprotein (LDL) cholesterol 4.5mmol/L (<2)
- Triglycerides 3.0 mmol/L (<2.3)
- Cholesterol/HDL ratio 6.8
- Urine albumin: creatinine ratio 2.4 mg/mmol (<3.0)

Q9 Which antihypertensive agents would be most appropriate for Mr KB and why?
Q10 Would you make any adjustment to Mr KB's pain relief therapy at this stage?
Q11 What other drug therapy should be initiated?
Q12 What monitoring would be necessary and when would you do this?
Q13 Is self-monitoring of blood glucose (SMBG) appropriate? How would you explain the benefits of SMBG to Mr KB?

Month 4 Mr KB attended for his 3-month review. His current medication was:

- Aspirin dispersible 75 mg orally daily
- Simvastatin 40 mg orally at night
- Ramipril 5 mg orally daily
- Paracetamol 1 g orally four times daily

His BP had reduced and was now 144/88 mmHg. His weight had reduced to 101 kg. His HbA_{1c} was 8.2%. He admitted to stopping simvastatin after 5 days as his legs were aching. He said he would prefer to lower his cholesterol by modifying his diet, and felt that he was already taking 'enough' tablets.

Q14 How can the risks and benefits of statins be explained to Mr KB so that he can make an informed choice about taking the drug?
Q15 Which oral hypoglycaemic agent would you recommend for Mr KB and why?

Month 10 Mr KB's HbA_{1c} was now 7.5%, his total cholesterol was 4.8 mmol/L and his weight 92 kg. He had made many dietary changes and was now more active, walking for at least 30 minutes every day. He had given up smoking and cut down his alcohol intake to 28 units per week. He complained of a dry cough, which had persisted for the last few weeks.

His current medication was:

- Aspirin dispersible 75 mg orally daily
- Metformin 1 g orally twice daily
- Ramipril 10 mg orally daily

- Simvastatin 40 mg orally at night
- Paracetamol 1 g orally four times daily

Q16 What could be causing Mr KB's cough, and what action would you take?
Q17 Which oral antidiabetic agent would you add in at this stage and why?

Year 5 Mr KB attended for his annual review. His BP was 148/86 mmHg and his HbA_{1c} 8.0%. His weight had increased to 97 kg. He had struggled to maintain his weight loss as he found it hard to stop snacking now that he was no longer smoking. He was worried that he might be started on insulin at this appointment.

His current medication was:

- Aspirin dispersible 75 mg orally daily
- Simvastatin 40 mg orally at night
- Metformin 1 g orally twice daily
- Gliclazide 160 mg orally twice daily
- Ramipril 10 mg orally daily
- Bendroflumethiazide 2.5 mg orally each morning
- Paracetamol 1 g orally four times daily

Q18 What further treatment options could Mr KB try before starting insulin?
Q19 What else could be added to Mr KB's antihypertensive regimen to achieve optimum control?
Q20 What are the benefits and risks of starting insulin in the patient, and how would you allay his fears?
Q21 What insulin preparation would you recommend for Mr KB?

Answers

What risk factors does Mr KB have for the development of type 2 diabetes?

A1 **Mr KB's risk factors are his age, obesity, family history and lifestyle.**

Type 2 diabetes is most commonly diagnosed in people over the age of 40, although it is now not unusual in younger people owing to the rise in obesity. Obese individuals usually develop insulin resistance, where the normal biological response to insulin in liver, muscle and fat cells is impaired, resulting in high circulating glucose levels. The pancreas over-compensates by producing more insulin, but eventually cannot keep up with demand, so glucose levels remain high despite higher than normal insulin levels (hyperinsulinaemia).

Lifestyle factors are particularly important, as the consumption of excess calories from food and alcohol, combined with a lack of physical activity, will inevitably lead to weight gain and subsequent obesity.

The strong genetic link with type 2 diabetes is well documented.

What are the management priorities for Mr KB?

A2 The management priorities are:

(a) Reduce his blood sugars.
(b) Treat his hypertension.
(c) Encourage him to stop smoking.
(d) Help him to lose weight.
(e) Lower his cholesterol levels.
(f) Monitor and prevent the development of complications.

A diagnosis of type 2 diabetes has a major impact on lifestyle, health, psychological wellbeing and life expectancy. It is a chronic and progressive long-term condition with a multitude of influential components that will dictate whether an individual will go on to develop serious complications. The National Service Framework for Diabetes (NSF, 2001) aimed to raise the standards of diabetes care and improve consistency in care regardless of the geographical area where it is provided. Standard 4 of the NSF sets out 'key interventions' to help reduce the development of microvascular (retinopathy, neuropathy and nephropathy) and macrovascular (cardiovascular) complications. These can be summarised as follows:

(a) Improve blood glucose control.
(b) Control raised BP.
(c) Reduce raised cholesterol levels.
(d) Encourage smoking cessation.
(e) Regular recall and review.

It can be a challenge to prioritise these recommendations, as the UK Prospective Diabetes Study (UKPDS) showed that tight control of BP may be more important than blood glucose control in reducing cardiovascular disease, but that microvascular disease could be prevented by tight blood glucose control. Smoking cessation is frequently cited as being even more important than both of these factors. This is due to the significant increased risks associated with smoking of developing both microvascular and macrovascular complications.

As it is not possible to address all risk factors at the same time, it is essential that the individuals' beliefs and expectations are taken into account at an early stage. There is little benefit in persevering with a smoking cessation attempt if the patient is not ready to give up, whereas the provision of information to help lower blood sugars to help improve the physical symptoms of diabetes (e.g. thirst, polyuria, tiredness) will have a greater impact on the patient's wellbeing and may help to make them feel more in control of their condition.

Type 2 diabetes is a complex long-term condition that a patient may well have been suffering from unknowingly for some years prior to diagnosis, so there is no urgency to address everything immediately. However, it is vital that newly diagnosed patients are made aware of all the risks and benefits of interventions at the outset, to help them make informed choices about their condition.

Outline a pharmaceutical care plan for the initial management of Mr KB.

A3 The pharmaceutical care plan for Mr KB should include the following:

(a) Ensure that appropriate prophylactic (aspirin and statin) and therapeutic (antihypertensives, oral hypoglycaemics) medications are prescribed at the optimal dosages.
(b) Review current prescription and non-prescription medications for drugs that may now be contraindicated (e.g. non-steroidal anti-inflammatory drugs (NSAIDs) in deteriorating renal function), or cause blood sugars to rise (e.g. corticosteroids, thiazide diuretics, glucosamine).
(c) Monitor outcomes of drug therapy for efficacy and side-effects. Specifically, monitor BP, sodium, potassium and estimated glomerular filtration rate (eGFR) (antihypertensive therapy), and serum lipids and liver function (cholesterol-lowering therapy).
(d) Counsel Mr KB on his prescribed medicines. Support this with appropriate written information, e.g. medication reminder chart and relevant patient information leaflets. This will ensure his full understanding and help support adherence.
(e) Address Mr KB's concerns and anxieties about his diagnosis and treatment.
(f) Discuss how Mr KB can reduce his risk factors for developing complications of diabetes (smoking, obesity, high salt/sugar/fat intake, lack of physical activity).
(g) Ensure Mr KB understands what follow-up care will be required.

What dietary advice would you give to Mr KB?

A4 Mr KB should be advised to reduce his sugar, fat and salt intake. He should include starchy carbohydrate foods (especially wholegrain), eat more fruit and vegetables, oily fish at least

twice a week, increase his fibre intake and drink alcohol in moderation.

People with type 2 diabetes can eat the same healthy diet as recommended for everyone. They do not need to eat a restricted diet, and certainly do not need to purchase special 'diabetic' or 'slimming' foods, which are expensive and offer no benefit over ordinary foods. Mr KB will still be able to eat sweet foods as an occasional treat, but he should opt for no-added-sugar or sugar-free (diet) drinks wherever possible.

Mr KB should be advised to eat regular meals throughout the day and aim for at least five portions of fruit and vegetables daily. He should aim to eat only healthy snacks, such as a piece of fruit or a handful of nuts, and to increase his fibre intake, which will help keep his digestive system healthy and improve satiety. He will need to reduce the fat in his diet (especially saturated fats) by choosing low-fat dairy products, spreads containing monounsaturated oils such as olive or rapeseed oils, removing excess fat from meat, and using low-fat cooking methods. He should aim to eat two to three portions of oily fish such as salmon, mackerel, sardines, trout, kippers, herring or pilchards each week. Mr KB should use herbs and spices to flavour his food instead of adding salt. Finally, he should be advised to reduce his alcohol intake to a maximum of 28 units per week.

Mr KB is trying to lose weight, so he should reduce his daily calorie intake by eating more healthily, reducing his portion sizes and moderating his alcohol consumption. He should also aim to drink at least eight cups of fluid per day, e.g. water, squash, tea, diet drinks, as keeping hydrated may help to suppress his appetite.

Would it be appropriate to prescribe Mr KB an anti-obesity drug?

A5 **Yes, it would be appropriate to prescribe an anti-obesity drug such as orlistat.**

Orlistat, which reduces the absorption of dietary fat, could be prescribed for Mr KB as he fulfils the NICE criteria with a BMI $\geq$ 28 kg/m^2 in the presence of other risk factors such as type 2 diabetes, hypertension or hypercholesterolaemia. Orlistat would need to be used in conjunction with dietary modification, and stopped if he did not lose at least 5% of his starting body weight at 12 weeks. Mr KB should be warned about the unpleasant side-effects associated with the drug, especially steatorrhoea, flatulence, faecal urgency or incontinence, which usually occur as a result of not adhering to a low-fat diet. He should also be advised to contact the patient support programme provided by the manufacturer.

Sibutramine, a centrally acting appetite suppressant, would not be suitable for Mr KB as it is contraindicated in those with uncontrolled hypertension.

What information would you give Mr KB about alcohol consumption now that he has type 2 diabetes?

A6 **Mr KB does not need to give up alcohol completely, but should moderate his intake to a maximum of three to four units per day.**

The recommendations for alcohol intake for people with type 2 diabetes are the same as for the general population, i.e. 2–3 units/day for women and 3–4 units/day for men. Alcoholic drinks should preferably be taken before, during, or shortly after a meal, and never on an empty stomach to prevent hypoglycaemia (most likely in patients on sulphonylureas or insulin). Low-calorie beers or cider offer no benefit over standard drinks owing to their higher alcohol content, and low-alcohol wines, sweet sherries and liqueurs will have a higher sugar content so should also be limited.

How would you explain to Mr KB why giving up smoking is so important, and how could you help him to achieve this?

A7 **Mr KB should be advised that by stopping smoking he will dramatically reduce the risk of developing diabetes-related complications (heart attack, stroke, kidney damage, nerve damage). He should be offered nicotine replacement therapy (NRT) with regular follow-up for support.**

Smoking is known to promote atherosclerosis, increase BP, reduce oxygen supplies to the body's tissues, and may stimulate stress hormones, which in turn can raise blood glucose levels. People with diabetes already have up to a fivefold increased risk of developing cardiovascular complications compared to those without diabetes. Smoking further increases this risk, as well as the risk of developing nephropathy and neuropathy.

Mr KB's smoking history should be assessed and the pros and cons of different NRT products explained to enable him to choose the most appropriate. He should be reviewed on a regular basis and NRT continued for the recommended period (usually a minimum of 12 weeks). It is worth reinforcing healthy eating advice at this stage, because of the fear of weight gain, which often occurs as a result of giving up smoking.

Bupropion would not be appropriate for Mr KB as it should not be prescribed to patients with other risk factors for seizures, such as diabetes. Varenicline may be considered if NRT fails, but should be used with caution in patients with a history of psychiatric illness, including depression.

How long should Mr KB be given to improve his glycaemic control through lifestyle measures before starting an oral hypoglycaemic agent?

A8 Mr KB should be allowed up to 3 months to improve his glycaemic control.

The current recommendations are that a person newly diagnosed with type 2 diabetes should be encouraged to try diet and exercise for up to 3 months in order to control their blood sugars. This should be reviewed 6 weeks after diagnosis to check whether symptoms have improved. If not, the patient should be given the option of whether to start oral hypoglycaemic agents or to continue with lifestyle modifications for a further 6 weeks. The latter is preferred, but not all patients will be willing or able to achieve this, and further consultations may be warranted. The importance of reducing glycated haemoglobin (HbA_{1c}) is demonstrated in UKPDS where, for every 1% reduction, there was an associated risk reduction of 21% for any diabetes-related endpoint and 37% for microvascular endpoints.

It is possible for >50% of patients with a new diagnosis of type 2 diabetes to achieve optimal glycaemic control without the use of oral hypoglycaemic agents even if their starting sugars are as high as 20 mmol/L. Studies are currently in progress looking at the effects of intensive diet and/or physical activity input on maintaining optimal blood glucose control in the 18 months after diagnosis. However, it is important to bear in mind the progressive nature of diabetes, so lifestyle modifications will only act by delaying and not preventing the use of medication in the future.

Which antihypertensive agents would be most appropriate for Mr KB and why?

A9 An angiotensin-converting enzyme inhibitor (ACEI) is an appropriate first-line antihypertensive for Mr KB.

NICE guidelines recommend an ACEI as first-line antihypertensive treatment for a patient like Mr KB (see Chapter 1). The BP target for patients with diabetes is <140/80 mmHg unless there is kidney, eye, or cerebrovascular damage, when the target is lowered to 130/80 mmHg.

ACEIs are known to have renoprotective effects that can prevent or slow the progression of renal disease. Where microalbuminuria is present an ACEI should be prescribed even in normotensive patients, as this will confer some benefit. Caution should be exercised in patients with suspected renovascular disease or where creatinine is already raised. Serum creatinine and electrolytes should be monitored within 1–2 weeks of starting an ACEI and after each dose increase. The ACEI should be stopped if a creatinine rise of >20% persists, or if hyperkalaemia occurs despite withdrawal of other suspect drugs, e.g. potassium-sparing diuretics. Angiotensin receptor blockers (ARBs) should only be used in place of an ACEI where 'continuing intolerance' other than hyperkalaemia or deterioration in renal function occur. In some cases it may be reasonable to try an alternative ACEI before changing to an ARB.

Would you make any adjustment to Mr KB's pain relief therapy at this stage?

A10 Yes. His diclofenac should be stopped and replaced by a non-nephrotoxic analgesic such as paracetamol.

NSAIDs can precipitate renal failure, especially in patients with renal impairment or renovascular disease (see also Chapter 8 on Acute renal failure). They can also cause fluid retention, which will counteract the effect of antihypertensive therapy. It is therefore recommended that the concomitant use of ACEIs and NSAIDs be avoided. Mr KB's omeprazole therapy should also be stopped as it will no longer be necessary.

Long-term diclofenac therapy at the dose taken by Mr KB is also associated with a small increase in thrombotic events.

What other drug therapy should be initiated?

A11 Aspirin and statin prophylaxis should be initiated.

The NSF and NICE recommend primary prevention with antiplatelet agents for patients over 50 years of age, or younger patients with significant cardiovascular risk. Low-dose aspirin (75 mg) daily should be initiated only when BP is <145/90 mmHg. Clopidogrel 75 mg daily may be considered only where true aspirin intolerance has been demonstrated. Co-prescription of a proton pump inhibitor may be warranted in patients at higher risk of gastrointestinal side-effects from aspirin.

It is also recommended that all diabetic patients over the age of 40 should have simvastatin 40 mg daily irrespective of the starting cholesterol level. With a cholesterol:HDL ratio of 6.8 Mr KB already has an increased cardiovascular risk and should start simvastatin 40 mg daily, which should be titrated until a total cholesterol of <4 mmol/L is reached (NICE CG 66). He should be advised to take this either after his evening meal or at bedtime, as the body's natural cholesterol production occurs during this time. It is also important to mention that he must avoid grapefruit juice, as this can raise statin plasma concentrations.

Mr KB also has a raised triglyceride level, which should be monitored and a fibrate started if it does not reduce to <2.3 mmol/L despite a statin and lifestyle modifications. Highly concentrated omega-3 fish oils may also be an option to help lower his triglyceride levels.

What monitoring would be necessary and when would you do this?

A12 Mr KB should be warned about potential side-effects of the medications and asked to return in 1 month for review and in 3 months for blood tests.

Mr KB should be warned about the potential gastrointestinal side-effects of aspirin and advised not to take it on an empty stomach. It may be necessary to reinstate omeprazole if he is unable to tolerate aspirin alone. He should also be advised about the side-effects of statins, most commonly nausea and muscle aches or cramps. He should be asked to contact the surgery immediately should he develop any muscle problems because of the small risk of myositis.

Mr KB should have a blood test in 1 month to re-check his HbA_{1c} (i.e. 3 months after his diagnosis and previous test). NICE guidelines recommend this should be <6.5%, otherwise oral hypoglycaemic agents should be started. He should also have routine blood tests for his serum lipids and liver function in 3 months' time.

Is self-monitoring of blood glucose (SMBG) appropriate? How would you explain the benefits of SMBG to Mr KB?

A13 Not at this stage, as Mr KB is being treated by diet alone. If medication is started there is a role for self-monitoring, particularly with sulphonylureas, which can cause hypoglycaemia. It is essential with insulin therapy.

Urine testing is no longer considered of any benefit as it does not identify hypoglycaemia, can only detect levels above the renal threshold (usually 10 mmol/L), and does not provide any information about current blood levels. Blood glucose testing is now the preferred method of monitoring glycaemic control.

Despite the current lack of evidence SMBG is considered beneficial in conjunction with education and support. Patients should be taught when and how to test, and how to interpret and use the results to modify diet and lifestyle. The healthcare professional can use the results in conjunction with the HbA_{1c} (which provides an average over the previous 2–3 months) to adjust medication doses and provide tailored dietary advice.

People with type 2 diabetes should generally test up to twice weekly, but there may be circumstances when they may need to test more often, for example before driving, during a period of illness, pregnancy, postprandial hyperglycaemia, loss of hypoglycaemic awareness (if on insulin), or if there is a change in diet, physical activity or medication regimen. SMBG may improve Mr KB's confidence and motivation as well as providing him with reassurance about controlling his diabetes.

How can the risks and benefits of a statin be explained to Mr KB in order that he can make an informed choice about taking the drug?

A14 Mr KB should be given information about the well-documented cardiovascular protection benefits of statins as well as their potential side-effects.

It is often helpful to show patients the cardiovascular disease risk tables that clearly demonstrate the benefits of lowering cholesterol levels. It will help to reassure the patient if you check his liver function and creatine kinase levels to demonstrate that he has come to no harm from the medicine. Repeating his cholesterol level will also allow him to recognise that diet alone is usually not sufficient to improve cholesterol levels. Starting at a lower dose and reviewing it after a few weeks may give him the confidence to restart the simvastatin. If this does not succeed it may be necessary to try an alternative statin, again titrating from a lower dose.

Which oral hypoglycaemic agent would you recommend for Mr KB and why?

A15 Metformin is recommended as the first-line treatment for Mr KB, especially as his BMI is >25 kg/m^2.

The UKPDS study clearly demonstrated that metformin is the drug of first choice in all type 2 diabetics unless contraindicated. Mr KB has a creatinine level within the normal range and is overweight, so metformin should be started and titrated over time until the diabetic control is good or the maximum tolerated dose has been achieved. The commonest side-effects that interrupt this are diarrhoea and abdominal discomfort. If this occurs the dose should be reduced to the previously tolerated dose, or the modified-release formulation could be tried. Metformin should be stopped if Mr KB's serum creatinine rises above 150 micromol/L or the eGFR falls to <30 mL/min/1.73 m^2 or during intercurrent illness where dehydration is likely, due to the rare side-effect of lactic acidosis.

At this stage Mr KB should be advised to inform the DVLA that he has been started on medication for diabetes, and if he were under 60 he would now be entitled to free prescriptions.

Mr KB should have his HbA_{1c} checked every 2–6 months until good glycaemic control is achieved, i.e. HbA_{1c} 6.5–7.5%.

What could be causing Mr KB's cough, and what action would you take?

A16 **Ramipril is likely to be causing Mr KB's cough. Either an alternative ACEI should be tried or he should be changed to an ARB.**

It is important to consider other causes of chronic cough, particularly in an ex-smoker, and a full history and examination, possibly including X-ray, should be undertaken. However, it is likely to be the ACEI causing the dry cough as it is a well-documented side-effect, occurring in 10–20% of patients owing to the inhibition of the breakdown of bradykinins, which stimulate the synthesis of nitric oxide leading to inflammatory effects on bronchial epithelial cells. The possible risks and benefits in changing his antihypertensive medication should be discussed with Mr KB. If he elects to try an alternative medication then an ARB would be the most appropriate choice. Mr KB should be warned that the cough may not completely resolve for up to 2–3 months after the ACEI has been stopped.

Which oral antidiabetic agent would you add in at this stage, and why?

A17 **A sulphonylurea such as gliclazide is an evidence-based second-line treatment.**

NICE recommends a sulphonylurea as the second-line drug of choice, either in combination with metformin or alone. Mr KB should be warned that because of its mode of action this drug frequently causes weight gain, and he should be reminded of the need to adhere to his diet and lifestyle measures. He should also be educated about how to recognise and manage hypoglycemia, which is a common side-effect of sulphonylureas. Self-monitoring of blood glucose should be started at this point so that Mr KB can check his sugar levels, especially prior to driving or operating heavy machinery. This will help to avoid unexpected hypoglycaemia.

An alternative option at this stage is a rapid-acting insulin secretagogue, such as nateglinide or repaglinide, which can be taken shortly before each main meal, thereby offering greater flexibility for those with irregular lifestyles. If hypoglycaemia is a particular problem with sulphonylureas then a thiazolidinedione or a dipeptidyl peptidase type 4 (DPP-4) inhibitor can be substituted at this stage.

What further treatment options could Mr KB try before starting insulin?

A18 **A thiazolidinedione such as pioglitazone.**

The thiazolidinediones, also referred to as glitazones, reduce peripheral insulin resistance by making muscle and adipose cells more sensitive to insulin. They also suppress hepatic glucose production. Glitazones can be used as adjunct therapy and very occasionally have a place in triple therapy if it is essential to avoid insulin. If Mr KB has an HGV licence he may, after counselling, prefer to try this until his retirement, when he can give up his HGV driving. Glitazones should not be started if there is any evidence of heart failure or a higher risk of failure. Rosiglitazone is now contraindicated in patients with acute coronary syndrome, and not recommended for use in patients with ischaemic heart disease or peripheral arterial disease. Mr KB should be warned that glitazones can also cause weight gain, usually as a result of significant fluid retention, and if he chooses to start a glitazone, advised to seek medical advice if this occurs. Liver toxicity is rare; however, it would be prudent to check liver function before and 1 month after a glitazone is initiated.

Acarbose, an inhibitor of intestinal alpha-glucosidases, delays the digestion of starch and sucrose, which can lower postprandial hyperglycaemia. It may be an option for patients unable to tolerate other agents, as it can reduce HbA_{1c} by 0.5–1%, although in practice its use tends to be limited by the high incidence of gastrointestinal side-effects, such as flatulence and abdominal discomfort.

More recently newer agents have been included in NICE guidelines which work by enhancing the natural incretin hormone glucagon-like peptide 1 (GLP-1). DPP-4 inhibitors (or 'gliptins'), for example sitagliptan and vildagliptan, work by inhibiting the enzyme (DPP-4) responsible for the breakdown of GLP-1 in the small intestine. GLP-1 works by stimulating glucose-dependent insulin sectretion as well as suppressing glucagon levels, delaying gastric emptying and reducing appetite. Gliptins are now recommended as second-line therapy particularly where 'there is a significant risk of hypoglycaemia (or its consequences)'. They are 'weight neutral' and have been shown to reduce HbA_{1c} by approximately 0.5%.

The other new agent, exenetide, is a peptide that mimics GLP-1, and is given as a twice-daily subcutaneous injection. It not only lowers blood glucoase levels with a low risk of hypoglycaemia, but also has a highly advantageous weight-lowering effect. It can be added to metformin and a sulphonylurea when HbA_{1c} ≥7.5% and BMI ≥ 35 kg/m^2 in people of European descent (with adjustment for other ethnic groups) and problems associated with high weight, or if BMI < 35 kg/m2 and insulin is unacceptable due to occupation, or weight loss would benefit other comorbidities.

What else could be added to Mr KB's antihypertensive regimen to achieve optimum control?

A19 A calcium-channel blocker could be added to help lower Mr KB's BP further.

Mr KB is already on the maximum doses of an ACEI and diuretic, so the next choice, as suggested by NICE guidelines, would be a calcium-channel blocker. There are other drugs that would be regarded as third-line choices, and the decision may be guided by the individual patient and any additional symptoms. For example, if the patient has established ischaemic heart disease a beta-blocker is indicated, or if they have urinary symptoms such as frequency it may be appropriate to consider an alpha-blocker. However, it is important first to check that Mr KB is actually taking his medication as prescribed, before adding another agent, as non-adherence may explain his uncontrolled BP.

What are the benefits and risks of starting insulin in this patient, and how would you allay his fears?

A20 **Mr KB has had type 2 diabetes for 5 years and his control is not optimal. Current recommendations are that he should be considered for insulin therapy.**

Most patients are initially frightened at the thought of starting insulin. The benefits to Mr KB will need to be explained in clear terms, detailing the reduction in his risk of developing the complications of diabetes. Perversely, many patients gain weight on insulin, and this should be explained to allow the patient to adapt their diet if possible and to manage their expectations. If possible, the concept of insulin should be introduced at an early stage in the course of the disease to help patients to come to terms with this. Dummy insulin pens should be demonstrated, and needles shown and even tried so that the patient can gain a better understanding of the process and dispel the myths about injecting. It is important to remember that this is not a medical emergency, and the clinician has time to address the patient's anxieties before commencing insulin.

Mr KB would need to monitor his blood glucose levels for a period before converting to insulin, so that the pattern of highs and lows can be established. It may also be necessary at this stage to refer him back to a dietitian to optimise his diet. A decision can then be made about which insulin regimen is most suitable. The usual options will be a once-daily injection of an intermediate-acting insulin or a long-acting analogue insulin, or a twice-daily injection of biphasic insulin.

What insulin preparation would you recommend for Mr KB?

A21 **A once-daily injection of either an intermediate-acting or a long-acting insulin would be ideal.**

Insulins are broadly divided into five categories, depending on their duration of action:

(a) Rapid acting.

(b) Short acting.
(c) Intermediate acting.
(d) Long acting.
(e) Biphasic.

Mr KB has not achieved optimum glycaemic control on maximum oral therapy and so should be offered insulin as the next step, unless his lifestyle or beliefs prohibit this. Local experience, patient preference and relative costs will guide the choice of insulin and regimen. Mr KB should be allowed to choose a pen device that suits his needs and that he feels comfortable using; this will then dictate which insulin can be used.

At this point the patient must be confident with home monitoring of blood sugars and have received clear guidance on altering the insulin dose appropriately. In general, 10 units of intermediate- or long-acting insulin is a good starting point, with dose increases every 3 days to achieve optimal fasting sugars between 4 and 6 mmol/L. Mr KB should be advised how to recognise and manage hypoglycaemia, and ensure that he carries glucose tablets or Glucogel at all times.

It is recommended that oral treatment be continued when insulin is started, especially metformin, as this will help reduce some of the weight gain associated with insulin use. Mr KB could reduce the dose of gliclazide once his sugars have improved, with a view to stopping completely as it is unlikely to be having any effect at this stage; however, if his sugars deteriorate dramatically after its withdrawal then gliclazide can always be reinstated. Mr KB should have regular follow-ups during his insulin titration, some of which can be via the telephone, as it may take several consultations to achieve good control.

Further reading

Bandolier. *Pharmacist Case Management of Type 2 Diabetes*. May 2005; 135–137. www.bandolier.com

Cantrill JA, Wood J. Diabetes mellitus. In: *Clinical Pharmacy and Therapeutics*. R Walker, C Edwards, eds. Churchill Livingstone, Edinburgh, 2003: 657–677.

Charbonnel B, Karasik A, Liu J *et al*. Efficacy and safety of the dipeptidyl peptidase-4 inhibitor sitagliptan added to ongoing metformin therapy in patients with type 2 diabetes inadequately controlled with metformin alone. *Diabetes Care* 2006; **29**: 2683–2643.

Clinical Knowledge Summaries. *Diabetes – glycaemic control*. Available from URL: http://cks.library.nhs.uk

Department of Health. *National Service Framework for Diabetes*. Department of Health, London, 2001.

Department of Health. *Improving Diabetes Services: The NSF Four Years On. The Way Ahead: The Local Challenge*. Department of Health, London, 2007.

Diabetes Control and Complications Trial. The effect of intensive treatment of diabetes on the development and progression of long-term complications in insulin dependent diabetes. *N Engl J Med* 1993; **329**: 977–986.

Diabetes UK Position Statement. *Self-monitoring of blood glucose*. Diabetes UK, London, 2006.

Diabetes UK. *Weight management. Managing diabetes in primary care*. Diabetes UK, London, 2004.

Drug and Therapeutics Bulletin. Pioglitazone and Rosiglitazone for diabetes. *Drug Ther Bull* 2001: **39**: 65–68.

Early ACTID study. Available from URL: www.bristol.ac.uk/earlyactid.

Mackinnon M. *Providing Diabetes Care in General Practice – a practical guide for integrated care*. Class Publishing, London, 2002.

National Institute for Health and Clinical Excellence. CG66. *The Management of Type 2 Diabetes*. NICE, London, 2008.

National Institute for Health and Clinical Excellence. CG43. *Obesity*. NICE, London, 2006.

National Institute for Health and Clinical Excellence. CG34. *Hypertension: Management of Hypertension in Adults in Primary Care*. NICE, London, 2006.

National Institute for Health and Clinical Excellence. CG67. *Cardiovascular Risk Assessment and the Modification of Blood Lipids for the Primary and Secondary Prevention of Cardiovascular Disease*. NICE, London, 2008.

National Institute for Health and Clinical Excellence. CG87. *Type 2 Diabetes: Newer Agents (partial update of CG66)*. NICE, London, May 2009.

National Prescribing Centre. MeReC Briefing. *Type 2 Diabetes (Part 1): The Management of Blood Glucose*. 2004. Issue No. 25.

Royal Pharmaceutical Society of Great Britain. *Practice Guidance on the Care of People with Diabetes*. RPSGB, London, 2004.

Scottish Intercollegiate Guidelines Network. *Management of Diabetes*. SIGN, Edinburgh, 2001.

UK Prospective Diabetes Study Group. Tight blood pressure control and risk of macrovascular and microvascular complications in Type 2 diabetes. UKPDS 38. *Br Med J* 1998; **317**: 713–720.

UK Prospective Diabetes Study Group. Intensive blood glucose control with sulphonylureas or insulin compared with conventional treatment and risk of complications in patients with Type 2 diabetes. UKPDS 33. *Lancet* 1998; **352**: 837–853.

UK Prospective Diabetes Study Group. Effect of intensive blood glucose control with metformin on complications in overweight patients with Type 2 diabetes. UKPDS 34. *Lancet* 1998; **352**: 854–865.

8

Acute renal failure

Caroline Ashley

Case study and questions

Day 1 Mrs NC, a 69-year-old woman, was admitted urgently at the request of her general practitioner (GP). His letter detailed the following history: Mrs NC had collapsed at the supported living complex where she lived. The warden said she had been complaining of nausea and loss of appetite for 2 or 3 days (her current weight was 51 kg) and had vomited two or three times in the previous 24 hours. She had fallen 2 days ago but had recovered quickly.

She had a long history of biventricular cardiac failure which had been controlled for some time with furosemide 80 mg in the morning, isosorbide mononitrate 20 mg twice daily and ramipril 5 mg once daily, although a degree of ankle oedema had recently necessitated an increase in the dose of furosemide to 120 mg in the morning. However, this increase had precipitated gout, which had been manifested by pain in the distal interphalangeal joint of both great toes. The pain had been treated with diclofenac 50 mg three times daily for the previous 21 days.

The patient herself was a poor historian. On examination she was pale and tired looking, with sunken eyes. Her pulse rate was 120 beats per minute (bpm) and her blood pressure was 105/70 mmHg lying and 85/60 mmHg standing. Ankle oedema was absent and there was no evidence of pulmonary oedema. Her extremities were cold and there was a marked reduction in skin turgor.

Mrs NC's serum biochemistry results were:

- Sodium 131 mmol/L (reference range 135–150)
- Potassium 5.5 mmol/L (3.5–5.0)
- Bicarbonate 17 mmol/L (22–31)
- Creatinine 312 micromol/L (60–110)
- Urea 27.2 mmol/L (3.2–6.6)
- Glucose 4.8 mmol/L (3.5–6.0)
- Mean cell volume 71 fL (77–91)
- Osmolarity 306 mmol/kg (275–295)

A diagnosis of sodium and water depletion with consequent renal hypoperfusion was made. An infusion of 1 L sodium chloride 0.9% every 4–6 hours was prescribed, and the following investigations were requested: full blood count; culture and sensitivity of blood and urine; 24-hour urine collection for determination of creatinine clearance; urinary sodium, urea and osmolarity; chest and abdominal X-ray.

Q1 Could Mrs NC's drug therapy have contributed to her renal problems?
Q2 What is the aim of intravenous (IV) sodium chloride 0.9% therapy?
Q3 What would you include in a pharmaceutical care plan for Mrs NC?
Q4 Which methods of assessing and monitoring Mrs NC's status would you recommend?

Day 2 The 24-hour urine collection yielded a volume of only 290 mL. Other data obtained from analysis of Mrs NC's urine included:

- Sodium 43 mmol/L
- Urea 117 mmol/L
- Creatinine 20.12 mmol/L
- Osmolarity 337 mmol/kg

The low urine volume obtained despite the concurrent volume expansion indicated that further measures were required to prevent the development of acute tubular necrosis, and so furosemide 250 mg was administered by slow IV infusion. A further dose of 500 mg was administered after 6 hours, but neither produced an increase in urine production. A diagnosis of established acute tubular necrosis causing acute renal failure (ARF) was made. The following recommendations were proposed: daily fluid charts; daily weights; daily serum urea and electrolyte estimations; dietary restrictions (consult dietitian).

Q5 Would mannitol have been an appropriate alternative to high-dose furosemide therapy?
Q6 Would you have recommended the use of high-dose IV furosemide at this point?
Q7 Would you have used dopamine in this patient?
Q8 What dietary considerations are necessary for Mrs NC?

Day 4 Mrs NC complained of having muscle cramps at night, with the result that quinine sulphate 300 mg at night was prescribed. She also complained of diarrhoea, which was described by the nursing staff as black and tarry in appearance. A full blood count revealed a normochromic and normocytic anaemia with a haemoglobin of 8.1 g/dL (12–16 g/dL). Omeprazole 20 mg at night was prescribed.

Serum biochemistry results revealed the following:

- Sodium 137 mmol/L (135–150)
- Albumin 34 g/L (33–55)

- Potassium 7.1 mmol/L (3.5–5.0)
- Calcium 2.04 mmol/L (2.25–2.6)
- Bicarbonate 19 mmol/L (22–31)
- Phosphate 1.8 mmol/L (0.9–1.5)
- Urea 31.7 mmol/L (3.2–6.6)
- Creatinine 567 micromol/L (60–110)
- pH 7.28 (7.36–7.44)

A 10 mL bolus dose of calcium gluconate 10% was administered IV, followed immediately by an IV injection of 10 units of soluble insulin with 50 mL of 50% glucose solution; the latter was written up for three further administrations over the next 12 hours. Therapy with Calcium Resonium 15 g orally four times daily was also initiated. A monitor was ordered to observe for cardiac toxicity, but no electrocardiogram (ECG) changes were apparent.

Q9 Would you have recommended quinine sulphate 300 mg at night to treat Mrs NC's nocturnal cramps?
Q10 What factors may have contributed to Mrs NC's low haemoglobin? Is omeprazole therapy appropriate?
Q11 Is Mrs NC's hyperkalaemia being treated appropriately? Should her hypocalcaemia, hyperphosphataemia and acidosis be treated at this point?
Q12 What factors should be considered when initiating drug therapy for a patient in ARF?

Day 5 Mrs NC complained of breathlessness which was increased on lying flat, and examination revealed crepitations in both lung bases. She complained of nausea and was noted to be drowsy and to have developed a flapping tremor.

Her serum biochemistry results included:

- Potassium 6.6 mmol/L (3.5–5.0)
- Bicarbonate 17 mmol/L (22–31)
- Urea 40.5 mmol/L (3.2–6.6)
- Creatinine 588 micromol/L (60–110)
- pH 7.24 (7.36–7.44)

It was decided to treat Mrs NC by haemodialysis, and arrangements were made for the insertion of a temporary central dialysis catheter.

Q13 What were the indications for dialysis in Mrs NC?
Q14 What forms of dialysis therapy are available, and what are their advantages and disadvantages?
Q15 What factors affect drug therapy during dialysis?

Day 10 Mrs NC developed a temperature of 39.6°C and a tachycardia of 120 bpm. Subjectively she complained of headache and feeling 'awful'. A full blood count revealed a neutrophil count of 10.5×10^9/L ($2.2–7.0 \times 10^9$). A diagnosis of septicaemia was made, and blood samples were sent for culture and sensitivity. All indwelling catheters were removed and the following therapy was written up:

- Cefotaxime 1 g IV every 12 hours
- Gentamicin 80 mg IV every 24 hours
- Metronidazole 500 mg IV every 8 hours

Q16 Is this therapy appropriate for Mrs NC's septicaemia?
Q17 What are the dangers associated with prescribing gentamicin for Mrs NC? How should her gentamicin therapy be monitored?

Day 11 Mrs NC complained of acute abdominal pain, with non-specific findings on physical examination. The decision was made to send her for a computed tomography (CT) scan of her abdomen with contrast enhancement, so she was prescribed sodium bicarbonate 1.26% IV, 500 mL prior to the scan and another 500 mL afterwards.

Q18 Why was Mrs NC prescribed the sodium bicarbonate? What else can be used for the same indication?

Day 12 Microbiological assays revealed the infective organism to be *Staphylococcus aureus*. Gentamicin and metronidazole therapy was discontinued and, as Mrs NC was clinically much improved, cefotaxime was continued as sole antibiotic therapy.

Day 17 Mrs NC reported that she was starting to pass increasing volumes of urine again.

Day 19 Mrs NC, now free of infection, passed over 4 L of urine. It was felt that she was over the worst and that she would continue to improve.

Q19 Did Mrs NC follow the normal course of ARF? What is her prognosis?

Answers

Could Mrs NC's drug therapy have contributed to her renal problems?

A1 **Yes. Mrs NC's furosemide and/or diclofenac therapy may have contributed to her admission.**

Mrs NC demonstrates many of the traditional signs of sodium and water depletion, including tachycardia, hypotension, postural hypotension, reduced skin turgor, reduced ocular tension (the cause of the sunken eyes), collapsed peripheral veins and cold extremities. Evidence that Mrs NC had suffered some degree of renal impairment can be seen by the elevation in her serum urea and creatinine levels, together with the other biochemical abnormalities. The symptoms Mrs NC suffers which cannot be explained by the sodium and water depletion (nausea, loss of appetite and vomiting) can be attributed to her high blood urea level (uraemia). acute renal failure (ARF) is defined as a rapid deterioration (several hours to several days) of renal function associated with the accumulation of nitrogenous waste in the body that is not due to pre- or post-renal factors.

One of the physiological responses to sodium and water depletion is a reduction in renal perfusion, which may in turn lead to intrinsic renal damage with a consequent acute deterioration in renal function. The condition may be caused by any significant haemorrhage, or by septicaemia, in which the vascular bed is dilated, thereby reducing the circulating volume. It may also be caused by excessive sodium and water loss from the skin, urinary tract or gastrointestinal tract. Excessive loss through the skin by sweating occurs in hot climates and is rare in the UK, but it also occurs after extensive burns. Gastrointestinal losses are associated with vomiting or diarrhoea. Urinary tract losses often result from excessive diuretic therapy but may also occur with the osmotic diuresis caused by hyperglycaemia and glycosuria in a diabetic patient (for this reason a random blood glucose level was measured for Mrs NC).

Mrs NC had vomited two or three times, but at a late stage in her illness. Although it was more likely to be a symptom of her condition rather than the cause, it was probably the final insult that led to her collapse. The most likely explanation is that her plight has been brought about by the diuresis induced by her recently increased furosemide therapy, plus the co-prescribing of diclofenac.

Despite a large blood supply, the kidneys are always in a state of incipient hypoxia because of their high metabolic activity, and any condition that causes the kidney to be underperfused may be associated with an acute deterioration in renal function. However, such a deterioration may also be produced by nephrotoxic agents, including drugs. Non-steroidal anti-inflammatory drugs (NSAIDs) in particular are associated with renal damage, and even a short course of an NSAID (such as diclofenac) has been associated with ARF, especially in older patients. The main cause of NSAID-induced renal damage is inhibition of prostaglandin synthesis in the kidney, particularly prostaglandins E_2, D_2 and I_2 (prostacyclin). These are all potent vasodilators, and consequently produce an increase in blood flow to the glomerulus and the medulla. In normal circumstances they do not play a large part in the maintenance of the renal circulation; however, in patients with increased amounts of vasoconstrictor substances (such as angiotensin II) in the blood, vasodilatory prostaglandins become important in maintaining renal blood flow. The maintenance of blood pressure in a variety of clinical conditions, such as volume depletion (which Mrs NC has), biventricular cardiac failure (which she had also had) or hepatic cirrhosis with ascites, may rely on the release of vasoconstrictor substances. In these circumstances, inhibition of prostaglandin synthesis may cause unopposed renal arteriolar vasoconstriction, which again leads to renal hypoperfusion. NSAIDs thus impair the ability of the renovasculature to adapt to a fall in perfusion pressure or to an increase in vasoconstrictor balance.

Angiotensin-converting enzyme inhibitors (ACEIs) and angiotensin receptor blockers (ARBs) may also produce a reduction in renal function by preventing the angiotensin II-mediated vasoconstriction of the efferent glomerular arteriole, which contributes to the high-pressure gradient across the glomerulus. This problem is important only in patients with renal vascular disease, particularly those with bilateral stenoses, and is consequently rare. Its aetiology is as follows: when there is a significant degree of renal artery stenosis, renal perfusion falls. To maintain the pressure gradient across the glomerulus, efferent arteriolar resistance must rise. This is predominantly accomplished by angiotensin-induced efferent vasoconstriction. If ACEIs are administered this system is rendered inoperable, and there is no longer any way of maintaining effective filtration pressure. This leads to a fall in glomerular filtration rate (GFR) and ARF. In these circumstances deterioration in renal function is seen shortly after ACEI initiation. As Mrs NC has been taking her ramipril therapy for a while, it is unlikely to have contributed to her current problems.

Iatrogenic factors, including fluid and electrolyte imbalance and drug nephrotoxicity, can be identified in over 50% of cases of hospital-acquired ARF and also play a large role in many cases of community-acquired ARF. It has been estimated that up to 20% of individuals over the age of 65 are prescribed diuretics, with a lesser number receiving NSAIDs; consequently, there is a large population of elderly patients susceptible to renal damage in the event of any insult to the kidney. ARF that requires dialysis is fortunately rare, with only 50–70 patients per million of the population affected annually, but less severe degrees of impairment may occur in up to 5% of hospital inpatients.

What is the aim of intravenous (IV) sodium chloride 0.9% therapy?

A2 The aim of therapy is to restore her extracellular fluid volume.

The initial therapeutic aim in the management of ARF is immediate correction of reversible causes. Support of renal perfusion, with either volume infusion or therapeutics that improve renal oxygen delivery, should be considered before any attempt to improve urinary flow. The fluid infused should mimic the nature of the fluid lost as closely as possible, and should therefore be blood, colloid or saline. Patients should be observed continuously and the infusion stopped when features of volume depletion have been resolved, but before volume overload has been induced.

A diagnosis of acute deterioration of renal function due to renal underperfusion carries with it the implication that restoration of renal perfusion will reverse the renal impairment. Mrs NC is depleted of both water and sodium ions. Sodium chloride 0.9% is therefore an appropriate choice of IV fluid, as it replaces both water and sodium ions in a concentration approximately equal to that of plasma. Situations occasionally arise where a patient is hyponatraemic but not water depleted, as a result of either sodium depletion or water retention; such a condition may be treated with an infusion containing sodium chloride in excess of its physiological concentration, e.g. sodium chloride 1.8% or higher. Similarly, should water depletion with hypernatraemia occur, isotonic solutions that are either free of, or low in, sodium are available, e.g. glucose 5%, or sodium chloride 0.18% with glucose 4%. Possibly the most common cause of ARF is the peripheral vasodilation that occurs in septic shock. In such cases it would be appropriate to infuse a colloid as well as sodium chloride, as this would help restore the circulating volume. It is important to remember, however, that not all shocked patients are hypovolaemic and some, notably those in cardiogenic shock, could be adversely affected by a fluid challenge.

The effect of fluid replacement therapy on urine flow and central venous pressure (CVP) should be carefully monitored. CVP provides a guide to the degree of fluid deficit and reduces the risk of pulmonary oedema resulting from over-rapid transfusion. If the kidneys do not respond to replacement treatment, the probable diagnosis is acute tubular necrosis, but it is common practice – albeit often not correct practice – to try other measures, such as treatment with mannitol and loop diuretics, to try to turn the condition towards recovery.

What would you include in a pharmaceutical care plan for Mrs NC?

A3 The pharmaceutical care plan for Mrs NC should include the following:

(a) Her drug therapy must be reviewed to ensure that any agents that might be contributing to her condition are discontinued.
(b) It must be ensured that the optimum drug therapy is prescribed to achieve the desired therapeutic outcome.
(c) All drug therapy should be monitored for efficacy and safety.

(d) Adjust the doses of any medications according to the degree of renal impairment, if appropriate.
(e) It is essential that, when it becomes appropriate, Mrs NC is counselled about her prescribed medicines and any other factors that might affect her in the future (e.g. avoidance of over-the-counter NSAIDs).
(f) Mrs NC must be assessed to ensure she can manage her prescribed medication on discharge. Further counselling or compliance aids must be given if appropriate.
(g) Steps must be taken to ensure that prescribed therapy is continued after discharge.

Which methods of assessing and monitoring Mrs NC's status would you recommend?

A4 **(a) Creatinine clearance (CrCl).**

Creatinine is a byproduct of normal muscle metabolism and is formed at a rate proportional to the mass of muscle. It is freely filtered by the glomerulus, with little secretion or reabsorption by the tubule. When muscle mass is stable, any change in plasma creatinine reflects a change in its clearance by glomerular filtration. Consequently, measurement of CrCl gives an estimate of the GFR. The ideal method of calculating CrCl is by performing an accurate collection of urine over 24 hours and taking a plasma sample midway through this period. The following equation may then be used:

$$\text{CrCl} = \frac{U \times V}{P}$$

where U = urine creatinine concentration (micromol/L), V = urine flow rate (mL/min), P = plasma creatinine concentration (micromol/L). This provides an accurate measure of GFR provided all of the urine over the 24-hour period is collected. Using this formula, it is possible to calculate Mrs NC's CrCl as 13 mL/min.

A quicker and less cumbersome method is to measure the plasma creatinine concentration and collect those patient factors that affect the mass of muscle, i.e. age, sex and weight (preferably ideal body weight). This allows an estimation of CrCl to be made from average population data. The equation of Cockcroft and Gault is a useful way of making such an estimation:

$$\text{CrCl} = \frac{F \times (140 - \text{age}) \times \text{weight (kg)}}{\text{plasma creatinine (micromol/L)}}$$

where F = 1.04 (females) or 1.23 (males).

Assuming the normal CrCl to be 120 mL/min, this enables classification of renal impairment as follows: mild, GFR 20–50 mL/min; moderate, GFR 10–20 mL/min; severe, GFR <10mL/min. Using the method of Cockroft and Gault, Mrs NC's CrCl can be estimated as 12 mL/min and her renal impairment could thus be classified as moderate verging on severe.

There are, however, limitations to using this equation, and in the following situations caution needs to be exercised when interpreting the assessment:

(i) Obesity: use ideal body weight (IBW).
(ii) Muscle wasting: CrCl will be overestimated.
(iii) Oedematous patients: use IBW.
(iv) Ascites: use IBW and consider the dilutional effect on serum creatinine.
(v) ARF: when two serum creatinine levels measured in 24 hours differ by >40 micromol/L this may represent non-steady-state serum creatinine levels, therefore the degree of renal impairment may be underestimated.

The latest means of estimating a patient's renal function is to calculate the eGFR (estimated GFR) from the MDRD (Modified Diet in Renal Disease) equation. This is now quoted by most clinical chemistry laboratories, and can be easily calculated via the internet, using the patient's age, serum creatinine, gender and race. It should be noted that the eGFR is a normalised value, in that it reports renal function in units of mL/min/1.73 m^2. Hence, for greater accuracy it needs to be corrected for an individual patient's actual body surface area. Mrs NC is calculated to have an eGFR of 14 mL/min/1.73 m^2.

(b) Urine analysis.

A healthy kidney that is underperfused will attempt to compensate for the condition by retaining sodium and water, a response mediated by aldosterone and antidiuretic hormone. Thus, the urine produced will be low in sodium (<10 mmol/L) but otherwise concentrated, with a high urea (>250 mmol/L) and osmolarity (>500 mmol/kg). However, damaged kidneys fail to reabsorb sodium adequately, which results in high urinary sodium concentrations (>30 mmol/L). In addition, the urea concentration mechanisms fail, which results in reduced urinary urea (<150 mmol/L). Urine osmolarity also falls close to that of plasma. It therefore follows that examination of the urine enables assessment of the renal state. Various indices using these data have been produced, but their value is more theoretical than practical.

(c) **Serum urea levels.**

These are commonly used to assess renal function; however, the rate of production of urea is considerably more variable than that of creatinine, and it fluctuates throughout the day in response to the protein content of the diet. It may also be elevated by dehydration or an increase in protein catabolism, such as occurs with haemorrhage into the gastrointestinal tract or body tissues, severe infections, trauma (including surgery) and high-dose steroid therapy. The serum urea level is therefore an unreliable measure of renal function, but it is often used as a crude test because it does give information on the patient's general condition and state of hydration.

(d) **Fluid charts and weight.**

Fluid charts are frequently used in patients with sodium and water depletion, but they are often inaccurate and should not be relied upon exclusively. Records of daily weight are more reliable but are rarely available before renal failure is diagnosed.

(e) **Central venous pressure.**

This is of value in assessing circulating volume. The normal range is 10–15 cmH_2O.

(f) **Serum electrolyte levels.**

Plasma potassium should be measured regularly because hyperkalaemia, which occurs in ARF, may be fatal.

Would mannitol have been an appropriate alternative to high-dose furosemide therapy?

A5 No. Mannitol is inappropriate because it can be nephrotoxic.

The rationale for using mannitol arises from the theory that tubular debris may contribute to the oliguria of ARF by causing mechanical obstruction, and that the use of an osmotic diuretic may wash out the debris. A dose of 0.5–1.0 g/kg as a 10–20% infusion used to be recommended, but only after the circulating volume had been restored (this caution holds true for any diuretic therapy). However, before producing a diuresis, IV mannitol will cause a considerable increase in the extracellular fluid volume by attracting water from the intracellular compartment. This expansion of the extracellular volume is potentially dangerous for patients with cardiac failure, especially if a diuresis is not produced.

In addition, mannitol has no renoprotective effects and can cause significant renal impairment by triggering osmotic nephrosis. It may also increase tubular workload by increasing solute delivery. Hence its use has now been discredited.

Would you have recommended the use of high-dose IV furosemide at this point?

A6 Yes, provided Mrs NC was euvolaemic before it was started.

As well as producing substantial diureses, all loop diuretics have been shown to increase renal blood flow, probably by stimulating the release of renal prostaglandins. This haemodynamic effect can be inhibited by diclofenac and other NSAIDs. It has been argued that furosemide, especially at high doses, may convert oliguric ARF to non-oliguric ARF and thus reduce the requirement for dialysis. However, meta-analysis has shown that furosemide is not effective in the prevention and treatment of ARF in adults. It does not reduce mortality, the requirement for dialysis, the proportion of patients remaining oliguric (urine output <500 mL/day) or the length of hospital stay.

As furosemide is excreted largely unchanged in the urine and influences tubular reabsorption from the luminal side, it is the urinary excretion of the drug and not its plasma concentration that determines the efficacy of its diuretic action. Non-oliguric ARF is generally associated with a better prognosis than oliguric ARF, and studies have shown that patients who have a diuretic response to furosemide have less severe ARF and so are more likely to recover anyway. However, it is undeniable that any increase in urine volume produced will simplify the future management of Mrs NC by reducing the risk of fluid overload and hyperkalaemia.

The patient must be euvolaemic before furosemide is considered, or diuresis could lead to severe cardiovascular volume depletion. Doses of up to 1 g may be given IV at a rate of not more than 4 mg/min, as higher infusion rates may cause transient deafness. The addition of metolazone orally may also be considered. Metolazone, which is by itself a weak diuretic, has been shown to act synergistically with loop diuretics to produce a more effective diuresis. If fluid repletion followed by furosemide challenge fails to achieve a diuresis this therapy should be discontinued, as the kidneys are evidently incapable of mounting any response, and further doses of furosemide could cause increased nephrotoxicity and ototoxicity.

Would you have used dopamine in this patient?

A7 **No.**

Dopamine has been used for many years as a renoprotective agent, but numerous clinical trials have now shown that the use of a low-dose dopamine infusion is of no benefit in patients with acute renal dysfunction and systemic inflammatory response syndrome. The theory behind its use was that dopamine at low doses (e.g. 1–5 micrograms/kg/min) has a vasodilator effect on the kidney. At slightly higher doses (e.g. 5–20 micrograms/kg/min) inotropic effects on the heart produce an increase in cardiac output. This dual effect increases renal perfusion. However, at even higher doses (e.g. 20 micrograms/kg/min and above) dopamine also acts on α receptors, causing peripheral and renal vasoconstriction which results in impairment of renal perfusion. As with furosemide, dopamine may produce increases in urine volume even in those patients who progress to ARF; however, dopamine also has a number of potential disadvantages. Even at low doses it may increase cardiac contractility and systemic resistance, and it has been reported to cause tissue necrosis. It has also been suggested that desensitisation of renal dopaminergic receptors occurs with prolonged administration.

What dietary considerations are necessary for Mrs NC?

A8 **In a patient with ARF the aim is to provide sufficient nutrition to prevent the breakdown of body tissue, especially protein, and to enhance wound healing and resistance to infection.**

The diet should provide all the essential amino acids in a total protein intake of about 0.6 g/kg body weight/day. This should reduce the symptoms of uraemia, such as nausea, vomiting and anorexia. A higher intake of protein stimulates its use as an energy source, which results in increases in blood urea concentrations, whereas any further reduction in protein intake brings about endogenous protein catabolism, again causing blood urea to increase. Fat and carbohydrate should be given to maintain a high energy intake of about 2000–3000 kcal/day or more in hypercatabolic patients, as this helps prevent protein catabolism and promotes anabolism. However, it should be borne in mind that any excessive amounts of carbohydrate can increase the production of carbon dioxide and induce respiratory failure in these patients. Finally, to avoid the commonly encountered problem of hyperkalaemia, potassium intake should be kept as low as possible. Sodium and phosphorus intake should also be limited.

Would you have recommended quinine sulphate 300 mg at night to treat Mrs NC's nocturnal cramps?

A9 **Yes.**

Muscle cramps are common in patients with renal failure, probably as a result of electrolyte imbalances, and patients are often prescribed quinine salts in doses of 200–300 mg at night. The efficacy of this form of treatment is dubious, and few comparative trials have been performed. Nonetheless, some patients insist that it does work, and as it poses no risk to renal patients it may be worth trying. The dose of quinine does not require alteration in renal failure.

What factors may have contributed to Mrs NC's low haemoglobin? Is omeprazole therapy appropriate?

A10 **Mrs NC's low haemoglobin may be a result of reduced erythropoietin secretion, but it is more likely to be the result of gastrointestinal bleeding, and so omeprazole therapy is appropriate.**

Erythropoietin, the hormone that stimulates production of red blood cells, is produced almost exclusively by the kidney and a normochromic normocytic anaemia due to reduced erythropoietin secretion is a very common symptom of chronic renal failure. However, the time course of ARF is often too short for this type of anaemia to become a problem, and although it may be present in a patient on the verge of chronic renal failure who has an acute crisis, this does not appear to be the case with Mrs NC.

Anaemia may also arise if there is a haemolytic element to the condition (e.g. severe septicaemia) or if a haemorrhage occurs, either as the cause of the ARF or as a result of it. Although stress ulcers are not uncommon in acutely ill patients, uraemic gastrointestinal haemorrhage is a recognised consequence of ARF. It probably occurs as a result of reduced mucosal cell turnover owing to high circulating levels of uraemic toxins. Gastrointestinal haemorrhage is also a well-recognised consequence of treatment with NSAIDs such as diclofenac, which Mrs NC had been taking prior to admission.

Mrs NC has passed melaena (black, tarry stools) and has been diagnosed as having had a gastrointestinal bleed. This is therefore the most likely cause of her low haemoglobin. Proton pump inhibitors or H_2-receptor antagonists are effective in this situation, and it is unlikely that any one would be more advantageous than another. Omeprazole was thus an appropriate choice of treatment, and because it is metabolised in the liver to inactive metabolites it was appropriate to prescribe it at the normal therapeutic dose, even though Mrs NC's estimated GFR was <10 mL/min at this stage in her illness.

Is Mrs NC's hyperkalaemia being treated appropriately? Should her hypocalcaemia, hyperphosphataemia and acidosis be treated at this point?

A11 Yes. The methods used to treat Mrs NC's hyperkalaemia are appropriate. However, Mrs NC's calcium and phosphate levels and serum pH, although abnormal, are not sufficiently deranged to warrant treatment yet.

(a) **Hyperkalaemia.** Hyperkalaemia is a particular problem in ARF, not only because of reduced urinary potassium excretion, but also because of potassium release from cells. Particularly rapid rises are to be expected when there is tissue damage, as in burns, crush injuries and sepsis, although this is not the case for Mrs NC. She is, however, acidotic, and this aggravates the situation by provoking potassium leakage from healthy cells. It is worth noting that ACEIs and ARBs can increase serum potassium levels; however, in this case it is much more likely to be due to the ARF, as Mrs NC has been on ramipril for some time.

Hyperkalaemia may be life-threatening as a result of causing cardiac arrhythmias and, if untreated, may result in asystolic cardiac arrest. Emergency treatment is necessary if the serum potassium is >7.0 mmol/L (as in Mrs NC's case) or if there are ECG changes. Emergency treatment consists of:

(i) 10–20 mL of calcium gluconate 10% IV. This has a stabilising effect on the myocardium but no effect on the serum potassium concentration.

(ii) 10 units of soluble insulin plus 50 mL of 50% glucose. The insulin stimulates potassium uptake into cells, thereby removing it from the plasma. The glucose counteracts the hypoglycaemic effects of the insulin.

(iii) Calcium Resonium 15 g three or four times a day, orally or by enema. This ion-exchange resin binds potassium in the gastrointestinal tract, releasing calcium in exchange. It is used to lower serum potassium over a period of hours or days, and is required because the effect of insulin and glucose therapy is only temporary. Both the oral and the rectal routes of administration have disadvantages. Administration of large doses by mouth may result in faecal impaction, which is why it is recommended that lactulose should be co-prescribed. The manufacturer recommends that the enema be retained for 9 hours: retaining it is not usually the problem, rather the reverse. Oral therapy is not contraindicated after a gastrointestinal bleed, so this is probably more appropriate for Mrs NC. Using a calcium-exchange resin is also appropriate as she is hypocalcaemic. She, and the nursing staff, should be counselled not to mix it with orange juice to improve the taste, as this is also high in potassium.

(iv) 200–300 mL of sodium bicarbonate 1.26% or 1.4% IV may be used in addition to insulin and glucose therapy. As well as stimulating potassium reuptake by cells, this helps to correct the acidosis of ARF. However, its use can be limited in ARF as there are potential problems with volume overload.

(b) **Hypocalcaemia.** Calcium malabsorption, probably secondary to disordered vitamin D metabolism, often occurs in ARF. However, it usually remains asymptomatic, as tetany of skeletal muscles and convulsions do not usually occur until plasma concentrations are as low as 1.6–1.7 mmol/L. Should it become necessary, oral calcium supplementation with calcium gluconate or lactate is usually adequate. Although vitamin D may be used to treat the hypocalcaemia of ARF, it rarely has to be prescribed. Effervescent calcium tablets should be avoided as they invariably contain a high sodium and potassium load. It should also be noted that correction of acidosis can lead to symptoms of hypocalcaemia developing (see **(d)**). Ionised calcium is important for cellular activation of the membrane potential, and when acidosis is corrected ionised calcium drops, which causes symptomatic hypocalcaemia. There is a realistic and fairly often-seen phenomenon in which giving sodium bicarbonate corrects acidosis but lowers ionised calcium, which may lead to fitting.

(c) **Hyperphosphataemia.** Phosphate is normally excreted by the kidney. Phosphate retention and hyperphosphataemia may also occur in ARF, but usually only to a slight extent, and the condition rarely requires treatment. Should it become necessary, phosphate-binding agents may be used to retain phosphate ions in the gut. The most common agents are calcium-containing agents, e.g. Calcichew (calcium carbonate) or Phosex (calcium acetate). Aluminium hydroxide is infrequently prescribed, although it is an excellent phosphate binder. This is for two reasons: there is a slight risk that aluminium may be absorbed from the gut and deposited in bones to give a severe form of fracturing bone disease; also, aluminium accumulation over long periods of time is associated with the risk of dementia. Aluminium levels can be monitored to minimise these risks. More recently, calcium-based phosphate binders have been associated with reports of calciphylaxis and calcium–phosphate complexes being deposited in the organs and blood vessels. This has led to the development of non-calcium, non-aluminium-containing phosphate binders, e.g. Renagel (sevelamer hydrochloride) and Fosrenol (lanthanum carbonate).

(d) **Acidosis.** Metabolic acidosis in ARF results from increased acid production, reduced renal reabsorption of bicarbonate, and an inability of the kidney to excrete hydrogen ions. In itself this is generally not a serious problem, although it may contribute to hyperkalaemia. It may be treated orally with sodium bicarbonate 1–6 g/day in divided doses, although if elevations in plasma sodium preclude the use of sodium bicarbonate, extreme acidosis (plasma bicarbonate <10 mmol/L) is best treated by dialysis.

Although Mrs NC does not currently require treatment for her electrolyte abnormalities, it is essential that she is carefully monitored for any further derangement.

What factors should be considered when initiating drug therapy for a patient in ARF?

A12 How the drug to be prescribed is absorbed, distributed, metabolised and excreted, and whether it is intrinsically nephrotoxic, are all factors that must be considered. The pharmacokinetic behaviour of many drugs may be altered in renal failure.

(a) **Absorption.** Oral absorption in ARF may be reduced because of vomiting or diarrhoea, although this is of limited clinical significance, and by slowing of the gastrointestinal tract as a result of 'soggy gut' syndrome.

(b) **Metabolism.** The main hepatic pathways of drug metabolism appear to be unaffected in renal impairment. The kidney is also a site of metabolism in the body, but the effect of renal impairment is clinically important in only two cases:

(i) Vitamin D. The conversion of 25-hydroxycholecalciferol to 1,25-dihydroxycholecalciferol (the active form of vitamin D) occurs in the kidney and the process is impaired in renal failure. Patients in ARF therefore occasionally require vitamin D replacement therapy, and this should be in the form of 1-hydroxycholecalciferol (alfacalcidol) or 1,25-dihydroxycholecalciferol (calcitriol).

(ii) Insulin. The kidney is the major site of insulin metabolism and the insulin requirements of diabetic patients in ARF are often reduced.

(c) **Distribution.** Changes in distribution may be altered by fluctuations in the degree of hydration or by alterations in tissue or plasma protein binding. The presence of oedema or ascites tends to increase the volume of distribution, whereas dehydration tends to reduce it. In practice, these changes are only significant if the drug's volume of distribution is small (<50 L).

Plasma protein binding may be reduced, owing either to protein loss or to alterations in binding because of uraemia. For certain highly bound drugs the net result of reduced protein binding is an increase in free drug, so care must be taken when interpreting plasma concentrations of such drugs. Most analyses measure total plasma concentration, i.e. free plus bound drug. A drug level may therefore fall within the accepted concentration range but still result in toxicity because of the increased proportion of free drug. However, this is usually only a temporary effect. As the unbound drug is now available for elimination, its free concentration will eventually return to its original value, albeit with a lower total bound plus unbound level. As a consequence, the total drug concentration may fall below the therapeutic range although therapeutic effectiveness is maintained. It must be noted that the time required for the new equilibrium to be established is about four or five elimination half-lives of the drug, and this itself may be altered in renal failure. Some drugs that show reduced plasma protein binding include diazepam, morphine, phenytoin, L-thyroxine, theophylline and warfarin. Tissue binding may also be affected. For example, the displacement of digoxin from skeletal and cardiac muscle-binding sites by metabolic waste products results in a significant reduction of its volume of distribution in renal failure.

(d) **Excretion.** Alterations in the renal clearance of drugs in renal impairment are by far the most important parameter to consider when making dosing decisions. Generally, a fall in renal drug clearance indicates a decline in the number of functioning nephrons. The GFR, of which CrCl is an approximation, can be used as an estimate of the number of functioning nephrons. Thus, a 50% reduction in GFR will suggest a 50% decline in renal clearance.

Renal impairment often necessitates drug-dosing adjustments; however, loading doses of renally excreted drugs are often necessary in renal failure because the prolonged elimination half-life leads to a prolonged time to reach steady state. The equation for loading dose is the same in renal disease as used normally:

$$\text{Loading dose (mg)} = \text{target conc. (mg/L)} \times \text{vol. of distribution (L)}$$

The volume of distribution may be altered (see above) but generally remains unchanged.

It is possible to derive other formulae for dosage adjustment in renal impairment. One of the most useful is:

$$DR_{rf} = DR_n \times [(1 - F_{eu}) + (F_{eu} \times RF)]$$

where DR_{rf} = dosing rate in renal failure, DR_n = normal dosing rate, RF = extent of renal impairment (i.e. patient's creatinine clearance in mL/min divided by the ideal creatinine clearance of 120 mL/min) and F_{eu} = fraction of drug normally excreted unchanged in the urine. For example, if $RF = 0.2$ and $F_{eu} = 0.5$, DR_{rf} will be 60% of normal.

An alteration in total daily dose can be achieved by altering either the dose itself, the dosage interval, or a combination of both as appropriate. Unfortunately, for this method it is not always possible readily to obtain the fraction of drug excreted unchanged in the urine. In practice it is therefore often simpler to use the guidelines to prescribing in renal impairment found in standard references such as the *Renal Drug Handbook* or *Drug Prescribing in Renal Failure*.

(e) **Nephrotoxicity.** Some drugs are known to be capable of damaging the kidney by a variety of mechanisms. The commonest forms of damage are interstitial nephritis (hypersensitivity reaction with inflammation affecting those cells lying between the nephrons) and glomerulonephritis (thought to be caused by the passive trapping of immune complexes in the glomerular tuft eliciting an inflammatory response). The list of potentially nephrotoxic drugs is long, but the majority cause damage by producing hypersensitivity reactions and are quite safe in most patients. Some drugs, however, are directly nephrotoxic and their effects on the kidney are consequently more predictable. Such drugs include the aminoglycosides, amphotericin, colistin, the polymyxins and ciclosporin. The use of any drug with recognised nephrotoxic potential should be avoided in any patient if at all possible. This is particularly true in patients with pre-existing renal impairment or renal failure, such as Mrs NC. Inevitably, occasions will arise when the use of potentially nephrotoxic drugs becomes necessary, and on these occasions constant monitoring of renal function is essential.

In conclusion, the simplest solution to prescribing in renal failure is to choose a drug that:

(a) Is <25% excreted unchanged in the urine.

(b) Is unaffected by fluid balance changes.
(c) Is unaffected by protein-binding changes.
(d) Has a wide therapeutic margin.
(e) Is not nephrotoxic.

What were the indications for dialysis in Mrs NC?

A13 **Her severe uraemic symptoms (nausea, reduced consciousness, flapping tremor) and evidence of pulmonary oedema indicate that dialysis would be of value for Mrs NC.**

Dialysis should be started in a patient with ARF when there is: hyperkalaemia >7 mmol/L; increasing acidosis (pH <7.1 or plasma bicarbonate of <10 mmol/L); severe uraemic symptoms such as impaired consciousness; fluid overload with pulmonary oedema; or any combination of the above that may threaten life.

What forms of dialysis therapy are available, and what are their advantages and disadvantages?

A14 **There are traditionally two types of dialysis: haemodialysis and peritoneal dialysis. Both put the patient's blood on one side of a semipermeable membrane and a dialysate solution on the other. Exchange of metabolites occurs across the membrane. In haemodialysis, blood is diverted out of the body, passed through an artificial kidney (dialyser) and returned to the patient, whereas in peritoneal dialysis the fluid is run in and out of the patient's abdominal cavity, and the peritoneum itself acts as the semipermeable membrane. Other options for Mrs NC are haemofiltration and haemodiafiltration.**

In haemodialysis, blood is taken from an arterial line, heparinised, actively pumped through a dialyser where diffusion and ultrafiltration occur, and returned to the patient via the venous line. The dialyser contains synthetic semipermeable membranes which allow the blood to come into close proximity with the dialysate. Metabolites and excess electrolytes pass from the blood to the dialysate, and by increasing the pressure of the blood, water can also be removed from the patient. Haemodialysis is performed three times a week and the duration of a single dialysis is usually about 4 hours. One disadvantage of haemodialysis is its dependence on expensive technology. The capital cost is considerable and the technique requires specially trained staff, so it is seldom undertaken outside a renal unit. Haemodialysis also produces rapid fluid and electrolyte shifts, which may be dangerous. However, it does treat renal failure and reverse metabolic abnormalities much more rapidly than peritoneal dialysis, and is therefore essential in hypercatabolic renal failure, where urea is produced faster than peritoneal dialysis can remove it.

Peritoneal dialysis is a technique whereby pre-warmed dialysate is run into the peritoneum via an indwelling catheter, where it dwells for a variable length of time before being drained out and fresh fluid run in. Both haemodialysis and continuous ambulatory peritoneal dialysis (CAPD) have been used for acute renal replacement therapy (RRT), although haemodialysis or a continuous RRT modality such as haemofiltration or haemodiafiltration are now the mainstays of treatment for ARF, and are usually used in an intensive care setting.

Haemofiltration is the process of convection and ultrafiltration by which water and solutes (including drugs) are removed from the blood through a highly permeable membrane when pressure is applied.

The rate of blood flow past the membrane generates hydrostatic pressure, which forces plasma water across the membrane dragging various solutes with it. The solution produced containing this solute is called ultrafiltrate or haemofiltrate. Excess fluid is best removed by haemofiltration, but large volumes of fluid need to be removed if solutes are to be cleared effectively from the plasma.

Haemodiafiltration is a process that combines dialysis with large-volume ultrafiltration and diffusion to remove water and solutes. Dialysis fluid is introduced through the filter in a counter current direction to the blood flow in order to create a concentration gradient (between the blood compartment and the dialysis fluid compartment) across the semi-permeable membrane. Dialysis fluid is usually introduced at a rate of 1–2 L/h, depending on the efficiency of the system

Both haemofiltration and haemodiafiltration are continuous, well tolerated haemodynamically, and avoid the 'peaks and troughs' in metabolic, electrolyte, acid–base and volume control which are a feature of intermittent dialysis treatments.

What factors affect drug therapy during dialysis?

A15 Whether or not the drug is significantly removed by dialysis.

Drugs that are not removed will require dose reductions in order to avoid accumulation and possible toxic effects. In general, because haemodialysis, haemofiltration and haemodiafiltration depend on filtration, the processes can be considered analogous to glomerular filtration. Thus, drug characteristics that favour clearance by the glomerulus are similar to those that favour clearance by dialysis or haemofiltration. They include low molecular weight, high water solubility, low protein binding, small volume of distribution and low metabolic clearance. With continuous haemofiltration the situation is more manageable than in intermittent processes, as there are fewer oscillations in drug elimination.

Unfortunately, a number of other factors that depend on the dialysis process itself also affect clearance by dialysis. These include the duration of the dialysis procedure, the rate of blood flow to the dialyser, the surface area and porosity of the dialyser, and the composition and flow rate of dialysate.

Thus it is usually possible to predict whether or not a drug will be removed by dialysis, but it is very difficult to quantify the process, except by direct measurement, and this is rarely practical. Limited data for specific drugs are available in the literature, and many drug manufacturers have information on the dialysability of their products, some of which is included in the summary of product characteristics. In addition, standard reference texts such as the *Renal Drug Handbook* or *Drug Prescribing in Renal Failure* contain the information required for safe and effective prescribing of drugs in patients undergoing RRT.

Is this therapy appropriate for Mrs NC's septicaemia?

A16 **No. Cefotaxime should be replaced by an agent with broader activity against Gram-positive organisms, such as a penicillin (e.g. ampicillin, amoxicillin or co-amoxiclav).**

Patients in ARF are prone to infection and septicaemia and this is a common cause of death in this population. Between 50% and 80% of all dialysis patients are carriers of *Staphylococcus aureus* and/or *Staphylococcus epidermidis*. Bladder catheters and IV lines should therefore be used with care in order to reduce the chance of bacteria gaining access to the patient. Leukocytosis is sometimes seen in ARF and does not necessarily imply infection, but when seen in conjunction with pyrexia, as in Mrs NC, simple caution mandates aggressive treatment. Samples of blood, urine, sputum and any other material should be sent for culture before antibiotic therapy is started. Therapy should be prescribed to cover as wide a spectrum as possible until a causative organism is identified.

Aminoglycoside therapy is appropriate for Mrs NC as this class of compounds is highly active against most Gram-negative organisms as well as having useful activity against *S. aureus*. Gentamicin is also inexpensive. Metronidazole is highly active against anaerobic organisms. Cefotaxime is a 'third-generation' cephalosporin with increased sensitivity against Gram-negative organisms, although this is balanced by reduced activity against some Gram-positive organisms, notably *S. aureus*. It can be useful when given in combination with an aminoglycoside, but it would be more advantageous to Mrs NC to use an agent with greater activity against Gram-positive organisms, e.g. ampicillin or one of its analogues such as amoxicillin or co-amoxiclav. All penicillins may cause renal damage, most commonly acute interstitial nephritis, but the damage is a hypersensitivity reaction and therefore unpredictable, and it is not an absolute contraindication to penicillin use.

What are the dangers associated with prescribing gentamicin for Mrs NC? How should her gentamicin therapy be monitored?

A17 **Gentamicin can cause nephrotoxicity and toxicity to the eighth cranial nerve. Regular monitoring for these side-effects, and of Mrs NC's gentamicin serum levels, is essential.**

Treatment with an aminoglycoside is justified for the reasons given in **A16**; however, all aminoglycosides are potentially nephrotoxic, being associated with damage to the proximal tubule. Aminoglycosides can also precipitate ARF. Because of this, they should generally be avoided in renal impairment; however, their bactericidal activity against an extremely broad spectrum of Gram-negative organisms means that they are often prescribed for seriously ill patients with systemic infections. They are excreted solely by the kidney, so accumulation may lead to a vicious circle of increasing drug levels causing further renal deterioration and hence further accumulation. The risk of nephrotoxicity is increased when their use is combined with other nephrotoxic drugs, notably the loop diuretics. Mrs NC was prescribed the loop diuretic furosemide at an early stage of this admission, but her diuretic therapy has now been discontinued; however, if it is required again, the doses of aminoglycoside and loop diuretic must be staggered as much as possible.

In addition to being nephrotoxic, aminoglycosides are toxic to the eighth cranial nerve and may produce vestibular symptoms (i.e. loss of sense of balance) or adversely affect hearing. Such symptoms should therefore be checked for on a regular basis.

Traditionally aminoglycosides have been given in two to three divided doses over 24 hours; however, there is now a large body of evidence that administration once a day reduces the risk of toxicity while maintaining superior efficacy. Also, owing to its accumulation in renal failure, gentamicin may only need to be administered every 24 hours, or even less frequently. Other practical advantages include simplified dose calculation, a reduction in personnel time for drug administration and lower consumables costs. In practice, many renal units give 'stat' doses of gentamicin, e.g. 80 mg or 2 mg/kg to patients with moderate to severe renal impairment. The levels are monitored, and when the level is <2 mg/L the dose is re-administered. Alternatively, the *Renal Drug*

Handbook gives recommendations for once-daily gentamicin dosing according to GFR.

In general, it is thought that the risk of nephrotoxicity and eighth cranial nerve toxicity is associated with peak serum concentrations persistently >10 mg/L and, perhaps more importantly, troughs persistently >2 mg/L, although persistently low levels do not guarantee freedom from nephrotoxicity.

Why was Mrs NC prescribed the sodium bicarbonate? What else can be used for the same indication?

A18 She was prescribed sodium bicarbonate to prevent contrast-induced nephropathy. Alternatives would be sodium chloride 0.9% or *N*-acetylcysteine infusions.

Contrast-induced nephropathy (CIN) is defined as a creatinine level increased by at least 40 micromol/L, or more than 25%, above baseline. Renal impairment usually peaks within 3–5 days after completion of the diagnostic procedure and is usually self-limiting. Contrast agents, in particular non-ionic (iodine-based) contrast media, cause nephropathy primarily through renal ischaemia and, possibly, through direct toxicity to tubular epithelial cells. After contrast is injected, renal blood flow transiently increases. There is then a prolonged decrease caused by renal vasoconstriction, suggesting that renal ischaemia is a major factor in the pathogenesis of CIN. Pre-existing renal insufficiency is the single greatest risk factor for CIN, occurring in an estimated 60% of patients with CIN. The more severe the baseline renal insufficiency, the greater the risk that a patient will develop CIN, but anyone with a GFR <60 mL/min is considered to be at risk.

The best strategy to avoid the development of CIN is for patients to receive hydration therapy, starting 2–4 hours before the administration of contrast, during the radiographic procedure and continuing for 4–6 hours afterwards. Various solutions have been used, including IV sodium chloride 0.9% or sodium bicarbonate 1.26% or 1.4%. A typical regimen for sodium chloride 0.9% would be 1–2 L beginning at least 3 hours before the procedure at a rate of 100–150 mL/h, and continuing at least 6–8 hours post procedure at a slower rate depending on the patient's clinical status.

Sodium bicarbonate is believed to work by alkalising the tubular environment, thereby reducing the formation of free radicals, and it has been shown to be more effective than sodium chloride in this respect. A typical hydration regimen is 3 mL/kg/h for 1 hour prior to the procedure, followed by 1 mL/kg/h for 6 hours afterwards.

An alternative to sodium bicarbonate is the administration of *N*-acetylcysteine solution, where the mechanism of action is considered to be the trapping and destruction of free radicals. Despite several single studies and several meta-analyses, the true benefit of *N*-acetylcysteine is still unclear; however, it is used in some centres, with typical doses being either 600 mg orally or IV every 12 hours the day before and repeated the day after the procedure, or 1 g IV given both before and after the procedure.

Did Mrs NC follow the normal course of ARF? What is her prognosis?

A19 Yes. Mrs NC's illness followed the typical course of ARF and her survival to this stage is a good prognostic sign.

Acute tubular necrosis, the commonest form of ARF, usually occurs as a consequence of severe shock or as a result of sodium and water depletion giving rise to hypotension and generalised vasoconstriction, which in turn give rise to renal ischaemia. This was the sequence that resulted in Mrs NC's ARF. Acute tubular necrosis may also develop in the absence of any circulatory disturbance, e.g. through direct damage to the renal parenchyma that can result from toxic or allergic reactions to drugs or other substances.

The course of ARF may be divided into two phases. The first is the oliguric phase, where both the glomerulus and the renal tubule are no longer able to function properly. It is characterised by a urine volume of only 200–400 mL in 24 hours, a volume at which the kidney is unable adequately to excrete the products of metabolism. This inevitably leads to uraemia and hyperkalaemia unless adequate management is provided. This phase usually lasts no longer than 7–14 days, but may last for up to 6 weeks. If the patient does not die in this period, he or she will enter the second phase, where the glomerulus recovers and is now able to filter, but the tubule has not recovered sufficient function to properly reabsorb solutes and concentrate the urine. This phase is characterised by a urine volume that rises over a few days to several litres in a 24-hour period. This, the diuretic phase, lasts for up to 7 days, and patients who survive into this phase, as Mrs NC has, have a relatively good prognosis. Recovery of renal function takes place slowly over the following months, although the GFR rarely returns to its initial level. The elderly recover function more slowly and less completely.

The mortality for ARF varies according to the cause, but overall is about 50%. Death due to uraemia and hyperkalaemia is rare nowadays. The major causes of death are septicaemia and, to a lesser extent, gastrointestinal haemorrhage. Death is more common in patients aged over 60.

Acknowledgement

I would like to thank Alexander Harper who wrote the original chapter and Kate Richardson, who wrote the last revision, for giving permission for the material to be used as the basis for this update.

Further reading

Albright RC. Acute renal failure: a practical update. *Mayo Clin Proc* 2001; **76**: 67–74.

Aronoff GR, ed. *Drug Prescribing in Renal Failure*, 5th edn. American College of Physicians, Philadelphia, PA, 2007.

Ashley C, Currie A. *The Renal Drug Handbook*, 3rd edn. Radcliffe Medical Press, Oxford, 2008.

Davison AM, Cameron JS, Grunfeld J-P *et al*., eds. *Oxford Textbook of Clinical Nephrology*, 3rd edn. Oxford University Press, Oxford, 2005.

Dishart MK, Kellum JA. An evaluation of the pharmacological strategies for the prevention and treatment of acute renal failure. *Drugs* 2000; **59**: 79–91.

Levy J, Morgan J, Brown E. *Oxford Handbook of Dialysis*. Oxford University Press, 2nd edn. Oxford, 2004.

Mueller C. Prevention of contrast-induced nephropathy with volume supplementation. *Kidney Int* 2006; **69**: S16–S19.

Slack A, Ho S, Forni LG. The management of acute renal failure. *Medicine* 2007; **35**: 434–437.

Stevens P. Assessment of patients presenting with acute renal failure (acute kidney injury). *Medicine* 2007; **35**: 429–433.

Warrell DA, Cox TM, Firth JD *et al*., eds. *Oxford Textbook of Medicine*, 4th edn. Oxford University Press, Oxford, 2003.

9

Chronic renal failure managed by automated peritoneal dialysis

Aileen D Currie

Case study and questions

Day 1 Mr FB, a 52-year-old insulin-dependent diabetic with established renal failure (ERF) managed by automated peritoneal dialysis (APD), was admitted to the renal ward with a 2-day history of abdominal pain and malaise. He had noticed that his peritoneal dialysis (PD) effluent had become very cloudy over the previous 24 hours. It was his first admission to the renal unit at this hospital.

Mr FB had had insulin-dependent diabetes since childhood and had required PD for the last 10 years because of diabetic nephropathy. He continued to work as a personnel officer and had got married last year. He had recently been referred to the urology department for treatment of erectile dysfunction.

On admission Mr FB was noted to be unwell, with a pulse rate of 68 beats per minute (bpm), a blood pressure of 180/90 mmHg and a temperature of 38.9°C. His weight was 61 kg, which was slightly above his normal dry weight. Clinical examination revealed moderate hypertension, mild ankle oedema and abdominal tenderness.

His drug therapy at the time of admission was:

- Sevelamer 800 mg three tablets orally three times a day with meals
- Epoetin (NeoRecormon) 2000 IU twice weekly by subcutaneous injection
- Perindopril 2 mg orally daily
- Lactulose liquid 20 mL orally twice daily when necessary
- Co-dydramol, two tablets orally four times daily when necessary
- Clonazepam 0.5 mg orally at night, when required for restless legs
- Ispaghula husk, one sachet orally twice daily when necessary
- Insulin Human Mixtard 30 Penfill cartridge, 18 units subcutaneously each morning and 12 units subcutaneously each evening using the Novopen device

Mr FB's dialysis therapy consisted of a 15 L exchange overnight, using Physioneal 40, two bags of 2.5 L of 2.27% and four bags of 1.36%. He also had a daytime dwell with 2 L of Icodextrin. His serum biochemical and haematological results were as follows:

- Glucose 7.9 mmol/L (reference range 3.3–6.1)
- Potassium 4.2 mmol/L (3.6–5.4)
- Creatinine 800 micromol/L (50–140)
- Calcium 2.46 mmol/L (2.15–2.65)
- Phosphate 2.30 mmol/L (0.8–1.4)
- Sodium 134 mmol/L (133–144)
- Alkaline phosphatase 220 IU/L (70–300)
- Intact parathyroid hormone (iPTH) 85 pmol/L (0.8–5)
- Red blood cells (RBC) 3.23×10^{12}/L ($4.5–6 \times 10^{12}$)
- White blood cells (WBC) 8.1×10^{9}/L ($4–11 \times 10^{9}$)
- Haemoglobin (Hb) 8.8 g/dL (11.5–18)
- Haematocrit 0.258 (0.4–0.54)
- Serum ferritin 87 micrograms/L (25–350)

A sample of dialysate effluent was sent for microbiological screening.

Mr FB was diagnosed as having peritonitis. He was also fluid overloaded, hyperglycaemic, hyperphosphataemic, had hyperparathyroidism and anaemia, and was complaining of pruritus.

It was noted that his insulin doses were to be adjusted according to his measured blood sugars, as his requirements were likely to be altered by his infection and short-term changes to his dialysis regimen and it was documented that if he stopped eating he should be switched to a sliding-scale insulin regimen.

Q1 Should the results of the microbiological cultures be obtained before initiating antibiotic therapy?
Q2 What treatment would you recommend for Mr FB's peritonitis and why?
Q3 Why does Mr FB have renal bone disease and how would you recommend he be treated? What are the alternative therapeutic options?
Q4 Is clonazepam the best treatment for restless legs syndrome?
Q5 What are the reasons for pruritus in renal patients and what treatment would you recommend for Mr FB?

Mr FB was prescribed vancomycin 2 g and gentamicin 20 mg/L to be administered intraperitoneally (IP) via an extra daytime exchange which would have a dwell time of at least 6 hours (normally Mr FB would only have his Icodextrin in during the day, but because he had an infection he was to receive an extra daytime 1.36% glucose bag in order to receive his antibiotics). IP gentamicin was then to be continued once daily in his usual daytime exchange at a dose of 20 mg/L, starting 24 hours after the first IP dose. Heparin was also prescribed to be added at a dose of 1000 units/L to each antibiotic bag.

Q6 Why is heparin being added to Mr FB's PD bags?

Day 2 Mr FB's condition was still not improving and his weight was increasing. He was becoming slightly breathless and his ankle oedema was still present. The dialysis effluent remained cloudy and his abdomen tender. It was discovered that the heparin was not being added to the bags. The laboratory was phoned to try to expedite his culture results.

Day 3 Microbiological culture revealed infection with the Gram-negative organism *Proteus mirabalis*, which was sensitive to gentamicin and ceftazidime but not vancomycin. As a result, the IP gentamicin was continued in one exchange daily and intravenous (IV) ceftazidime was started. The vancomycin was discontinued, as the organism was not sensitive to it.

Q7 What dose of ceftazidime should be used to treat Mr FB's peritonitis, and can it be given IP?

Day 4 Mr FB's condition was beginning to improve. His bags were less cloudy and his abdominal pain was resolving. His weight was reducing, his ankle oedema improving, and he was less breathless. As this was Mr FB's first inpatient episode since starting dialysis it was decided to review all his medication during the evening ward round.

Q8 What information and recommendations would you prepare for the review with respect to Mr FB's:
(a) Phosphate binder?
(b) Analgesia?
(c) Laxative regimen?
(d) Antihypertensive therapy?
Indicate briefly other possible therapeutic options where appropriate.

Q9 What recommendations would you make for the treatment of Mr FB's anaemia?

Day 5 Mr FB's condition was still improving. His pulmonary and ankle oedema had resolved; his dialysate effluent was less cloudy, and his abdomen was less tender; however, he was having a problem with drainage of his dialysate exchanges. An abdominal X-ray was taken which revealed constipation.

As a result of the medication review his phosphate binder was changed to lanthanum and his analgesia was changed to paracetamol. Ispaghula husk therapy was discontinued and the lactulose liquid changed to Movicol one sachet twice daily, with senna tablets to be taken as required.

His dose of perindopril was increased.

Cinacalcet was initiated to control his renal bone disease as indicated by his high serum alkaline phosphatase and iPTH. He was also advised about the most appropriate way to take his phosphate binder and the importance of adhering to his therapy.

Day 13 Mr FB continued to improve. His APD effluent had now been clear for 6 days, so discharge was planned for the following day.

Day 14 His medication on discharge was:

- Lanthanum carbonate 1 g, chew one three times daily with food
- Perindopril 4 mg orally daily
- Ropinirole 0.25 mg orally at night for restless legs
- Cinacalcet 30 mg orally once daily
- Senna, two tablets orally at night when required
- Movicol sachets one twice daily
- Paracetamol 500 mg, two tablets orally four times daily when necessary for pain relief
- Insulin Human Mixtard 30 Penfill cartridges, 18 units subcutaneously each morning and 12 units subcutaneously each evening using the Novopen device
- Darbepoetin (Aranesp) 40 micrograms fortnightly
- Cetirizine 5 mg orally daily when required for relief from itch

An outpatient clinic appointment was made to check that his peritoneal fluid remained clear.

Q10 What are the key elements of a pharmaceutical care plan for Mr FB at discharge?

Day 21 Mr FB returned to clinic and mentioned that he had been started on sildenafil 25 mg orally for his erectile dysfunction. He also mentioned that his blood glucose monitoring strips had been changed, and since then he had noticed that his blood glucose levels were a bit high.

Q11 Outline the oral therapeutic options for erectile dysfunction. Which is most appropriate for Mr FB?

Q12 Are all blood monitoring strips suitable for PD patients?

Six months later Mr FB was admitted very unwell with abdominal pain. After repeated tests, including a computed tomography (CT) scan, he was diagnosed with encapsulating sclerosing peritonitis (ESP).

Q13 What treatment options are available to treat ESP?

Mr FB's catheter was removed and he was started on haemodialysis. His ESP was treated with tamoxifen and steroids, which controlled his disease. He received a renal transplant 6 months later.

Answers

Should the results of the microbiological cultures be obtained before initiating antibiotic therapy?

A1 Definitely not.

A delay in treatment can lead to the infection, which is usually confined to the peritoneal cavity, becoming systemic. Infection can also damage the peritoneum, reducing its efficiency as a dialysis membrane in the long term. Empirical antibiotic therapy should therefore be started as soon as peritonitis is clinically diagnosed.

What treatment would you recommend for Mr FB's peritonitis and why?

A2 The concomitant use of intraperitoneal (IP) vancomycin and gentamicin in accordance with the local, clinically audited protocol. The antibiotics should be added to PD bags instead of infusion fluids, and administered via the dialysate so that they can exert a local effect on the peritoneum. Intravenous (IV) antibiotic therapy is not warranted for Mr FB as a systemic infection is unlikely.

Recurrent episodes of peritonitis can lead to damage of the peritoneum and result in PD treatment failure and the patient needing to commence haemodialysis.

An antibiotic regimen that is effective against all the major Gram-positive and Gram-negative pathogens, in particular *Staphylococcus* and *Pseudomonas* species and *Enterobacteriaceae*, is required. Gram-positive organisms cause 60% of all cases of peritonitis, 20% are caused by Gram-negative organisms, 5% are fungal, and in 15% of cultures no growth is found. Evidence to date favours the IP route of drug administration. This route enables precise therapeutic and non-toxic concentrations of the antibiotics to be delivered directly to the site of infection.

Vancomycin has excellent antimicrobial activity against Gram-positive *Staphylococcus* and *Streptococcus* species, the most common causative organisms of PD peritonitis. Gentamicin has excellent antimicrobial activity against a broad range of Gram-negative organisms and some Gram-positive organisms.

The local protocol for a patient such as Mr FB would be as follows:

Days 1–2 Empirical therapy. Sample of dialysis effluent sent to pathology for culture and sensitivity tests. Vancomycin 2 g and gentamicin 20 mg/L to be administered IP by adding both drugs to the dialysis fluid and instilling for a 6-hour dwell time. Thereafter, gentamicin 20 mg/L to be given IP once daily, starting 24 hours after the first IP dose. Heparin 1000 units/L should be added to each antibiotic bag. If after the culture results the vancomycin is to be continued, then it should be given at weekly intervals depending on levels.

Day 3 The results of the microbiological culture of the sample of drained dialysis fluid taken on day 1 should be known. IP antibiotic therapy should be adjusted as follows:

Gram-positive organism sensitive to vancomycin and gentamicin: maintain on both antibiotics. If sensitive to only one, stop the prescription for the other.

Gram-negative organism: continue on gentamicin only, if sensitive. If not, give the appropriate antibiotic either orally, IP or IV.

Culture negative: maintain on vancomycin only, although in some circumstances gentamicin may also be continued. However, it is best to limit the use of gentamicin to minimise the risk of ototoxicity and nephrotoxicity. If the fluid is not clearing after 5 days of treatment the catheter should be removed. The use of heparin 1000 units/L in the antibiotic bag should be continued if the bags are still cloudy.

Days 4–6 **Review.** If the bags are still cloudy add another antibiotic (depending on reported sensitivities). Continue with gentamicin 20 mg/L IP daily as above, if indicated.

Day 7 Gentamicin 20 mg/L IP should be continued as above, if indicated. If a further dose of vancomycin is required levels should be taken. Another dose should not be given until the vancomycin trough level is <10 mg/L.

Vancomycin has been shown to be relatively stable (<10% loss in potency) in PD fluid for at least 24–48 hours. Aminoglycosides are much less stable in the low pH of glucose-containing PD fluids. It is advisable to add the two antibiotics to 'weak' rather than 'strong' dialysis bags, as the latter tend to have a more acidic pH. Although not relevant in Mr FB's case, if the dialysis effluent had still not been clearing after 14 days, PD catheter removal would usually be indicated.

When given by the IP route both vancomycin and gentamicin are absorbed systemically, particularly through an infected and inflamed peritoneal membrane. This may lead to potentially ototoxic and nephrotoxic serum levels after an extended course of treatment (the latter being relevant for patients who still have some remaining renal function).

Accumulation of vancomycin and gentamicin to potentially toxic levels does not occur in patients with ERF after 14 days' therapy.

Netilmicin, although more expensive than gentamicin, is reported to be the least toxic of the aminoglycosides and is an alternative to gentamicin.

There are many other reported regimens for the effective treatment of PD peritonitis, including the use of oral quinolones such as ciprofloxacin. Cephalosporins and aminoglycosides have a synergistic activity and can also be used to treat peritonitis very effectively.

In cases of fungal peritonitis, IP fluconazole and oral flucytosine (available on a named-patient basis) are generally used, although catheter removal is usually also required.

Why does Mr FB have renal bone disease and how would you recommend he be treated? What are the alternative therapeutic options?

A3 **Renal bone disease occurs because of the reduced synthesis of calcitriol (the physiologically active form of vitamin D) in the failing kidney, which in turn results in reduced serum calcitriol levels and reduced calcium absorption from the gut. This, together with hyperphosphataemia and reduced bone resorption, causes hypocalcaemia. Mr FB requires cinacalcet. Alternative therapeutic options are oral or parenteral alfacalcidol, calcitriol or paricalcitol, although because Mr FB is a PD patient parenteral therapy is not recommended.**

Hypocalcaemia and a reduction in the direct suppressive action of calcitriol on the parathyroid gland results in an increased secretion of iPTH. Uraemia reduces the sensitivity of the parathyroid gland to calcium, and inhibition of binding of calcitriol to receptors in the parathyroid gland also leads to raised iPTH levels. As it is not possible for the failing kidney to increase synthesis of calcitriol in response to the increased serum iPTH levels (which would result in a reduction in iPTH levels in a patient with normal renal function) the serum iPTH levels remain chronically elevated and hyperplasia of the parathyroid glands occurs. The resultant secondary hyperparathyroidism is central to the development of renal osteodystrophy.

Renal osteodystrophy covers the four main types of bone disease: secondary hyperparathyroidism, osteomalacia, mixed renal osteodystrophy and adynamic bone disease. Renal osteodystrophy results in a reduction in bone mineral density, osteopenia and metastatic calcification. It is due to reduced phosphate excretion and reduced vitamin D production.

If Mr FB was hypocalcaemic he would be treated with oral alfacalcidol, which is metabolised to calcitriol in the liver. An initial dose of 0.5 micrograms three times a week would be appropriate and can be adjusted according to response. During alfacalcidol therapy serum calcium levels should be monitored regularly. If the patient becomes hypercalcaemic, stopping the alfacalcidol should quickly result in a reduced serum calcium level. Significant hyperphosphataemia should always be corrected before correcting hypocalcaemia, as elevated phosphate and calcium levels can result in metastatic calcification of soft tissue.

The administration of calcitriol or alfacalcidol results in a rise in serum calcitriol and calcium, which suppresses iPTH secretion to some extent. To suppress serum iPTH to normal levels, large doses of calcitriol (or alfacalcidol) would have to be given and hypercalcaemia would quickly ensue. Hypercalcaemia is the rate-limiting step to treatment of hyperparathyroidism. It has been shown that giving alfacalcidol at a higher dose (1–4 micrograms) as a pulsed (three times a week) regimen causes greater suppression of iPTH by downregulation of iPTH receptors without as great an increase in calcium levels. Giving the dose of alfacalcidol at night has also been shown to be better, as less calcium is absorbed. It is important not to over-suppress iPTH, as this can lead to adynamic bone disease: an iPTH level of two to four times the normal level should be aimed for.

Paricalcitol is now available in both IV and oral formulations. It reputedly has the advantage over alfacalcidol and calcitriol of not increasing calcium and phosphate levels to the same extent, which in turn could lead to increased survival.

Cinacalcet is also available to treat hyperparathyroidism, although NICE has put limitations on its use and it can only be used in patients with an iPTH >85 pmol/L, who are hypercalcaemic or have a normal calcium and are unfit for surgery.

Cinacalcet is a calcimimetic that binds to the calcium receptor in the parathyroid gland and increases the sensitivity of the parathyroid glands to calcium, thereby switching off parathyroid hormone (PTH) production. It has the advantage that it can lower levels of both calcium and phosphate. Close monitoring of calcium is essential, as patients can become hypocalcaemic very quickly after starting therapy, and may also need their phosphate binders stopped or reduced. Cinacalcet has also been shown to reduce the risk of hospitalisation for fractures and cardiovascular disease.

Parathyroidectomy is not normally required until the iPTH is >100 pmol/L. This is referred to as tertiary hyperparathyroidism, when the iPTH remains elevated despite normal calcium and phosphate levels.

Is clonazepam the best treatment for restless legs syndrome?

A4 **No. Restless legs is a condition that affects many dialysis patients and tolerance to treatment can be a problem, so a drug holiday is sometimes required. First-line therapy should be with one of the agents used to treat Parkinson's disease.**

Restless legs syndrome is characterised by the involuntary jerking of the legs during sleep or rest, and can be as disturbing for the patient's partner as it is for them.

The cause of restless legs is unknown, although various hypotheses have been put forward, for example iron-deficiency anaemia and uraemic polyneuropathy. It can be exacerbated by phenytoin, neuroleptics and antidepressants.

First-line treatment should now be with the Parkinson's drugs such as ropinirole or pramipexole (both of which are licensed for restless legs) or the unlicensed alternatives co-beneldopa and co-careldopa. These types of drug are now preferred over clonazepam because of the addictive potential of the benzodiazepines.

Clonazepam, however, can still be used at a dose of 0.5 mg at night, increasing gradually to 4 mg, although in practice doses above 1 mg can cause daytime drowsiness and are rarely used. Dependence may become a problem, and treatment should be withdrawn gradually if a treatment-free period is required or when changing to an alternative treatment. Other alternatives are carbamazepine 100 mg at night increasing to 300 mg at night, or chlorpromazine, cabergoline, naloxone, clonidine, propranolol, tricyclic antidepressants, haloperidol, baclofen and even a tot of brandy.

In Mr FB's case his risk factors for restless legs would be chronic kidney disease and iron-deficiency anaemia. Although at the moment his clonazepam is working, it would be a good idea to try to wean him off it and use one of the licensed alternatives. As Mr FB has been on clonazepam for a few years, it should be withdrawn gradually.

What are the reasons for pruritus in renal patients, and what treatment would you recommend for Mr FB?

A5 **Pruritus is common in renal failure due to uraemia, iron deficiency, hyperparathyroidism, dialysis itself, hyperphosphataemia and dry skin. The release of histamine from mast cells causes itching; also, high histamine levels have been found in patients with chronic kidney disease and have been linked with uraemic pruritus. First-line treatments include antihistamines and topical agents.**

Mr FB has poorly controlled phosphate levels which may be the main reason for his pruritus, so he should be counselled on the effects of high phosphate levels. In renal failure the itch can be very difficult to treat, so a combination of systemic and topical agents tends to be used. The topical agents include moisturising lotions and creams containing urea or menthol. Sedative antihistamines tend to work better than the non-sedative ones and have the advantage of helping the patient sleep at night, when the itch tends to be worse; however, as Mr FB works he wants a non-sedative alternative. The drug of choice tends to be cetirizine at a dose of 5 mg daily or loratadine 10 mg daily. It is best to avoid the antihistamines which may cause an increased risk of arrhythmias, as renal patients are prone to rapid electrolyte changes. Other drugs that can be tried are naltrexone injection and thalidomide capsules, although they are not commonly used. It is also important to treat some of the other causes of Mr FB's pruritus, namely his iron deficiency and renal bone disease.

Why is heparin being added to Mr FB's PD bags?

A6 **Heparin is being added to one bag of PD fluid daily to help break down the fibrin that appears in the peritoneum as a result of peritonitis and which contributes to the cloudy appearance of the PD effluent. The breakdown of the fibrin helps prevent blockage of the PD catheter. The heparin should be added to the daytime dwell with the gentamicin unless his fluid is very cloudy, when it should also be added to his night-time bags.**

Heparin additions should continue until the PD effluent becomes clear. The dose of heparin per bag varies considerably between renal units and is somewhat empirical.

In this unit the addition of 1000 units/L of heparin per bag has been found to be a simple and effective regimen. Although not the case with Mr FB, a proportion of patients always have a cloudy fibrinous PD effluent that is not associated with peritonitis. These patients add heparin to each of their PD bags routinely.

What dose of ceftazidime should be used to treat Mr FB's peritonitis, and can it be given IP?

A7 **Sensitivities have shown that the organism is sensitive to ceftazidime, so a dose of 500 mg every 24 hours IV is appropriate. Ceftazidime can also be given IP.**

As Mr FB is not improving he should be started on a course of IV ceftazidime at a dose of 500 mg every 24 hours. Cephalosporins, and especially ceftazidime, can be very neurotoxic in renal patients, and as they are renally excreted a marked dose reduction is required to prevent drug accumulation. Ceftazidime can also be given IP at a dose of 125 mg/L.

What information and recommendations would you prepare for the review, with respect to Mr FB's (a) Phosphate binder? (b) Analgesia? (c) Laxative regimen? (d) Antihypertensive therapy? Indicate briefly other possible therapeutic options where appropriate.

A8 **(a) Phosphate binder.**

Lanthanum may be a more appropriate phosphate binder for Mr FB than sevelamer.

Serum phosphate levels rise in patients with renal failure once the glomerular filtration rate (GFR) is <50 mL/min, owing mainly to the reduced renal excretion of phosphate. The resulting hyperphosphataemia plays a major role in the development of secondary hyperparathyroidism and hence renal osteodystrophy, because excessive PTH release is stimulated by the hyperphosphataemia-induced hypocalcaemia and hypocalcitriolaemia.

Management of hyperphosphataemia centres on a combination of dialysis and the binding of orally ingested phosphate in the gut to prevent its systemic absorption. A phosphate-binding agent is usually the salt of a di- or trivalent metallic ion. The advantages and disadvantages of the available phosphate binders are summarised below.

Aluminium hydroxide used to be widely used as a phosphate binder; however, aluminium is systemically absorbed and is toxic, causing encephalopathy, osteomalacia, proximal myopathy and anaemia. The latest K-DOQI Guidelines recommend that it is used for as short a time as possible to reduce accumulation. Aluminium salts also cause constipation, which can quickly lead to drainage problems in PD patients. Aluminium absorption can also be increased if patients take ulcer-healing drugs concurrently, as ulcer-healing agents raise the pH of the gut.

(a) Aluminium hydroxide should be taken 5–10 minutes before food to ensure an optimal phosphate-binding effect and to reduce aluminium absorption.

(b) Calcium carbonate has been used with success in chronic dialysis patients. The dose required to control serum phosphate in PD patients is generally lower than for patients on haemodialysis, probably owing to the continuous removal of serum phosphate by this method of dialysis; however, unpredictable episodes of hypercalcaemia due to systemic calcium absorption are often a problem in this patient group. Calcium carbonate should be taken 5–10 minutes before food to ensure an optimal phosphate-binding effect, and also to reduce calcium absorption.

(c) Calcium acetate (Phosex). The acetate salt of calcium has a stronger phosphate-binding effect and less calcium is absorbed than from the carbonate formulation. Calcium acetate should be taken with meals, which may also help to remind patients to take it. It is of most use in people with calcium levels at the higher end of the normal range.

(d) Sevelamer (Renagel) has the advantage of being a non-absorbed phosphate-binding poly(allylamine hydrochloride) polymer which is free of aluminium and calcium. It should be taken with food to optimise the phosphate-binding effect and to reduce nausea. The product has a further advantage in that it can reduce low-density lipoprotein cholesterol levels by 20%; however, it does have the disadvantage that between one and five 800 mg tablets must be taken with each meal, and it is considerably more expensive than calcium-containing binders.

(e) Lanthanum is a heavy metal. It has the advantage that it can reduce tablet burden in patients, but is still considerably more expensive than calcium- and aluminium-based binders. Nausea can be a major problem, especially if the drug is taken without food, so it should also be taken with meals. As lanthanum is a heavy metal found near barium in the periodic table it can be seen distributed throughout the body if the patient requires an X-ray.

Renal units now often calculate the product of the calcium and phosphate levels (Ca × P), as this gives a more accurate measurement of total body calcium content than serum measurements of calcium or phosphate alone. Ca × P products >4.5 $mmol^2/L^2$ may lead to an increased incidence of soft tissue and vascular calcification, left ventricular hypertrophy and sudden cardiac death. For such patients there is increasing interest in the use of non-calcium-containing phosphate binders such as sevelamer and lanthanum as a way of minimising calcium intake. Mr FB's Ca × P product is 5.65 $mmol^2/L^2$.

Mr FB's compliance with his phosphate binders should be queried, as tablet burden can be a problem for renal patients. Sevelamer in high doses also has a side-effect of causing bowel obstruction in PD patients, so it may not be the best choice for him. Lanthanum may thus be an option so as both to avoid calcium absorption and also to reduce the number of tablets Mr FB has to take. Following any change in therapy his serum phosphate and calcium levels should be monitored regularly.

(b) Analgesia.

Co-dydramol therapy should be discontinued and replaced by paracetamol 500 mg, up to two tablets four times daily when necessary. If Mr FB's pain is continuous, regular therapy should be recommended.

Co-dydramol (containing paracetamol 500 mg and dihydrocodeine 10 mg) is not commonly used. Dihydrocodeine and its active metabolites accumulate in renal failure, enhancing side-effects such as constipation and sedation. This has probably contributed to Mr FB's feeling of lethargy and his need for laxatives. There is no conclusive evidence that co-dydramol is a significantly stronger analgesic than paracetamol alone.

If pain relief is not achieved with paracetamol, an NSAID could be considered, although such a drug may cause gastrointestinal bleeding and reduce any residual renal function Mr FB may have. Co-codamol 8/500 could also be considered as an alternative, but sedation and constipation can also occur with this compound.

(c) Laxative regimen.

Factors that are probably contributing to Mr FB's constipation are:

(i) The use of an analgesic containing dihydrocodeine, a synthetic narcotic analgesic with morphine-like action.
(ii) Inappropriate 'when-necessary' use of his prescribed laxatives. The concomitant use of ispaghula husk sachets is illogical and can even lead to constipation.
(iii) Fluid restriction.
(iv) A low-fibre diet. Renal patients are usually restricted in their fruit and vegetable intake owing to restrictions on potassium intake.

The ispaghula husk sachets and lactulose should be discontinued, and senna and Movicol sachets should be commenced. Movicol is slightly more effective than lactulose in diabetic patients. Senna is a stimulant laxative and can be used on a 'when-required' basis combined with regular Movicol to maintain adequate bowel movements.

Constipation in PD patients can lead to obstruction of drainage of the dialysate from the peritoneum. In PD patients with resistant constipation Picolax is sometimes required if the catheter is not working.

(d) Antihypertensive therapy.

Mr FB's perindopril therapy should be increased to 4 mg daily.

Hypertension in ERF is attributed to either increased cardiac output or increased peripheral vascular resistance, or both. Increased cardiac output reflects volume expansion secondary to sodium and water retention and/or the anaemia of chronic renal failure. Increased peripheral resistance may reflect an increase in circulating renin and angiotensin II or, possibly, reduced levels of vasodilators such as prostaglandins, bradykinin and renal medullary lipids. Hypertension is occasionally controlled by dialysis, but most patients, including Mr FB, need antihypertensive medication.

Although there is no absolute contraindication to beta-blocker therapy in Mr FB, it is not the treatment of choice as he suffers from erectile dysfunction. If a beta-blocker was desired, metoprolol therapy would be most appropriate. Beta-blockers have the potential to affect diabetics by increasing the frequency of hypoglycaemic attacks, by delaying the rate of recovery, and also by impairing carbohydrate tolerance. This risk is reduced by the use of the more cardioselective beta-blockers such as atenolol or metoprolol. Small initial doses are advised in renal failure.

An appropriate antihypertensive for Mr FB from a pharmacological viewpoint is an angiotensin-converting enzyme inhibitor (ACEI), which causes vasodilation and reduced sodium retention by reducing the amount of circulating angiotensin II. There have also been some studies showing that ACEIs can preserve residual renal function in PD patients.

The kidney is the major route of excretion of most ACEIs. To prevent accumulation and consequent hypotension and other adverse drug reactions in the renally impaired, therapy should be initiated with small doses, which should then be increased until the desired hypotensive effect is achieved. Although clinically there is little to choose between the newer and the older ACEIs, perindopril, fosinopril and some of the newer agents offer the potential of once-daily dosing as well as being either hepatically or dual metabolised, which prevents the problem of accumulation in renal failure When renal patients first start one of the newer ACEIs they take the first dose at night: a patient on haemodialysis would be advised to take the first dose at night on a non-dialysis day. ACEIs are very effective in the management of hypertension in patients with renal failure. Furthermore, there are reports that ACEIs reduce thirst, which is potentially useful in those dialysis patients who have a tendency to fluid overload as a result of excessive drinking. A first step to control Mr FB's hypertension is therefore to optimise the use of perindopril by increasing the dose to 4 mg daily.

Angiotensin receptor blockers can also be used in renal failure, either instead of an ACEI if there have been problems with side-effects such as cough, or in combination with ACEIs in patients with very resistant hypertension.

A calcium-channel blocker would also be a possibility, although ankle swelling can be a problem.

Other options are alpha-blockers such as doxazosin, or centrally acting drugs such as moxonidine.

The sensitivity of patients to all these drugs is increased in ERF and, if used, therapy must be initiated with small doses.

What recommendations would you make for the treatment of Mr FB's anaemia?

A9 **Mr FB is being treated with subcutaneous recombinant human erythropoietin (epoetin), a bioengineered form of the hormone. His iron deficiency should also be treated with IV iron therapy. It is likely that he is not complying with his epoetin injections as he says that he keeps 'forgetting' them, therefore an option is to change him to a product he can administer once a fortnight in an attempt to encourage him to comply.**

Mr FB's anaemia is probably the major contributor to his continuous feeling of lethargy and fatigue. The anaemia of chronic renal failure is caused mainly by a deficiency in the renal production of the hormone erythropoietin, which results in reduced bone marrow erythropoiesis. Other contributing factors include the inhibition of erythropoiesis by uraemic toxins, a shortening of red cell survival, uraemic bleeding, iron deficiency, aluminium toxicity and hyperparathyroidism.

Before the introduction of epoetin, red blood cell transfusions were the cornerstone of management of the anaemia of chronic renal failure, but erythroid marrow suppression, human leukocyte-associated antigen (HLA) antibody induction and iron overload made this treatment very unpopular. There are now a number of erythropoietin products to choose from. They include:

(a) Epoetin alpha (Eprex) has now got its subcutaneous licence back after concerns about pure red cell aplasia. It is given to PD patients at an initial dose of 50 units/kg twice weekly.
(b) Epoetin beta (Neorecormon) is licensed to start at a dose of 20 units/kg three times a week, although in practice the same starting dose as for Eprex is used.
(c) Further options collectively known as biosimilars (see manufacturer's data sheets).
(d) Darbepoetin alpha (Aranesp) stimulates erythropoiesis in the same way as epoetin therapy. It has a half-life three times as long as the endogenous protein and the epoetins owing to the presence of an extra two sugar residues on the molecule, which causes a reduction in its hepatic metabolism. Because of its longer half-life, darbepoetin only has to be administered once weekly or once a fortnight. The starting dose is 0.45 micrograms/kg/week as a subcutaneous or IV injection.
(e) Mircera, which is related to epoetin beta, has the advantage that it can be administered monthly. It has a starting dose of 0.6 micrograms/kg every fortnight. Once the patient is stable the frequency can be reduced to monthly.

IV administration of epoetin is effective but requires a higher dose than via the subcutaneous route to achieve the same rise in haemoglobin, thereby reducing the cost-effectiveness of this route. The newer products darbepoetin and Mircera can be given by the IV route at the same dose as for subcutaneous administration, but this is not feasible for PD patients.

For all products the dose should be increased by 25% monthly until the target haemoglobin level is reached. A slow rise in haemoglobin (not more than 1–2 g/dL/month) should minimise aggravation of Mr FB's hypertension and avoid other reported haemodynamically induced side-effects, such as seizures and clotting of vascular access. The hypertension sometimes seen during erythropoietic stimulating agent (ESA) therapy is probably due to a reverse of the vasodilation caused by chronic anaemia. Mr FB's blood pressure should be regularly monitored and, if necessary, controlled by adjusting his antihypertensive therapy. The improved appetite that accompanies ESA therapy can also increase potassium intake, which in turn can necessitate the institution of some dietary control.

Pure red cell aplasia is a very rare condition/side-effect of ESA that results in failure of the production of erythroid elements (i.e. red blood cell precursors) in the bone marrow, which leads to profound anaemia. This is possibly due to an immune response to the protein backbone of the molecule. The antibodies formed as a result of this immune response render the patient unresponsive to the therapeutic effects of epoetin alpha, epoetin beta and darbepoetin, or any other erythropoietic product.

Depletion of available iron is common during ESA therapy because of the greatly increased marrow requirements. Mr FB's iron status should be regularly monitored and IV iron administered if his serum ferritin is <100 micrograms/L, so as to maintain an effective response to ESA therapy. It takes 20 micrograms/L of ferritin to increase a patient's haemoglobin concentration by 1 g/dL, therefore patients on ESA therapy require higher than normal iron stores to achieve an adequate response. Ferritin is not an ideal measurement of iron status as it can be increased during infective or inflammatory periods; therefore, in people with high ferritin levels it is best also to measure transferrin saturation, which should be >20%, or the percentage of hypochromic red blood cells, which should be <10%. The percentage of hypochromic red blood cells is a measure of the number of individual red blood cells with a haemoglobin content of <28 g/dL.

As Mr FB's ferritin is only 87 micrograms/L he should be started on an accelerated course of IV iron sucrose once he is free from infection, as IV iron treatment is associated with an increased risk of infection. The total dose of iron he requires can be calculated from the following equation:

$$\text{Body weight (kg)} \times (13 - \text{actual Hb}) \times 2.4 + 500 \text{ (storage iron)}$$

He should receive this at a dose of 200 mg once weekly, possibly at a nurse-led clinic. Once his iron stores are replete, he should receive a dose of 200 mg iron sucrose at each clinic visit, which he will attend every 2–3 months. Giving IV iron can reduce the dose of ESA required to achieve the desired haemoglobin and result in cost savings. An alternative to iron sucrose is CosmoFer, a new formulation of iron dextran which can be given as a total-dose infusion and can be useful for patients who live some distance from the renal unit, or who have very fragile veins. This new formulation of iron dextran has a smaller molecule size and therefore fewer anaphylactic reactions occur. A new single-dose preparation is now also available called ferric carboxymaltose (Ferinject), which can be administered as an IV bolus.

Iron tablets are not ideal in dialysis patients because of the increased risk of gastrointestinal side-effects, poor bioavailability, and interactions with phosphate binders leading to reduced efficacy of both drugs. As a result, iron tablets are rarely used.

Our target haemoglobin level is 10–12 g/dL (haematocrit 0.30–0.40). Once this target has been reached, the dose of ESA is reduced and adjusted to maintain the haemoglobin at this desired level.

What are the key elements of a pharmaceutical care plan for Mr FB at discharge?

A10 The key elements are to ensure that Mr FB understands the reasons for the changes in his drug regimen and can comply with his prescribed medication when at home, and that there is full communication with the Primary Care Team who will share his care after discharge. This communication should include details of his drug therapy and the monitoring required to ensure the desired therapeutic outcomes are met.

Although Mr FB's oral drug regimen is relatively simple, it is good clinical practice to counsel him before discharge. He should be informed that his new phosphate binder, lanthanum, should be chewed before swallowing and taken with meals, and that he should take his new laxative regularly. He should be told about the change to his ESA treatment and reminded of the importance of it and the implications of anaemia. His general practitioner (GP) or practice nurse will measure Mr FB's haemoglobin, and the results will be analysed in the hospital. He should be advised that if the ropinirole for his restless legs does not work then he can go back to his

GP and the dose can be increased. Mr FB should be reminded not to take any other drugs, either purchased or prescribed, without first checking with the renal unit.

This unit issues a printed medication record card to help communicate information on medication at discharge with the Primary Care Team. At discharge, Mr FB's GP should be sent a discharge letter which includes his up-to-date medication record, together with information on his ESA therapy. Mr FB should also be given a copy of the information to give to his community pharmacist.

Outline the oral options available for erectile dysfunction. Which is most appropriate for Mr FB?

A11 **As a renal dialysis patient, Mr FB is entitled under Schedule 11 to receive oral treatment for his erectile dysfunction. Sildenafil 25 mg initially is an appropriate choice for him.**

Mr FB could be suffering from erectile dysfunction due to his diabetes, hypertension, chronic renal failure or anaemia. His anaemia and hypertension are already being treated, but this has not solved his problem. It is important to avoid beta-blockers and alpha-blocker therapy for his hypertension as they can cause erectile dysfunction. However, ACEIs have also been implicated.

Sildenafil inhibits phosphodiesterase type 5, causing an increase in cyclic GMP levels which results in corporal smooth muscle relaxation. This restores natural erectile function in response to sexual stimulation. It has a 56% success rate in diabetics and a 71% success rate in PD patients. As Mr FB is not on anginal medication he is eligible for sildenafil. He should be advised to take it on an empty stomach, 30 minutes to 4 hours prior to sexual intercourse. In renal failure an initial dose of 25 mg should be used and slowly increased as required. Sildenafil is relatively well tolerated in renal failure.

Although both tadalafil and vardenafil are options, sildenafil may be slightly safer for renal patients as it has the shortest half-life.

Are all blood monitoring strips suitable for PD patients?

A12 **No.**

It has been discovered that test strips using the enzyme glucose dehydrogenase pyrroloquinolinequinone (GDH-PQQ) can cause an overestimation in blood glucose readings in patients using Icodextrin or other products which are metabolised to maltose, xylose or galactose. This would include Roche Accu-check and Abbott Diabetes Care Freestyle meters and strips. It should therefore be ensured that Mr FB uses another brand, such as Ascensia or Contour.

What treatment options are available to treat encapsulating sclerosing peritonitis (ESP)?

A13

ESP is irreversible sclerosis of the peritoneal membrane and usually occurs after patients have been on PD for a long time. It can be related to continual inflammation, and the risk increases after 4 years on PD. It can be difficult to detect, and CT and ultrasound scans are required. Chlorhexidine gluconate, which can be used to cleanse the exit site, and long-term damage to the peritoneum by advanced glycation end-products (AGEs), have been implicated.

Treatment can be with 0.5 mg/kg/day prednisolone and 10–40 mg tamoxifen daily, and/or other anti-inflammatory or immunosuppressive drugs such as azathioprine, or by surgery.

Removal of the catheter is essential and PD must be discontinued, as the condition can be fatal.

Acknowledgements

The author wishes to thank Raymond Bunn for giving permission for his original chapter to be used as the basis for this revised case.

Further reading

Ashley C, Currie A. *The Renal Drug Handbook*, 3rd edn. Radcliffe Medical Press, Abingdon, 2008.

Ashley C, Morlidge C. *Introduction to Renal Therapeutics*. Pharmaceutical Press, London, 2008.

Casadevall N, Nataf J, Viron B *et al.* Pure red cell aplasia and antierythropoietin antibodies in patients treated with recombinant erythropoietin. *N Engl J Med* 2002; **346**: 469–475.

Cunningham J, Danese M, Olson K *et al.* Effects of the calcimimetic cinacalcet HCl on cardiovascular disease, fracture, and health-related quality of life in secondary hyperparathyroidism. *Kidney Int* 2005; **68**: 1793–1800.

Del Peso G, Bajo MA, Aguilera A *et al.* Clinical experience with tamoxifen in peritoneal fibrosing syndromes. *Adv Perit Dial* 2003; **19**: 32–35.

Evrenkaya TR, Atasoyu EM, Unver S *et al.* Corticosteroid and tamoxifen therapy in sclerosing encapsulating peritonitis in a patient on continuous peritoneal dialysis. *Nephrol Dial Transplant* 2004; **19**: 2423–2424.

Flood TA, Veinot VP. Test and teach. Diagnosis: Sclerosing encapsulating peritonitis. *Pathology* 2008; **40**(6): 629–631.

Gokal R. Peritoneal dialysis in the 21st century: An analysis of current problems and future developments. *J Am Soc Nephrol* 2002; **13**: S104–S116.

Lo WK. Latest strategy in renal anemia management in peritoneal dialysis patients. *Perit Dial Int* 2008; **28** (Suppl 3): S76–80.

Moe SM, Drüeke T. Improving global outcomes in mineral and bone disorders. *Clin J Am Soc Nephrol* 2008; **3** (Suppl 3): S127–130.

National Institute for Clinical Excellence. CG39. *Anaemia Management in People with Chronic Kidney Disease*. NICE, London, 2006.

Piraino B, Bailie GR, Bernardini J *et al.* ISPD Guidelines/Recommendations: Peritoneal dialysis-related infections recommendations – 2005 update. *Perit Dial Int* 2005; **25**: 107–131.

Teng M, Wolf M, Lowrie E *et al.* Survival of patients undergoing hemodialysis with paricalcitol or calcitriol therapy. *N Engl J Med* 2003; **349**(5): 446–456.

10

Renal transplantation

Caroline Ashley

Case study and questions

Day 1 (am) Mr JO, a 38-year-old man, was urgently admitted from home for a cadaveric renal transplant. He had a 6-year history of renal impairment, having first presented to his general practitioner (GP) with persistent headaches. He had also complained of weakness, fatigue and generally 'not feeling well', and on investigation was found to have a markedly elevated serum creatinine. He had been diagnosed as having chronic kidney disease (CKD). For the 5 years prior to this admission he had been in end-stage renal failure (CKD5), receiving intermittent haemodialysis three times a week while awaiting a transplant. A donor kidney was now available.

His drug therapy on admission was:

- Calcichew (calcium carbonate 1250 mg), two tablets three times daily
- Alfacalcidol 1 microgram three times a week
- Folic acid 5 mg daily
- Ketovite, one tablet daily
- Amlodipine 10 mg twice daily
- Perindopril 4 mg daily
- Venofer 100 mg intravenously (IV) once a month
- Erythropoietin 4000 IU subcutaneously three times a week

Mr JO was a non-smoker who rarely drank alcohol. He was married with an 8-year-old daughter and worked as a draughtsman, although he had recently been having difficulty maintaining his job owing to the frequent dialysis sessions.

On examination Mr JO was reported to be pale, but generally quite well. He was mildly hypertensive (blood pressure 135/85 mmHg) and had a pulse of 70 beats per minute (bpm), with no oedema or signs of cardiac failure. His urine output was <50 mL/day and he weighed 72 kg.

His serum biochemistry and haematology results were:

- Creatinine 672 micromol/L (reference range 60–120)
- Potassium 4.0 mmol/L (3.5–5.0)
- Calcium 2.44 mmol/L (2.1–2.6)
- Urea 12.8 mmol/L (3.0–6.5)
- Haemoglobin 10.2 g/dL (13.5–18.0)
- Phosphate 1.66 mmol/L (0.8–1.4)
- Sodium 140 mmol/L (135–146)
- White blood cells (WBC) 5.2×10^9/L ($4–10 \times 10^9$)
- Liver function tests within normal limits

Day 1 (pm) Mr JO was prepared for transplant. One hour before the operation he was given 20 mg basiliximab IV, 5.5 mg tacrolimus (approximately 0.075 mg/kg) orally, 1 g mycophenolate mofetil orally, 500 mg methylprednisolone IV, and 1.2 g co-amoxiclav IV. The latter was given to cover the surgery and insertion of a central line.

Q1 How should these injections be administered?
Q2 What are the therapeutic aims on return from theatre?
Q3 Which immunosuppressant(s) would you recommend be prescribed subsequently, and why?

On return to the renal unit later that evening, Mr JO was started on:

- Tacrolimus 5.5 mg orally, to be repeated every 12 hours
- Mycophenolate mofetil 1 g orally, to be repeated every 12 hours
- Prednisolone 20 mg orally, to be repeated once each day

Q4 How should therapy with a calcineurin inhibitor such as ciclosporin or tacrolimus be monitored?
Q5 Are there any parameters that should be monitored when mycophenolate mofetil (MMF) is prescribed?

Hourly fluid balance charts, temperature, blood pressure and respiration rate monitoring were started. Mr JO initially had a urine output of 40 mL/h. He was given Monosol (an electrolyte replacement solution containing glucose, calcium, sodium, magnesium, chloride and lactate), 1 L IV, plus the replacement volume to match his urine output each hour, using the central venous pressure (CVP) as a guide to fluid balance. The kidney initially failed to diurese, so an infusion of furosemide (10 mg/h) was set up.

Mr JO's blood pressure was noted to be 125/95 mmHg, but in order to keep the transplanted kidney well perfused, it was decided that antihypertensive therapy was not necessary. He was, however, started on omeprazole to prevent stress ulceration.

Two hours postoperatively, serum biochemistry and haematology results were:

- Sodium 139 mmol/L (135–146)
- Urea 8.3 mmol/L (3.0–6.5)
- Creatinine 412 micromol/L (60–120)
- Potassium 3.6 mmol/L (3.5–5.0)
- Haemoglobin 9.0 g/dL (13.5–18.0)
- WBC 5.8×10^9/L ($4.0–10.0 \times 10^9$)

Q6 What other medications should be prescribed for Mr JO and why?

Day 3 Mr JO was well, apyrexial, and his urine output was good (approximately 150 mL/h). Serum biochemistry and haematology results were:

- Creatinine 208 micromol/L (60–120)
- WBC 6.5×10^9/L ($4.0–10.0 \times 10^9$)
- Tacrolimus 10.2 nanograms/mL (target level 5–15 by HPLC of whole blood)

Amlodipine 10 mg orally when required was prescribed as an antihypertensive, to be used if Mr JO's diastolic blood pressure was >100 mmHg.

Q7 Would you have recommended amlodipine as an antihypertensive for Mr JO?

Day 4 Serum biochemistry and haematology results were:

- Creatinine 215 micromol/L (60–120)
- WBC 6.1×10^9/L ($4.0–10.0 \times 10^9$)

Day 5 Mr JO became pyrexial with a temperature of 37.5°C and the kidney site was slightly tender. His blood pressure was 130/100 mmHg.

Serum biochemistry and haematology results were:

- Creatinine 270 micromol/L (60–120)
- WBC 6.4×10^9/L (4.0–10.0)
- Lymphocytes 3.2×10^9/L (1.0–3.5)
- Tacrolimus 9.9 nanograms/mL (5–15)

A MAG3 (^{99m}Tc mercapto acetyl triglycene) scan showed reduced perfusion of the kidney, and it was decided that Mr JO was suffering from an episode of acute rejection, which was confirmed by renal biopsy.

Q8 How should Mr JO's acute rejection episode be managed?

Day 8 Mr JO was looking better. His serum creatinine level had fallen to 143 micromol/L and the graft site was no longer tender. His tacrolimus level (trough) was 10.3 nanograms/mL.

Day 12 Mr JO again became pyrexial, and the transplant had become tender and increased in size. There was no obvious infection.

Serum biochemistry and haematology results were:

- Creatinine 378 micromol/L (60–120)
- WBC 5.6×10^9/L ($4.0–10.0 \times 10^9$)
- Lymphocytes 3.9×10^9/L ($1.0–3.5 \times 10^9$)
- Tacrolimus 10.1 nanograms/mL (5–15)

Renal biopsy showed severe acute vascular rejection, and it was decided that Mr JO required further immunosuppression with anti-thymocyte immunoglobulin (ATG).

Q9 What precautions should be taken when starting ATG?
Q10 How should the dose be calculated?
Q11 How should ATG be administered?
Q12 Should the doses of his other immunosuppressants be adjusted during ATG therapy?

Day 12 A subclavian line was inserted and a 7-day course of ATG started. The initial dose was 125 mg (approximately 1.5 mg/kg).

Day 13 Lymphocytes 1.09×10^9/L, dose of ATG = 125 mg.

Day 14 Lymphocytes 0.31×10^9/L, dose of ATG = 75 mg.

Day 15 Lymphocytes 0.15×10^9/L, dose of ATG = 75 mg.

Day 16 Lymphocytes 0.07×10^9/L, dose of ATG omitted.

Day 17 Lymphocytes 0.14×10^9/L, dose of ATG = 75 mg.

Day 18 Lymphocytes 0.26×10^9/L, dose of ATG = 125 mg.

Day 19 Mr JO was showing a marked improvement, with increased renal perfusion shown by a MAG3 scan.

His serum biochemistry and haematology results were:

- Creatinine 131 micromol/L (60–120)
- WBC 3.1×10^9/L (4.0–10.0)
- Tacrolimus 9.8 nanograms/mL (5–15)

Mr JO was now well, with good renal function, and so he was discharged home. He was to attend outpatients three times a week initially so that his progress could be closely monitored.

Q13 What pharmaceutical care plans should be made in preparation for Mr JO's discharge?

Mr JO was discharged on the following medication:

- Tacrolimus 4 mg orally twice daily
- Prednisolone 15 mg orally each morning
- Omeprazole 20 mg orally once daily
- Mycophenolate mofetil 1 g orally twice daily
- Amphotericin lozenges, one to be sucked four times each day
- Aspirin 75 mg once daily
- Co-trimoxazole 480 mg once daily

Q14 How long should Mr JO remain on immunosuppressants?
Q15 How long is Mr JO likely to require concomitant prophylactic therapy?
Q16 What points would you cover when counselling Mr JO about his medication?

Day 35 Mr JO became pyrexial again, but this time the transplant site was not tender. He had developed a dry cough, had some shortness of breath and exhibited a marked deterioration in blood oxygen saturation on exertion. He had also developed a swinging fever, and a chest X-ray showed diffuse interstitial shadowing.

His serum biochemistry and haematology results were:

- Creatinine 118 micromol/L (60–120)
- WBC 3.9×10^9/L ($4.0–10.0 \times 10^9$)
- Platelets 129×10^9/L (140–400)
- Tacrolimus 9.2 nanograms/mL (5–15)

Blood and midstream urine samples were sent to microbiology and virology for culture.

Q17 What has predisposed Mr JO to infection?
Q18 What types of infection is Mr JO susceptible to?

Mr JO was diagnosed as having a pneumonitis due to cytomegalovirus (CMV).

Q19 What course of treatment would you recommend?

Over the next 14 days Mr JO's temperature returned to normal and he appeared to be progressing well. His urine output was approximately 2 L/24 h and his blood gases were improving.

At 3 months post transplant Mr JO was discharged back to the care of his GP, attending the hospital for transplant outpatient appointments every 3 months.

Day 122 Mr JO presented to the renal unit as an emergency. He mentioned that he had recently been treated by his GP with clarithromycin for a chest infection. His urine output had fallen to 750 mL in the last 24 hours and he had become oedematous. He was prescribed IV furosemide 40 mg twice daily to relieve the oedema. A MAG3 scan showed deterioration of renal perfusion, but a biopsy of the transplant showed no evidence of rejection. Tacrolimus nephrotoxicity was diagnosed.

Serum biochemistry and haematology results were:

- Creatinine 380 micromol/L (60–120)
- WBC 5.3×10^9/L ($4.0–10.0 \times 10^9$)
- Tacrolimus level 27 nanograms/mL (5–15)

Q20 What could have caused tacrolimus toxicity?
Q21 Which drugs interact with tacrolimus?
Q22 How can tacrolimus nephrotoxicity be differentiated from rejection?

Day 540 Mr JO attended the transplant outpatient clinic for a routine 3-monthly check-up.

Serum biochemistry results were:

- Creatinine 197 micromol/L (60–120)
- Tacrolimus level 6.5 nanograms/mL (5–15)

He was admitted for a renal transplant biopsy, which showed evidence of chronic allograft nephropathy (CAN). The decision was made to change Mr JO's immunosuppression regimen and convert him from tacrolimus to sirolimus.

Q23 Why is sirolimus an appropriate immunosuppressive agent to use now?

Mr JO was prescribed a loading dose of 6 mg sirolimus orally, followed by a maintenance dose of 3 mg once daily. Concurrently, his tacrolimus dose was halved for 1 week, then stopped completely.

Q24 When should blood levels of sirolimus be measured?

Answers

How should these injections be administered?

A1 (a) **Basiliximab 20 mg in 50 mL sodium chloride 0.9% or glucose 5% over 20–30 minutes.**

Basiliximab should be reconstituted with 2.5 mL Water for Injection and then further diluted to be given by IV infusion. An alternative method of administration is by slow IV bolus injection over 2–3 minutes. The first dose should be given within the 2 hours prior to surgery, and the second 4 days after transplantation.

(b) **Co-amoxiclav 1.2 g in 100 mL sodium chloride 0.9% over 30–40 minutes.**

Again, an alternative method is by reconstitution with 20 mL Water for Injection, followed by administration by slow bolus injection over 3–4 minutes.

(c) Methylprednisolone 500 mg in 100 mL glucose 5% infused over at least 30 minutes.

The reconstituted solution may also be diluted with sodium chloride 0.9% or glucose/saline. It must be given slowly to minimise the cardiac arrhythmias, circulatory collapse and cardiac arrests associated with rapid infusions.

What are the therapeutic aims on return from theatre?

A2 **(a) Volume expansion using a combination of crystalloid fluids and blood/colloids.**

The latter are given to maintain a high central venous pressure (CVP). Clear fluids are given to replace the urine output volume for volume. HSA (human serum albumin) or Gelofusine are usually given as the colloid.

(b) Maintain good renal perfusion, using furosemide (10 mg/h) if the urine output is <50 mL/h and ensure Mr JO is volume replete.

Mannitol has been used in the past to obtain a diuresis, but it has been shown to have an osmotic effect on renal tubules, is itself nephrotoxic, and exacerbates the nephrotoxicity of tacrolimus and ciclosporin.

(c) Control any post-operative hypertension.

This will reduce the risk of fitting and/or renal damage.

(d) Treat any systemic vasoconstriction using vasodilators.
(e) Maintain adequate immunosuppression to prevent rejection.
(f) Avoid infection.
(g) Recheck plasma electrolytes (risk of rapidly rising potassium levels) and haemoglobin (to ensure Mr JO is not bleeding) on return from theatre.

Which immunosuppressant(s) would you recommend be prescribed subsequently, and why?

A3 **Mr JO should receive combined immunosuppressive therapy with tacrolimus, mycophenolate mofetil (MMF) and corticosteroids.**

Combining immunosuppressants provides a synergistic effect, allowing lower doses of each agent and a lower incidence of toxicity and rejection. Most centres use 'triple therapy' according to NICE guidelines, employing a combination of immunosuppressive agents, typically a calcineurin inhibitor (ciclosporin or tacrolimus) plus an anti-proliferative agent (azathioprine or MMF) plus steroids (prednisolone).

Rejection occurs when Mr JO's grafted kidney is recognised as 'foreign' and is attacked by his immune system. On recognition of the 'foreign' tissue, the lymphokine interleukin (IL-2) causes T lymphocytes in his lymph nodes to differentiate into T helpers (lymphocytes that provide information to B lymphocytes about the antigens), T-cytotoxic cells (killer lymphocytes that cause direct damage to 'foreign' cells) and T suppressors (which suppress B lymphocytes and prevent multiplication and antibody formation). Sensitised lymphocytes return to the graft site in large numbers, reacting with the antigenic material and releasing lymphokines ('messenger' substances), which attract macrophages to the site. These, together with T-cytotoxic cells, destroy the grafted kidney.

The risk of acute rejection is greatest in the first 3–6 months. After this period some kind of adaptive process appears to occur, although a patient may experience a rejection episode any time during the life of the transplant, especially if they omit to take their immunosuppressive medication. Once the risk of acute rejection is less, the doses of the immunosuppressive drugs are usually reduced down to maintenance levels. This reduces the incidence and severity of side-effects without compromising graft function.

Immunosuppression either reduces to ineffectiveness the number of cells reacting against the transplanted organ or it inhibits their normal function.

Prophylactic regimens against rejection vary between transplant centres. The main immunosuppressants used are ciclosporin; tacrolimus; azathioprine; prednisolone; MMF; sirolimus; polyclonal antibodies such as anti-thymocyte globulin (ATG); monoclonal antibodies such as basiliximab, alemtuzumab and OKT_3.

(a) **Ciclosporin.** This appears to act primarily by blocking the production of IL-2 by T-helper (Th) cells through inhibition of their messenger RNA. Unlike azathioprine it is not myelosuppressive. Ciclosporin is used initially at oral doses of 5–10 mg/kg/day (it has an oral bioavailability of the order of 30%), reducing over several months to maintenance doses as low as 3 mg/kg/day without an apparent increase in graft rejection. Individual patient handling of ciclosporin is very variable and doses must be tailored according to ciclosporin levels. Toxic effects include nephrotoxicity and hypertension as well as hirsutism, acne and gum hypertrophy.

(b) **Tacrolimus (FK506).** This is a macrolide immunosuppressant that suppresses T-cell activation and T-helper cell-dependent B-cell proliferation, as well as the formation of lymphokines such as IL-2 and IL-3, and beta-interferon through similar mechanisms to ciclosporin.

Oral absorption is estimated to be approximately 20% in kidney transplant patients. An initial dose of 0.1 mg/kg/day in two divided doses is generally used, again with the dose being adjusted according to blood levels. As with ciclosporin, the side-effects of tacrolimus include nephrotoxicity and hypertension; however, it does not cause the other more cosmetic side-effects of ciclosporin, and if anything may be associated with causing alopecia.

Studies comparing ciclosporin with tacrolimus as primary immunosuppressants following renal transplantation have shown tacrolimus to be the more potent of the two, and to be associated with a lower incidence of acute allograft rejection. Tacrolimus has been shown to cause nephrotoxicity, neurotoxicity and cardiotoxicity, although the incidence of these side-effects is much less with the lower doses now used in clinical practice.

(c) **Azathioprine.** This is metabolised to 6-mercaptopurine, which disrupts purine metabolism and consequently interferes with DNA synthesis and cell proliferation, thereby reducing lymphocyte function.

(d) **MMF.** This is a prodrug of mycophenolic acid, and acts by inhibiting the intracellular *de novo* pathway for purine synthesis. Most cells also possess a salvage pathway, but T lymphocytes do not, thereby rendering them unable to synthesise purines, which in turn prevents successful cell replication. MMF is therefore similar to azathioprine, but is more selective in its pharmacological effect. Its main side-effects are gastrointestinal upsets and increased susceptibility to infections, especially viral illnesses. Another formulation, mycophenolate sodium EC, is now available. It is purported to have a lower incidence of gastrointestinal side-effects, although the evidence does not support this claim.

(e) **Corticosteroids.** These have several possible mechanisms of action, which include anti-inflammatory activity (which profoundly alters the effector phases of graft rejection, including macrophage function), blocking the production of IL-1 and IL-2 (lymphokines), and causing the sequestration of circulating lymphocytes and monocytes in lymphoid tissue, particularly the bone marrow.

Adverse effects are commonly encountered and include cushingoid appearance, hypertension, hyperglycaemia, weight gain, increased susceptibility to infection and personality changes. Long-term complications include skin and muscle atrophy and avascular necrosis of bone.

(f) **Sirolimus** is a novel immunosuppressive agent that inhibits T-cell proliferation by inhibiting cytokine-mediated signal transduction pathways. It has been used in combination with ciclosporin and prednisolone to lower the incidence of early acute rejection. However, its place in therapy has now been defined by NICE guidelines as in the treatment of chronic rejection, or CAN. Side-effects include hyperlipidaemia, anaemia and severe aphthous ulceration.

(g) **Monoclonal antibodies**, e.g. basiliximab (chimeric) and daclizumab (humanised). These bind to the CD25 antigen on human T lymphocytes to prevent them from expressing IL-2, thereby inhibiting the activation of T-cytotoxic cells and hence effectively hiding the graft from the recipient's immune system, resulting in a reduced incidence of acute rejection. These agents are very expensive, but NICE guidelines recommended that they be given to all renal transplant recipients. OKT3 is a murine monoclonal antibody used only for the treatment of severe acute rejection unresponsive to other therapies. It is associated with side-effects such as rigors, high fever, abdominal pain and pulmonary oedema, and is rarely used nowadays. Alemtuzumab, a drug originally developed for the treatment of patients with B-cell chronic lymphocytic leukaemia (B-CLL), has also been used as part of the pre-conditioning regimen for bone marrow transplantation, and there is now increasing evidence that it can be successfully used at a low dose as induction therapy prior to solid organ transplantation. It is associated with side-effects such as infusion reaction and profound immune system suppression, with an increased susceptibility to infection.

(h) **Polyclonal antibodies**, e.g. ATG (rabbit). ATG removes circulating T lymphocytes and blocks their formation and proliferation in response to antigenic stimuli. It reacts with a wide variety of receptors on T cells. Before the advent of the newer monoclonal antibodies a 10-day course of low-dose ATG was given as induction therapy after a 'high-risk' transplant, but its use now tends to be reserved for salvage therapy in patients whose acute vascular rejection episodes are not responding to high-dose steroids.

How should therapy with a calcineurin inhibitor such as ciclosporin or tacrolimus be monitored?

A4 **By regular review of blood levels of the drug itself, glucose and potassium levels, liver function tests, plasma lipid levels, and blood pressure.**

(a) **Drug level monitoring.** Ciclosporin levels may be monitored in two ways:

(i) Trough levels should be taken before the morning dose every 2–3 days until therapy is stabilised, then monthly, or 2–3 days after any dosing change. Times to achieve peak levels are variable (1–6 hours after oral dosing); 12-hour trough levels provide more consistent results. The risk of rejection is greatest shortly after transplant, and pathophysiological changes occur rapidly. The half-life of ciclosporin has been reported to be 5–20 hours, and hence 2–3 days is the time usually required to achieve steady-state concentrations.

(ii) Profiling of the absorption of ciclosporin is a concept of therapeutic drug monitoring designed to further optimise the clinical efficacy of the drug while at the same time minimising adverse effects. A trough (C_0), followed by a single blood concentration measured 2 hours after ciclosporin administration (C_2) to determine the area under the curve (AUC) has been shown to be a significantly more accurate predictor of total drug exposure than trough concentrations alone. Although this would be the ideal way to monitor exposure to ciclosporin in all transplant patients, in practice it is difficult to achieve this in the outpatient clinic as it requires two blood samples to be taken exactly 2 hours apart. Hence its use is often restricted to the inpatient setting when initiating therapy.

Ciclosporin in blood distributes between erythrocytes (50%), leukocytes (10%) and plasma (40%). Whole blood, plasma or serum samples may be used, but quoted therapeutic ranges differ depending on the sample type and the assay method.

Several assay techniques are available: high-performance liquid chromatography (HPLC) is regarded as the gold standard, but is laborious and costly. Immunoassays such as EMIT and ELISA have been developed in order to measure microamounts of drugs in human biological fluids. Using a standard triple-therapy immunosuppression regimen, it is usual to aim for 12-hour ciclosporin trough levels of 250–350 nanograms/mL for the first 2 months, reducing to a target level of 150–250 nanograms/mL for the next 4–6 months. Thereafter, in a stable graft, levels of 100–150 nanograms/mL or less are acceptable. These levels vary according to local protocols.

(iii) Tacrolimus trough level (C_0) monitoring provides a good correlation with the AUC, although research has also been carried out to see whether C_2, C_3, C_4 and C_5 monitoring can provide a better correlation. In practice, 12-hour trough levels are routinely measured for tacrolimus, with most units aiming for whole blood levels of 10–15 nanograms/mL for the first 2 months post transplant, reducing over the following year so that by 12 months post transplant levels of 5–10 nanograms/mL are achieved. The half-life of tacrolimus has been reported to be 12–16 hours, so again 2–3 days is the time usually required to achieve steady-state concentrations, both on initiating therapy and after each dose change.

(b) **Liver function tests.** Reversible dose-related hepatotoxicity may be seen with both drugs, resulting in increases in serum bilirubin and liver enzymes.
(c) **Serum glucose levels.** Hyperglycaemia may develop as a result of ciclosporin, tacrolimus or concomitant corticosteroid therapy.
(d) **Serum potassium levels.** Toxic levels of ciclosporin or tacrolimus are often associated with hyperkalaemia.
(e) **Blood pressure monitoring.** Hypertension is frequently observed and has been associated with seizures. It is not generally dose related, but may result from the vasoconstrictive effects of these drugs.
(f) **Plasma lipid levels.** As ciclosporin and tacrolimus can both cause reversible increases in plasma lipids, serum cholesterol and triglycerides should be regularly monitored.

Are there any parameters that should be monitored when mycophenolate mofetil (MMF) is prescribed?

A5 MMF therapy is associated mainly with dose-dependent reversible bone marrow suppression, and with disturbances of the gastrointestinal tract.

Because of the risk of developing neutropenia, the patient should have a full blood count taken once a week for the first month of therapy, then every 2 weeks for months 2 and 3 of therapy, then monthly for the rest of the first year. If the patient develops neutropenia (defined as a neutrophil count $<1.3 \times 10^3$/microL), it may be appropriate to interrupt or discontinue MMF therapy. Patients should also be monitored for signs of infection, unexpected bruising, bleeding, or any other manifestations of bone marrow suppression.

MMF therapy is also associated with an increased risk of bacterial and fungal infection, especially viral infections. In addition, the patient will be more susceptible to opportunistic infections such as cytomegalovirus (CMV), and so should be appropriately monitored for signs of infection, e.g. by measuring CMV viral load by the quantitative Polymerase Chain Reaction (PCR) method.

Mycophenolate is well known to cause adverse effects such as nausea, vomiting and diarrhoea. There is also an increased risk of further gastrointestinal tract adverse events such as ulceration, haemorrhage and perforation.

Blood levels of the metabolite mycophenolic acid may be measured, although this is not routine practice in all transplant units. Typically a 12-hour trough level is measured, the therapeutic range being 2–4 micrograms/mL.

What other medications should be prescribed for Mr JO, and why?

A6 **As well as the immunosuppression therapy to prevent graft rejection, Mr JO will also require prophylactic therapy.**

Most transplant units have their own standard prophylaxis regimen, although they are all variations on an original theme. Typically, patients will be prescribed aspirin 75 mg daily, as there is evidence that the antiplatelet effect of low-dose aspirin helps to prevent thrombosis of the transplanted renal artery, thereby maintaining good perfusion of the transplanted kidney. Most units will also prescribe some form of gastric mucosal protection, either as ranitidine or as a proton pump inhibitor, as patients are initially on a relatively high dose of steroids and are also at increased risk of developing stress ulceration.

Other therapies that are frequently used include antifungal prophylaxis with either nystatin or amphotericin mouthwash or lozenges, and co-trimoxazole 480 mg daily for the prevention of *Pneumocystis carinii* (*Pneumocystis jirovici*) infection.

Some units maintain patients on vitamin D (alfacalcidol) therapy and erythropoietin injections for a month or so post transplant, as the synthetic functions of the kidney may take a while to work at full capacity and the patient may be at risk of exacerbating their renal bone disease or their renal anaemia. However, this practice is not universal, and other units stop these drugs immediately after transplantation. Many transplant patients will require statin therapy to reduce cholesterol levels. Concomitant therapy with a calcineurin inhibitor and a statin carries an increased risk of myositis or rhabdomyolysis, so the lowest possible dose of statin should be used and the patient carefully monitored for adverse effects.

Would you have recommended amlodipine as an antihypertensive for Mr JO?

A7 **Yes.**

Renal patients often have high renin profiles, resulting in systemic vasoconstriction and hypertension. Vasoconstriction may also be catecholamine mediated, and this may also partly explain the hypertension associated with ciclosporin therapy. Vasodilators are probably the most appropriate method of reducing the blood pressure acutely.

Amlodipine is a vasodilator and does not require dosage adjustment in renal failure. It has a longer duration of action than nifedipine, and tends not to be associated with some of the undesirable effects that nifedipine can cause, such as severe headache.

Research has indicated that calcium-channel blockers may cause increases in glomerular filtration rate (GFR) and renal blood flow, despite a substantial reduction in blood pressure. As vasoconstriction appears to play a role in acute as well as chronic ciclosporin-induced renal dysfunction, amlodipine may counteract these effects on renal vasculature. However, some patients on calcium-channel blockers develop marked vasodilation-dependent oedema, which may cause alarm by suggesting renal impairment.

IV antihypertensives such as glyceryl trinitrate, hydralazine and labetalol are usually reserved for more severe hypertension. Overzealous treatment of hypertension could compromise the function of the transplanted kidney by reducing renal perfusion.

How should Mr JO's acute rejection episode be managed?

A8 **Methylprednisolone 500 mg to 1 g IV in 100 mL of either glucose 5% or sodium chloride 0.9%, administered over 60 minutes once daily for 3 days.**

Acute rejection is most commonly seen 5–10 days post transplant. The three agents most frequently used to treat acute rejection are methylprednisolone and both monoclonal and polyclonal antibodies.

(a) **Methylprednisolone.** This is the cheapest alternative and has been demonstrated to reverse 72–83% of first allograft rejections. Up to two consecutive rejection episodes may be treated with this drug. Thereafter, concern for the cumulative corticosteroid dose given increases and other strategies need to be considered, depending on the degree of severity of the rejection as determined by transplant renal biopsy.

(b) **Monoclonal (OKT3) and polyclonal (ATG) antibodies**. These are very expensive and their use tends to be reserved either for third or subsequent rejection episodes, or for severe acute rejection not responsive to IV methylprednisolone. It should be noted that the chimeric/humanised monoclonal antibodies basiliximab and daclizumab are ineffective in the treatment of an established severe rejection episode.

Methylprednisolone 750 mg/day for 3 days is thus the preferred option for Mr JO's first rejection episode.

What precautions should be taken when starting ATG?

A9 (a) **A test dose of ATG (5 mg diluted in 100 mL 0.9% sodium chloride administered over 1 hour) is often given first. This is to check Mr JO's tolerance, as ATG has been associated with anaphylaxis, due to allergy to rabbit protein.**
(b) **Ensure that IV epinephrine (adrenaline), hydrocortisone and chlorphenamine are available and ready for use during administration of the first dose, in case they are required urgently.**
(c) **Administer ATG via a large vein, preferably a central line, to avoid thrombophlebitis and localised pain.**

How should the dose be calculated?

A10 **The initial dose is 1.5–2.5 mg/kg ATG (Genzyme brand) per day until the biological signs and symptoms improve. A typical course would be 5–10 days in duration. Each subsequent day's dosage is determined by monitoring the patient's full blood count, including WBC and lymphocytes. The aim is to maintain a WBC count of 2–4 × 10^9/L and a total lymphocyte count of 0.1–0.4 × 10^9/L. ATG dosing schedules vary with local protocols.**

Some centres administer ATG using alternate-day regimens to minimise the risk of neutropenia. If the total WBC is <3 x 10^9/L but >2 × 10^9/L , the next dose of ATG should be halved, but if the total WBC is <2 × 10^9/L, the next dose of ATG should be omitted.

Platelets should be similarily monitored during treatment and any thrombocytopenia <100 000/mm^3 necessitates halving the dose; a count <50 000/mm^3 will require interruption of treatment.

How should ATG be administered?

A11 **Each 25 mg vial should be diluted in 50 mL 0.9% sodium chloride, but in practice, on the prescriber's responsibility, a higher concentration (e.g. 1 mg/mL) may be administered, so that the sodium and fluid load is not too great for the patient.**

Alternatively, glucose 5% may be used as the diluent. The infusion should be administered over not less than 6 hours (usually 8–12 hours) via a large vein (preferably via a central line). A 0.22 micrometre inline filter should be used to avoid the inadvertent administration of particulate matter following reconstitution. Any associated fever or shivering may be relieved by administering chlorphenamine or hydrocortisone IV 1 hour prior to the infusion.

Should the doses of his other immunosuppressants be adjusted during ATG therapy?

A12 **Mr JO's MMF therapy should be reduced or stopped while the ATG course is in progress. Both drugs are myelosuppressive, and concurrent use may cause a marked leukopenia, necessitating the withdrawal of the ATG. The prednisolone and tacrolimus doses should initially be unchanged; however, 2 days before the end of the ATG course the prednisolone dose should be doubled, as practice has shown that episodes of acute rejection may occur shortly after stopping ATG.**

Immediately the ATG course finishes the MMF should be restarted at a reduced dose, which should be gradually increased (e.g. weekly) if the WBC count remains stable. The prednisolone therapy is then reduced back to the maintenance dose of 20 mg each morning. The tacrolimus should remain at the current dose, provided blood level monitoring indicates that this is still appropriate.

What pharmaceutical care plans should be made in preparation for Mr JO's discharge?

A13 **The pharmaceutical care plan for Mr JO should include the following:**

(a) Ensure there is agreement as to who will be responsible for Mr JO's community care. Some units continue to care for transplant patients, including the prescribing of all transplant medication for the first 3 months after discharge, whereas others transfer care back to the community immediately, in the context of a shared care protocol. If Mr JO's care is to be fully managed in the community it is essential that there is sufficient liaison with his local (regular) community pharmacist to ensure continuity of medication supply, and that there is a suitable shared care protocol in place which ensures that his GP is aware of Mr JO's current medication, the monitoring required, and of any clinically important drug interactions. Mr JO, his GP and his community pharmacist should be given information on how to obtain specialist advice, either from the renal pharmacy specialist or from the hospital renal team.

(b) Mr JO should receive appropriate discharge medication counselling to ensure that he understands the purpose of, and the directions given with, his medication. It is good practice for patients to be given an accurately written treatment record card. The packaging of the medication should be appropriate to Mr JO's needs. It is important to check whether any adherence aids are necessary.

How long should Mr JO remain on immunosuppressants?

A14 **Immunosuppressive therapy can rarely be stopped completely after transplant. Even the briefest cessation may precipitate an acute rejection episode; however, intensive immunosuppression is usually only required for the first few weeks post transplant or during a rejection crisis. Subsequently the graft may often be maintained on much lower doses of immunosuppressive drugs, and hence fewer adverse drug effects are experienced by the patient.**

In addition, the aim of immunosuppressive therapy nowadays is to tailor the drug regimen to the needs of the individual patient, in order to maximise efficacy and at the same time minimise side-effects. Although acute rejection episodes are not as common and are easily treated, even modern immunosuppressive agents appear to have little effect on chronic rejection – or, as it is now known, chronic allograft nephropathy (CAN). The precise mechanism of this process is not fully understood, but there is some evidence that long-term use of some immunosuppressive drugs such as ciclosporin or tacrolimus may contribute to the process. Long-term use of these agents is also known to be nephrotoxic, so there is now a move to switch patients to agents with an antiproliferative effect, such as sirolimus or mycophenolate, which theoretically will prevent the histological changes seen in CAN and so prolong the life of a transplanted kidney.

How long is Mr JO likely to require concomitant prophylactic therapy?

A15 **Omeprazole therapy is likely to continue while Mr JO remains on high-dose prednisolone. Some units discontinue such therapy once the patient is down to a maintenance dose of 5 mg daily, whereas others continue with therapy indefinitely. Other prophylactic agents such as amphotericin and co-trimoxazole are likely to be stopped 3–6 months post transplant, once the patient is on lower doses of maintenance immunosuppression. Prophylactic oral amphotericin may be needed if Mr JO requires any further courses of antibiotics.**

What points would you cover when counselling Mr JO about his medication?

A16 **In addition to explaining the purpose of each drug the following information should be given:**

(a) MMF:

(i) Although it was initially recommended that MMF be taken on an empty stomach, this is now not thought to be as important, and indeed, many patients take their MMF after food to minimise gastrointestinal adverse effects. In addition, as the most common side-effect of MMF is diarrhoea, many patients have found it useful to split the dose and take it as 500 mg four times daily, to minimise the incidence of diarrhoeal episodes.

(ii) Mr JO should report any unusual bleeding or bruising, as this could indicate bone marrow suppression.

(b) **Tacrolimus:**

(i) Try to maintain a consistent schedule with regard to the time of day the tacrolimus is taken. Ideally, twice-daily regimens should be taken at regular 12-hourly intervals. Maximal absorption is achieved if tacrolimus is taken on an empty stomach; however, many patients find this difficult and prefer to take their doses with meals. This is acceptable, provided the patient is consistent and always takes their tacrolimus either on an empty stomach or after a meal. The capsules should be swallowed with fluid, preferably water. Grapefruit juice should be avoided as it contains the flavonoid naringenine, which inhibits cytochrome P450 3A4, thereby increasing blood tacrolimus levels.

(ii) Try to make early morning clinic appointments if tacrolimus blood levels are to be monitored. Do not take that morning's dose until the blood sample has been taken. This will ensure a trough serum level is measured.

(c) **Prednisolone:**

(i) Take at approximately the same time each day, preferably in the morning in order to mimic diurnal production of endogenous steroids.

(ii) Always carry a steroid card. It must also be ensured that Mr JO understands the written instructions on the card.

(d) **Omeprazole:** Take one dose daily, either in the morning or at night.

(e) **Amphotericin lozenges:** Take at regular intervals throughout the day. Suck the lozenges slowly, and if taken near to meal times, suck after meals rather than before.

(f) **Aspirin:** Take one tablet each day, with or after food. The tablet may be dispersed in water, or can be swallowed whole, whichever the patient finds easiest.

(g) **Co-trimoxazole:** Take one tablet each day until advised by the renal unit that treatment is no longer necessary.

(h) **General:** Do not discontinue any of the medication unless advised by the doctor.

Mr JO should be particularly advised to seek further expert advice, either from the community pharmacist or from the hospital specialists if over-the-counter medications are required. He should keep all his medication out of the reach of children and report to the doctor any signs of infection, including sore throats.

What has predisposed Mr JO to infection?

A17 **Corticosteroids, MMF and tacrolimus all increase Mr JO's susceptibility to infection. In addition, Mr JO had recently undergone a course of ATG, which would impair his lymphocyte function and hence his resistance to infection for several months afterwards.**

What types of infection is Mr JO susceptible to?

A18 **During the first 1 or 2 months post transplantation patients are susceptible to most opportunistic infections.**

Mr JO could develop fungal infections (e.g. *Candida, Aspergillus*), protozoal infection (e.g. *Pneumocystis carinii* pneumonia (PCP)), viral infection (e.g. CMV, herpes) or common or uncommon bacterial infections (including reactivation of past tuberculosis). He could also contract common illnesses such as flu more easily than usual, and find it harder to recover from such infections.

CMV disease is very common in renal transplant patients, especially in the first few months. It is characterised by a swinging fever and can manifest as pneumonitis, accompanied by breathlessness and blood oxygen desaturation, interstitial shadowing on the chest X-ray, and a reduced platelet and WBC count. Other organs that can be affected are the liver (causing CMV hepatitis, with raised liver enzymes), the gastrointestinal tract (causing acute diarrhoea) and the bone marrow (resulting in severe bone marrow depression).

What course of treatment would you recommend?

A19 **CMV disease may be treated with either IV ganciclovir or with oral valganciclovir. Foscarnet is extremely nephrotoxic and should not be used unless the patient has failed to respond to a prolonged course of ganciclovir therapy. Ganciclovir is renally excreted, so the dose will have to be adjusted according to Mr JO's renal function.**

Estimating Mr JO's creatinine clearance does not pose quite the same problems as in the immediate post-transplant period, as his serum creatinine results now appear more stable. However, the Cockcroft and Gault formula is not always accurate in transplant patients, because they have only one functioning kidney. Mr JO's estimated creatinine clearance is 76 mL/min, but a 24-hour urine collection measured his GFR as 63 mL/min.

For patients with this level of renal function it is recommended that the appropriate dose of ganciclovir is 5 mg/kg twice a day, given IV in 100 mL sodium chloride 0.9% over 1 hour. As treatment will last at least 14 days, insertion of a central line may be advisable. If Mr JO was well enough to be treated as an outpatient, he might be prescribed valganciclovir 900 mg twice daily orally (unlicensed indication). During treatment, Mr JO's renal function and full blood count should be closely monitored to detect signs of ganciclovir toxicity. It would also be wise to reduce temporarily or to discontinue the dose of MMF, as its use can hinder the immune response to viruses, making it much harder to eradicate them effectively.

What could have caused tacrolimus toxicity?

A20 **Co-administration of clarithromycin and tacrolimus.**

Acute reversible nephrotoxicity has been associated with tacrolimus levels >20 nanograms/mL, although it can occur at levels much lower than this. Mr JO's tacrolimus levels may have been increased by concomitant clarithromycin therapy. Studies in healthy adults suggest that clarithromycin can substantially reduce the plasma clearance of tacrolimus, by inhibition of the cytochrome P450 3A4 system. Patients who experience tacrolimus toxicity often exhibit a fine tremor and are found to be hypertensive, owing to vasoconstriction within the kidney. It is also worth noting that it is most unlikely that the administration of IV furosemide 40 mg worsened Mr JO's established tacrolimus nephrotoxicity. Only diuretic doses large enough to cause a marked hypovolaemia would be likely to have such an adverse effect.

Which drugs interact with tacrolimus?

A21 (a) **Drugs reported to increase the nephrotoxicity of tacrolimus include aciclovir, ganciclovir, aminoglycosides, amphotericin B, co-trimoxazole, ciprofloxacin, furosemide (and other potent diuretics), cephalosporins, vancomycin, gyrase inhibitors and non-steroidal anti-inflammatory drugs.**

(b) **Drugs reported to increase tacrolimus levels, by inhibition of metabolism, include clarithromycin, erythromycin, ketoconazole, fluconazole, itraconazole, methylprednisolone, protease inhibitors, tamoxifen, omeprazole, danazol, diltiazem and verapamil.**

(c) **Drugs reported to reduce tacrolimus levels, by induction of metabolism, include phenytoin, phenobarbital, carbamazepine, rifampicin, metamizole and isoniazid.**

(d) **Tacrolimus is extensively bound to plasma proteins, so there is the possibility of interactions with other drugs known to have high affinity for plasma proteins, e.g. oral anticoagulants and oral antidiabetic agents.**

How can tacrolimus nephrotoxicity be differentiated from rejection?

A22 Tacrolimus nephrotoxicity is difficult to differentiate from organ rejection.

Differentiation is necessary to determine whether an increased or reduced dose of immunosuppressants is required.

Rejection is usually associated with fever, low urine output, a rapidly rising serum creatinine level, graft tenderness or enlargement and MAG3 scans that show reduced renal perfusion. Tacrolimus levels are usually low or within the trough reference range, and on further reduction of the dose there is either no change or a worsening of renal function.

Tacrolimus toxicity is usually associated with an afebrile patient, low urine output, slowly or rapidly increasing creatinine levels, non-tender grafts and MAG3 scans that show reduced renal perfusion. Serum potassium levels may be high and the patient may be hypertensive. Tacrolimus levels are usually high (>15–20 nanograms/mL) and reduction of the tacrolimus dose improves renal function.

The differentiation of the two is, however, often unclear and histological examination is frequently required. This may reveal renal tubular atrophy and interstitial scarring in the case of tacrolimus toxicity. Small blood vessels (arterioles) may show nodular thickening. The mechanism for tacrolimus nephrotoxicity is unclear, but one proposal is that the drug reduces renal perfusion by interfering with renal prostaglandin release, which may explain any accompanying hyperkalaemia. Tacrolimus toxicity usually responds to a reduction in dose; however, if it appears that the patient is exhibiting signs of toxicity even though the blood levels are not particularly high, then the intolerant patient may be switched to an alternative agent, e.g. sirolimus.

Why is sirolimus an appropriate immunosuppressive agent to use now?

A23 Sirolimus is a second-generation immunosuppressant. It is an mTOR (mammalian Target of Rapamycin) inhibitor which is also known as rapamycin. Despite its similar name, it is not a calcineurin inhibitor (CNI) like tacrolimus or ciclosporin. However, it has a similar suppressive effect on the immune system. Sirolimus

inhibits the response to interleukin-2 (IL-2) and thereby blocks the activation of T and B cells. In contrast, tacrolimus and ciclosporin inhibit the production of IL-2.

As CAN evolves there are two distinct phases. The initial phase shows early tubulointerstitial damage from ischaemic injury, evidence of prior severe rejection and subclinical rejection; the later phase is characterised by microvascular and glomerular injury. Progressive luminal narrowing, increasing glomerulosclerosis and additional tubulointerstitial damage are associated with the use of CNIs. Once this damage is established it is irreversible, resulting in declining renal function and ultimately graft failure.

The chief advantage of sirolimus over the calcineurin inhibitors is that it is not toxic to kidneys. Because of its antiproliferative effects it can impair wound healing and cause wound dehiscence, so it tends not to be used in the immediate post-transplant period; however, there is now a large body of evidence which demonstrates that switching from a CNI-based to a sirolimus-based immunosuppression regimen can impede the progression of CAN, and in some cases even reverse some of the damage to the graft. NICE guidance stipulates that these are exactly the circumstances under which sirolimus is to be prescribed. As Mr JO is exhibiting signs of CAN, switching him from tacrolimus to sirolimus would be a logical decision in an attempt to preserve the function of his graft.

When should blood levels of sirolimus be measured?

A24 **Sirolimus has a long half-life (53–63 hours), so it will take approximately 1 week to reach steady state.**

It is recommended that when initiating therapy, and after each dose change, a minimum of 7 days elapse before blood levels are checked. Levels should then be checked at weekly intervals until the patient is in the desired therapeutic range. Once the patient has been stabilised on this therapy, levels need only be checked at each clinic visit. As with other immunosuppressive agents, trough levels are measured: in this case 24-hour trough levels, as sirolimus is taken once daily. Again, Mr JO should be advised not to take his sirolimus on the days he is coming to clinic until he has had his blood tests taken.

Further reading

Andrews PA. Renal transplantation. *Br Med J* 2002; **324**: 530–534.

Ashley C, Currie A. *Renal Drug Handbook*, 3rd edn. Radcliffe Medical Press, Oxford, 2008.

British Transplantation Society. *Guidelines for the Prevention and Management of Cytomegalovirus Disease after Solid Organ Transplantation,* 2nd edn. British Transplantation Society, London, 2004.

British Transplantation Society. *Standards for Solid Organ Transplantation in the United Kingdom.* British Transplantation Society, London, 2003.

Dantal J, Soulillou JP. Immunosuppression drugs and the risk of cancer after organ transplantation. *N Engl J Med* 2005; **352**: 1371–1373.

Djamali A, Samaniego M, Muth B *et al.* Medical care of kidney transplant recipients after the first post-transplant year. *J Am Soc Nephrol* 2006; **1**: 623–640.

Fellstrom B. Risk factors for and management of post-transplant cardiovascular disease. *BioDrugs* 2001; **15**: 261–278.

Halloran PF, Melk A. Tailoring therapy: balancing toxicity and chronic allograft dysfunction. *Transplant Proc* 2001; **33**(suppl. 3A): 7S–10S.

Hariharan S, McBride MA, Cherikh WS *et al.* Post-transplant renal function in the first year predicts long-term kidney transplant survival. *Kidney Int* 2002; **62**: 311–318.

Nankivell BJ, Borrows RJ, Fung CLS *et al.* The natural history of chronic allograft nephropathy. *N Engl J Med* 2003; **349**: 2326–2333.

National Institute for Health and Clinical Excellence. TA85: *Immunosuppressive Therapy for Renal Transplantation in Adults.* NICE, London, 2004.

Pascal M, Theruvath T, Kawai T *et al.* Strategies to improve long-term outcomes after renal transplantation. *N Engl J Med* 2002; **346**: 580–590.

Taber DJ, Dupuis RE. Solid organ transplantation. In: *Applied Therapeutics: The Clinical Use of Drugs,* 8th edn. MA Koda-Kimble, LY Young, WA Kradjan *et al.,* eds. Lippincott Williams & Wilkins, Philadelphia, 2004: 35.1–35.50.

Tsunoda SM, Aweeka FT. Drug concentration monitoring of immunosuppressive agents. *BioDrugs* 2000; **14**: 355–369.

11

Asthma

Helen Thorp and Toby Capstick

Case study and questions

Day 1 Miss SN, a 24-year-old beauty therapist, was brought in at 11 am by ambulance from her place of work. On admission she was severely short of breath, drowsy, and unable to speak more than a couple of words at a time.

Miss SN had been complaining of flu-like symptoms and a worsening cough for the past few days. That morning she had started to complain of increasing difficulty in breathing. She had been seen to use her inhalers several times, and had started to panic and then collapsed. The paramedic diagnosed an asthma attack and administered a 2.5 mg dose of salbutamol via a nebuliser, with some improvement in shortness of breath, and 35% oxygen via a face mask.

Miss SN was able to confirm that she had a past medical history of asthma. On examination she was tachypnoeic (respiratory rate of 28 breaths per minute) and tachycardic (140 beats per minute (bpm)). Her blood pressure was 150/95 mmHg with no paradoxus. On auscultation her chest was almost silent. Her peak expiratory flow (PEF) was unrecordable. Chest X-ray showed no areas of consolidation and excluded a diagnosis of pneumothorax. After 15 minutes of 35% oxygen in the ambulance her oxygen saturation (SpO_2) was 85% and her arterial blood gases were:

- PaO_2 6.7 kPa (reference range 10.0–13.3)
- $PaCO_2$ 3.7 kPa (4.67–6.0)
- pH 7.47 (7.35–7.45)
- HCO_3 22 mmol/L (22–26)

Neurological observations were normal, as was her temperature (36.6°C). Her white cell count was 6.5×10^9/L ($4–10 \times 10^9$/L).

Miss SN was immediately given 60% oxygen via a high-flow mask and an intravenous (IV) sodium chloride 0.9% drip was started. She was moved to an acute medical ward and the following drugs were prescribed:

- IV hydrocortisone 200 mg immediately, then 100 mg 6-hourly
- Salbutamol 5 mg nebulised six times a day with 6 L oxygen/min
- Ipratropium 500 micrograms nebulised four times a day, with 6 L oxygen/min
- IV co-amoxiclav 1200 mg three times a day
- IV aminophylline 250 mg immediately followed by 1 g in 1 L sodium chloride 0.9% to run over 24 hours

Q1 What important signs and symptoms of a life-threatening exacerbation of asthma does Miss SN exhibit?
Q2 Outline a pharmaceutical care plan for Miss SN.
Q3 Did the treatment received by Miss SN comply with current guidelines regarding the management of life-threatening asthma? Would you recommend any adjustments or alterations to her prescribed therapy?
Q4 Which parameters would you want to monitor during the acute phase of Miss SN's asthma attack?

The patient's mother arrived on the ward and was able to expand on Miss SN's past medical history and the events that had resulted in her being admitted to hospital.

The family had a history of atopy, with Miss SN's father and brother both having asthma. Miss SN had been well until the last few days, when she had complained of feeling 'fluey' and had suffered from a barking cough, especially during the night. She also sometimes found it difficult to catch her breath, especially after exercise. She had bought some cough medicine which had no real effect, and so had seen her general practitioner (GP) who had prescribed a green inhaler. She commented that Miss SN had previously been given a brown inhaler by her GP, which she had refused to take as she had heard that steroids can cause weight gain and thinning of bones and skin.

Q5 Was it appropriate for Miss SN's GP to prescribe a salmeterol inhaler?

By 8 pm Miss SN was feeling better and was able to give a history. She could remember feeling very short of breath that morning, and using both her salmeterol inhaler and her salbutamol inhaler several times with no effect. She said that she had been using her salbutamol inhaler at least 10 times a day in the last week or so. Her PEF was now 140 L/min. Miss SN had never monitored her PEF at home. Her oxygen saturation was 92% and her arterial blood gases were now:

- PaO_2 10.7 kPa (10.0–13.3)
- $PaCO_2$ 4.7 kPa (4.67–6.0)
- pH 7.44 (7.35–7.45)
- HCO_3 23 mmol/L (22–26)

Q6 Was Miss SN correct to administer several doses of her inhalers as her attack worsened?

Q7 What is a PEF, and what is its role in the management of an asthmatic patient?
Q8 Can a 'normal' PEF be predicted for Miss SN?

Day 2 The junior doctor decided to restart a beclometasone inhaler. Her pre-nebuliser PEF was 120 L/min, compared to 220 L/min 15 minutes after her 6 am nebulised therapy. It was therefore decided to continue ipratropium and aminophylline for at least another 12 hours. Following continuous administration of 60% oxygen her oxygen saturation was now 98%, so the oxygen prescription was changed to 'when required'. Miss SN was now on the following:

- IV hydrocortisone 100 mg 6-hourly
- Salbutamol 5 mg nebulised six times a day using a compressor
- Ipratropium 500 micrograms nebulised four times a day using a compressor
- Beclometasone (Qvar) metered-dose inhaler (MDI) 50 micrograms/puff, two puffs twice a day
- IV aminophylline 1 g over 24 hours
- 60% oxygen when required

Her theophylline level was reported as 23 mg/L (10–20 mg/L).

Q9 What alterations would you recommend be made to Miss SN's acute therapy now?
Q10 Is the initial choice of beclometasone inhaler more appropriate than other inhaled corticosteroids (ICSs) for Miss SN?
Q11 How can the pharmacist contribute to optimising the administration of inhaled therapy?
Q12 How would you address Miss SN's concerns about the risks of ICSs so that she can make a more informed decision about taking her preventer therapy?

Later that afternoon the junior doctor rang to say that the IV aminophylline was being discontinued. He asked what oral dose he should prescribe.

Q13 What advice would you offer?

Day 3 Miss SN felt much better, almost back to her normal self. Her PEF was coming up but still showed quite a difference between pre- and post-nebuliser therapy (255 and 325 L/min, respectively). On the ward round, the new Registrar asks how they should step up her therapy.

Q14 What are the roles of long-acting beta$_2$-agonists (LABAs), leukotriene receptor antagonists and increasing doses of ICSs in the treatment of asthma?
Q15 What would you recommend be prescribed for Miss SN?

Day 5 Miss SN's PEF continued to improve and stabilised around 460 L/min. She felt completely back to normal and was eager to go home. On the ward round there was discussion as to whether a Symbicort maintenance and reliever regimen (Symbicort SMART) would be appropriate for Miss SN.

Q16 Is it appropriate that Miss SN be allowed home now?
Q17 Would you recommend Symbicort maintenance and reliever therapy (Symbicort SMART) as a suitable option for Miss SN?

Day 6 Miss SN was allowed home after being back on her inhaled bronchodilator therapy for 24 hours. An asthma action plan was discussed with her before she left. Her discharge prescription was:

- Salbutamol MDI 100 micrograms/puff, two puffs four times daily and when required
- Seretide 125 MDI, two puffs twice daily via spacer
- Prednisolone 40 mg each morning for 5 more days, then stop
- Peak flow meter and chart

Q18 What are the key elements of an asthma action plan?
Q19 How would you counsel Miss SN on her discharge medication?
Q20 How should Miss SN's pharmaceutical care be continued over the next few months?

Answers

What important signs and symptoms of a life-threatening exacerbation of asthma does Miss SN exhibit?

A1 **An unrecordable peak expiratory flow (PEF), a near-silent chest and severe hypoxia despite 35% oxygen therapy.**

The British Thoracic Society/Scottish Intercollegiate Guidelines Network (BTS/SIGN) guidance on the management of asthma aims to alert doctors to the importance of recognising the key features of the condition and to respond appropriately with optimum treatment. These guidelines are summarised in the latest *British National Formulary* (BNF).

Many, if not most, hospital admissions for acute severe asthma are preventable, as are most asthma deaths (1381 reported in 2004 in the UK). The severity of an asthma attack is often underestimated by the patient, their relatives and/or their doctors, largely because of failure to make objective measurements. In many cases the patient will have been deteriorating over the preceding few days: this is typically seen as a reduction in PEF measurement, an increase in diurnal variation of the PEF (particularly morning 'dipping'), and an increase in symptoms such as shortness of breath and cough.

Miss SN exhibited all the features of acute severe asthma (PEF <50% predicted, tachypnoea, tachycardia and inability to complete sentences), but the presence of one or more additional factors leads to a diagnosis of a life-threatening attack. First, her PEF was unrecordable. Patients often say they are too short of breath to perform a PEF and then, when encouraged, produce a reasonable result. A PEF should always be taken, even if it is unrecordable, as this is a valuable clinical indicator of attack severity. However, this should not delay urgent therapy. A silent chest indicates poor air entry into the lungs (as a result of bronchoconstriction). Despite 35% oxygen therapy, Miss SN was hypoxic on admission although she had not progressed to retaining CO_2, which can result from exhaustion and failing respiratory effort. Instead, her $PaCO_2$ was slightly low, denoting hyperventilation.

Outline a pharmaceutical care plan for Miss SN.

A2 **The pharmaceutical care plan for Miss SN should include the following:**

(a) Optimise initial medical management of her life-threatening exacerbation of asthma as outlined in the BTS/SIGN guidelines, by advising the medical staff on the following:

(i) Appropriate dosage regimen of nebulised bronchodilators
(ii) Role and choice of antibiotics
(iii) Appropriate dosage calculation and administration of IV aminophylline
(iv) Therapeutic drug monitoring of aminophylline and appropriate dosage adjustment
(v) Prescribing and administration of other medications for the treatment of a life-threatening exacerbation of asthma.

(b) Advise the nursing staff on the following:

(i) Administration of nebulised bronchodilators
(ii) Administration of IV antibiotics
(iii) Administration of IV aminophylline.

(c) Monitor Miss SN's response to treatment (see **A4**).
(d) Monitor for signs of adverse drug reactions.
(e) Review and advise on maintenance therapy once Miss SN is over the acute exacerbation.

(f) Provide information and education to Miss SN on all aspects of asthma and her medication:

(i) Use of preventer and reliever inhalers
(ii) Inhaler technique
(iii) Asthma action plans and use of PEF meters
(iv) Lifestyle advice, such as allergen avoidance, coping with coughs, colds and hay fever.

Did the treatment received by Miss SN comply with current guidelines regarding the management of life-threatening asthma? Would you recommend any adjustments or alterations to her prescribed therapy?

A3 Miss SN's initial treatment partly complied with current recommendations.

The current BTS/SIGN guideline recommends appropriate prescriptions for life-threatening asthma. Miss SN's therapy should be compared with them.

(a) **Oxygen.** Death as a consequence of an asthma exacerbation is most commonly due to hypoxaemia and should be rapidly corrected. High concentrations of oxygen (usually 40–60% using a high-flow mask) should be administered, as there is little danger of causing hypercapnia (which might occur in chronic obstructive pulmonary disease). The nebuliser should also be driven by oxygen, rather than air. If arterial blood gases had revealed hypercapnia this would indicate the development of near-fatal asthma and the need for emergency intervention and consideration for ICU admission. Miss SN remained hypoxic despite 35% oxygen in the ambulance, so it was vital that a higher percentage was administered on admission. The 60% oxygen started in A&E was appropriate. Oxygen saturations above 94–98% should be aimed for.

(b) **Beta$_2$-agonist bronchodilators** should be administered immediately in high doses (e.g. nebulised salbutamol 5 mg or terbutaline 10 mg) and repeated 4–6-hourly. The aim is to rapidly relieve bronchospasm. In mild to moderate exacerbations of asthma there is no difference in efficacy between repeated administration of inhaled beta$_2$-agonist via an MDI with a large-volume spacer compared to nebulised administration; however, if there are life-threatening features, nebulised administration should be used and IV beta$_2$-agonists should be reserved for patients in whom inhaled therapy cannot be reliably used, such as when patients are coughing excessively. Patients with severe asthma (PEF or forced expiratory volume in one minute (FEV_1) <50% best or predicted) who have responded poorly to an initial bolus dose of beta$_2$-agonist should be considered for continuous nebulisation. However, there is no evidence that this is likely to be more effective in relieving acute asthma.

(c) **Corticosteroids** should be administered in adequate doses for all patients with acute asthma because they reduce mortality, relapse rates, subsequent hospital admissions and the requirement for beta$_2$-agonist therapy. The earlier they are given in an acute attack, the better the outcome. There is no difference in efficacy between oral and parenteral steroid treatment, so steroid tablets should be used in all patients who are able to swallow and retain them and have no problems with absorption. Prednisolone 40–50 mg daily or hydrocortisone 100 mg every 6 hours should be prescribed for at least 5 days, or until recovery. The dose does not need to be tapered unless the patient has been taking steroids for more than 3 weeks or has been taking a maintenance dose of steroids. IV hydrocortisone may be appropriate initially if Miss SN is so breathless that she has difficulty swallowing, but this should be switched to oral prednisolone as soon as possible.

There is no benefit in adding high doses of inhaled corticosteroids (ICSs) to the systemic steroid prescription, although any usual ICS therapy should be continued or restarted as soon as possible to ensure that the long-term asthma management plan is adhered to.

(d) **Ipratropium bromide** is not as effective as beta$_2$-agonists as an initial bronchodilator and may not be beneficial in mild exacerbations of asthma; however, it should be prescribed in combination with beta$_2$-agonists in patients with acute severe or life-threatening asthma, or those with a poor initial response to beta$_2$-agonist therapy, as greater bronchodilation may be achieved than with a beta$_2$-agonist alone.

(e) **IV magnesium sulphate** (1.2–2 g over 20 minutes) has been shown in a placebo-controlled trial to produce significant improvements in mean FEV$_1$ in patients with severe asthma exacerbations, but not in those with mild exacerbations, although it does not affect airway hyperresponsiveness. IV magnesium should be given to patients with acute severe asthma with a poor initial response to inhaled bronchodilator therapy, and to those with life-threatening or near-fatal asthma. Miss SN should therefore be prescribed IV magnesium.

(f) **IV aminophylline** is unlikely to provide any additional bronchodilation compared to treatment with inhaled bronchodilators and steroids, and has many undesirable adverse effects. However, some patients with life-threatening or near-fatal asthma may gain some additional benefit, so it may be justified for Miss SN. However, the dose prescribed is not appropriate. Unless the patient takes maintenance oral therapy a 5 mg/kg loading dose given over 20 minutes should be prescribed. This ensures that a steady-state concentration of theophylline is achieved rapidly. The loading dose should be followed by a continuous infusion of 500–700 micrograms/kg/h, adjusted according to daily serum theophylline levels. It is therefore important that Miss SN's weight is known, or at least estimated with a high degree of confidence, to ensure that an appropriate dose is prescribed.

(g) **Antibiotics** are not routinely indicated for acute asthma because infections that precipitate an acute attack are likely to be viral. Miss SN is apyrexial, has a normal white cell count, and has no signs of consolidation on the chest X-ray. Therefore the prescription of co-amoxiclav is inappropriate and should be challenged.

Which parameters would you want to monitor during the acute phase of Miss SN's asthma attack?

A4

(a) PEF before and after nebulised or inhaled beta$_2$-agonist therapy, at least four times a day, throughout her hospital stay.

(b) Arterial blood gases. These should be repeated within 30–60 min of starting treatment, as the initial PaO_2 is <8 kPa, and again if not improved 4–6 hours later.

(c) Oxygen saturation by oximetry to maintain SpO_2 >94–98%.

(d) Blood theophylline level, aiming for a concentration of 10–20 mg/L. The level can be measured 6 hours after the loading dose to ensure it is not toxic, then daily thereafter to ensure therapeutic efficacy and absence of toxicity.

(e) Blood potassium level: steroids, beta$_2$-agonists and aminophylline therapy can all cause hypokalaemia.

(f) Blood glucose level: this may be elevated by corticosteroids in susceptible individuals.

(g) Pulse and respiratory rate.

Was it appropriate for Miss SN's GP to prescribe a salmeterol inhaler?

A5 **No.**

It is not appropriate to prescribe a long-acting beta$_2$-agonist (LABA) such as salmeterol without also prescribing an inhaled steroid. A large multicentre study compared the safety of salmeterol to usual care in 26 355 asthma patients who had not previously received salmeterol. The study was terminated early when an interim analysis revealed a small but statistically significant increased risk of respiratory-related and asthma-related deaths in patients who had been treated with salmeterol compared to those who had been treated with placebo. The Commission on Human Medicines (CHM) advise that LABAs should:

(a) Be added only if regular use of standard-dose ICSs has failed to control asthma adequately.
(b) Not be initiated in patients with rapidly deteriorating asthma.
(c) Be introduced at a low dose and the effect properly monitored before considering a dose increase.
(d) Be discontinued in the absence of benefit.
(e) Be reviewed as clinically appropriate: stepping down therapy should be considered when good long-term asthma control has been achieved.

Miss SN was starting to show signs of uncontrolled asthma, with recent onset of night-time symptoms and worsening of daytime symptoms. Such patients are at significant risk of developing acute severe asthma. According to the BTS/SIGN guidelines Miss SN had previously been managed at Step 1, i.e. occasional use of relief bronchodilators. As her control had begun to deteriorate, her GP should have stepped up her treatment and the logical action would have been to add an inhaled steroid (Step 2). The current guidelines recommend a starting dose of 400 micrograms daily of beclometasone given via an MDI or equivalent in adults with mild to moderate asthma.

It is possible that the GP's decision to prescribe salmeterol had been influenced by the fact that Miss SN had previously refused to use an ICS because of her perception of weight gain and thinning of bones and skin with these medicines. It would have been more appropriate to allay her fears through education about the low risk of systemic adverse effects from ICS and the benefits of treatment. It is clear that this has not happened, and that she failed to understand that her asthma was deteriorating. Her GP should perhaps have also initiated regular PEF monitoring, and a short course of oral steroids might have been valuable in preventing this acute episode.

Was Miss SN correct to administer several doses of her inhalers as her attack worsened?

A6 Yes, but only of her salbutamol inhaler.

The BTS/SIGN guidelines recommend the administration of 4–10 puffs (given one at a time) of a short-acting beta$_2$-agonist MDI via a large-volume spacer, using tidal breathing repeated at intervals of 10–20 minutes. The patient's response to this treatment should be monitored to determine the next appropriate course of action, such as prescribing a short course of prednisolone or admission to hospital for further treatment and observation.

The use of repeated doses of salmeterol will not be helpful because there is no additional benefit achieved by increasing the dose above 50 micrograms twice daily, although adverse effects will be increased.

It is clear that Miss SN did not recognise the severity of her condition and had not sought urgent medical attention. One of the elements of an asthma action plan (see **A18**) should address this issue.

What is a PEF, and what is its role in the management of an asthmatic patient?

A7 **The PEF is the highest flow achieved from a maximum forced expiratory manoeuvre started without hesitation from a position of maximal lung inflation. Changes in PEF are an important indicator of an asthmatic patient's clinical status and as such are a key element of any asthma action plan.**

It is important that the patient is encouraged to produce the maximal force of expiration that she can manage, otherwise inaccurate values may be recorded. PEF monitoring can easily be undertaken by the patient at home using a PEF meter (prescribable on FP10) and provides a useful self-assessment tool. Measurements should be undertaken twice a day, morning and evening, before inhaled therapy. The results should be recorded on a peak flow monitoring chart (FP1010, available from nhsforms.co.uk) or a PEF diary (available from Asthma UK) which can then be reviewed by the doctor. Patients should be taught to recognise signs of deteriorating asthma, namely a sustained reduction in PEF value and/or a 25% or greater diurnal variation between morning and evening values, with the lower reading occurring characteristically in the morning (morning 'dipping'). Such changes are often the first signs that a patient's asthma is becoming uncontrolled.

Can a 'normal' PEF be predicted for Miss SN?

A8 **It is not possible to predict a 'normal' PEF for an asthmatic patient.**

The 'predicted normal' PEF for a non-asthmatic person is related to height, age and gender, and can be obtained from various 'predicted normal' PEF charts; however, an asthmatic patient of the same height, age and gender may have a best PEF considerably lower than the values in the chart. It is therefore important for asthmatic patients to establish their own record of monitoring so that comparisons to their own best recording can be made. In the newly diagnosed asthmatic the 'predicted normal' PEF can be used as a level to aim for. For a known asthmatic, predicted PEF should only be used if the recent best (within 2 years) is unknown.

What alterations would you recommend be made to Miss SN's acute therapy now?

A9 (a) **Change her steroid therapy from the IV to the oral route.**
(b) **Adjust the dose of IV aminophylline to bring it into the therapeutic range and thus avoid the development of symptoms of toxicity.**

Miss SN is now much improved after 24 hours in hospital. She no longer needs to be given IV steroids and should be converted to a once-daily dose of oral prednisolone (40–50 mg) in the morning: in fact, this change could have taken place the previous evening.

Miss SN's plasma theophylline level is slightly high, although she is not showing any symptoms of theophylline toxicity. Theophylline exhibits first-order pharmacokinetics, so it is possible to calculate a dose to bring the theophylline level into the therapeutic range using the formula:

$$\frac{S \times F \times \text{dose}}{T} = C_{SS} \times CL$$

where S = salt factor (0.79 for aminophylline), dose = dose (in mg), F = bioavailability factor, T = dosage interval (in hours), C_{SS} = average plasma concentration at steady state and CL = clearance.

In this case F is a constant (with a value of 1) because the drug is being given IV, therefore:

$$\frac{0.79 \times 1 \times 1000 \text{ mg}}{24} = 23 \text{ mg/L} \times CL$$

thus CL = 1.43 L/h (for this patient).

To give an average theophylline concentration of 15 mg/L then:

$$\frac{0.79 \times 1 \times \text{dose}}{24} = 15 \times 1.43$$

thus the dose = 652 mg/24 h. This could be rounded down to 650 mg for ease of administration.

Alternatively, it should be realised that as S, F, T, and CL are all constant, the above formula can be rearranged to:

$$\frac{\text{dose}}{C_{SS}} = \frac{CL \times T}{S \times F}$$

Therefore, the calculation for the new infusion rate can be simplified to:

$$\frac{\text{dose}_1}{C_{SS_1}} = \frac{\text{dose}_2}{C_{SS_2}}$$

where dose_1 and C_{SS_1} refer to the current infusion rate and serum theophylline level, and dose_2 and C_{SS_2} refer to the required infusion rate and target serum theophylline level. Therefore:

$$\text{dose}_2 = \frac{\text{dose}_1 \times C_{SS_2}}{C_{SS_1}} = \frac{1000 \times 15}{23} = 652 \text{ mg/24 h.}$$

The need for continued nebulised ipratropium and IV aminophylline should also be reviewed as these two drugs can often be discontinued once the patient has recovered significantly from the acute event.

Is the initial choice of beclometasone inhaler more appropriate than other inhaled corticosteroids (ICSs) for Miss SN?

A10 To date, no significant clinical advantages between different ICS have been demonstrated. The choice of ICS needs to be made on an individual patient basis, taking into consideration the choice of inhaler device and cost.

Meta-analysis of ICS use has shown that Qvar beclometasone is dose equivalent to fluticasone and mometasone but requires half the dose of budesonide and chlorofluorocarbon (CFC)-beclometasone to provide equal clinical activity. The difference between Qvar beclometasone and CFC-beclometasone is due to the delivery of smaller particles, which improves lung deposition. This is not true for all non CFC-beclometasone products. Some meta-analyses have demonstrated small improvements in FEV_1 and morning PEF with fluticasone, but the clinical significance of this is not clear. The 2008 NICE appraisal concluded that when comparing ICS at equivalent low or high doses there was no difference between them in terms of effectiveness.

It is appropriate to start Miss SN on Qvar beclometasone as a first-line ICS at Step 2 of the BTS/SIGN guidelines, provided she can use the device effectively.

How can the pharmacist contribute to optimising the administration of inhaled therapy?

A11 The pharmacist can have a key role in the selection of the most appropriate inhaler device for each individual patient and in counselling on its correct use.

Many studies have shown that inhaler technique is frequently poor, even after verbal instruction and demonstration.

Patients with asthma should only be prescribed inhalers after they have received training and education on how to use them and have demonstrated satisfactory technique, as this will ensure that they obtain maximum benefit from therapy. Inhaler counselling requires patience and tact, and the patient's beliefs and opinions should be respected when deciding on the appropriate device to prescribe.

In order to obtain the maximum benefit from different inhaler devices it is important to ensure that each patient can achieve the optimum inspiratory flow rate for their inhaler. This can be determined using an In-Check DIAL inspiratory flow meter (Clement Clarke Ltd, Harlow, UK), which mimics the internal resistance of a range of inhaler devices, allowing the measurement of inspiratory flow rate and ensuring the patient can inhale through a device at its optimal inspiratory flow rate. Optimum inspiratory flow rates for common devices are:

(a) MDIs 25–90 L/min.
(b) Turbohalers 60–90 L/min.
(c) Accuhalers 30–90 L/min.

A frequent error made by 26–70% of patients using MDIs is failure to inhale slowly and deeply: increasing inspiratory flow rate from 37 to 151 L/min using an MDI reduces total lung deposition from 11.2% to 7.2%. Conversely, reducing the inspiratory flow rate through a turbohaler from 60 to 30 L/min will reduce lung deposition by 50%.

Inhaler technique is not solely dependent on inspiratory flow. Use of an MDI requires the patient to remember to shake the canister, and to have good coordination and dexterity to ensure that actuation, inhalation and breath-holding occur in the correct sequence. Patients with poor coordination, or who are unable to hold their breath, or who cough while using their MDI (the 'cold Freon' effect caused by the impact of the cold propellant on the back of their throat), should use a large-volume spacer. This can increase lung deposition, reduce coughing and overcome problems with breath-holding by acting as a holding chamber for the aerosol. This allows the patient to inhale their medication over several breaths, which also makes coordination less of an issue. However, spacers can be large and cumbersome and make the patient feel conspicuous, and so they may not use them.

Dry powder devices are often easier to use and frequently preferred by patients, although they are generally more expensive than MDIs and require the patient to hold their breath. Other devices that can be used to assist inhaler technique training include the 2-Tone Trainer (Canday Medical Ltd), Turbohaler Trainer Whistles (Astra Zeneca), the MAG-FLO inhaler trainer (Fyne Dynamics), or the aerosol inhalation monitor (AIM) machine (Vitalograph Ltd).

When ICS are inhaled it is important that the patient is advised to rinse their mouth with water to prevent local adverse effects such as oral candidiasis. The use of the MDI with a large-volume spacer will also reduce oropharyngeal deposition, which further reduces the risk of oral candidiasis, particularly when large doses are required.

How would you address Miss SN's concerns about the risks of ICSs so that she can make a more informed decision about taking her preventer therapy?

A12 It is important to discuss with Miss SN the benefits of ICS against their potential risks.

There is little evidence that doses below 800 micrograms (CFC-beclometasone or equivalent) per day cause any short-term detrimental effects apart from dysphonia and oral candidiasis, side-effects that can be minimised by following the advice in A11. The possibility of long-term side-effects from ICS is still unknown. Higher doses of ICS have been associated with a low but increased risk of systemic adverse effects such as adrenal suppression (<1/10 000), but the extent of such effects is poorly quantified. Systemic effects are much less likely with ICS than with repeated doses of oral steroids for asthma exacerbations. The need for oral steroids should also be reduced by the use of ICS as a preventer. To minimise risks Miss SN's ICS should be titrated to the lowest dose that controls her asthma.

What advice would you offer?

A13 There is no indication to convert Miss SN to oral theophylline at this stage.

Oral theophylline should initially be considered in patients who need to move up to Steps 4–5 of the BTS/SIGN guidelines, i.e. when asthma is not adequately controlled on a combination of an ICS (800 micrograms daily of beclometasone CFC-MDI) and an additional drug, usually a long-acting beta$_2$-agonist. Occasionally oral theophylline may be prescribed at Step 3 of the BTS/SIGN guidelines if a patient's asthma is not adequately controlled on ICS (800 micrograms daily), and has failed to respond at all to a long-acting beta$_2$-agonist.

The junior doctor should be advised to reduce the aminophylline infusion rate slowly over the next few hours.

What are the roles of long-acting beta$_2$-agonist (LABAs), leukotriene antagonists and increasing doses of ICSs in the treatment of asthma?

A14 **LABAs (salmeterol/formoterol) are synthetic sympathomimetic bronchodilators. They are structurally and pharmacologically similar to the short-acting beta$_2$-agonist salbutamol and are licensed for the treatment of reversible airway obstruction in patients with asthma who are inadequately controlled on ICSs.**

Leukotriene antagonists (montelukast/zafirlukast) selectively block the action of leukotrienes on the respiratory tract, resulting in an anti-inflammatory and a bronchodilator action. Evidence supports their use as potential add-on agents in asthma uncontrolled by inhaled steroids.

LABAs have a prolonged duration of action of 12 hours, compared to 4–6 hours for salbutamol. A meta-analysis demonstrated that the addition of a LABA to a low-dose ICS reduced the risk of exacerbations by 19%, improved lung function, increased the number of symptom-free days and reduced the requirement for rescue short-acting beta$_2$-agonist therapy. The addition of a LABA achieves a similar reduction in the risk of exacerbations as increasing the ICS dose, but results in a greater improvement in lung function, an increased number of symptom-free days, and a reduced requirement for rescue short-acting beta$_2$-agonist therapy. As discussed earlier, LABAs are not a replacement for inhaled steroids and nor should they be used for the relief of acute attacks. An important counselling point to discuss with patients receiving LABAs is the differences between these and salbutamol.

Leukotriene receptor antagonists are more effective than placebo, but should be prescribed in combination with an ICS. A meta-analysis comparing leukotriene receptor antagonists with ICSs demonstrated that patients taking the former were 65% more likely to experience asthma exacerbations, although a similar benefit on improved lung function, symptoms and reduced rescue medication use was observed. The addition of leukotriene receptor antagonists to ICSs produces modest improvements in lung function; however, LABAs produce greater benefit and have a 17% lower risk of exacerbation than leukotriene receptor antagonists. In aspirin-allergic asthmatics improvements in pulmonary function and symptoms may be achieved when montelukast is added to inhaled steroids. Leukotriene receptor antagonists used in combination with intranasal corticosteroids may also be effective for symptomatic relief of seasonal allergic rhinitis.

In summary, asthmatic patients who are inadequately controlled on low-dose ICSs should also be prescribed a LABA (Step 3 of the BTS/SIGN guidelines). If asthma control remains suboptimal the inhaled steroid dose should then be increased before treating at Step 4. If there is no response to the LABA, it should be stopped and the inhaled steroid dose increased; consideration can also be given to adding in a leukotriene receptor antagonist.

What would you recommend be prescribed for Miss SN?

A15 There is unlikely to be a definite correct answer to this question. A combination of ICS and LABA may well be appropriate.

Prior to the onset of Miss SN's symptoms of deteriorating asthma control she was prescribed only a salbutamol inhaler at Step 1 of the BTS/SIGN guidelines. Therefore, it could be argued that she has not yet been treated with an ICS and so should continue on Qvar (Step 2 of the BTS/SIGN guidelines) and her symptom control and treatment reviewed in the outpatient clinic after discharge. However, it is important to prescribe treatment that is appropriate to the severity of a patient's asthma symptoms, with the aim of achieving early control before stepping down when control is good. Consequently, it may be more appropriate to prescribe treatment for Miss SN at Step 3 of the BTS/SIGN guidelines, and step-down if control is achieved and sustained over a few months.

Using this rationale Miss SN should be prescribed a combination inhaler containing an ICS and a LABA. The choice of which of the available products to prescribe (Seretide, Fostair or Symbicort) will depend on her ability to use the device, her preference and the cost. There is little evidence to support the addition of a leukotriene receptor antagonist at this stage. Approximately 3 months is an appropriate period to review the control of her asthma (preferably by using PEF and symptom diaries) before considering whether to step down her treatment. Polypharmacy should be avoided wherever possible, as it may adversely affect adherence.

Is it appropriate that Miss SN be allowed home now?

A16 No. Patients should not usually be discharged from hospital until their symptoms have cleared and their PEF has stabilised.

A guide to this is when the PEF is >75% of the predicted or best value, diurnal variability is <25% and there are no nocturnal symptoms. Patients should also be on the medical therapy they will continue at home. As Miss SN has obviously improved it would be appropriate to discuss changing her nebulised therapy back to standard inhaler devices at this time.

Would you recommend Symbicort maintenance and reliever therapy (Symbicort SMART) as a suitable option for Miss SN?

A17 Possibly not at this stage.

The basis for prescribing Symbicort maintenance and reliever therapy (Symbicort SMART) relies on the fact that formoterol has an onset of action (3–5 mins) that is comparable to that of salbutamol and, unlike salmeterol with an onset of action of 15–30 minutes, can thus be used as a reliever medicine. A comparison of fixed-dose Seretide plus salbutamol as needed versus Symbicort SMART (200/6, one or two inhalations twice daily plus one inhalation as needed) in 2143 asthmatic patients demonstrated that Symbicort SMART significantly reduced the annual exacerbation rate compared to regular Seretide use. Despite the fact that patients can use additional doses of their Symbicort as needed, the mean equivalent ICS dose was not significantly different between the two groups, and there was less need for rescue medication in the Symbicort SMART group. Consequently, Symbicort SMART is a cost-effective treatment regimen.

However, it is important that patients who are prescribed Symbicort SMART are carefully selected and receive clear education. There are several groups of patients for whom this treatment regimen may be inappropriate, for example those who may be poorly adherent to their medication (particularly if they worry about side-effects from their ICSs). Patients who are unable to monitor their asthma control adequately are unlikely to be able to adjust the dose of their Symbicort independently, and patients who overuse their short-acting $beta_2$-agonist because of poor perception of their symptoms should not use this regimen.

Symbicort SMART may be inappropriate for Miss SN because she has previously been poorly adherent with her prescribed asthma treatment and has been reluctant to use her ICS.

What are the key elements of an asthma action plan?

A18 The key elements to an asthma action plan are:

(a) Instructions on how to recognise symptoms of good, worse and severe asthma
(b) Instructions on when to use a reliever inhaler (e.g. short-acting $beta_2$-agonist) and, if necessary, when to increase the dose of the preventer inhaler (e.g. ICS) as symptom control starts to worsen
(c) Instructions on the prompt use of a reliever inhaler and when to take a course of oral corticosteroids at the onset of severe symptoms
(d) Instructions on how to monitor response to treatment

(e) Information on when to seek assistance or follow-up review to assess asthma control
(f) Useful contact numbers (e.g. doctor or nurse).

All patients admitted to hospital with an exacerbation of their asthma should be offered a written, personalised asthma action plan. Asthma action plans have been shown to reduce hospital admissions, emergency room visits, days off work or school, nocturnal asthma symptoms, and to improve quality of life.

There is no consensus about the exact components of an asthma action plan, although the key elements above are frequently suggested. It is important for the plan to be discussed with, and individualised for, each patient.

The patient should be advised of the aims of asthma treatment in terms of symptom control and their best peak-flow readings. Patients should check and record their peak flow regularly, as this helps to give an objective measure of asthma control, and the severity of an exacerbation can then be determined by expressing their peak flow as a percentage of their best value. Action plans need to instruct patients on the action to take following worsening symptoms, or when their peak flow has dropped below a pre-specified value. A final important component of an action plan is to advise the patient to seek urgent medical attention when treatment is not working.

A number of generic asthma action plans are available, e.g. 'Be in Control' Asthma UK.

How would you counsel Miss SN on her discharge medication?

A19 Miss SN should by now have received extensive counselling from the multidisciplinary team, including the pharmacist, caring for her in the hospital. There are, however, some specific points related to her medication that should be discussed at discharge.

(a) It should be emphasised that Miss SN is being asked to use her reliever (salbutamol) regularly four times a day and also when required for an initial short period of time following discharge. This regular use of her reliever should be reviewed after a suitable period. If Miss SN responds well to the Seretide inhaler she may only need to use her reliever intermittently and prophylactically, e.g. before exercise.

(b) It should be explained that the spacer used with Miss SN's Seretide (preventer) may be used with the salbutamol reliever during an acute exacerbation in conjunction with her asthma action plan (see **A18**). However, it should be stressed that this is not a substitute for seeking urgent medical attention.

(c) The need to complete the course of oral steroids should be emphasised. Prednisolone should be taken for 5 days or until recovery, therefore it is reasonable for Miss SN to be discharged with a short course. This treatment should be explained in light of the co-prescription of inhaled steroids. Any worries regarding the safety or adverse effects from short courses of oral steroids should be addressed.

(d) The importance of regular use (twice a day) of her preventer Seretide inhaler should be reiterated.

(e) It should be checked that Miss SN knows how to use the PEF meter and chart.

How should Miss SN's pharmaceutical care be continued over the next few months?

A20 **By ensuring good communication between secondary and primary health carers, continual assessment of her condition, and by reinforcing education as necessary.**

Good communication with Miss SN's GP is essential. Information supplied to her GP should include PEFs on admission and discharge, details of medication changes and treatment to be continued at home, plus a copy of any asthma action plan discussed in the hospital. All patients should be followed up in a hospital clinic within 1 month of discharge, in addition to follow-up by the GP or asthma nurse within 2 working days.

Community and hospital outpatient pharmacists are in an ideal position to offer reinforcement of education to patients such as Miss SN when they return for repeat inhaler prescriptions.

Miss SN is currently being managed according to Step 3 of the BTS/SIGN guidelines, but continual assessment of her asthma control is essential, not only to ensure stepping up of treatment if necessary, but also to review stepping down when possible. The BTS/SIGN guidelines emphasise the importance of considering stepping down treatment in well-controlled patients to ensure that they are not inappropriately overtreated. In particular, patients should be maintained on the lowest possible dose of corticosteroid: a reduction in dose should be considered every 3 months, reducing the dose by approximately 25–50% each time.

Further reading

Asthma UK. www.asthma.org.uk

Adams N, Lasserson TJ, Cates CJ *et al. Fluticasone versus Beclometasone or*

Budesonide for Chronic Asthma in Adults and Children. Cochrane Database of Systematic Reviews 2007, Issue 4.

Braganza G, Thomson NC. Acute severe asthma in adults. *Medicine* 2008; **36**: 209–212.

British Thoracic Society. *Burden of Lung Disease*, 2nd edn. A report compiled by the Lung and Asthma Information Agency, St George's, University of London, 2006. Available from www.brit-thoracic.org.uk

British Thoracic Society/Scottish Intercollegiate Guidelines Network. British Guideline on the management of asthma. June 2009. Available from www.brit-thoracic.org.uk

Capstick T. What do respiratory function tests tell us? *Pharm Pract* 2007; **17**: 233–237.

Cochrane MG, Bala MV, Downs KE *et al*. Inhaled corticosteroids for asthma therapy: Patient compliance devices and inhalation technique. *Chest* 2000; 117: 542–550.

Commission on Human Medicines. *Asthma: Long-Acting Beta2 Agonists*. Safety information published online and available from www.mhra.gov.uk.

Corrigan C. Mechanisms of asthma. *Medicine* 2008; **36**: 177–180.

Ducharme FM, Di Salvio F. *Anti-Leukotriene Agents Compared to Inhaled Corticosteroids in the Management of Recurrent and/or Chronic Asthma in Adults and Children*. Cochrane Database of Systematic Reviews 2004, Issue 1.

Ducharme FM, Lasserson TJ, Cates CJ. *Long-Acting Beta2-Agonists versus Anti-Leukotrienes as Add-On Therapy to Inhaled Corticosteroids for Chronic Asthma*. Cochrane Database of Systematic Reviews 2006, Issue 4.

Ducharme F, Schwartz Z, Kakuma R. *Addition of Anti-Leukotriene Agents to Inhaled Corticosteroids for Chronic Asthma*. Cochrane Database of Systematic Reviews 2004, Issue 1.

Gibbs KP, Cripps D. Asthma. In: *Clinical Pharmacy and Therapeutics*, 4th edn. R Walker, C Whittlesea, eds. Churchill Livingstone, Edinburgh, 2007: 367–385.

Gibson PG, Powell H, Coughlan J *et al*. *Self-Management, Education and Regular Practitioner Review for Adults with Asthma*. Cochrane Database of Systematic Reviews 2002, Issue 3.

Gibson PG, Powell H, Ducharme F. *Long-Acting Beta2-Agonists as an Inhaled Corticosteroid-Sparing Agent for Chronic Asthma in Adults and Children*. Cochrane Database of Systematic Reviews 2005, Issue 4.

Haldar P, Pavord ID. Diagnosis and management of adult asthma. *Medicine* 2008; **36**: 201–208.

Lenny J, Innes JA, Crompton GK. Inappropriate inhaler use: assessment of use and patient preference of seven inhalation devices. *Resp Med* 2000; **94**: 496–500.

Lenny W. Asthma in Children. *Medicine* 2008; **36**: 196–200.

Miller MR, Hankinson J, Brusasco V *et al*. Standardisation of Spirometry. *Eur Respir J* 2005; **26**: 319–338.

Murphy A. *Asthma in Focus*. Pharmaceutical Press, London, 2007.

National Institute for Health and Clinical Excellence. TA138. *Inhaled Corticosteroids for the Treatment of Chronic Asthma in Adults and in Children Aged 12 Years and Over*. NICE, London, 2008.

Nelson HS, Weiss S T, Bleeker ER *et al.* The Salmeterol Multicentre Asthma Research Trial: A comparison of usual pharmacotherapy for asthma or usual pharmacotherapy plus salmeterol. *Chest* 2006; **129**: 15–26.

Newman S, Steed K, Hooper G *et al.* Comparison of gamma scintigraphy and pharmacokinetic technique for assessing pulmonary deposition of terbutaline sulphate delivered by pressurized metered dose inhaler. *Pharm Res* 1995; **12**: 231–236.

Ni Chroinin M, Greenstone IR, Danish A *et al. Long-Acting Beta2-Agonists versus Placebo in Addition to Inhaled Corticosteroids in Children and Adults with Chronic Asthma*. Cochrane Database of Systematic Reviews 2005, Issue 4.

O'Driscoll BR, Howard LS, Davidson AG on behalf of the British Thoracic Society. BTS guideline for emergency oxygen use in adult patients. *Thorax* 2008; **63**(suppl 6): vi1–vi68.

Vogelmeier C, D'Urzo A, Pauwels R *et al.* Budesonide/formoterol maintenance and reliever therapy: an effective asthma treatment option? *Eur Respir J* 2005; **26**: 819–828.

12

Chronic obstructive pulmonary disease

Anna Murphy

Case study and questions

Day 1 Mr LT, a 68-year-old man, attended his general practitioner's (GP's) surgery for a routine check-up. He had been diagnosed with asthma 5 years earlier when he had first become short of breath on exertion (although there was no record of any objective testing having been carried out). He had had no history of breathing problems as a child but had been a heavy smoker, smoking approximately 20 cigarettes a day since he was 14 years old, although he had stopped completely 2 years earlier. He lived with his wife in a bungalow and had retired from his job as a factory storekeeper at the age of 60.

Since his diagnosis his condition had deteriorated. He became short of breath after he had walked only 500 metres or climbed one flight of stairs, and he had a chronic cough that produced approximately one tablespoon of sputum on a daily basis. Mr LT had recently had a chest infection that had been successfully treated with a course of antibiotics.

His current drug treatment was:

- Montelukast 10 mg once daily at night
- Co-amilofruse 5/40 two tablets once daily
- Beclometasone dipropionate chlorofluorocarbon (CFC)-free (Clenil) 100 microgram metered-dose inhaler (MDI), two puffs twice daily
- Salbutamol 100 microgram MDI, two puffs when required for shortness of breath
- Simple Linctus, 5 mL when required

His surgery had contacted him to review his condition, prompted by the fact that he had requested four salbutamol inhalers every month for the last year and had not used his beclometasone inhaler for several months. Spirometry was performed. His spirometry results were as follows:

- Forced expiratory volume (FEV_1) 0.95 L
- Predicted FEV_1 2.70 L
- FEV_1 % predicted 35%
- Forced vital capacity (FVC) 1.53 L
- FEV_1/FVC 0.62 (62%)
- FEV_1 post salbutamol 0.99 L

In view of his spirometry results, symptoms and history, Mr LT was diagnosed with chronic obstructive pulmonary disease (COPD).

Q1 What are the clinical similarities and differences between a patient with asthma and one with COPD?
Q2 What factors do you think contributed to Mr LT's developing COPD?
Q3 A person's smoking history can be quantified by calculating their pack years. What is Mr LT's smoking history in pack years?
Q4 What do Mr LT's spirometry results tell us about his disease?
Q5 In light of Mr LT's revised diagnosis would you recommend any changes to his therapy?
Q6 How would you decide if an intervention to his therapy had helped?

Mr LT was started on ipratropium 20 micrograms, 2 puffs four times a day via an MDI with a spacer device. Mr LT questioned whether this would be better given to him via a nebuliser.

Q7 Many COPD patients ask for home nebulisers. What is the place of nebulisers in the management of COPD?

Day 30 Mr LT struggled to the surgery for his follow-up appointment. He admitted to having felt unwell for the last 5 days, with increasing dyspnoea and wheeze. He had a cough productive of yellow/green sputum and swelling of the ankles. His wife said he had become too breathless to speak or eat, and today had been delirious. He could not walk further than from the chair to the toilet.

His GP referred him to the hospital and he was admitted to a medical ward via A&E. On examination he was centrally cyanosed. His chest was initially silent, but after one dose of salbutamol 5 mg by nebulisation coarse crackles could be heard at the right base. He was diagnosed as having a right basal pneumonia with deterioration of his COPD. An arterial blood sample was sent for analysis of blood gases, with the patient breathing 35% oxygen by face mask.

Mr LT's blood gas results were:

- Blood pH 7.26 (reference range 7.32–7.42)
- $PaCO_2$ 10.21 kPa (4.5–6.1)
- PaO_2 10.23 kPa (12–15)
- Standard bicarbonate 29.2 mmol/L (21–25)

The following drug therapy was written up:

- Intravenous (IV) aminophylline 1 g in 1 L sodium chloride 0.9% to be given by continuous infusion over 24 hours
- Salbutamol 5 mg every 4 hours via a nebuliser
- Ipratropium bromide 500 micrograms every 4 hours via a nebuliser
- Hydrocortisone 100 mg IV every 6 hours
- Ceftriaxone 2 g IV once daily

Serum biochemistry and haematology results were:

- Sodium 141 mmol/L (137–150)
- Potassium 5.2 mmol/L (3.5–5.0)
- Urea 5.4 mmol/L (2.5–6.6)
- Haemoglobin 17.7 g/dL (14–18)
- White blood cells (WBC) 18.1×10^9/L ($4–11 \times 10^9$)

Mr LT was thought to be fluid depleted and was prescribed 1 unit of polygeline IV infusion to be given over 30 minutes, followed by 2 L of glucose/saline infusion, each litre to be given over 8 hours.

Q8 What do Mr LT's history, symptoms and blood gases indicate about his respiratory disease?
Q9 What are the immediate therapeutic priorities for Mr LT?
Q10 Outline the key elements of a pharmaceutical care plan for Mr LT.
Q11 Do you agree with the choice of agents to treat Mr LT's respiratory condition? Comment on the doses prescribed.
Q12 What would you tell a nurse who had never administered salbutamol or ipratropium by nebuliser before?

Day 32 (Inpatient day 2) Mr LT's condition started to improve, with little breathlessness and wheezing at rest, minimal coughing and sputum production, and no cyanosis. Following continuous administration of 28% oxygen his arterial oxygen concentration was 12 kPa, so the oxygen prescription was changed to 'when required'. He was apyrexial and only scattered rhonchi could now be heard in both lungs. A repeat chest X-ray still showed some increased shadowing at the right base. Aminophylline was continued by the IV route, with the infusion rate unchanged. The patient was noted to be shaking.

Q13 Could Mr LT's drug therapy be causing his tremor?

Day 33 (Inpatient day 3) On the ward round Mr LT's salbutamol dosage was reduced as suggested to 2.5 mg by nebuliser every 6 hours.

His serum theophylline concentration was reported to the ward as 15.8 mg/L (10–20). His IV aminophylline therapy was stopped and oral theophylline was prescribed.

Q14 How would you recommend IV aminophylline be converted to oral theophylline?

Day 35 (Inpatient day 5) Mr LT was now on the following regimen:

- Prednisolone 30 mg once daily every morning
- Salbutamol nebuliser solution, one 2.5 mg nebule four times daily via a nebuliser
- Salbutamol 100 microgram MDI, two puffs when required
- Ipratropium nebuliser solution, one 500 microgram nebule four times daily via a nebuliser
- Theophylline 400 mg slow-release tablets, one tablet twice daily
- Amoxicillin 500 mg three times daily for 7 days
- Tiotropium 18 micrograms once daily via a handihaler device

Q15 Is the prescribing of a long-acting anticholinergic appropriate for Mr LT? Is there any therapy that should be discontinued?

Day 37 (Inpatient day 7) Because a degree of cor pulmonale was present, with ankle oedema and ECG (electrocardiogram) abnormalities (large P waves and right axis deviation), Mr LT was started on furosemide 40 mg, one tablet each morning. His oxygen saturations were noted to be 91% on air.

Q16 Is this treatment appropriate for Mr LT's cor pulmonale? What alternative therapies could be prescribed?

Day 40 (Inpatient day 10) A pre-dose serum theophylline level was reported as 19.6 mg/L (10–20). Mr LT was noted to have a significant tremor.

Q17 Would you recommend any change in his theophylline dosage?

Day 41 (Inpatient day 11) Mr LT's respiratory condition was greatly improved and his ankle swelling had diminished significantly on furosemide. He was discharged on the following medication:

- Furosemide 40 mg once daily in the morning
- Prednisolone 10 mg once daily in the morning for 7 days, then stop
- Theophylline 300 mg slow-release tablets one twice daily
- Salbutamol 100 microgram MDI, two puffs when required
- Tiotropium 18 micrograms daily via a handihaler device
- Salbutamol 2.5 mg four times daily via a nebuliser PRN

He was given an outpatient appointment for 6 weeks later.

Q18 Would there be any advantage in continuing Mr LT's oral steroid therapy long term? Would inhaled steroid therapy be more appropriate?

Q19 What points would you discuss with Mr LT when counselling him on his take-home medication?

Day 70 Mr LT attended the outpatient department. He was reasonably well, able to walk around the house, and dress and wash himself. He was still short of breath on exertion, with some ankle oedema and a few rhonchi at both bases. The doctor prescribed a further inhaler containing both a steroid and a long-acting beta$_2$-agonist, and Mr LT was advised to use this on a regular basis twice a day. He was warned that he might need antibiotics should he get another chest infection, and the nurse provided him with a self-management plan to guide him should he have another exacerbation of his COPD.

Q20 How should Mr LT be advised on the self-management of his COPD?

Q21 Would you recommend that Mr LT receive continuous antibiotic prophylaxis? If so, which agents would you recommend, and at what dose?

Answers

What are the clinical similarities and differences between a patient with asthma and one with COPD?

A1 **Both asthma and COPD are major chronic obstructive airways diseases that involve underlying airway inflammation. They can present in similar ways, but it is important to distinguish between the two as the pharmacological management is very different.**

COPD is characterised by airflow limitation that is not fully reversible, is usually progressive, and is associated with an abnormal inflammatory response of the lungs to noxious particles or gases. In COPD there is permanent damage to the airways. The narrowed airways are 'fixed', and so symptoms are chronic (persistent). In contrast, episodes of asthma are usually associated with widespread but variable airflow obstruction which is often reversible. In asthma, symptoms come and go and are of varying severity. Many asthmatics are completely asymptomatic for much of the time. Table 12.1 will help to explain the differences between asthma and COPD.

If the features above are considered alongside Mr LT's history it can be seen that he exhibits a picture of COPD rather than asthma. He was a heavy smoker and his symptoms started later in life, at the age of 63, after

Table 12.1 Clinical features differentiating COPD and asthma

Feature	*COPD*	*Asthma*
Smoker or ex-smoker	Yes, nearly all	Maybe
Chesty child	Maybe	Often
Symptoms under the age of 35	Rare	Often
Chronic productive cough	Common	Uncommon
Breathlessness	Persistent and progressive	Variable
Onset of breathlessness	Gradual	Paroxysmal
Night time waking with breathlessness and/or wheeze	Uncommon	Common
Significant diurnal or day-to-day variability of symptoms	Uncommon	Common
Eczema and rhinitis	No correlation	Common, especially in children

having had no breathing problems as a child. In addition, his condition has deteriorated over the years, with a gradual and persistent increase in breathlessness and now the production of sputum on a daily basis.

What factors do you think contributed to his developing COPD?

A2 **Mr LT has a significant smoking history, and this is most likely to have led to the development of his COPD. His occupation should also be explored in more detail, as this too may have contributed to his disease.**

COPD is overwhelmingly smoking related. Although it can occur in non-smokers, this is rare. A significant smoking history for COPD is 15–20 pack years. However, not all smokers are at risk. The popular perception that only 15–20% of smokers develop COPD is being challenged, and the proportion may actually be as high as 50%. What determines whether people are affected or not is still not understood. The number of cigarettes smoked is important, and people who start smoking early seem more likely to develop COPD. It is likely that an individual's genetic make-up is one of the contributory factors.

One inherited cause of COPD is deficiency of the protective enzyme α-antitrypsin. This deficiency renders the individual susceptible to the damaging effects of cigarette smoke; however, it is rare and accounts for <1% of all cases of COPD. Other identified risk factors are unlikely to cause clinically significant, symptomatic COPD on their own, but when combined with smoking in a susceptible individual may compound the risk. These include occupational exposure to dusts and fumes, for example factory workers (such as Mr LT) or coal miners; recurrent lower respiratory tract infection in childhood; and low birthweight.

A person's smoking history can be quantified by calculating their pack years. What is Mr LT's smoking history in pack years?

A3 Mr LT's pack-year history is 52 years.

Lifetime smoking exposure is quantified in 'pack years', where one 'pack year' is 20 cigarettes smoked per day for 1 year. Therefore:

Number of pack years = (Number of cigarettes smoked per day × Number of years smoked)/20 (the number of cigarettes in a pack)

Mr LT's pack year history is:

$$\frac{20}{20} \times 52 \text{ (started at age 14 and stopped at 66) years} = 52 \text{ pack years}$$

Quantification of pack years smoked is important in clinical care, where the degree of tobacco exposure is closely correlated to the risk of disease. There is a strong dose–response relationship between the number of pack years smoked and the risk, severity and mortality associated with COPD.

What do Mr LT's spirometry results tell us about his disease?

A4 Mr LT has a reduced FEV_1 (35% of predicted (normal >80%)) and a reduced FEV_1/FVC ratio (62%). The results confirm a diagnosis of obstructive pulmonary disease. The fact that there is very little reversibility following salbutamol therapy makes the diagnosis of COPD most likely.

Spirometry is performed by asking the patient to exhale as hard and as quickly as possible after a full deep inspiration until there is no breath left in the lungs. Two measurements are of particular interest; forced expiratory volume in the first second (FEV_1) and forced vital capacity (FVC). The FEV_1 is the volume of air expelled in the first second of a forced expiration starting from full inspiration, and the FVC is the maximum volume of air in litres that can be forcibly and rapidly exhaled following a maximum inspiration. Individual performance is compared with population norms standardised for height, age and race, and is expressed as a percentage of the predicted value.

In an obstructive lung disease such as COPD in which the airways are narrowed, FEV_1 is predominately reduced and the FVC is normal or only slightly reduced, making the FEV_1/FVC ratio lower than normal (i.e. a ratio of <70%). FEV_1 is preferred to peak expiratory flow (PEF) as a measure of airflow in patients with COPD because it more reliably measures the extent of airway obstruction.

Categorisation of the severity of COPD varies between countries and clinical guidelines. NICE has graded the severity of airflow limitation in COPD as follows:

Mild:	FEV_1 50–80% of predicted value.
Moderate:	FEV_1 30–49% of predicted value.
Severe:	FEV_1 <30% of predicted value.

Using these definitions, Mr LT can be classed as having moderate COPD; however, the severity of a patient's disease should not be based simply on their airflow limitation. Assessment of COPD severity should consider the level of their symptoms, the degree to which the symptoms affect daily life, the severity of the spirometric abnormality, and the presence of complications such as respiratory failure, cor pulmonale, weight loss, and arterial hypoxemia.

Mr LT's airways showed little reversibility after a dose of salbutamol. Measurement of the degree of reversibility using bronchodilators or corticosteroids has traditionally been used to confirm the diagnosis of COPD, and in particular to try to separate COPD patients from those with asthma.

The recent NICE COPD guideline recommends against the use of routine spirometric reversibility testing as part of the diagnostic process, as the two diseases can usually be distinguished on the basis of history and examination. If diagnostic doubt remains, or both COPD and asthma are present, a large (>400 mL) response to bronchodilators should be used to help identify asthma.

Spirometric staging is therefore a pragmatic approach to guide care, and should only be regarded as an educational tool and a general indication to the initial approach to patient management.

In light of Mr LT's revised diagnosis, would you recommend any changes to his therapy?

A5 Yes. Mr LT has been treated as an asthmatic and his medicines need to be reviewed in order to manage his COPD. COPD is not synonymous with asthma and should be approached and treated differently.

The pharmacological management of a patient with asthma is very different from that of one with COPD, although similar drugs may be used for both. Asthma should be regarded as a separate condition from COPD, with different causes, different cellular mechanisms and different responses to treatments.

Comparison of tissues sampled from the airways of non-smoking asthmatics with reversible disease and smokers with COPD, in whom there is 'fixed' airflow obstruction, demonstrates that although both conditions are associated with chronic inflammation, their pathologies are distinct. In COPD the abnormal inflammatory response involves macrophages, neutrophils and CD8+ T cells and results in structural changes and fixed narrowing of the airways, with destruction of the lung parenchyma. In the bronchial wall of patients with asthma there is frequently a prominent eosinophil infiltrate which is readily damped down by corticosteroids. Neutrophils are relatively insensitive to corticosteroids. The airway lumen in asthma patients is normally maintained, although it may be plugged with mucus. In contrast, in COPD the bronchiole wall is considerably thickened with extensive fibrosis and an inflammatory infiltrate, and the lumen may be collapsed, with reduced alveolar wall attachments (the latter normally hold the walls of the small airways open).

Not surprisingly, COPD patients do not respond as well to treatments as do asthmatics, and this frequently leads to unnecessary escalation of treatment while other important management issues are overlooked. It looks as if this has happened in Mr LT's case. Now his correct diagnosis has been established he can be given the correct medication regimen, more realistic expectations about the outcomes of treatment, advice regarding his lifestyle and more appropriate and holistic management.

The following changes should be made to his therapy:

(a) Montelukast, a leukotriene receptor antagonist, is not licensed for the management of COPD. It has no proven role in the management of COPD and should be stopped.

(b) Beclometasone diproprionate CFC-free or any inhaled corticosteroid is not licensed for patients with COPD (unless prescribed in combination with a long-acting beta$_2$-agonist). Managing COPD as asthma may lead to overuse of steroids. Inhaled steroids are indicated for nearly all asthmatics, but only for COPD patients with moderate or severely reduced FEV_1 (defined as FEV_1 <50%) with frequent exacerbations. Mr LT had not been using his beclometasone as he perceived no benefit from it. As he appears not to be experiencing frequent exacerbations it could be removed from his repeat prescription at present. However, it is important to question him carefully about his exacerbation history: more than half of COPD patients fail to report life-threatening exacerbations. In addition, his currently prescribed dose of inhaled beclometasone would not be high enough to manage his COPD and reduce the risk of exacerbations. The benefits of inhaled corticosteroids in patients with COPD have only been observed using high-range dosing (e.g. fluticasone 1000 micrograms daily or budesonide 800 micrograms daily).

An inhaled corticosteroid may be an appropriate option for Mr LT later in the course of his disease.

(c) Bronchodilators may be underused if patients with COPD are managed as asthmatics. In symptomatic patients the cornerstone of management of breathlessness in COPD is inhaled bronchodilation. Although they do not significantly improve lung function (FEV_1), bronchodilators improve breathlessness, exercise capacity and quality of life.

Short-acting bronchodilators such as salbutamol, terbutaline or ipratropium are given for relief of intermittent breathlessness and can be used regularly throughout the day, often at higher than licensed doses. This level of bronchodilator use in patients with asthma would be regarded as a sign that the asthma is poorly controlled and the patient's treatment may need optimising. Indeed, the surgery had asked Mr LT to make an appointment for a review of his 'asthma' as he was 'overusing' his salbutamol inhaler (four each month). Furthermore, in contrast to asthma, anticholinergic drugs such as ipratropium are as effective as or more effective than $beta_2$-agonists and are thus indicated in the management of stable COPD. It would be logical to prescribe regular ipratropium therapy for Mr LT, with salbutamol added on a 'when required' basis to supplement this if necessary.

(d) There may also be underuse of non-pharmacological methods to manage Mr LT's condition, especially pulmonary rehabilitation and vaccination.

  (i) Exercise programs are beneficial to COPD patients at all stages of the disease and can improve quality of life, sexual function and pulmonary function tests, and also reduce oxygen requirements if regular oxygen therapy is required. Mr LT should be referred to a local pulmonary rehabilitation class.
  (ii) COPD patients are at increased risk of mortality and morbidity from respiratory infections. It is important that Mr LT receive pneumococcal and annual influenza vaccines.

(e) Advice about nutrition may be appropriate for Mr LT. Weight loss is common in people with advanced COPD, and being underweight is clearly associated with a higher risk of dying. People with COPD work harder to breathe and burn more calories at rest than individuals without COPD, making nutritional supplementation an important non-pharmacologic treatment modality. However, obesity increases breathlessness, and such patients should be encouraged to lose weight. Dietary advice can help to maintain an ideal weight and is most effective when combined with exercise training that builds muscle mass.

How would you decide if an intervention to his therapy had helped?

A6 Assessment of effectiveness should be based on both objective and subjective measures.

The effectiveness of bronchodilator therapy should be assessed using a variety of factors, including lung function, improvement in symptoms and exercise capacity. Asking Mr LT some simple questions can help to determine whether a treatment has helped. For example:

(a) How often does he tend to use his salbutamol inhaler? An increase in use indicates poor symptom control.
(b) Does he think his treatment has helped in any way:
   (i) Has it made a difference to his life?
   (ii) Is his breathing easier?
   (iii) Can he do things now that he was unable to do before, or the same things but faster?
   (iv) Can he do the same things as before but is now less breathless doing them?
   (v) Has his sleep improved?

Table 12.2 MRC dyspnoea scale

Grade	*Level of activity*
1	Not troubled by breathlessness except during strenuous exercise
2	Short of breath when hurrying or walking up a slight hill
3	Walks slower than contemporaries on the level because of breathlessness, or has to stop for breath when walking at own pace
4	Stops for breath after walking about 100 m or after a few minutes on the level
5	Too breathless to leave the house or breathless when dressing or undressing

Recording his Medical Research Council (MRC) dyspnoea scale score (see Table 12.2) is a useful measure of his exercise tolerance. Also, checking how many exacerbations he has had during the last year (as a minimum), or longer if recorded or he can remember, can help to assess whether drugs such as long-acting bronchodilators or inhaled corticosteroids have helped.

Many COPD patients ask for home nebulisers: what is the place of nebulisers in the management of COPD?

A7 **In the majority of cases an MDI (plus spacer) is either as good as or better than a nebuliser. NICE guidance restricts the prescribing of nebulisers, and only recommends consideration of a nebuliser for patients with distressing or disabling breathlessness despite maximal therapy using inhalers.**

Most patients achieve maximum possible bronchodilation with drugs administered by conventional inhalers. This statement is supported by clinical trials, as there is no evidence to suggest superiority of nebulised therapy over the use of an MDI with a spacer. However, nebuliser therapy is popular with patients because it requires no effort, and many patients derive subjective benefit from the moistening or cooling effects of the aerosol generated by the nebuliser. Often this can be achieved by recommending that the patient uses a fan. Nebulisers also have a mystique for patients and their families which ensures that their reputation often outweighs the reality. Compressors to drive nebulisers are relatively cheap, but the drug costs are high and patients may experience more systemic side-effects. Other disadvantages are listed in Table 12.3.

For all these reasons patients should be encouraged to use spacer devices with MDIs before considering the use of nebulisers. Certainly, a formal assessment should be made before long-term, regular nebuliser therapy is initiated. The assessment should confirm that one or more of the following occurs:

(a) A reduction in symptoms.
(b) An increase in the ability to undertake activities of daily living.
(c) An increase in exercise capacity.
(d) An improvement in lung function.

Nebulised therapy should generally be reserved for patients with severe COPD. It is likely that such patients will have some contact with a specialist respiratory team who are usually best placed to arrange appropriate supply, proper use and maintenance of the device.

Table 12.3 Advantages and disadvantages of nebuliser therapy

Advantages	*Disadvantages*
No inspiratory effort is required	Time consuming (at least 15 minutes per dose)
No breath coordination required	Requires an electricity supply
High doses of drugs can be delivered	Must be cleaned and maintained regularly
	Expensive compared to other inhaled formulations
	Source of infection
	Few patients benefit from the high dose delivered
	Not very portable, and can unnecessarily tie a patient to home
	Nebulised short-acting beta$_2$-agonist (e.g. salbutamol) can worsen the condition by reducing arterial oxygen tension in individuals who are severely hypoxaemic
	Patients become psychologically dependent on nebulisers

What do Mr LT's history, symptoms and blood gases indicate about his respiratory disease?

A8 **Mr LT's rapidly increasing dyspnoea and general disability over the past few days suggest that his respiratory condition has deteriorated because of an acute event. His productive cough and discoloured sputum make a chest infection the most likely cause. His symptoms of cyanosis show that his lungs are failing to provide efficient gaseous exchange and that he is in respiratory failure.**

This can be confirmed by the blood gas results. Mr LT was given 35% oxygen on admission, before the first blood gases were measured. Usually a lower oxygen concentration (24%) is used, in order to avoid inhibiting the hypoxic ventilatory drive often present in COPD patients. The high oxygen concentration administered to Mr LT initially may have contributed to his carbon dioxide retention. There is little point raising the

PaO_2 >8–9 kPa, as the increase in oxygen saturation achieved will not be worthwhile (from about 90% to 95%) when balanced against the risk of raising the $PaCO_2$.

Mr LT's $PaCO_2$ is markedly raised, which means that he has type 2 (ventilatory) failure, where alveolar ventilation is insufficient to prevent a rise in $PaCO_2$. This is in contrast to type 1 (oxygenation) failure, where the PaO_2 falls below 8 kPa, but a rise in $PaCO_2$ is counteracted by increased respiratory muscle drive. The accumulation of carbon dioxide leads to respiratory acidosis with a low blood pH. When this becomes a chronic condition, as in Mr LT's case, the kidneys compensate by excreting more hydrogen ions into the urine at the expense of potassium ions and returning more bicarbonate ions to the circulation, thereby causing a rise in plasma bicarbonate.

What are the immediate therapeutic priorities for Mr LT?

A9 **The immediate therapeutic aims are:**

(a) Correction of acute respiratory failure.
(b) Treatment of infection.

Outline the key elements of a pharmaceutical care plan for Mr LT.

A10 **The pharmaceutical care plan for Mr LT should include the following:**

(a) Advise medical staff on: choice of antibiotics and formulary restrictions; dosage regimens of bronchodilators; therapeutic drug monitoring of aminophylline/theophylline; treatment options for cor pulmonale.
(b) Advise nursing staff on: administration of IV antibiotics; administration of nebulised bronchodilators.
(c) Monitor Mr LT's therapy for efficacy and toxicity of antibiotics, bronchodilators and diuretics.
(d) Monitor theophylline serum concentration measurements.
(e) Review therapy prescribed for his acute condition, assessing the suitability of each drug for long-term maintenance therapy.
(f) Assess the suitability of the patient's own drugs (PODs) belonging to Mr LT for use in hospital, and remove those no longer appropriate, after discussion with the patient or his relatives.
(g) Counsel Mr LT on the use of his medication, with particular emphasis on his inhaled therapy.
(h) Ensure that any of Mr LT's own drugs used during his stay are still current and suitably labelled before discharge, and check that any medicines at home are still appropriate for his use.

(i) Consider issuing a Patient Medication Record to the patient, his carer, his GP and/or a community pharmacist of his choice.
(j) Consider non-drug factors that may be important, e.g. if he had still been smoking, would referral to a smoking cessation clinic have been appropriate?
(k) Consider whether the patient is suitable for long-term oxygen therapy.
(l) Consider referral to a local pulmonary rehabilitation programme.
(m) Consider referral to a dietitian.

Do you agree with the choice of agents to treat Mr LT's respiratory condition? Comment on the doses prescribed.

A11 **(a) Antibiotic therapy.**

An antibiotic with a narrower spectrum of activity would have been more appropriate.

The Department of Health recommends prudent antibiotic prescribing to reduce the use of broad-spectrum antibiotics, such as ceftriaxone, to help prevent and control *Clostridium difficile* infection. Many clinical areas have introduced a narrow-spectrum antibiotic policy.

The cause of Mr LT's acute respiratory failure is infection, so treatment with an appropriate antibiotic is very important. Sputum and blood samples should be sent for culture and sensitivity, but the most likely causative organisms are *Haemophilus influenzae* and *Streptococcus pneumoniae*. Amoxicillin, erythromycin, tetracycline or trimethoprim would therefore usually be adequate; however, up to 10% of *H. influenzae* strains are now resistant to amoxicillin, and, bearing in mind the severity of Mr LT's condition, the use of these agents is probably not appropriate without a sensitivity report. Co-amoxiclav at a dose of 1.2 g 8-hourly would have been a more suitable alternative for Mr LT, as it is effective against penicillinase-producing bacteria that are resistant to amoxicillin. In a patient with a severe community-acquired pneumonia such as Mr LT, the British Thoracic Society (BTS) guidelines recommend a combination of a broad-spectrum beta-lactamase antibiotic such as co-amoxiclav, cefuroxime or ceftriaxone, together with a macrolide antibiotic such as erythromycin or clarithromycin. This would then cover for Legionnaire's disease and other atypical organisms.

Use of a macrolide would also be appropriate if Mr LT had recently returned from a foreign holiday. Additionally, penicillin-resistant pneumococci are becoming much more common, particularly in certain parts of Europe, South Africa and South America, and recent travel to these areas could justify the use of ceftriaxone.

A urine test is available for pneumococcal and Legionella antigens, which could have confirmed or eliminated the presence of these organisms in 15 minutes.

(b) Bronchodilator therapy.

It was appropriate to prescribe three bronchodilators for Mr LT, but a loading dose of aminophylline should have been given.

Much of the airways obstruction of COPD is not reversible by bronchodilator therapy as it is caused by mucus plugs and bronchiolar inflammation. Airway obstruction leads to excess air being trapped in the lungs during exhalation. This is a primary cause of breathlessness and often restricts a patient's ability to perform daily activities. Although bronchodilators cannot reverse the effects of COPD, their efficacy as a treatment lies in their ability to act on the airway smooth muscle, widening the airways and reducing dynamic hyperinflation during exercise and at rest. Although only a small objective improvement can be measured, this may be significant in someone with extremely poor respiratory function.

The mode of action of beta$_2$-agonists is to increase smooth-muscle-cell cyclic adenosine monophosphate (AMP) levels and stabilise mast cells. Salbutamol or terbutaline in nebulised form are routinely prescribed in hospital for patients with an acute severe COPD exacerbation, even though as discussed earlier an MDI and spacer may be as effective. The decision as to what method to use will depend on the need for expedient treatment and the availability of staff to aid the administration. The dose equivalent to 5 mg of salbutamol delivered by nebuliser is 8–10 puffs of 100 micrograms salbutamol by MDI and spacer. The maximum recommended dose for nebulised salbutamol is 5 mg four times daily, but because in severe airways obstruction the quantity of drug reaching the site of action may be limited, a smaller dose given more frequently can be more successful. NICE guidance on COPD points out that the dose–response curve for salbutamol given by nebuliser in largely or completely irreversible COPD is almost flat. The response is slower in COPD than in asthma, and there is little benefit in giving doses larger than 1 mg salbutamol. The mode of delivery should be changed to an MDI with a spacer device or a dry powder inhaler within 24 hours of the initial dose of nebulised bronchodilator, unless the patient remains severely ill.

Ipratropium bromide is an anticholinergic agent which blocks the cholinergic reflex that causes bronchospasm. It is particularly useful in combination with beta$_2$-agonists in COPD patients, producing slightly greater bronchodilation than either agent alone. The onset of action of ipratropium is slower than for the short-acting beta$_2$-agonists and the duration of action is longer. The peak effect is noted between 1 and 2 hours after the dose. The maximum recommended dose of nebulised ipratropium is 500 micrograms four times daily, and in view of its longer duration of action than salbutamol there is unlikely to be any advantage in giving it more frequently than this. Rationalising the use of ipratropium nebules in this way can also result in a significant cost saving.

In addition to causing relaxation of bronchial smooth muscle, there is some evidence that theophylline may have other beneficial actions in COPD. It is thought to act as a respiratory stimulant, reduce respiratory muscle fatigue, improve right ventricular performance and increase mucociliary clearance. Another advantage is that, unlike the other two bronchodilators in the regimen, IV aminophylline does not depend on penetration of the obstructed bronchioles to exert its effect. However, the use of a methylxanthine drug such as aminophylline as an additional bronchodilator during an acute exacerbation is not well supported by evidence. A recent systematic review on the use of methylxanthines in acute COPD exacerbations found no evidence to support their routine use, particularly for clinical situations involving mild to moderate and/or non-acidotic acute exacerbations.

Although clinical evidence for the benefits of methylxanthines is inconclusive, IV aminophylline should be added to the bronchodilator therapy of a COPD patient such as Mr LT, who has severe acute respiratory failure. In such circumstances the benefits of respiratory stimulation and any effect on respiratory muscles may be more important than bronchodilation *per se*. However, the aminophylline dosage regimen prescribed for Mr LT was not optimal. He was given an arbitrary maintenance dose (MD) of 42 mg/h. As he was not taking oral theophylline or aminophylline before admission, he should have received a loading dose (LD) in order to achieve a therapeutic concentration rapidly. The normal half-life of theophylline in adults is 8 hours, and so steady state without an LD can only be achieved after approximately 32 hours. With a suitable LD of 5 mg/kg (or worked out by pharmacokinetic calculation) administered over 20–30 minutes, a therapeutic concentration would have been achieved far more rapidly. After loading is completed, the MD should be started. Ideally the MD should be determined using pharmacokinetic calculation, which takes into account those factors that affect theophylline clearance, such as smoking history.

The plasma concentration of theophylline should then be monitored to maintain therapeutic levels between 10 and 20 mg/L. As no LD was given, the earliest time usefully to measure Mr LT's plasma concentration is 12–20 hours after starting the infusion, which represents twice the normal half-life. Even at this time the concentration can only be a guide as to whether the dose is too high or too low, as steady state will not have been reached. If an LD had been given, it would have been worth checking the level after 6–8 hours and adjusting the dose up or down as necessary.

(c) Corticosteroid therapy.

The use of IV and oral corticosteroids in the short term in Mr LT's condition is normal practice and makes theoretical sense, as eosinophilic inflammation is thought to play a significant part in airways obstruction during an acute exacerbation. Steroids do seem to improve several outcomes during an acute COPD exacerbation, including hastening resolution and reducing the likelihood of relapse. Even though the optimal dose and duration of therapy have not been established, a 7–14-day course of prednisolone 30 mg daily would be appropriate for most patients. The dose of hydrocortisone prescribed for Mr LT is one that is commonly used and should be reduced as his condition improves, with a change to prednisolone as soon as he can take oral medication.

What would you tell a nurse who had never administered salbutamol or ipratropium by nebuliser before?

A12 **(a) Volume of nebulised solution.**

Nebulisers have a dead volume of usually just under 1 mL which will not be available to the patient, so the larger the fill volume, the greater the fraction of drug released. However, increasing the volume increases the time for nebulisation. In hospital a volume of 4–5 mL is an acceptable compromise, producing an administration time of 15–30 minutes. As Mr LT is written up for 5 mg salbutamol (one 2.5 mL nebule) and 500 micrograms ipratropium (one 2 mL nebule) every 4 hours, it is convenient to mix the two in the nebuliser, making a total volume of 4.5 mL. This is common practice on wards, although the stability of the two solutions combined has not been fully evaluated. Unpublished work carried out on the stability of the mixture using the preserved formulations suggested that they would be compatible when mixed in this way, but both formulations are now preservative free, which could theoretically affect the results. Where the volume of fluid is insufficient and dilution is required, sodium chloride 0.9% should be used, as hypotonic solutions may provoke bronchospasm.

A combination product, Combivent nebules, is available, which contains ipratropium bromide 500 micrograms plus salbutamol 2.5 mg in 2.5 mL saline. This may be used as an alternative where the dose of each drug prescribed is equivalent, bearing in mind the above considerations. However, the need for these drugs to be prescribed together should be considered carefully in each case, particularly in long-term maintenance therapy. Combivent MDI inhaler has been discontinued as the company was unable to reformulate it as CFC free.

(b) Driving gas.

The driving gas for nebulisers may be air or oxygen at a rate of 6–8 L/min. In patients with COPD who may have low oxygen tolerability the driving gas should be air using a nebuliser compressor. If supplementary oxygen is required a safe approach would be to use air as the driving gas for administration of bronchodilators and to administer oxygen via a nasal cannula.

Could Mr LT's drug therapy be causing his tremor?

A13 **Yes.**

Salbutamol is known to cause a fine tremor of skeletal muscle, along with other manifestations of sympathetic stimulation such as an increase in heart rate and peripheral vasodilation. These effects occur particularly when large doses are inhaled. Aminophylline can also cause tremor, but in most cases only at plasma concentrations above the therapeutic range.

How would you recommend IV aminophylline be converted to oral theophylline?

A14 **(a) Convert the hourly infusion rate of aminophylline to the total amount administered in 24 hours by multiplying the hourly dose by 24.**

(b) In order to calculate the equivalent theophylline dose, multiply this total aminophylline dose by 0.8, which is the salt correction factor.

(c) Divide this total amount by the dosing interval for oral administration, e.g. by 2 for twice-daily dosing. It is assumed that the oral product is completely absorbed, i.e. the bioavailability is 100%.

(d) A suitable theophylline dosing regimen could be Uniphyllin Continus 400 mg twice daily.

Mr LT has received 1008 mg (dose 42 mg/h) of aminophylline (a combination of theophylline and ethylenediamine) in 24 hours:

1008 mg aminophylline = 1008 × 0.8 (salt factor) = 806 mg theophylline daily

When calculating a convenient dose for Mr LT it is advisable to round the dose downwards, because in some patients theophylline exhibits zero-order kinetics in the upper half of the therapeutic range and a small increase in dose may produce a large increase in plasma concentration.

As his reported plasma concentration was in the middle of the therapeutic range, conversion to an equivalent oral regimen is appropriate. The infusion has been running for over 48 hours at a constant rate, so steady state has been achieved, and as it is a continuous IV infusion the sampling time is not critical. As always, when interpreting drug-level data the result should be judged in the light of the patient's clinical response: if the current dose had been ineffective or toxicity had occurred, a change of dose should have been considered even if the reported level was in the therapeutic range.

When changing a patient's therapy from IV aminophylline to oral therapy with either theophylline or aminophylline, the bioavailability and the salt equivalence should be considered. The salt factor for aminophylline is approximately 0.8 (i.e. the amount of a labelled dose of aminophylline that comprises theophylline is about 80%). It is often not possible to achieve a dose that is exactly the same when converting from IV to oral therapy. The nearest practical dose should therefore be used. This is rarely a problem, as pharmacokinetic and drug-assay variability means that measured theophylline levels are often not the same as predicted levels anyway.

When treatment is changed from IV to oral therapy, the maintenance infusion should be stopped and oral therapy should be begun immediately.

Is the prescribing of a long-acting anticholinergic appropriate for Mr LT? Is there any therapy that should be discontinued?

A15 **Yes, a long-acting anticholinergic should be started to try to improve his symptoms. It may also help to reduce his risk of exacerbations. It would be appropriate to substitute tiotropium for ipratropium at this stage while continuing 'when required' salbutamol.**

In patients with persistent breathlessness regular bronchodilation with a long-acting anticholinergic agent such as tiotropium (or a long-acting $beta_2$-agonist) can improve lung function, reduce dynamic hyperinflation of the lungs, and hence reduce the work of breathing and improve exercise capacity. Long-acting bronchodilators also reduce the frequency of exacerbation rates in patients with COPD, and NICE guidance recommends that they should be used in patients who have two or more exacerbations per year.

Tiotropium is more effective than ipratropium in COPD. It has been shown to reduce exacerbations and related hospitalisations compared to placebo and ipratropium therapy. It also improves health-related quality-of-life and symptom scores in patients with moderate and severe disease, and may slow the decline in lung function. Further randomised controlled trials (RCTs) are required to assess the effectiveness of tiotropium in mild and very severe COPD. Until then, ipratropium continues to be recommended as first-line treatment for patients with COPD with intermittent symptoms.

The UPLIFT (Understanding Potential Long-term Impacts on Function with Tiotropium) study was a 4-year prospective double blind RCT ($n = 5993$) which compared tiotropium with placebo in patients with COPD. It did not show a benefit in its primary outcome of reducing the rate of lung function decline (as measured by FEV_1). However, there was a small reduction in exacerbations (about 12 fewer for every 100 patients per year) but no reduction in exacerbations leading to hospitalisation, total number of exacerbations or number of days in hospital. A recent meta-analysis and observational study has signalled the possibility of an increased risk of cardiovascular (CV) events with inhaled anticholinergics in people with COPD. UPLIFT provides limited reassurance about these CV risk signals for tiotropium. In the UPLIFT study there were no statistically significant differences in the risk of myocardial infarction or stroke compared with placebo; however, the trial was not designed to look at any CV endpoints, so there may have been differences in how these outcomes were reported. Uncertainty still exists regarding the cardiovascular safety of inhaled anticholinergics in people with COPD. A long-term RCT specifically designed to look at CV outcomes is necessary to confirm and quantify any possible increased CV risk.

INSPIRE, a study comparing the long-acting anticholinergic bronchodilator tiotropium against a combination of the long-acting $beta_2$-agonist salmeterol and inhaled steroid fluticasone in 1323 patients, found little to choose between the two treatments. However, they did appear to work in different ways, thus suggesting there may be benefit from combining all three. Indeed, the combination of salmeterol, fluticasone propionate and tiotropium are commonly used treatments in COPD, but there are few data on their effectiveness when used together. Adequately powered long-term studies of the benefits of triple therapy on exacerbation rates and other clinical endpoints are now needed to justify this approach in clinical practice.

The co-administration of tiotropium bromide with other anticholinergic-containing drugs has not been studied and is therefore not recommended. Both tiotropium and ipratropium are antagonists of three muscarinic receptor subtypes: i.e. M1, M2 and M3. Blockade of these receptors in the smooth muscle of the airways inhibits the activity of acetylcholine, which reduces cyclic guanosine monophosphate levels to yield bronchodilation. Tiotropium's differences in receptor association and dissociation rates distinguish its pharmacology from that of ipratropium. Tiotropium dissociates most rapidly from the M2 receptors. Stimulation of the M2 receptors reduces acetylcholine release; blockade may result in further bronchoconstriction. Tiotropium's long duration of action is likely to be a result of its slower dissociation from the M1 and M3 receptors. This selective pharmacology at M2 is theoretically lost when both agents are used together. Furthermore, there may potentially be an increase in anticholinergic adverse effects from the administration of both agents (e.g. dry mouth, blurred vision).

Is this treatment appropriate for Mr LT's cor pulmonale? What alternative therapies could be prescribed?

A16 **The treatment is appropriate provided Mr LT's serum potassium level is checked first. Treatment of the respiratory failure, supplementation with oxygen, and diuretic therapy are the mainstays of the treatment of cor pulmonale. Other drugs such as vasodilators may be helpful as second-line agents.**

Cor pulmonale is fluid retention and heart failure associated with diseases of the lung. It is initiated by pulmonary artery hypertension, which produces a high afterload and hence right ventricular hypertrophy. There is no intrinsic abnormality of the heart, and initially there may be sufficient functional reserve to maintain cardiac output at normal values; however, the right ventricle eventually fails to compensate for the hypertension and venous pressure becomes elevated. There is also evidence that the oedema associated with COPD may be partly due to poor water handling by hypoxic kidneys and may occur without raised atrial pressure, i.e. before pulmonary hypertension has occurred.

It is now believed that pulmonary hypoxic vasoconstriction, rather than anatomical damage to the capillary bed, causes the rise in pulmonary artery pressure. Erythrocytosis, occurring as a response to hypoxia and causing a rise in haematocrit, increased resistance to flow and an increase in red-cell clumping, can also play a part. As hypoxia is the causative factor, treatment of Mr LT's respiratory failure is vital. Episodes of frank heart failure frequently appear during infective episodes. Supplementation with oxygen reduces hypoxia and there is now good evidence that long-term oxygen therapy reduces mortality, morbidity and frequency of hospital admission in such patients. Current guidelines recommend that long-term oxygen therapy (LTOT) is prescribed for patients with COPD who, when stable, have a resting PaO_2 <7.3 kPa, or between 7.3 and 8.0 kPa with at least one of the following: secondary polycythaemia, nocturnal hypoxaemia (oxygen saturation of arterial blood (SaO_2) <90% for more than 30% of the time), peripheral oedema or evidence of pulmonary hypertension. To obtain the benefits of LTOT, patients should breathe supplemental oxygen for at least 15 hours per day. Mr LT's oxygen saturations (SaO_2), as measured by a pulse oximeter, were recorded as 91% before discharge. Oxygen saturations can be used to select patients who require further blood analysis. If the SaO_2 is >92%, assessment with arterial blood gases is not indicated. If SaO_2 <92% on two occasions 2–3 weeks apart, referral for an LTOT assessment is indicated. Patients should not be assessed for LTOT during an acute exacerbation of their disease or for 1 month afterwards. LTOT assessment consists of arterial blood gas analysis on air on two separate occasions at least 3 weeks apart. It is important that Mr LT is assessed again when he is stable before oxygen therapy is started.

Diuretic therapy will reduce oedema, improve peripheral circulation, and may improve gaseous exchange in the lungs if pulmonary congestion is present. It should be remembered that as Mr LT recovers from the acute exacerbation of his pulmonary disease, the cor pulmonale is also likely to improve and his diuretic requirement may therefore decrease.

The potency of a loop diuretic will be valuable in the acute treatment of Mr LT's cor pulmonale. In addition, as he had a raised serum potassium on admission, the greater capacity of loop diuretics for lowering potassium levels acutely may be a further advantage. During long-term use, however, thiazides have a greater potential for causing hypokalaemia, and as patients with COPD tend to have low total body potassium, a loop diuretic would also appear to be more appropriate as long-term therapy. Furthermore, a potassium-sparing diuretic can be added to the treatment to avoid exacerbation of this problem. Spironolactone has traditionally been used in severe heart failure and is theoretically appropriate, as raised aldosterone levels are frequently present owing to hepatic congestion. Amiloride is a suitable alternative, but before either of these drugs is prescribed it is important to check that Mr LT's serum potassium has returned to normal. Whichever diuretics are chosen, it is important that their effect on Mr LT's electrolyte balance is monitored.

Digoxin is thought to be of little value in cor pulmonale unless atrial fibrillation needs to be controlled. Pulmonary vasodilators are theoretically useful additions to therapy, but are not yet of proven value: hydralazine, calcium-channel blockers and angiotensin-converting enzyme inhibitors (ACEIs) are examples.

Although ACEIs are first-line therapy in many forms of heart failure, there is no evidence of their benefit in cor pulmonale. This group of drugs is beneficial in patients who have left ventricular failure, which is not the case in cor pulmonale, where left ventricular function is usually not severely impaired. If there is a more complex aetiology, such as a history of ischaemic heart disease, there may be a place for an ACEI.

Would you recommend any change in his theophylline dosage?

A17 **Yes. Mr LT's dose of slow-release theophylline should be reduced to 300 mg twice daily, given every 12 hours.**

The serum theophylline sample was taken on the third day after changing to slow-release tablets, so steady state had been reached. As the level is from a pre-dose or trough sample it is likely that the peak theophylline concentration is >20 mg/L. This observation, combined with Mr LT's continued tremor, which is a side-effect associated with high serum theophylline levels, leads to the recommendation for dosage reduction. A suitable dose could be more accurately determined by pharmacokinetic calculation. His serum theophylline level should then be re-checked at his first outpatient appointment, or preferably earlier by his GP. The sample should ideally be taken 8 hours post dose, giving a mean steady-state concentration for a 12-hourly regimen, but this is unlikely to be practicable in an outpatient setting and the actual time of sampling must be taken into account when interpreting the result.

Would there be any advantage in continuing Mr LT's oral steroid therapy long term? Would inhaled steroid therapy be more appropriate?

A18 **No. Indefinite continuation of Mr LT's systemic corticosteroid therapy would not be appropriate. However, inhaled corticosteroid therapy could be considered.**

Oral corticosteroids are beneficial in the management of exacerbations of COPD. They shorten recovery time, improve lung function (FEV_1) and hypoxaemia (PaO_2), and may reduce the risk of early relapse, treatment failure, and duration of hospital stay. However, they have only a limited role in the management of stable COPD and few data suggest which patients (if any) derive benefit from long-term use. Indeed, oral corticosteroids have been shown to increase mortality in patients with advanced disease. However, for some severely affected patients with advanced airflow obstruction it is difficult to stop oral corticosteroids after an exacerbation, and it might be necessary for patients to continue on them at the lowest possible dose (e.g. prednisolone 2.5–5 mg/day) to minimise adverse effects.

Abrupt withdrawal of doses of up to 40 mg daily of prednisolone, or equivalent, which have been taken for up to 3 weeks is unlikely to lead to clinically relevant hypothalamopituitary–adrenal (HPA) axis suppression in the majority of patients. Therefore, for most patients treated for an exacerbation of COPD with prednisolone 30 mg daily for 7–14 days the tablets can be stopped abruptly. There is no need for gradual tapering.

Regular treatment with inhaled corticosteroids does not modify the long-term decline of lung function in patients with COPD. However, there is good evidence to suggest that it reduces the frequency of exacerbations and thus improves health status for symptomatic COPD patients with moderate/severe disease (FEV_1 <50% predicted) who suffer from repeated exacerbations. The role of corticosteroids in milder disease is, however, less clear.

Prior to admission Mr LT had been prescribed a beclometasone inhaler, but he had not used it for several months because he felt it did not help. This is a common observation by patients with COPD (and asthma), but is very misleading. On further questioning it can frequently be established that the patient did not realise that regular, continuous therapy was required for benefit, and that he or she had stopped using it because no immediate relief was obtained on a 'when required' basis. As mentioned previously, the dose of inhaled corticosteroid may have been too low (400 micrograms beclometasone daily) to have a therapeutic effect on his COPD. The dose required to achieve a beneficial effect with minimal adverse effects is not known, and more data are needed. Many trials in the treatment of COPD have only used maximum daily doses. As a consequence, Mr LT should be prescribed regular, high-dose inhaled corticosteroid therapy. He certainly fulfils NICE criteria for an inhaled corticosteroid: FEV_1 32% with at least two exacerbations in the last 12 months.

The only formulations of inhaled steroids currently licensed for the treatment of COPD are the inhalers that contain both a corticosteroid and a long-acting beta$_2$-agonist. One of these should be added to Mr LT's regimen. The choice depends on Mr LT's inhaler technique and preference, local prescribing guidelines and cost.

What points would you discuss with Mr LT when counselling him on his take-home medication?

A19 **(a) Salbutamol.**

The nebulised therapy is the most complex part of his treatment and must be explained to Mr LT in detail if he is to continue using it long term, with emphasis on the importance of using the correct fill volume, cleaning and maintenance. If possible, Mr LT should be observed using his own equipment. He must understand when he is to use his nebuliser rather than administering salbutamol via his inhaler. Nebulisers are not routinely recommended, as discussed earlier, for the management of stable COPD but some patients may keep one at home to use in the event of an exacerbation. He must also know who to contact if the machine breaks down, and arrange to have it serviced at least annually.

(b) Prednisolone.

Confirm that Mr LT understands that he is to stop taking this drug after 1 week.

(c) Furosemide.

The dose should be taken regularly in the morning and Mr LT should continue taking these tablets until told otherwise.

(d) Theophylline.

The tablets should be swallowed whole, at regular intervals, and preferably after food with a cold drink. The concept of sustained release should be explained. Mr LT should realise that this therapy will continue indefinitely, and that he will need occasional blood tests to check that the dose is right for him. He should be aware that a number of other medicines, including some antibiotics, affect the level of theophylline and he should remind his doctor that he is on theophylline when his treatment is changed. This is also important when buying over-the-counter medicines.

(e) Tiotropium.

The effect of this medicine lasts for 24 hours, so it should be taken just once a day. It may take several days before full benefits occur, and this should be explained to Mr LT. He should be told about the incidence of it causing a dry mouth, and should be advised to rinse his mouth after using the inhaler to help prevent dryness and relieve throat irritation. It is important to check he can use his inhaler by asking him to demonstrate this to you. The patient information leaflet provided with the medication is useful to help guide your counselling.

How should Mr LT be advised on the self-management of his COPD?

A20 **The vital components of a COPD self-management plan have yet to be determined, and there is no evidence that asthma self-management plans are helpful. However, the NICE guideline suggests that self-management or exacerbation action plans look to be promising.**

The plan should cover:

(a) How to recognise when the COPD is getting worse (breathlessness, more sputum, coloured sputum, and/or fever).
(b) How to first increase the use of short-acting bronchodilators, and, if there is no response, when to contact a primary healthcare professional.
(c) If oral corticosteroid or antibiotic therapy is held in reserve by the patient:
    (i) When to start oral corticosteroids (if there is no improvement after 1–2 days with a maximum dose of bronchodilator treatment).
    (ii) When to start antibiotics (if sputum becomes discoloured and/or increases in volume).
    (iii) When to contact a primary healthcare professional (if they are concerned or not responding to treatment).

The aim of self-management plans is to prevent exacerbations by promoting lifestyle adaptation and the acquisition of skills to treat exacerbations early so as to reduce hospitalisation and morbidity.

Patients with chronic illness who participate in self-management have better outcomes, including reduced healthcare costs, than those who do not. This includes people with COPD.

In patients with COPD most exacerbations evolve over days rather than hours, but even small changes can precipitate a major deterioration in functional status. The traditional approach to exacerbations of moderate to severe COPD has been admission to hospital. The concept of self-management plans for patients with COPD is derived from their success in asthma management, when they are used to indicate doses and medications to take for maintenance therapy and during exacerbations. Instructions for crises are often also included. Clinical trials are currently ongoing to support the routine use of self-management plans in patients with COPD.

Would you recommend that Mr LT receive continuous antibiotic prophylaxis? If so, which agents would you recommend, and at what dose?

A21 **No. Prophylactic antibiotics are not recommended for people with stable COPD, because of concerns about antibiotic resistance and potential adverse effects.**

Antibiotics have been given 'prophylactically' with the aim of preventing infections and thereby reducing the number of exacerbations. The antibiotics are usually administered daily, particularly in the winter months, although other regimens have been used. The use of prophylactic antibiotics (e.g. routine continuous or intermittent antibiotics) in patients with COPD was studied extensively in the 1950s and 1960s. These studies were small, used less effective antibiotics than those available today, and generally showed no benefit. Because of these poor results and the concern about promoting resistance with widespread antibiotic use and the increased incidence of adverse effects, prophylactic antibiotics are not recommended. NICE guidance states that there is insufficient evidence to recommend prophylactic antibiotic therapy in the management of stable COPD. In contrast to prophylactic antibiotics, influenza vaccination is clearly effective at reducing influenza as a cause of acute exacerbation of COPD. Mr LT is in the group of patients highly vulnerable to influenza and he should be vaccinated annually. Pneumococcal pneumonia is also a significant risk, and COPD patients should receive the pneumococcal vaccine at least once.

Acknowledgement

This case study was based on a case originally written by Peter Bramley and Susan Brammer.

Further reading

British Lung Foundation. *Lost in Translation: Bridging the Communication Gap in COPD*. British Lung Foundation, London, 2006.

British Thoracic Society. 2004 update of BTS pneumonia guidelines: what's new? *Thorax* 2004; **59**: 364–366

British Thoracic Society. Guidelines for the management of community acquired pneumonia. *Thorax* 2001; **56**(suppl. IV): IV1–IV63.

Cochrane Library. *Combined Corticosteroid and Long Acting Beta-Agonist in One Inhaler for Chronic Obstructive Pulmonary Disease*. The Cochrane Library 2004, Issue 3.

Cochrane Library. *Ipratropium Bromide versus Long-Acting Beta-2 Agonists for Stable Chronic Obstructive Pulmonary Disease*. The Cochrane Library 2006, Issue 3.

Cochrane Library. *Tiotropium for Stable Chronic Obstructive Pulmonary Disease*. The Cochrane Library, 2005, Issue 2.

Duffy N, Walker P, Diamantea F *et al.* Intravenous aminophylline in patients admitted to hospital with non-acidotic exacerbations of chronic obstructive pulmonary disease: a prospective randomised controlled trial. *Thorax* 2005; **60**(9): 713–717.

GOLD. *Global Strategy for the Diagnosis, Management, and Prevention of Chronic Obstructive Pulmonary Disease*. December 2007 [www.goldcopd.com].

Hurst JR, Wedzicha JA. Chronic obstructive pulmonary disease: the clinical management of an acute exacerbation. *Postgrad Med J* 2004; **80**: 497–505.

Inhaled Corticosteroids Reduce the Progression of Airflow Limitation in Chronic Obstructive Pulmonary Disease: A Meta-analysis. Database of Abstracts of Reviews of Effects (DARE), 2005.

Long-Term Effects of Inhaled Corticosteroids on FEV_1 *in Patients with Chronic Obstructive Pulmonary Disease: A Meta Analysis*. Database of Abstracts of Reviews of Effects (DARE), 2006.

National Institute for Clinical Excellence. Chronic obstructive pulmonary disease: national clinical guideline on management of chronic obstructive pulmonary disease in adults in primary and secondary care. *Thorax* 2004; **59**(Suppl 1): 1 – 19.

Nici L, Donner C, Wouters E *et al.* American Thoracic Society/European Respiratory Society statement on pulmonary rehabilitation. *Am J Respir Crit Care Med* 2006; **173**: 1390–1413.

O'Driscoll BR, Howard LS, Davison AG on behalf of the British Thoracic Society (BTS). Emergency oxygen use in adult patients. *Thorax* 2008; **63** (Suppl 6):

Winter ME. Basic *Clinical Pharmacokinetics*, 4th edn. Applied Therapeutics, Vancouver, 2003.

13

Peptic ulcer

Andrew Clark

Case study and questions

Day 1 Mrs GE, an 86-year-old Caucasian woman, was taken to A&E from her care home. She had a 1-week history of tiredness, weakness, and some epigastric discomfort and nausea. She had had one episode of malaena the previous day and coffee ground vomit earlier today. Her past medical history included osteoarthritis, gout, hypertension, and resting tremor secondary to anxiety. She had no known drug allergies and was taking the following prescription drugs:

- Propranolol 40 mg up to three times daily when required
- Arthrotec (diclofenac 50 mg + misoprostol 200 micrograms) tablets twice daily
- Indometacin 25 mg three times daily
- Allopurinol 100 mg daily
- Ramipril 10 mg daily
- Simvastatin 40 mg at night

Her haematology and biochemistry results on admission were:

- Haemoglobin 8.3 g/dL (reference range 11–13)
- Packed cell volume (PCV) 0.275 (0.360–0.470)
- Mean cell volume (MCV) 75 fL (80–100)
- Mean cell haemoglobin (MCH) 25 pg (27–32)
- Platelets 264 × 10^9/L (150–400)
- Haematocrit 0.31 (0.36–0.46)
- C-reactive protein 45 mg/L (0–4)
- International normalised ratio (INR) 1.01
- Sodium 141 mmol/L (135–145)
- Potassium 4.0 mmol/L (3.5–5)
- Creatinine 105 micromol/L (45–84)
- Urea 20.3 mmol/L (1.7–8.3)

Her blood pressure was recorded as 115/59 mmHg, her respiratory rate was 24 and her pulse rate 155 beats per minute (bpm). A provisional diagnosis of upper gastrointestinal (GI) bleeding was made and she was admitted to the ward.

Q1 How serious is the bleed?
Q2 What immediate treatment options should be considered?

Q3 How would you treat this patient's (a) shock and (b) symptoms?
Q4 How would you suggest Mrs GE's current drug therapy be managed acutely?
Q5 What is the mechanism for non-steroidal anti-inflammatory (NSAID)-induced ulcers?
Q6 How effective is misoprostol at preventing NSAID-induced peptic ulcers?
Q7 How can the cause of the bleed be confirmed, the bleeding stopped, and re-bleeding prevented?

An urgent endoscopy was arranged for Mrs GE.

Q8 Is endoscopic treatment of the bleed more effective than drug treatment?
Q9 What is the likelihood of the patient suffering a re-bleed?
Q10 What test should be performed on Mrs GE during the endoscopy?

An endoscopy was performed and active duodenal bleeding was noted and treated. Following the procedure Mrs GE was admitted to the medical high-dependency unit. The consultant wanted an acid-suppressing drug to be prescribed.

Q11 Which acid-suppressing drug, and what dose regimen and route would you suggest? What evidence is there to support your recommendation? What alternatives could be used?

Mrs GE was prescribed omeprazole 80 mg intravenously (IV) to be given immediately, followed by an 8 mg/h omeprazole infusion for 72 hours, then omeprazole 40 mg orally twice daily for 5 days. Her *Helicobacter pylori* test was reported as positive.

Q12 Does infection with *H. pylori* predispose to NSAID-induced damage to the GI mucosa?
Q13 What other factors could have contributed to Mrs GE's duodenal ulcer, and might potentially increase the chances of relapse?

Mrs GE's consultant wanted to eradicate the bacteria.

Q14 When should *H. pylori* eradication begin?

The consultant prescribed omeprazole 20 mg daily to continue for 2 months. After a week of observation in hospital the patient's symptoms had resolved and her blood results were normalising. She was discharged back to her care home to complete the treatment.

Q15 Outline a pharmaceutical care plan for Mrs GE's further treatment.
Q16 In the patient's discharge letter, what would you recommend the general practitioner (GP) prescribes to eradicate the *H. pylori*?

Q17 Should Mrs GE be prescribed iron therapy, and if so, for how long?
Q18 What counselling should Mrs GE be given in preparation for discharge to optimise successful treatment and adherence to treatment?

Mrs GE completed the *H. pylori* eradication therapy and remained well and symptom free. Her care home arranged for her to be reviewed by her GP.

Q19 Should the GP check to see whether the *H. pylori* eradication was successful? If so, how?
Q20 How long does Mrs GE need to be prescribed a proton pump inhibitor (PPI)?

Mrs GE told the nursing staff in her home that her knees were painful, and that she was worried that the gout in her toe would return.

Q21 How would you recommend her GP manages her osteoarthritis?
Q22 How would you recommend her GP manages her gout?

Answers

How serious is the bleed?

A1 **Her initial (pre-endoscopy) Rockall score is 3. This means that Mrs GE has an 11% risk of mortality from this bleed.**

Upper GI bleeding is a common cause of emergency hospital admission. An upper GI bleed can range in severity from insignificant bleeds that resolve spontaneously to major bleeds which lead to a huge loss of blood and death. There have been various attempts to predict the seriousness of a bleed from the patient's observations on admission, with the aim of focusing emergency treatment on those who really need it, thereby reducing unnecessary hospital admissions and allowing patients with minor bleeds to return home and be treated as an outpatient within 24–48 hours. The most widely used scoring system is the Rockall score, which predicts death and re-bleeding rates pre and post endoscopy (Tables 13.1 and 13.2).

In this case the bleed is serious and the patient should be admitted for treatment as soon as possible. It is worth noting that her pulse rate was 155 bpm despite the beta-blocker therapy (assuming she was taking this medicine).

Table 13.1 The pre-endoscopy Rockall score

Variable/ score	*0*	*1*	*2*	*3*
Age (years)	<60	60–79	>80	
Shock	No shock (SBP >100 mmHg, Pulse <100 bpm)	Tachycardia (SBP >100 mmHg, Pulse >100 bpm)	Hypotension (SBP <100 mmHg, Pulse >100 bpm)	
Comorbidity	Nil major		Heart failure, ischaemic heart disease, any major comorbidity	Renal failure, liver failure, disseminated malignancy

SBP, systolic blood pressure; bpm, beats per minute

Table 13.2 Percentage mortality associated with each Rockall score

Score	0	1	2	3	4	5	6	7
Mortality (%)	0.2	2.4	5.6	11.0	24.6	39.6	48.9	50.0

What immediate treatment options should be considered?

A2 **The immediate treatment options are to:**

(a) Treat shock
(b) Stop bleeding/prevent re-bleeding
(c) Confirm the cause/source of bleed
(d) Treat symptoms.

How would you treat this patient's (a) shock and (b) symptoms?

A3 **Treat the shock with plasma expansion and her nausea with metoclopramide.**

(a) **Shock.** Mrs GE urgently requires plasma expanders, preferably whole blood. Her low MCV indicates there has also been some chronic blood loss. Sodium chloride 0.9% (or another isotonic crystalloid) is an appropriate interim intravenous (IV) fluid as it expands the extracellular fluid volume. The addition of potassium to the IV fluids is not advisable at this point, as whole blood can contain large amounts of this ion from lysed cells.

(b) **Symptom control.** It is important to control Mrs GE's symptom of nausea. Metoclopramide is an effective antiemetic as it increases gastric emptying and also acts centrally at the chemoreceptor trigger zone to relieve vomiting. It is available in parenteral and oral formulations.

How would you suggest Mrs GE's current drug therapy be managed acutely?

A4 Stop her non-steroidal anti-inflammatory drugs (NSAIDs) and antihypertensives.

The potential for NSAIDs to induce mucosal damage is well recognised.

Recent epidemiological studies as well as large case–control studies and case reports have all demonstrated a link between NSAIDs and serious upper GI tract disease, including peptic ulcer, bleeding and perforation. In the UK the GI side-effects of this group of drugs probably account for around 1200 deaths per year. The complications may appear soon after the initiation of therapy. Mrs GE's other risk factors for NSAID-induced bleeds include being aged over 60, and the use of two concurrent NSAIDs. Other risks include concomitant use of steroids or anticoagulants, a previous history of peptic ulcer disease (PUD), and the use of high doses of NSAIDs. Risk rises significantly with age. For example, in patients over 75 approximately one in 100 will suffer a bleed, and in one in 650 this will lead to death. The risk also varies according to the individual NSAID used. Large population studies in the UK and Italy have documented differing absolute values of risk, but the trend towards which were the safer/riskier NSAIDs was similar: ibuprofen is considered the 'safest', and ketorolac and azapropazone the highest risk. In Mrs GE's case she was on diclofenac and indometacin, which are both classed as 'intermediate' risk, along with naproxen and fenoprofen. Diclofenac and indometacin have a relative risk compared to ibuprofen of 1.4 (0.7–2.6) and 1.3 (0.7–2.3), respectively, according to the UK study, and a relative risk compared to placebo of 2.7 (1.5–4.8) and 5.4 (1.6–18.9), respectively.

NSAIDs also appear to increase the chance of complications such as bleeding in patients with underlying ulcer disease. NSAIDs lead to between a three- and a tenfold increase in ulcer complications, hospitalisation and death from ulcer disease.

Mrs GE is also taking propranolol for her tremor related to anxiety and ramipril for hypertension. She has lost blood, and is exhibiting some signs of shock that require correction. To help maintain her blood pressure, and prevent worsening of any shock that would be associated with re-bleeding, both drugs should be temporarily stopped. It should be noted that this patient is tachycardic (pulse of 155 bpm) even though she has been prescribed a potentially rate-controlling beta-blocker for her anxiety symptoms. Although the dose prescribed is probably too low to affect her heart rate greatly, it would be useful to check her care home medication records to see whether she has actually been receiving doses of propranolol and ramipril in the last few days: her recent vomiting and epigastric pain may have meant that she did not receive them.

What is the mechanism for NSAID-induced ulcers?

A5 **NSAIDs cause inhibition of prostaglandin synthesis.**

Preclinical studies suggest that two factors contribute to the pathogenesis of NSAID-associated ulcers. First, the inhibition of prostaglandin synthesis impairs mucosal defences and leads to an erosive breach of the epithelial barrier. Second, acid attack deepens the breach into frank ulceration, and low pH encourages passive absorption of the NSAID so it is trapped in the mucosa.

How effective is misoprostol at preventing NSAID-induced peptic ulcers?

A6 **Misoprostol is effective at preventing chronic NSAID-related gastric and duodenal ulcers. It is less effective than proton pump inhibitors (PPIs) at preventing duodenal ulcers, but at least as effective at preventing gastric ulcers. It is less well tolerated than PPIs and its use is often limited by diarrhoea.**

Various trials of the prostaglandin analogue misoprostol have proved the drug's effectiveness at preventing peptic ulcers in patients taking NSAIDs. The Cochrane Collaboration conducted a meta-analysis of 22 studies that assessed the long-term effect of misoprostol on the prevention of NSAID-induced ulcers. Eleven of the studies, which together included 3641 patients, compared the incidence of ulcers seen endoscopically after at least 3 months of NSAID plus misoprostol, to that of NSAID plus placebo. The cumulative incidence of gastric and duodenal ulcers with placebo was 15% and 6%, respectively. Misoprostol therapy significantly reduced the relative risk of gastric and duodenal ulcers by 74% and 53%, respectively. The problem with applying this meta-analysis to the choice of misoprostol for Mrs GE is that the trials used variable doses, with some using 200 micrograms four times daily and some 200 micrograms three times daily. Only six of the 11 studies used the 200 micrograms twice-daily dose that Mrs GE was receiving (as part of a combination tablet containing diclofenac 50 mg). When misoprostol total daily doses of 800 micrograms/day and 400 micrograms/day were analysed separately, both doses significantly reduced the risk of endoscopic ulcers compared to placebo, with the higher dose demonstrating statistically significant better prophylaxis against endoscopic gastric ulcers than 400 micrograms/day ($P = 0.0055$), but this was not seen for duodenal ulcers.

There is less evidence to say how effective misoprostol is compared to PPIs. The Cochrane Collaboration analysed two trials of 838 patients which compared the ulcer-preventing effects of PPIs to those of misoprostol in patients taking NSAIDs. One compared low-dose misoprostol (400 micrograms/day) daily to omeprazole 20 mg daily, the other compared high-dose misoprostol (800 micrograms/day) to lansoprazole 15 or 30 mg daily. Overall, when both trials were compared together, PPIs were statistically superior to misoprostol for the prevention of duodenal but not gastric ulcers. In the trial looking at the dose of misoprostol Mrs GE was taking (400 micrograms/day), the estimated proportion of patients in remission from any type of ulcer at 6 months was 61% among those taking omeprazole 20 mg daily, compared to 48% among those taking misoprostol 200 micrograms twice daily ($P = 0.001$) and 27% among those taking placebo ($P < 0.001$ for the comparisons with omeprazole and misoprostol). Of patients taking placebo, 32% had gastric ulcers at relapse, compared to 10% of patients taking misoprostol and 13% of those taking omeprazole. Duodenal ulcers developed in 12% of patients given placebo, compared to 10% of those given misoprostol and 3% of those given omeprazole.

How can the cause of the bleed be confirmed, the bleeding stopped, and re-bleeding prevented?

A7 **Endoscopic investigation and treatment are indicated in this case.**

The Blatchford score states that if a patient fits all the criteria below, they are unlikely to require endoscopic treatment:

(a) Urea <6.5 mmol/L.
(b) Haemoglobin >13 g/dL (M), 12 g/dL (F).
(c) Systolic BP >110 mmHg.
(d) Pulse <100 bpm.

This system had a 99% sensitivity for predicting serious bleeds when trialled in 1748 patients.

The benefit of scoring patients to assess their need for endoscopy is to avoid any unnecessary associated risks, costs and staff time.

Mrs GE only has one of the four markers in range, so is therefore highly likely to require her bleed treating endoscopically.

Is endoscopic treatment of the bleed more effective than drug treatment?

A8 **Yes.**

In a trial comparing endoscopic haemostatic treatment with high-dose PPI treatment, the PPI group was associated with higher re-bleeding rates and longer duration of hospital stay.

What is the likelihood of the patient suffering a re-bleed?

A9 **As a result of the findings during endoscopy this patient now scores 6 on the post-endoscopy Rockall score, which means that she has a 32.9% chance of re-bleeding and a 17.3% mortality risk (Tables 13.3 and 13.4).**

The risk of re-bleeding or death is substantial for Mrs GE, even after her endoscopic treatment. She will require close monitoring, in a high-dependency ward if a bed is available.

Table 13.3 The post-endoscopy Rockall score

Variable/ score	*0*	*1*	*2*	*3*
Age (years)	< 60	60–79	>80	
Shock	No shock (SBP >100 mmHg, Pulse <100 bpm)	Tachycardia (SBP >100 mmHg, Pulse >100 bpm)	Hypotension (SBP <100 mmHg, Pulse >100 bpm)	
Comorbidity	Nil major		Heart failure, ischaemic heart disease, any major comorbidity	Renal failure, liver failure, disseminated malignancy
Diagnosis	Mallory–Weiss tear, no lesion and no SRH	All other diagnosis	Malignancy of upper GI tract	
Major stigmata of recent haemorrhage (SRH)	Non or dark spot		Blood in upper GI tract, adherent clot, visible or spurting vessel	

Table 13.4 Percentage risk of re-bleed and mortality associated with each Rockall score

Score	0	1	2	3	4	5	6	7	8+
Re-bleed (%)	4.9	3.4	5.3	11.2	14.1	24.1	32.9	43.8	41.8
Mortality (%)	0	0	0.2	2.9	5.3	10.8	17.3	27.0	41.1

What test should be performed on Mrs GE during the endoscopy?

A10 **A CLOtest should be performed for *Helicobacter pylori*.**

A CLOtest is a sealed plastic slide holding an agar gel which contains urea and a pH indicator. A 2–3 mm biopsy specimen from the stomach (usually the sump of the antrum) is added to the slide. If the urease enzyme of *H. pylori* is present, degradation of the urea causes the pH to rise and a corresponding change in the colour of the gel from yellow (negative) to purple (positive).

H. pylori is a highly motile Gram-negative bacterium that colonises the mucous layer of the stomach. It is one of the commonest pathogens in man, and has been recognised as the principal cause of PUD and the main risk factor in the development of gastric cancer. It is found in the gastric mucosal surface of 85–100% of patients with a duodenal ulcer and 70–90% of those with a gastric ulcer.

It is not known how *H. pylori* infection is usually acquired and its route of transmission is unknown, although gastro-oral or faeco-oral routes are probable. The prevalence of *H. pylori* infection increases with age in the developed world and is higher in developing countries, leading its acquisition to be linked with social deprivation. The poorer socio-economic conditions when this patient was born mean that she is much more likely to be infected than a child who is born in the UK today.

Infection with *H. pylori* initially induces an acute inflammatory gastritis which persists for life. A single patient may be infected with multiple strains of the organism (this is particularly common in the developing world), and in colonised hosts the organisms may mutate over decades. Different strains are now being linked with different gastric diseases, and in future genotyping could help identify people at risk of particular diseases. Some strains of *H. pylori* appear to exert a protective effect against certain diseases (gastro-oesophageal reflux, Barrett's oesophagus, adenocarcinoma of the oesophagus and gastric cardia), leading to controversy over when to eliminate the organism.

Around 15% of infected individuals will go on to develop PUD or gastric cancer. It is thought that in patients with *H. pylori*-induced antral gastritis there is a loss of regulatory feedback, together with an intact and undamaged acid-secreting gastric corpus, and that the consequent high acid load reaching the duodenum leads to duodenal gastric metaplasia. These 'islands' of gastric metaplasia are then colonised by *H. pylori*, which leads to duodenitis and a high risk of duodenal ulcer. In patients with pangastritis an inflamed corpus results in a loss of acid-secreting cells, which leads in turn to an increased risk of gastric ulcer and gastric cancer.

A CLOtest has a high specificity (90–95%) and sensitivity (90–95%) for detecting the presence or absence of infection in the gastric mucosa. Its sensitivity is higher than that of other biopsy methods; however, it is recommended that multiple biopsy specimens be taken to achieve the highest sensitivity, as infection is often patchy; up to 14% of infected patients do not have antral infection, but do have *H. pylori* elsewhere in the stomach.

A careful drug history should be taken from the patient before a CLOtest is performed. Antibiotics or bismuth salts taken in the 3 weeks prior to biopsy may suppress *H. pylori* growth, making the organism difficult to detect and leading to a false negative result. In contrast, a false positive result can occur if the patient has achlorhydria, e.g. after taking high doses of an H_2-receptor antagonist or a PPI. Alternatively, PPIs can affect the pattern of *H. pylori* colonisation of the stomach and compromise the accuracy of antral biopsy. For these reasons it is recommended that patients who have taken these drugs prior to endoscopy have multiple biopsies taken from the antrum and corpus for histology, plus either culture or urease testing, or are tested for *H. pylori* once the ulcer has been treated.

In primary care, when patients are exhibiting symptoms associated with *H. pylori*, but not actively bleeding, carbon-13 (^{13}C) urea breath testing (sensitivity 95%, specificity 96%) and stool antigen tests (sensitivity 95%, specificity 94%) can also be used to test for *H. pylori*. Serological testing (sensitivity 92%, specificity 83%) is less accurate and therefore not recommended.

Which acid-suppressing drug, and what dose regimen and route, would you suggest? What evidence is there to support your recommendation? What alternatives could be used?

A11 A high-dose IV bolus of the PPI omeprazole 80 mg should be given followed by an infusion of omeprazole 8 mg/h for 72 hours, followed by high-dose oral PPI therapy for 5 days. Alternative therapies include somatostatin and antifibrinolytics.

The effect of acid suppression in patients with active or recent ulcer bleeding has been widely studied. If intragastric pH can be maintained at 6 or above, peptic activity is reduced, platelet aggregation (clot formation) is improved, and clot lysis is inhibited. These effects should help to stabilise the clot over an ulcer, promoting healing and reducing the chance of the ulcer re-bleeding.

Meta-analysis of the effects of histamine H_2 antagonists on clinically important outcomes associated with duodenal ulcers showed no significant difference compared to placebo. This is likely to be because H_2 antagonists are not effective enough at increasing gastric pH above 6.

PPIs have been shown to reduce the rate of re-bleeding and the need for surgery in patients with peptic ulcer bleeding. For this reason they are the drug class of choice in this situation; however, PPIs do not significantly affect mortality in patients suffering from bleeding ulcers.

Both oral and IV PPIs have been shown to reduce re-bleeding and the need for surgery. In patients who have not had a major bleed requiring endoscopic treatment, an oral PPI would be an appropriate and cost-effective treatment. One trial showed that oral omeprazole 40 mg twice daily for 5 days reduced re-bleeding rates to 11% (vs 36% in the placebo group). In cases such as Mrs GE, where endoscopy is needed, high-dose IV treatment is required. Various regimens have been trialled, including high bolus doses or infusions, but none has been adequately powered to draw conclusions from head-to-head comparison of the different regimens. Omeprazole 80 mg IV stat, then 8 mg/h infusion for 72 hours has been shown to reduce recurrent bleeding to 6.8% vs 22.5% for placebo (NNT = 6), and blood transfusions to 2.7 units vs 3.5 units for placebo. This regimen is therefore considered the 'gold standard'. After 72 hours of PPI infusion a high-dose oral PPI should be prescribed. Again, various doses and frequencies have proved effective. Omeprazole 40 mg twice daily orally for 5 days after endoscopy has been shown to reduce re-bleeding to 7% vs 21% in the placebo group (NNT = 7); omeprazole 20 mg four times daily orally led to re-bleeding rates of 17% vs 33% in the placebo group (NNT = 6). It can be argued that twice-daily dosing is preferred by most patients and the nurses who have to administer the drugs.

Alternative therapies include somatostatin and antifibrinolytics such as tranexamic acid.

High-dose IV somatostatin suppresses acid secretion and splanchnic blood flow and is theoretically an attractive therapy; however, although a meta-analysis of available trials showed some benefit, the quality of much of the data was poor, and this drug is not routinely used for the management of bleeding peptic ulcers.

A meta-analysis of trials using tranexamic acid, which inhibits fibrinolysis, has demonstrated that the drug does not appear to reduce re-bleeding, but does reduce the need for surgical intervention and may reduce mortality. However, the overall benefits are unclear and further trials are needed.

Does infection with *H. pylori* predispose to NSAID-induced damage to the GI mucosa?

A12 There is now good evidence to suggest that the presence of *H. pylori* predisposes to NSAID-induced ulceration.

NSAID ingestion can lead to a variety of GI injuries, ranging from petechial haemorrhages to erosions and, occasionally, ulceration.

However, the move from erosion to ulceration is not necessarily inevitable, and endoscopic studies have shown that NSAID-induced erosions can appear and disappear over time, presumably as a result of adaptation and repair processes.

Investigations into the relationship between long-term NSAID use and *H. pylori* infection have concluded that NSAID-induced damage to the gastroduodenal mucosa does not increase susceptibility to *H. pylori* infection, but that ulcers are more likely to develop in long-term NSAID users who are infected with *H. pylori*, especially if they smoke.

Meta-analysis has suggested that both *H. pylori* infection and NSAID use independently and significantly increase the risk of peptic ulcer and ulcer bleeding. In addition, there is a synergy for the development of peptic ulcer and ulcer bleeding between *H. pylori* infection and NSAID use. The presence of *H. pylori* infection has been shown to increase the rate of PUD in NSAID takers 3.5-fold, compared with the risk associated with NSAIDs alone. The risk of ulcer bleeding with *H. pylori* and NSAID use separately was 1.8 and 4.6, respectively, this increased to 6.1 when both factors were present.

To try to establish whether eradication of *H. pylori* reduces the risk of NSAID-induced ulceration, a study of patients with a history of dyspepsia or PUD who were NSAID naive but *H. pylori* positive (via urea breath test) were randomised to either eradication therapy or PPI therapy alone for 1 week prior to commencement of the NSAID: 90% of patients in the treatment group had *H. pylori* eradicated. After 6 months' treatment with modified-release diclofenac 100 mg daily, five of 51 patients in the treated group and 15 of 49 of the group treated with omeprazole alone prior to therapy had ulcers. In another trial in patients with previous peptic ulcer and prescribed NSAIDs, *H. pylori* eradication reduced the recurrence of peptic ulcer from 18% to 10%.

In patients using NSAIDs without PUD, *H. pylori* eradication reduced the risk of a first occurrence of peptic ulcer: in a single trial of 8 weeks' duration, first occurrence was reduced from 26% to 7% of patients.

What other factors could have contributed to Mrs GE's duodenal ulcer, and might potentially increase the chances of relapse?

A13 Her age.

Mrs GE is over 60, which is a non-modifiable risk factor for PUD. Other risk factors (which do not apply to Mrs GE) for NSAID-induced bleeds include a previous history of PUD and concomitant use of steroids or anticoagulants. Cigarette smoking has been demonstrated in controlled trials to impair ulcer healing and promote ulcer recurrence. Many mechanisms have been suggested for this effect. Other possible lifestyle factors that have been implicated as predisposing to PUD include stress and a significant alcohol intake. Although it has been difficult to study these risk factors under controlled conditions there is mounting evidence that stress may function as a cofactor with *H. pylori*, either by stimulating the production of gastric acid or by promoting behaviour that causes a risk to health. Finally, genetic factors may determine susceptibility to PUD.

When should *H. pylori* eradication begin?

A14 **Eradication should take place after the ulcer has been healed. Full-dose PPI therapy should therefore continue for 2 months before *H. pylori* is eradicated.**

NICE recommends that patients with duodenal ulcer follow one of three pathways, depending on their *H. pylori* status and whether or not their ulcer is associated with NSAIDs. Patients who are *H. pylori* negative should receive 1–2 months of full-dose PPI, e.g. omeprazole 20 mg daily (or a histamine H_2 antagonist if a PPI is unsuitable), then be reviewed for response. This is sufficient to heal peptic ulcers in the majority of patients. Those who respond but remain symptomatic can continue on a low dose of PPI (e.g. omeprazole 10 mg daily) if/when required.

Those who have non-NSAID-related ulcers and who are *H. pylori*-positive should receive eradication therapy as soon as possible. *H. pylori*-eradication therapy increases duodenal ulcer healing in *H. pylori*-positive patients. After 4–8 weeks, patients receiving acid suppression therapy average 69% healing; eradication increases this by a further 5.4% (NNT = 18). *H. pylori* eradication therapy also reduces duodenal ulcer recurrence in *H. pylori*-positive patients. After 3–12 months, 39% of patients receiving short-term acid-suppression therapy are without ulcer; eradication increases this by a further 52% (NNT = 2).

In this case, where the ulcer is at least partly attributable to the NSAIDs but the patient is also *H. pylori* positive, the recommendation is to heal the ulcer with 2 months of full-dose PPI, then to eradicate the *H. pylori*. This is because in patients with peptic ulcer who are using NSAIDs, *H. pylori* eradication does not increase healing compared to acid-suppression therapy alone in trials of 8 weeks' duration; however, in patients using NSAIDs with a history of previous peptic ulcer, *H. pylori* eradication reduces the recurrence of peptic ulcer. In a single trial of 6 months' duration recurrence was reduced from 18% to 10%.

Outline a pharmaceutical care plan for Mrs GE's further treatment.

A15 The pharmaceutical care plan should include the following elements:

(a) Ensure appropriate therapy is prescribed to heal her ulcer and eradicate *H. pylori*.
(b) Ensure her analgesic therapies are reviewed and appropriate alternatives to NSAIDs prescribed for future use.
(c) Ensure her antihypertensive therapy is restarted when appropriate.
(d) Ensure that her gout and any new chronic conditions are managed appropriately in view of this new diagnosis.
(e) Review the need for oral iron therapy.
(f) Counsel Mrs GE on her medications (this will include ascertaining whether she manages her own medicines in her care home, or whether they are administered to her).
(g) Ensure her GP is clear about how to manage her therapies after discharge.

In the patient's discharge letter, what would you recommend the general practitioner (GP) prescribes to eradicate the *H. Pylori*?

A16 Triple therapy with a PPI, amoxicillin and clarithromycin 500 mg (PAC_{500} regimen). This comprises omeprazole 20 mg twice daily + amoxicillin 1 g twice daily + clarithromycin 500 mg twice daily for 7 days.

A PPI, metronidazole, clarithromycin 250 mg (PMC_{250}) regimen would be an appropriate alternative, especially if the patient was penicillin allergic.

The eradication of *H. pylori* can lead to a cure for patients with PUD. The National Institutes of Health consensus meeting in 1994 and the European Helicobacter Study Group in 1996 both recommended that the infection is eradicated in patients with active PUD and proven infection. Mrs GE falls into this category.

Eradication of *H. pylori* is a challenging task. Although many antibiotics are bactericidal to the organism *in vitro*, even high-dose regimens have proved ineffective *in vivo*. Possible reasons for this are that bactericidal concentrations are not achieved in the gastric mucosa; the drugs are inactivated or ineffective at low pH; or a combination of these factors. To be effective, antibiotic therapy must therefore be combined with either bismuth chelate or acid-suppressant therapy or both.

The rationale for the use of acid-suppressant therapy with antibiotics is to increase gastric pH, thereby inducing a favourable environment for antibiotic activity. In addition, omeprazole has been observed to reduce antral colonisation by *H. pylori*, presumably by disturbing its environment, although the effect is only temporary and colonisation returns to normal on cessation of therapy.

Many regimens have been evaluated for the eradication of *H. pylori*. Early dual therapies of omeprazole (40 mg daily) plus amoxicillin (750 mg twice daily) or clarithromycin (500 mg three times daily), although fairly well tolerated, led to mean eradication rates of only 50–60%. Bismuth chelate can lyse *H. pylori* in 30–90 minutes *in vitro*; however, it is not clear whether the compound is bactericidal or bacteriostatic to the organism *in vivo*. If bismuth chelate is used as sole therapy, *H. pylori* eradication rates are low; however, when combined with antibiotics, eradication levels are much higher. The mechanism for this synergistic effect is unclear. Triple therapies of bismuth chelate plus two antibiotics (metronidazole 400 mg three times daily plus amoxicillin or tetracycline 500 mg four times daily) raise the eradication rate to approximately 80%; however, the regimen is very complex to take and the side-effects can be considerable and frequent (seen in 20–50% of patients), which means that non-adherence, whether intentional or not, can lead to treatment failure. The addition of a PPI to this regimen (quadruple therapy) increases the eradication rate to >90%; however, side-effects and non-adherence remain significant issues, even in well-supported patients.

As a result, PPI-based triple therapy comprising a PPI plus two antibiotics has become the recommended first-line treatment for *H. pylori* eradication. It is simple, effective, and much better tolerated than earlier regimens. A 1-week course has a success rate of around 80–85%, and may also reduce the long-term risk of gastric cancer. In patients with diagnosed peptic ulcer, increasing the course to 14 days' duration improves the effectiveness of eradication by nearly 10%, but does not appear cost-effective. As the drugs need only be taken twice daily, adherence is easier. The PPI should be given at twice the therapeutic dose. The choice of antibiotic is usually clarithromycin twice daily; the dose is 250 mg (if with metronidazole) or 500 mg (if with amoxicillin). Either amoxicillin 1 g twice daily or metronidazole 400 mg twice daily is the second antibiotic. The choice will usually depend on local drug prices and the patient's allergy status, but is also influenced by antibiotic resistance. If amoxicillin or clarithromycin has been given to the patient for any infection in the last year, resistance may be present and the antibiotic should not be used as part of *H. pylori* eradication therapy.

Should Mrs GE be prescribed iron therapy, and if so for how long?

A17 Yes. Ferrous sulphate 200 mg twice daily for 1 month is appropriate.

Although Mrs GE's haemoglobin result is now almost normal, her admission haematology demonstrated a microcytic, hypochromic picture indicating that she had been bleeding chronically. As a result, her iron stores are now likely to be depleted. Approximately 120 mg of elemental iron daily in divided doses should ensure adequate iron absorption, and 1 month of therapy should be enough to replenish iron stores. If this form of iron is poorly tolerated, a formulation such as ferrous gluconate, which contains less elemental iron per tablet, could be tried, as GI toxicity appears to be in direct proportion to the concentration of iron in the gut.

What counselling should Mrs GE be given in preparation for discharge to optimise successful treatment and adherence to treatment?

A18 **(a) By providing appropriate discharge medications and counselling for each item prescribed.**
(b) By ensuring Mrs GE is clear about her future therapy needs.
(c) By reinforcing the general counselling and advice provided earlier in her hospital stay.

The extent of the counselling will depend upon whether or not Mrs GE manages her own medicines in her care home. If she does not, it is important that any counselling offered is tailored to her established needs and any necessary additional information provided with the medications for the care staff.

Non-adherence is an important reason for the failure of *H. pylori* eradication regimens. It is vital that Mrs GE understands the importance of completing this prescribed treatment. A medication record card plus any relevant information leaflets may help her if she is self-medicating after discharge. It is also vital that she understands how long each aspect of her treatment will be continuing.

Should the GP check to see whether the *H. pylori* eradication was successful? If so, how?

A19 **It is not necessary to recheck the patient's *H. pylori* status, unless she becomes symptomatic**

If patients with duodenal ulcer respond symptomatically to the ulcer healing dose of PPI and eradication therapy then there is no need to retest for *H. pylori* to ensure eradication. If the patient is anxious about the result, then a retest can be performed. Provided the patient adhered to the treatment regimen, remains symptom free and the NSAID has been stopped, there is no reason to believe that the patient has not been 'cured'. The major causes of the ulcer have been removed and the ulcer healed.

In patients who do not respond, or who relapse, retesting using carbon-13 urea breath testing is recommended; however non-adherence with treatment, surreptitious or inadvertent NSAID or aspirin use, and ulceration due to ingestion of other drugs should first be ruled out.

How long does she need to be prescribed a proton pump inhibitor (PPI)?

A20 The PPI should be prescribed for a maximum of 2 months.

Two months' treatment with a full dose of PPI has been shown to heal the majority of ulcers. Combined with stopping the NSAIDs and eradicating *H. pylori*, this should be considered adequate to prevent recurrence. If symptoms recur following the initial treatment, a PPI could be offered with the advice that it should be taken at the lowest dose possible to control symptoms, with a limited number of repeat prescriptions. There could also be a discussion with Mrs GE about using the treatment on an as-required basis to manage any symptoms.

How would you recommend her GP manages her osteoarthritis?

A21 Treat the osteoarthritis using paracetamol 1 g four times daily.

It is important to try to treat the pain associated with osteoarthritis but to avoid NSAIDs if possible. Paracetamol alone may control the pain, and is very well tolerated and 'safe' at licensed doses. Mrs GE may have a better analgesic affect if she takes it regularly four times a day than if she uses it just when required. If paracetamol alone is insufficient, low doses of a weak opioid (codeine or dihydrocodeine) could be added. The lowest effective dose should be found to avoid unnecessary opiate side-effects, constipation being most common in the elderly. Initially it might be helpful to prescribe small doses (15 mg four times daily when required) of dihydrocodeine or codeine to assess her requirements. Depending on the amounts Mrs GE needs, the prescription could be left to be taken when required, or given regularly either as separate drugs or as part of a 'co-analgesic' with the paracetamol, such as co-codamol or co-dydramol. It is important to assess the amount of opioid needed before starting a 'co-analgesic', as they offer no flexibility in the amount of opioid given: opioid cannot be omitted if side-effects are experienced without omitting all analgesia. Low-strength buprenorphine patches 5 micrograms/h offer similar amounts of opiate to the oral weak opiates codeine and dihyrocodeine, and may be easier for Mrs GE to use as they would reduce the number of tablets she needs to take each day. If constipation due to the oral opiates limits the effectiveness of analgesia she may tolerate the buprenorphine patches better.

How would you recommend her GP manages her gout?

A22 **Titrate her allopurinol dose upwards to 300 mg daily to prevent attacks. Acute attacks can be treated using oral colchicine or steroid injections.**

Mrs GE should avoid NSAIDs for preventing and treating her gout. If her attacks are not prevented by the allopurinol 100 mg daily that she is already taking, and she is avoiding any precipitating factors, the dose could be increased up to 300 mg daily. Acute attacks can be treated using colchicine if tolerated, and intra-articular steroid injections if necessary.

Further reading

Graham DY, Agrawal NM, Campbell DR *et al.* Ulcer prevention in long-term users of nonsteroidal anti-inflammatory drugs. *Arch Intern Med* 2002; **162**: 169–175.

Health Protection Agency & GP Microbiology Laboratory Use Group. *Diagnosis of* Helicobacter pylori *(HP) in Dyspepsia, Quick Reference Guide for Primary Care*. Health Protection Agency, London, 2008.

Lau JYW, Sung JJY, Lee KC *et al.* Effect of intravenous omeprazole on recurrent bleeding after endoscopic treatment of bleeding peptic ulcers. *N Engl J Med* 2000; **343**: 310–316.

Leontiadis GI, Sharma VK, Howden CW. Systematic review and meta-analysis of proton pump inhibitor therapy in peptic ulcer bleeding. *Br Med J* 2005; **330**; 568–572.

Levine JE, Leontiadis GI, Sharma VK, Howden CW. Meta-analysis: the efficacy of intravenous H_2-receptor antagonists in bleeding peptic ulcer. *Aliment Pharmacol Ther* 2002; **16**: 1137–1142.

Merki HS, Wilder-Smith CH. Do continuous infusions of omeprazole and ranitidine retain their effect with prolonged dosing? *Gastroenterology* 1994; **106**: 60–64.

National Institute for Health and Clinical Excellence. CG17. *Dyspepsia*. NICE, London, 2004.

Rostom A, Dube C, Wells G *et al. Prevention of NSAID-Induced Gastroduodenal Ulcers*. Cochrane Database of Systematic Reviews 2002, Issue 4.

Sung JJY, Chan FKL, Lau JYW *et al.* The effect of endoscopic therapy in patients receiving omeprazole for bleeding ulcers with nonbleeding visible vessels or adherent clots: a randomized comparison. *Ann Intern Med* 2003; **139**: 237–243.

14

Crohn's disease

Jackie Eastwood and Simon Gabe

Case study and questions

Day 1 Mr MA, a 25-year-old man, was admitted to the ward from A&E complaining of abdominal pain, frequent episodes of diarrhoea (six times per day) but with no blood or mucus. He reported weight loss, but was unsure of how much and when it started, and appeared lethargic.

He had no past medical history of any note and only took occasional analgesia when required. He reported smoking 20 cigarettes a day.

On abdominal palpitation his abdomen was soft, with no masses or organomegaly. A rectal examination showed no masses and there was no fresh blood.

His blood pressure was recorded as 125/74 mmHg, his pulse rate was 72 beats per minute (bpm) and his respiratory rate was 17. He was afebrile. His weight was 60 kg and his height 5′10″.

His haematology results were as follows:

- Haemoglobin 11.5 g/dL (reference range 13–16)
- Mean cell volume 101 fL (78–100)
- White cell count 12.2×10^9 (4.5–11.5)
- Erythrocyte sedimentation rate (ESR) 35 mm/h (0–8)
- C-reactive protein (CRP) 45 mg/L (<5)
- A stool sample for *C. Iostridium difficile* toxin was negative

A colonoscopy was performed which revealed patchy colitis and an inflamed ulcerated terminal ileum suggestive of Crohn's disease (CD). Biopsies were taken and the histology confirmed the diagnosis of CD.

Q1 What are the therapeutic aims of treatment for Mr MA?

Q2 What are the parameters that will indicate whether the aims of treatment are being met?

Q3 What are the options for treatment in the acute phase of the disease?

Q4 What are the first-line treatment options to prevent relapse once he is in remission?

Mr MA improved on hydrocortisone intravenously (IV) 100 mg four times a day. After 2 days this was converted to oral prednisolone 40 mg each day. A decision was made to start Mr MA on Pentasa 2 g twice a day.

Q5 How effective are 5-aminosalicylates (5ASAs) in treating CD?

Month 6 Mr MA was admitted to hospital with a significant flare-up. IV corticosteroids were again used to induce remission. Mesalazine was continued and a decision was made to start azathioprine therapy.

Q6 What tests need to be performed before starting a patient on azathioprine?
Q7 Outline your pharmaceutical care plan for Mr MA (after azathioprine).
Q8 Is azathioprine appropriate for achieving and maintaining remission in CD?
Q9 What monitoring should be undertaken for Mr MA now he is on azathioprine? How often should this be done and why?

Mr MA was discharged on:

- Prednisolone 40 mg daily for 2 weeks, then reduce by 5 mg/week until zero
- Azathioprine 150 mg daily
- Calcium carbonate 1500 mg and vitamin D 400 units, two tablets daily
- Pentasa 1 g three times daily

As Mr MA lived a 3-hour drive away from the hospital, his consultant asked his general practitioner (GP) if they would continue the prescribing of this treatment. The GP was concerned about prescribing azathioprine as it is an unlicensed use of a licensed medication. The GP was also unsure of the monitoring requirements, and what to do if Mr MA experienced any problems.

Q10 What can be put in place to help provide the GP with enough information to prescribe and monitor the azathioprine?

Month 7 After a month of azathioprine therapy Mr MA rang the hospital inflammatory bowel disease (IBD) nurse and said that he felt unwell and was suffering from nausea and malaise. He explained that he had tried stopping the azathioprine and found that these symptoms stopped, and then recurred when he started the azathioprine again. Mr MA was brought back to the outpatient clinic and changed to 6-mercaptopurine (6MP).

Q11 What is the rationale for changing to 6MP?

Month 18 Mr MA remained in remission on 6MP and was adherent with the medication and the monitoring schedule; however, he was again admitted to hospital with an acute flare. He had lost weight and was currently not eating much due to the nausea and vomiting he was experiencing.

Q12 What effect will the disease have on his nutritional status?
Q13 What nutritional input may be helpful at this stage?

Mr MA was started on oral supplements. He was asked to take three cartons per day of the supplement.

Q14 What are the treatment options for Mr MA at this stage in his disease?
Q15 What are the long-term options for this patient now?

Mr MA improved on steroids and was started on oral methotrexate 25 mg once a week and folic acid 5 mg once a week.

Q16 What counselling points would you discuss with Mr MA prior to discharge?
Q17 How quickly should the oral steroids be tapered down?

Month 19 Mr MA was seen in outpatients. He was not well on methotrexate and still had symptoms. A decision was made to try a biologic therapy. His current Crohn's Disease Activity Index (CDAI) was 310 (severe active disease score ≥300).

Q18 What biologic therapies are available for CD?
Q19 What are the doses and administration methods for these medications?
Q20 What are the advantages and disadvantages of these drugs that will affect the choice of which one to use?
Q21 What tests need to be done prior to commencing anti-TNF treatment?
Q22 Does Mr MA fulfil the criteria for using anti-TNF medication?

Mr MA had three doses of infliximab (IFX), and in clinic after the third infusion reported that his symptoms had improved and that he felt better. His clinical markers had also improved.

Q23 What are the options for treatment now?
Q24 What do you need to consider if Mr MA continues on IFX as maintenance therapy?
Q25 This is a step-up approach. Is there any benefit of using a step-down approach for these patients?

Answers

What are the therapeutic aims of treatment for Mr MA?

A1 The main aim of therapy at this time is to get Mr MA into remission so as to avoid complications and surgery. Once the patient is in remission the aim will be to maintain remission and prevent relapses.

Additional aims include the need to address his nutritional state and any deficiencies that may have occurred. He has a macrocytic anaemia which may be due to B_{12} deficiency and needs to be treated. He is also malnourished (body mass index (BMI) 19 kg/m^2) and needs nutritional support.

This man has been newly diagnosed with CD at the age of 25.

CD is most commonly diagnosed between the ages of 15 and 25. The prevalence is around 1:1000. Crohn's is an inflammatory disease that can affect any part of the intestine, from mouth to anus, and is also associated with extraintestinal manifestations (eyes, skin and joints). The cause is not yet known.

The main symptoms are abdominal pain, diarrhoea, tiredness and loss of weight. Patients are treated with drugs to reduce the inflammation and/or enteral feeds. Seventy-five percent of patients require an intestinal resection for complications related to stricturing or penetrating disease; 70% will require repeat surgery within 20 years.

The progression of the disease for this patient is hard to predict at this stage.

What are the parameters that will indicate if the aims of treatment are being met?

A2 His clinical signs and symptoms should be used to monitor his response to treatment.

The following improvements should occur:

(a) **Symptoms:** reduced frequency of diarrhoea, pain lessening.
(b) **Haematology:** indicators of an immune response should lessen. Inflammatory markers include white blood cell count, erythrocyte sedimentation rate (ESR) and C-reactive protein (CRP). CRP is a marker of inflammation which correlates well to disease activity.
(c) **Malnutrition:** his weight, BMI and muscle strength should be measured and seen to improve with increased nutritional support.
(d) **Anaemia:** folic acid and vitamin B_{12} should be given, and this should correct the macrocytic anaemia.

What are the options for treatment in the acute phase of the disease?

A3 **First-line treatment for the acute phase of CD is corticosteroids. If the flare is mild and the medication can be taken orally, prednisolone should be given. If the flare is severe, as with Mr MA, then intravenous (IV) hydrocortisone should be administered.**

Hydrocortisone is normally given at a dose of 100 mg four times a day. This should be reduced once the patient begins to improve. Once oral medication is recommenced he should be changed to oral prednisolone.

Prednisolone is normally given in doses >30 mg/day for at least 14 days. This should then be reduced slowly to prevent an addisonian crisis. Patients who are prescribed courses of corticosteroids should take calcium and vitamin D supplements if their oral intake is inadequate (1 g calcium per day and 800 units vitamin D per day). Treatment with bisphosphonates should also be considered. The current recommendations from the British Society of Gastroenterology (BSG) are:

(a) Patients under 65 years requiring steroids for more than 3 months should have a DEXA (dual energy X-ray absorptiometry) scan and start treatment with a bisphosphonate if the T-score is less than –1.5.
(b) For patients over 65, consider bisphosphonate when starting steroids.

What are the first-line treatment options to prevent relapse once he is in remission?

A4 **5-Aminosalicylates (5ASAs) are the mainstay of treatment for inflammatory bowel disease (IBD) to maintain remission. Their use is mainly in ulcerative colitis; however, they do have a role to play in the treatment of CD.**

The mode of action of 5ASAs is not well understood, but is thought to be a local effect on epithelial cells of the bowel through a number of mechanisms. The choice of agent depends on the location, severity and extent of the disease, as well as patient preference. The majority of 5ASA preparations are unlicensed for use in CD, and higher doses (>4 g/day) are often required (Table 14.1).

Pentasa was chosen as this preparation is thought to release the active ingredient in both the stomach and the small bowel.

Immunomodulators are not generally used as first-line maintenance treatment.

Table 14.1 Form and site of action of some 5ASA preparations

Drug	*Form*	*Site of initial release*
Asacol	Tablet of 5ASA coated with Eudragit S	Ileum
Pentasa	Microgranules of 5ASA coated with semipermeable ethylcellulose	Stomach
Salofalk	Tablet of 5ASA coated with Eudragit R	Jejunum
Sulfasalazine	5ASA molecule linked to sulfapyridine by azo bond	Colon
Olsalazine	Dimer of 5ASA linked with azo bond	Colon
Balsalazide	5ASA linked to inert carrier by azo bond	Colon
Mezavant XL	5ASA with milli matrix coating system	Colon

How effective are 5-aminosalicylates (5ASAs) in treating CD?

A5 **5ASAs are less effective in the treatment of CD than in ulcerative colitis; however, they do have a role in reducing the risk of relapse following bowel resection (40% reduction at 18 months).**

They are ineffective at maintaining remission in patients who have achieved remission using corticosteroids unless higher doses (>4 g/day) are used.

In one trial of patients with active ileocaecal disease, a greater reduction in the Crohn's disease activity index (CDAI) was seen in the mesalazine group than in the placebo group, but the clinical significance of this is unclear. The CDAI score incorporates measurements of bowel frequency, abdominal pain, wellbeing, symptoms and signs associated with CD, and laboratory indices.

What tests need to be performed prior to starting a patient on azathioprine?

A6 **A full blood count (FBC) and liver function tests (LFTs) should be carried out prior to starting Mr MA on azathioprine.**

Thiopurine methyl transferase (TPMT) is one of the enzymes that metabolises azathioprine and 6-MP to inactive metabolites: 90% of individuals have normal activity, 10% have intermediate activity (genetic heterozygotes) and 0.3% have low or no enzyme activity (homozygous for a mutant gene). Those with intermediate or low activity are more likely to develop accumulation of cytotoxic metabolites and suffer from severe haematopoietic toxicities; however, the BSG guidelines for the treatment of IBD from 2004 do not recommend the measuring of TPMT prior to starting therapy.

Outline your pharmaceutical care plan for Mr MA (after azathioprine).

A7
(a) **Ensure that appropriate doses of medication are being used in order to optimise treatment and reduce the risk of adverse effects.**
(b) **Ensure that the immunomodulator is appropriately monitored, either by primary or by secondary care.**
(c) **Provide information to the patient on his medication, including side-effects to look out for and the monitoring that needs to take place.**
(d) **Provide appropriate information on how to give up smoking.**
(e) **Ensure that secondary medications are started to prevent secondary complications of IBD.**

Smoking affects remission rate and disease activity in patients with CD. Patients who smoke require more surgery, and medications are often less effective. Patients should be advised to contact their primary care clinician for support, guidance and methods to give up smoking.

Side-effects that this patient should look out for include lethargy, bruising and sore throat.

Is azathioprine appropriate for achieving and maintaining remission in CD?

A8 **Thiopurines are unlicensed in the UK for the treatment of IBD, but are useful for achieving and maintaining remission in CD.**

Treatment with thiopurines should be considered in patients who have had more than two acute attacks within a year that required treatment with corticosteroids, or in those who are steroid dependent. Patients who have undergone surgery for complex CD should also be started on an immunomodulator.

What monitoring should be undertaken for Mr MA now that he is on azathioprine? How often should this be done, and why?

A9 **An FBC and LFTs should be carried out weekly for the first 8 weeks and then monthly after that.**

This is to ensure that the patient is tolerating the medication and not experiencing adverse effects of abnormal liver function or blood dyscrasias. Patients should also be advised to contact their clinician if a sore throat or infection develops.

What can be put in place to help provide the GP with enough information to prescribe and monitor the azathioprine?

A10 **A shared care protocol should be put in place.**

This should clearly state the roles and responsibilities of the hospital clinician and the GP; monitoring requirements and who is responsible for each aspect of the monitoring; possible side-effects and what to do if the patient suffers from them. Contact numbers for all secondary care clinicians should also be included in the document.

What is the rationale for changing to 6-MP?

A11 **Azathioprine is metabolised to 6-MP. Some patients who are intolerant to azathioprine find that they are able to tolerate 6-MP; however, if a patient has severe side-effects to a thiopurine the use of an alternate thiopurine should be avoided.**

What effect will the disease have on Mr MA's nutritional status?

A12 **Recurrent flares of CD and the current anorexia due to his illness will mean that Mr MA will lose weight with loss of fat and muscle mass. This will have an impact on his physical abilities, including his respiratory and cardiac function.**

In CD, there is evidence that artificial nutrition support does beneficially affect the inflammatory response, although the mechanism is unclear. The BSG guidelines for IBD state that nutrition is an integral treatment for all patients with CD and should be considered if there is malnutrition or failure to maintain body weight.

What nutritional input may be helpful at this stage?

A13 **At this stage, either oral supplements or nasogastric feeding should be started.**

In a Cochrane Review, 53–80% of patients achieved remission after 3–6 weeks of nutritional therapy. If Mr MA is unable to tolerate the oral supplement, then administration via a nasogastric tube could be considered while he is in hospital.

What are the treatment options for Mr MA at this stage in his disease?

A14 **To achieve remission he needs to restart corticosteroids and continue the oral supplements. Once he is in remission the steroids can be carefully reduced and then long-term therapy can be reconsidered.**

What are the long-term options for this patient now?

A15 **Treatment options once he is in remission are to switch to another immunomodulator such as methotrexate or tacrolimus, or to consider introducing a biologic therapy (anti-TNF-α medication such as infliximab (IFX) or adalimumab).**

If this patient just had terminal ileal disease, surgery could be considered; however, he also has colonic disease, so surgery would be extensive and should be a last resort.

What counselling points would you discuss with Mr MA prior to discharge?

A16 **Methotrexate is a dihydrofolate reductase inhibitor and must only be taken as a weekly dose. The patient must be told which day of the week to take the methotrexate, and that it should be the same day each week.**

The dose of methotrexate should be explained to the patient, in particular how many 2.5 mg tablets make up the total weekly dose. This information must be repeated on the medication label. Mr MA should be warned of the side-effects to look out for and what to do if they occur. In 2006, the National Patient Safety Agency produced guidance for patients on weekly methotrexate. This included patient information and a monitoring booklet. This booklet should be given to the patient and they should be made aware that it needs to be brought to each appointment and when collecting medication. Folic acid can be given once a week as rescue therapy. This should not be taken on the same day as the methotrexate.

How quickly should the oral steroids be tapered down?

A17 **There are no national guidelines for the reduction of steroid doses. Most clinicians will reduce by 5 mg each week until stopping. If a patient has previously relapsed on this regimen then the reducing regimen may be carried out more slowly. Too-rapid reduction of the steroid dose is associated with early relapse.**

What biologic therapies are available for CD?

A18 **Two anti-TNF-α inhibitors (anti-TNFs), infliximab (IFX) and adalimumab, are licensed in the UK at the time of writing.**

These are both monoclonal antibodies that bind to tumour necrosis factor-α (TNF-α). TNF-α is a proinflammatory cytokine that has been implicated in the pathophysiology of CD. There is evidence for the use of these therapies in both inflammatory and fistulating CD.

(a) **Efficacy in inflammatory CD.** A multicentre double-blind study in 108 patients with moderate to severe CD refractory to 5ASA, corticosteroids, and/or immunomodulators, demonstrated an 81% response rate at 4 weeks after 5 mg/kg IFX compared to 17% given placebo. The duration of response varied, but 48% who had received 5 mg/kg still had a response at week 12. The ACCENT-1 study was the definitive re-treatment trial. Maintenance of remission in 335 responders to a single infusion of IFX 5 mg/kg for active CD (out of an initial 573) was examined. The protocol was complex. In broad terms, patients were treated with placebo, 5 mg/kg or 10 mg/kg every 8 weeks until week 46. At week 30, 21% of the placebo-treated patients were in remission, compared to 39% of patients treated with 5 mg/kg infusions (P = 0.003) and 45% of those treated with 10 mg/kg infusions ($P = 0.0002$). IFX is licensed but not yet approved by NICE for maintenance therapy of CD in the UK.

(b) **Evidence for use in fistulating CD.** IFX is the first and only agent to show a therapeutic effect for fistulating CD in a controlled trial. Ninety-four patients with draining abdominal or perianal fistulae of at least 3 months' duration were treated: 68% in the 5 mg/kg group and 56% in the 10 mg/kg group experienced a 50% reduction in the number of draining fistulas at two or more consecutive visits, compared to 26% given placebo ($P = 0.002$ and $P = 0.02$, respectively). The problem is that the duration of this effect was in most cases limited to only 3 or 4 months. A large re-treatment trial for fistulating CD (ACCENT-II) has been conducted. A total of 306 patients with actively draining enterocutaneous fistulae were treated with three induction infusions of IFX 5 mg/kg at weeks 0, 2 and 6. Of the 306, 195 (69%) responded, and these were randomised to 5 mg/kg maintenance infusions or placebo every 8 weeks. Patients who lost response were switched from placebo to active treatment at 5 mg/kg, or the re-treatment dose was increased from 5 to 10 mg/kg. At the end of the 12-month trial, 46% of the patients on active re-treatment had a fistula response versus 23% of those on placebo ($P = 0.001$). Complete response (all fistulae closed) was observed in 36% of patients on active treatment, compared to 19% of those on placebo (P = 0.009). Treatment of fistulising CD with IFX is not currently approved by NICE unless criteria for severe active disease are also met.

What are the doses and administration methods for these medications?

A19 **IFX is given as an IV infusion and adalimumab as a subcutaneous injection. Both have an acute dosage regimen which may be followed by a maintenance regimen.**

IFX can be given as an initial dose of 5 mg/kg. If the condition responds the patient can either have another dose only if the symptoms recur, or have maintenance therapy of an infusion every 8 weeks.

The summary of product characteristics for IFX states that intervals between doses should not exceed 14 weeks because of the risk of formation of anti-IFX antibodies. The presence of these antibodies will result in the drug being less effective, resulting in breakthrough disease activity, or allergic reactions to the infusion may occur.

For adalimumab the initial dose is 160 mg, followed by 80 mg 2 weeks after the initial dose. Maintenance therapy at 40 mg every 2 weeks should start 2 weeks after the second dose. This can be increased to weekly injections if necessary.

What are the advantages and disadvantages of these drugs that will affect the choice of which one to use?

A20 **The key difference between the products is that IFX must be administered to the patient, whereas adalimumab may be self-administered.**

IFX is given as an IV infusion in an outpatient setting. Some patients suffer from allergic reactions to the drug, mainly due to the murine section of the antibody, so hospital-based administration is required. An additional benefit is that medication administration is ensured in poorly adherent patients.

Patients can be trained to self-administer adalimumab by subcutaneous injection at home, and in the UK the drug can be delivered by a homecare company direct to the patient's home. Patients are less likely to have a reaction to the medication as it is a humanised antibody.

What tests need to be done prior to commencing anti-TNF treatment?

A21 **Patients should have a chest X-ray to exclude past or present tuberculosis infection. There are limitations to tuberculin testing in these patients, as most will be on immunomodulators, and an immunomodulator will inhibit the patient's immune response to a tuberculin or Mantoux test.**

Does Mr MA fulfil the criteria for using anti-TNF medication?

A22 In the UK, NICE guidance governs the use of anti-TNF therapies in CD. Mr MA does fulfil the criteria as he has recurrent disease that is resistant to immunomodulators and his CDAI score is above NICE recommended guidelines.

NICE guidance states that IFX is recommended for patients who have severe active CD (CDAI ≥300) which is refractory to treatment with immunomodulators and in whom surgery is inappropriate.

What are the options for treatment now?

A23 The options are to continue on a maintenance therapy of IFX, change to adalimumab for maintenance therapy, or stop anti-TNF therapy altogether and only treat Mr MA again if his symptoms recur.

At this stage, Mr MA is having a good effect from the IFX induction regimen. It is therefore reasonable to continue this treatment. NICE guidance TA 40 does not cover maintenance therapy, and so some patients may receive IFX episodically. Adalimumab therapy could be considered if the patient preferred self-administration of the medication at home.

What do you need to consider if Mr MA continues on infliximab (IFX) as maintenance therapy?

A24 The long-term effects of maintenance therapy with IFX have not been completely ascertained. There have been reports of lymphomas in adolescent males, and there are concerns about how long this therapy should continue.

When starting anti-TNF therapy patients should remain on their immunomodulators; however, if the IFX is to continue, then Mr MA should stop the methotrexate at 6 months. There is evidence that no further benefit will be gained from using an immunomodulator with IFX compared to infliximab monotherapy.

This is a step-up approach. Is there any benefit of using a step-down approach for these patients?

A25 There is some evidence that more intensive treatment with combined immunosuppression using azathioprine and IFX earlier in the course of the disease may have advantages for some groups of patients.

This patient has had three admissions and six different medications since diagnosis. We currently use medication that we have had the most experience with and have evidence for. This normally means the use of corticosteroids, followed by immunomodulators and then biological therapy.

There is now evidence that early intervention with combined immunosuppression using azathioprine and IFX results in better outcomes in terms of patients in remission without corticosteroids or surgical resection than the use of conventional treatment of corticosteroids, azathioprine and IFX in sequence (60% vs 35.9% in remission). D'Haens has interpreted this result as showing that initiation of more intensive treatment early in the course of the disease could result in better outcomes.

Further reading

Brookes MJ, Green JRB. Maintenance of remission in Crohn's disease: Current and emerging therapeutic options. *Drugs* 2004; **64**: 1069–1089.

Carter MJ, Lobo AJ, Travis SPL *et al.* Guidelines for the management of inflammatory bowel disease in adults. *Gut* 2004; **53**(Suppl V): v1–v16. Also available from the BSG website (www.bsg.org.uk).

D'Haens G, Baert F, van Assche G *et al.* Early combined immunosuppression or conventional management in patients with newly diagnosed Crohn's disease: An open randomised trial. *Lancet* 2008; **371**: 660–667.

Hanauer SB, Feagan BG, Lichtenstein GR *et al.* Maintenance infliximab for Crohn's disease: The ACCENT 1 randomised trial. *Lancet* 2002; **359**: 1541–1549.

Lochs H, Dejong C, Hammarqvist F *et al.* ESPEN Guidelines on Enteral Nutrition: Gastroenterology. *Clin Nutr* 2006; **25**: 260–274. Also available from ESPEN website (www.espen.org).

Mpofu C, Ireland A. Inflammatory bowel disease – the disease and its diagnosis. *Hosp Pharm* 2006; **13**: 153–158.

National Institute for Clinical Excellence. TA40. *Guidance on the Use of Infliximab for Crohn's Disease.* NICE, London, 2002.

National Patient Safety Alert number 13. *Improving Compliance with Oral Methotrexate Guidelines*, London, June 2006.

Present DH, Rutgeerts P, Targan S *et al.* Infliximab for the treatment of fistulas in patients with Crohn's disease. *N Engl J Med* 1999; **340**: 1398–1405.

Sands BE, Anderson FH, Bernstein CN *et al.* Infliximab maintenance therapy for fistulizing Crohn's disease. *N Engl J Med* 2004; **350**: 876–885.

St Clair Jones A. Inflammatory bowel disease – drug treatment and its implications. *Hosp Pharm* 2006; **13**: 161–166.

Targan SR, Hanauer SB, van Deventer SJH *et al.* A short term study of chimeric monoclonal antibody cA2 to tumour necrosis factor α for Crohn's disease. *N Engl J Med* 1997; **337**: 1029–1035.

Van Assche G, Magdelaine-Beuzelin C, D'Haens G *et al.* Withdrawal of immunosuppression in Crohn's disease treated with scheduled infliximab maintenance: A randomised trial. *Gastroenterology* 2008; **134**(7): 1861–1868.

Van Dullemen HM, van Deventer SJH, Hommes DW *et al.* Treatment of Crohn's disease with anti-tumour necrosis factor chimeric monoclonal antibody (cA2). *Gastroenterology* 1995; **109**: 129–135.

15

Alcoholic liver disease

Sarah Knighton

Case study and questions

Day 1 Mrs CN, a 58-year-old retired pub landlady, was admitted to hospital having been referred by her general practitioner (GP) with haematemesis and melaena. She had been feeling unwell over the last few days and had passed fresh blood when going to the toilet. On the morning of admission her husband said she had vomited about 500 mL of fresh blood. She was known to have alcoholic liver disease and cirrhosis (Child–Pugh score B) and had been a heavy drinker for the past 15 years. She had recently been consuming approximately one large bottle of vodka a day. Her drug history on admission was spironolactone 100 mg daily, furosemide 20 mg daily and chlorphenamine 4 mg three times a day. She also occasionally took ibuprofen for back pain. Her husband admitted that she frequently forgot to take her medication.

On examination she was noted to smell strongly of alcohol. She was jaundiced and appeared slightly confused. She had spider naevi on her face and upper body, and showed signs of muscle wasting. Ascites was noted. Her blood pressure was 90/50 mmHg and her pulse rate was 115 beats per minute (bpm).

Her laboratory results were:

- Sodium 131 mmol/L (reference range 135–145)
- Potassium 3.5 mmol/L (3.5–5.0)
- Urea 4.1 mmol/L (3.3–6.7)
- Bilirubin 65 micromol/L (3–20)
- Alkaline phosphatase (ALP) 315 IU/L (30–130)
- Gamma-glutamyl transferase (GGT) 357 IU/L (1–55)
- Aspartate aminotransferase (AST) 180 IU/L (10–50)
- International normalised ratio (INR) 1.9 (0.9–1.2)
- Haemoglobin 6.8 g/dL (11.5–15.5)
- Creatinine 115 micromol/L (45–120)
- Platelets 90 × 10^9 L (150–450)
- Albumin 26 g/L (35–50)

Q1 What signs and symptoms of chronic liver disease is Mrs CN exhibiting?
Q2 What general pharmacokinetic and pharmacodynamic considerations need to be taken into account when prescribing for Mrs CN?
Q3 Outline a pharmaceutical care plan for Mrs CN.

Mrs CN vomited a further 500 mL of fresh blood and an emergency oesophagogastroduodenoscopy (OGD) was arranged.

Q4 What treatments should be given to Mrs CN to prepare her for the OGD?

Mrs CN was started on terlipressin. At endoscopy she was found to have three large oesophageal varices which were banded. There was still generalised oozing from the oesophagus, but the exact source could not be identified.

Q5 What is terlipressin and what is the rationale for prescribing it in this setting?
Q6 What advice would you give the medical and nursing staff with regard to using terlipressin in this patient?
Q7 What alternative treatments are there for acute variceal bleeding?

After the OGD Mrs CN was stabilised and transferred back to the ward.

Day 2 The 'nil by mouth' restriction was removed 24 hours after the OGD, and Mrs CN was allowed to start a soft oral diet. She was also prescribed the following additional therapies:

- Ciprofloxacin 500 mg orally twice daily
- Pabrinex (one pair of amps) intravenously (IV) three times daily
- Phytomenadione 10 mg intramuscularly once a day
- Lactulose 10 mL orally once a day
- Sucralfate 1 g orally four times daily
- Clomethiazole three capsules orally four times daily

Q8 What was the rationale for starting each of these drugs in Mrs CN?
Q9 What changes would you make to Mrs CN's prescriptions?

Day 5 Mrs CN was complaining of back pain and had requested ibuprofen, as she said she had found it to be effective in the past.

Q10 What advice would you give regarding the treatment of Mrs CN's back pain?

Day 6 Mrs CN was told that she would be started on a new tablet to help prevent her from having another variceal bleed.

Q11 What was the new tablet likely to be, and how should it be monitored?

Day 10 Mrs CN was ready for discharge home and said she was keen to abstain from alcohol.

Q12 What pharmacological treatments can be given to help Mrs CN abstain from alcohol?

Month 2 Mrs CN was readmitted to hospital from clinic with abdominal distension and bilateral ankle swelling. She was complaining of abdominal discomfort and pruritus. Her weight was now 68 kg, compared to 59 kg at her last admission. On examination she was jaundiced and had signs consistent with chronic liver disease. Her abdomen was grossly distended and she was found to have a moderate amount of ascites. On admission she was taking spironolactone 100 mg daily, chlorphenamine 4 mg three times a day, lactulose 20 mL twice daily, and propranolol 40 mg twice daily. She had also recently started taking magnesium trisilicate 10 mL four times a day for indigestion.

Her serum biochemistry results were:

- Sodium 133 mmol/L (reference range 135–145)
- Potassium 4.2 mmol/L (3.5–5.0)
- Urea 2.8 mmol/L (3.3–6.7)
- Bilirubin 54 micromol/L (3–20)
- Creatinine 75 micromol/L (45–120)
- Albumin 30 g/L (35–50)
- ALP 300 IU/L (30–130)
- GGT 255 IU/L (1–55)

Q13 What are the pharmacological options for treating Mrs CN's ascites and how should they be monitored?
Q14 What non-pharmacological options are available if Mrs CN fails to respond to drug treatment?

Day 1 Mrs CN had her spironolactone dose increased to 200 mg daily. She also had a diagnostic paracentesis performed.

Day 2 Mrs CN's weight was still 68 kg, so her dose of spironolactone was increased again to 200 mg twice daily. Her diagnostic paracentesis result showed a polymorphic nuclear count >250/mm^3.

Q15 What infection is Mrs CN suffering from, and what treatment should be given?

Day 4 Mrs CN's weight had been falling over the past few days and was now down to 63 kg. Her biochemistry results were:

- Sodium 128 mmol/L (reference range 135–145)
- Potassium 5.2 mmol/L (3.5–5.0)
- Creatinine 110 micromol/L (45–120)
- Urea 8.2 mmol/L (3.3–6.7)

Q16 How should Mrs CN's diuretic therapy be adjusted?

Days 5–13 Mrs CN began to feel better and no longer had any abdominal pain. Her weight stabilised at 62 kg and her biochemistry results normalised with the adjustments made to her diuretic therapy. She was still complaining of severe pruritus.

Q17 Do you agree with the choice of chlorphenamine for Mrs CN's pruritus? What other agents could be used?

Mrs CN was still suffering from acid reflux and requested magnesium trisilicate mixture.

Q18 What advice would you give regarding the treatment of her acid reflux?

Day 14 Mrs CN was discharged home on the following medications:

- Lactulose 20 mL orally twice a day
- Spironolactone 200 mg orally once daily
- Furosemide 40 mg orally once daily
- Norfloxacin 400 mg orally once daily
- Colestyramine 4 g orally twice a day
- Maalox 10 mL orally three times a day when required
- Propranolol 40 mg orally twice a day

Q19 What medication counselling points should be covered with Mrs CN before discharge?

Answers

What signs and symptoms of chronic liver disease is Mrs CN exhibiting?

A1 **Mrs CN has deranged liver function tests, coagulopathy and signs of decompensated liver disease.**

(a) **Raised aspartate aminotransferase (AST).** AST is one of the intracellular enzymes that is released as a result of liver cell (hepatocyte) damage. AST may be elevated in patients with liver disease, particularly those with acute hepatocellular damage. It is a common misconception that all patients with liver disease will have raised transaminase enzymes, but this is not true. For example, patients with established cirrhosis may not necessarily have raised transaminases. This is because in cirrhosis there will be a massive reduction in the number of functioning hepatocytes, which can lead to a false 'normal' result.

(b) **Raised alkaline phosphatase (ALP) and gamma-glutamyltransferase (GGT).** ALP and GGT are often termed hepatobiliary enzymes and may be elevated in patients with liver disease. ALP is mainly produced by bone and liver, and production is increased when there is damage to the biliary tree. A raised ALP in isolation is not commonly associated with liver dysfunction and may be due to other factors, such as Paget's disease.

GGT may be raised in all types of hepatic dysfunction. Levels may be raised by a high alcohol intake, or when taking enzyme-inducing drugs such as rifampicin and phenytoin.

(c) **Elevated INR.** Prothrombin time (PT) and the international normalised ratio (INR) form part of a clotting screen. Prothrombin is a vitamin K-dependent clotting factor produced in the liver which is essential for normal coagulation. Although not part of routine liver function tests, the clotting screen results provide key information on liver function. Deranged clotting, also known as coagulopathy, can indicate significant liver dysfunction so these parameters are useful in assessing the synthetic function of the liver. Increased PT and INR can be due to a deficiency of vitamin K (due to malabsorption, as it is a fat-soluble vitamin) or to impaired synthetic function of the liver. Vitamin K can be supplemented to see if the elevation is due to deficiency.

(d) **Low albumin.** Albumin is often low in liver disease. This is because the liver is the main site for plasma protein synthesis, so when hepatic dysfunction occurs protein synthesis is reduced. Albumin levels can thus be useful indicators of liver dysfunction.

All drugs metabolised by the liver are likely to be affected when the synthetic function of the liver is reduced, and this will result in an exaggerated clinical response to a drug or to a prolonged effect. The significance of this will depend on the drug and is difficult to predict. Lower doses are usually necessary, with close monitoring for therapeutic response and to avoid toxicity (see also **A2**).

(e) **Raised bilirubin and clinical jaundice.** Bilirubin is metabolised and excreted by the liver; therefore, when a patient has liver dysfunction this can be impaired. Accumulation of bilirubin manifests as jaundice (yellowing of the skin) which usually occurs when serum bilirubin is >50 micromol/L. Total bilirubin (conjugated and unconjugated) is measured as part of the standard liver function tests. However, an elevated bilirubin is not necessarily indicative of liver dysfunction and can be due to other causes, such as haemolytic anaemia.

(f) **Spider naevi.** These are formed of a central arteriole with radiating fine blood vessels which can look like a spider. They are found particularly on the face and upper trunk, and when a number are present they can indicate the presence of chronic liver disease.

(g) **Ascites.** Ascites is the presence of free fluid in the peritoneal cavity and occurs in patients with chronic liver disease. The precise mechanism by which ascites develops in chronic liver disease is unclear. Contributing factors include portal hypertension, reduced oncotic pressure and activation of the renin–angiotensin–aldosterone system.

(h) **Suspected gastro-oesophageal varices.** These are weak collateral vessels that can form anywhere in the gastrointestinal tract. They occur because of raised portal vein pressure (portal hypertension). In cirrhosis the normal liver architecture is destroyed by fibrosis, which results in an increased resistance to blood flow within the portal blood system.

(i) **Muscle wasting.** Malnutrition and muscle wasting are common in patients with chronic liver disease. They can be due to malabsorption, anorexia, vomiting and the increased metabolic rate associated with cirrhosis.

What general pharmacokinetic and pharmacodynamic considerations need to be taken into account when prescribing for Mrs CN?

A2 It is known that Mrs CN has cirrhosis of the liver and this will affect the pharmacokinetics of any drug that is hepatically metabolised. The pharmacodynamic consequences of liver disease will also make her more susceptible to adverse effects from a number of drug therapies.

Cirrhosis is a progressive disease defined as fibrosis and nodular regeneration resulting in disruption of the normal architecture of the liver. There is also a reduction in hepatic cell mass, with a corresponding decrease in the functional capacity of the liver. This is reflected in Mrs CN's low serum albumin level of 26 g/L (35–50) and raised INR.

The presence of liver disease will influence pharmacokinetic parameters such as absorption, metabolism, volume of distribution and the extent of hepatic extraction of a drug, but it is not possible quantitatively to predict the extent to which these variables will be affected in any one individual. In cirrhosis of the liver a reduction in intrahepatic blood flow plus the development of portosystemic shunts which divert blood from the liver to the systemic circulation result in the increased bioavailability of drugs that are highly extracted on the first pass through the liver (flow-limited drugs). Peak plasma concentrations of such drugs will be increased and their half-life will be prolonged. This may necessitate a reduction in dose and/or an increase in the dosage interval.

The reduced functional capacity associated with cirrhosis will cause an increase in the bioavailability of drugs with a high extraction ratio, owing to a reduction in first-pass metabolism. Reduced functional capacity and hence delayed elimination from the systemic circulation will also prolong the half-life of drugs with low hepatic extraction (capacity-limited drugs) which are dependent on the functional capacity of the liver for their clearance. In such cases, adjustment of the dosing interval will be necessary to avoid toxicity on repeated dosing.

Mrs CN's reduced albumin level will result in reduced plasma protein binding of drugs, which in turn will increase the concentration of free, active drug. In the presence of reduced hepatic blood flow, the bioavailability of drugs with a high hepatic extraction will be increased. For drugs that are poorly extracted by the liver at first pass, bioavailability will depend on the capacity of the liver to metabolise that drug. If liver function is not impaired, the increase in free drug concentration due to reduced protein binding will only be temporary, as a new equilibrium will develop.

In clinical practice it is important to account for pharmacodynamic variations associated with liver disease, as they can affect a patient's response to therapy. In patients with liver disease cerebral sensitivity to drugs with sedative and hypnotic effects is increased. Drugs with cerebral depressant activity should be prescribed with caution in severe liver disease, as there is a risk of precipitating hepatic encephalopathy. Care should also be taken when prescribing drugs that can cause constipation, as constipation can also precipitate encephalopathy in liver patients. An alternative agent that causes less constipation should be used, or lactulose can be co-prescribed. Drugs that may cause gastric irritation or an increase in bleeding tendency should be avoided, e.g. non-steroidal anti-inflammatory drugs (NSAIDs). NSAIDs can also cause deterioration in liver function, precipitate renal failure, and cause fluid retention, and are therefore contraindicated in patients with hepatic cirrhosis.

Outline a pharmaceutical care plan for Mrs CN.

A3 The pharmaceutical care plan for Mrs CN should include the following:

(a) Ensure appropriate drug therapy is prescribed in doses to be adjusted as necessary for Mrs CN.

(b) Monitor Mrs CN's prescriptions for drugs that may be contra-indicated or cause a deterioration in her condition.
(c) Ensure that the method of administration of parenteral therapy is appropriate.
(d) Monitor the outcomes of any prescribed drug therapy for efficacy and toxicity.
(e) Counsel Mrs CN on all aspects of her drug therapy.
(f) Counsel Mrs CN on her discharge medication and the likely duration of each therapy. Liaise with relatives/carers on the importance of continued medication, and arrangements for resupply where appropriate.

What treatments should be given to Mrs CN to prepare her for the OGD?

A4 **(a) Colloids and blood (packed red cells) for fluid resuscitation.**
(b) Fresh frozen plasma (FFP), platelets and vitamin K for correction of coagulopathy.
(c) Terlipressin for treatment of potential gastric or oesophageal varices.
(d) Midazolam as premedication for her endoscopy.

Mortality following the first variceal bleed is approximately 50%, therefore prompt treatment is key. Mrs CN needs urgent fluid resuscitation as she has suffered a large blood loss, and as a consequence has low blood pressure and a high pulse rate. This, along with protection of the airway to prevent aspiration, is the most important first step in the management of an acute variceal bleed. The circulating volume needs to be monitored carefully, preferably via a central venous catheter. Care needs to be taken not to fluid overload Mrs CN, otherwise further bleeding may be provoked. Volume replacement should be started with colloids such as Gelofusine, while transfusions are being prepared. Crystalloid fluids containing sodium chloride should be avoided as they can aggravate fluid retention in patients with chronic liver disease. Blood and coagulation factors (FFP) should be administered as required. Terlipressin should be started, as it can reduce the incidence of active bleeding at the time of endoscopy, and improves bleeding control in patients admitted with bleeding varices. Care needs to be taken with the dosing of midazolam as a premedication for OGD, as patients with chronic liver disease are more sensitive to the cerebral effects of sedatives. The metabolism of midazolam is likely to be reduced in Mrs CN, as she has reduced liver blood flow and poor synthetic function. Over-sedation may cause respiratory depression with a risk of aspiration, and can precipitate encephalopathy in these patients.

What is terlipressin, and what is the rationale for prescribing it in this setting?

A5 **Terlipressin is a synthetic analogue of vasopressin which causes vasoconstriction of blood vessels. Terlipressin has been shown to reduce bleeding and improve survival in patients with bleeding oesophageal varices.**

In cirrhosis the normal liver architecture is destroyed by fibrosis, which results in an increased resistance to blood flow within the portal blood system and portal hypertension. In normal individuals portal venous pressure is 7–12 mmHg: in portal hypertension this may increase to 30 mmHg or more. Increased portal pressure leads to the development of portosystemic collateral vessels, especially in the region of the stomach and oesophagus. These collateral veins become distended, forming varices, which may bleed if the pressure in the portal venous system increases. Bleeding varices can result in massive haemorrhage, and are associated with a mortality of up to 50% on the index (first) bleed and 30% for subsequent bleeds.

Terlipressin is a synthetic analogue of vasopressin. It has a biphasic action: the intact molecule has an immediate vasoconstrictive effect, reducing blood flow to varices through vasoconstriction of blood vessels. This is followed by a delayed portal haemodynamic effect caused by the slow transformation of terlipressin *in vivo* to lysine vasopressin. A meta-analysis of the three studies involving terlipressin showed a significant improvement in the rate of bleeding control and survival for patients treated with terlipressin compared to placebo.

What advice would you give the medical and nursing staff with regard to using terlipressin in this patient?

A6 **Terlipressin should be administered as an initial 2 mg intravenous (IV) bolus. Repeated IV injections of 1–2 mg should then be given every 4–6 hours until haemostasis is achieved. The patient's blood pressure, serum sodium, potassium and fluid balance should be checked and side-effects monitored while she is on therapy.**

Terlipressin's side-effects include coronary vasoconstriction and increases in arterial blood pressure. The drug should therefore be used with extreme caution in patients with a history of ischaemic heart disease. Although the coronary side-effects are less with terlipressin than with vasopressin, glyceryl trinitrate should be administered concurrently with terlipressin in those with a history of ischaemic heart disease. Other side-effects include ischaemic colitis, abdominal cramps and headaches. Therapy should be continued until haemostasis is achieved. Terlipressin is licensed to be given for up to 72 hours, but longer treatment may be required to prevent early rebleeding.

What alternative treatments are there for acute variceal bleeding?

A7 **A number of alternative treatments are available: other vasoactive agents such as vasopressin, somatostatin and octreotide; endoscopic band ligation or sclerotherapy; balloon tamponade; or transjugular intrahepatic portosystemic shunt (TIPS).**

Other vasoactive agents. Vasopressin was the first drug to be used to treat variceal bleeding and has been reported to be effective in approximately 50% of cases. It is the most potent vasoconstrictor and is administered by continuous IV infusion. Glyceryl trinitrate (40–400 micrograms/min by infusion or as a patch) has been used with vasopressin to help reduce coronary vasoconstriction, which is a side-effect of this therapy. The use of vasopressin has now virtually been abandoned because of its severe side-effects, such as decreased cardiac output and coronary blood flow.

Somatostatin is a vasoactive peptide hormone that causes selective splanchnic vasoconstriction and reduced portal pressure. It is free from any of the systemic adverse effects associated with vasopressin, but is not available in the UK. Octreotide is a derivative of somatostatin but is more potent and has a longer duration of action. The use of octreotide in this setting is controversial owing to conflicting evidence of its benefit. Octreotide, administered as an infusion at 25–50 micrograms/h, has been shown to be as effective as balloon tamponade in controlling bleeding in the acute situation and preventing rebleeding following injection sclerotherapy. However, in a large randomised clinical trial octreotide was not shown to improve survival or control of bleeding compared to placebo. Octreotide is not licensed for the treatment of bleeding oesophageal varices. It can cause tachyphylaxis and is only rarely used.

Endoscopic band ligation or sclerotherapy. Emergency endoscopy should be performed to identify the source of bleeding, and band ligation or sclerotherapy may be carried out. A meta-analysis of 10 randomised controlled trials showed an almost significant benefit of band ligation in the initial control of bleeding compared to sclerotherapy. Consensus guidelines recommend band ligation as the preferred form of endoscopic therapy, with sclerotherapy used when ligation is not technically feasible. Sclerotherapy involves the injection of a sclerosant – usually 5% ethanolamine oleate – in 1–2 mL boluses into the varix. Tissue adhesives and bovine thrombin have also been used to control bleeding gastric varices.

Balloon tamponade. Balloon tamponade controls bleeding by reducing inflow at the gastro-oesophageal junction and is effective in

80–90% of cases. It involves the insertion of a four-lumen tube (Sengstaken–Blakemore tube) through the mouth and into the stomach. The tube has an inflatable gastric balloon, an inflatable oesophageal balloon, and tubes through which to aspirate the stomach and oesophagus. Inflation of the gastric balloon is effective in controlling bleeding in most cases. Inflation of the oesophageal balloon should be considered as a last resort, because of the tendency of this strategy to cause oesophageal ulceration and perforation. Balloon tamponade is indicated in massive bleeding or as a bridge to other treatments.

Transjugular intrahepatic portosystemic shunt (TIPS). TIPS has been shown to be highly effective in the management of uncontrolled bleeding oesophageal varices when the first-line therapies discussed above have failed. The main problems are the limited availability of this procedure, the development of encephalopathy in up to 30% of patients, and occlusion of the shunt in up to 25% of cases. TIPS has largely replaced the surgical procedures that were performed in the past, such as oesophageal transection and portacaval shunts.

What was the rationale for starting each of these drugs in Mrs CN?

A8 (a) **Ciprofloxacin is used as antibiotic prophylaxis in patients with variceal bleeding as it has been shown to reduce the rate of infection and can improve survival.**

Bacterial infections occur in 35–66% of cirrhotic patients who have a variceal bleed. Antibiotic prophylaxis should always be given, as it has been shown in trials to reduce infection rates and improve survival. A 5–7-day course of antibiotic therapy is recommended. A number of different antibiotics have been shown to be of benefit in clinical trials, with quinolones being used most frequently. Broad-spectrum IV antibiotics are used in very sick patients and in those perceived to be at risk of aspiration pneumonia after endoscopy. It is important to check what the recommended antibiotic is at your hospital. This will be based on local resistance patterns. When using quinolones the adverse effect profile and the association with *Clostridium difficile* should be borne in mind.

(b) **Pabrinex is given to provide high doses of vitamins B and C. It contains thiamine (vitamin B_1), which is given to prevent the development of Wernicke–Korsakoff syndrome.**

Alcohol-dependent people tend to have an inadequate food intake and a diet that is high in carbohydrate and low in protein, vitamins and minerals. In addition, absorption of nutrients such as vitamins may be impaired owing to alteration of active transport and absorption in the intestinal mucosa. Pabrinex provides a source of high doses of vitamins B and C, including 250 mg of thiamine. Administration of thiamine is important, as thiamine deficiency can result in the development of Wernicke–Korsakoff syndrome. The acute component is Wernicke's encephalopathy, which is characterised by mental confusion, ataxia and ophthalmoplegia. Early administration of thiamine can reverse this encephalopathy and prevent the development of the irreversible amnesic syndrome, Korsakoff's psychosis.

(c) Phytomenadione (vitamin K_1) is given in an attempt to correct Mrs CN's coagulopathy.

The liver is responsible for the production of vitamin K-dependent clotting factors. Administration of vitamin K will help to correct a patient's INR if the patient is vitamin K deficient due to malabsorption or inadequate dietary intake; however, this approach is often ineffective because the liver is unable to produce clotting factors owing to underlying liver damage.

(d) Lactulose is given to prevent encephalopathy.

Acute or chronic encephalopathy is seen in patients with decompensated cirrhosis. It is thought to be associated with raised plasma concentrations of ammonia and other nitrogenous toxins, and can be precipitated by a number of factors, including constipation, gastrointestinal bleeding, diarrhoea and vomiting, infection, alcoholic binges, sedative and opiate drug therapy, electrolyte abnormalities, uraemia, dietary protein excess, surgery, and acute worsening of liver disease.

Following a gastrointestinal bleed there is an increased nitrogen load on the gastrointestinal tract, which can result in increased ammonia production by intestinal bacteria. This means that Mrs CN is at increased risk of encephalopathy. Lactulose is a disaccharide which is converted to lactic, acetic and formic acids by intestinal bacteria, thus changing the pH of the gut contents from 7 to 5. The acidic pH reduces the absorption of non-ionised ammonia and creates an environment more suitable for the growth of weak ammonia-producing organisms such as *Lactobacillus acidophilus*, rather than proteolytic ammonia-producing organisms such as *Escherichia coli*. The osmotic laxative effect of lactulose also speeds intestinal transit and so prevents constipation, reducing the time available for the absorption of potentially toxic nitrogenous compounds.

(e) Sucralfate is given as a mucosal protectant and helps to treat any ulceration caused by endoscopic banding.

(f) Clomethiazole is prescribed for the treatment of alcohol withdrawal.

Chronic excessive alcohol consumption can result in the development of withdrawal symptoms when a patient stops drinking. The symptoms can range from irritability, sweating, hypertension and tremor, to confusion, hallucinations, convulsions and dysrhythmias. Clomethiazole, a compound structurally related to thiamine, has hypnotic, sedative, anxiolytic and anticonvulsant properties. It can be given to prevent or control the symptoms of alcohol withdrawal.

What changes would you make to Mrs CN's prescription?

A9 **(a) The phytomenadione should be given IV rather than intramuscularly.**

Intramuscular injections should be avoided in patients with liver disease as they can lead to the development of a haematoma at the injection site in patients with a coagulopathy. Konakion MM is the IV product. It can be administered either as a 20–30-minute IV infusion diluted with 55 mL of glucose 5%, or as a slow injection (at a maximum rate of 1 mg/min). A dose of 10 mg daily for 3 days is usually given.

(b) The lactulose dose should be increased to a starting dose of at least 20 mL twice daily.

High-dose lactulose therapy is used to prevent encephalopathy. The dose should be titrated to produce two to three soft motions a day without diarrhoea.

(c) Chlordiazepoxide should be prescribed instead of clomethiazole. It should be given on an 'as-required' basis for 24 hours to assess the patient's requirements. The total dose administered over the 24 hours should then be divided by four to give a 6-hourly dose, which should be prescribed in a reducing regimen over 4–6 days.

Chlordiazepoxide is now considered the agent of choice for treating alcohol withdrawal because of concerns regarding the adverse effect profile of clomethiazole. Problems that have been documented with clomethiazole are a risk of respiratory depression, hypothermia, hypotension, coma and even death. Clomethiazole is particularly dangerous in an outpatient setting, where the patient may continue to drink alcohol. There is no specific antidote to clomethiazole, and hence there is a trend to switch to chlordiazepoxide, a long-acting benzodiazepine, for its equivalent efficacy and greater safety.

What advice would you give regarding the treatment of Mrs CN's back pain?

A10 Paracetamol should be given instead of ibuprofen as it is safer in patients with liver disease. If paracetamol alone is ineffective, dihydrocodeine can be added.

Paracetamol is the drug of choice and should be prescribed for Mrs CN initially. It is generally considered safe to use in the majority of liver patients at normal doses with no increased risk of hepatotoxicity. If paracetamol alone is not sufficient to control her pain then a weak opiate such as dihydrocodeine should be added. Like all other opiates dihydrocodeine can cause sedation and constipation, which may precipitate encephalopathy. It should be started at the lowest possible dose and titrated up according to her response.

NSAIDS drugs such as ibuprofen should be avoided in Mrs CN because of their adverse effect profile. The following adverse effects could be particularly problematic in liver patients: fluid retention and electrolyte abnormalities; gastrointestinal ulceration and bleeding; inhibition of platelet aggregation, and a reduction in glomerular filtration rate. Hepatotoxicity has also been associated with the use of NSAIDs. Gastrointestinal ulceration would be a particular problem for Mrs CN as she has a prolonged PT and is therefore at an increased risk of bleeding.

Strong opiates should be avoided unless absolutely necessary. In severe liver disease the metabolism and clearance of opiates such as morphine will be significantly reduced, and so low doses should be prescribed. The dosage interval will also need to be increased. If an opiate were to be required then doses should be titrated upwards gradually to achieve pain control. Opiates should always be prescribed with a laxative to prevent constipation, and naloxone to reverse dose-related side-effects.

Modified-release preparations of analgesics should always be avoided as they can accumulate significantly in liver disease.

What was the new tablet likely to be and how should it be monitored?

A11 The new tablet is likely to be propranolol, which is used as first-line therapy in the secondary prevention of variceal bleeding. It should be started at a low dose of 20 mg orally twice daily. The dose should then be titrated to the patient's blood pressure and pulse rate, which should be monitored during treatment.

Propranolol, a non-selective beta-blocker, reduces portal pressure by reducing splanchnic blood flow and the hyperdynamic circulation associated with cirrhosis. It has been shown in trials to reduce the risk of rebleeding from varices. This is important, as patients have a high risk of rebleeding, and it is therefore vital that preventative therapy is started to reduce the risk. Propranolol therapy has also been shown to be of benefit as primary prophylaxis in reducing the risk of the first variceal bleed in patients with cirrhosis who have moderate to large varices.

The drug is started at a low dose as it undergoes extensive first-pass metabolism. The dose should be titrated up as blood pressure tolerates, and the pulse rate should not be allowed to fall below 55 bpm. Portal pressure studies, which look at the pressure in the portal vein, can be performed to see if a patient has responded to propranolol therapy. The aim is to reduce the portal pressure below 12 mmHg, as the patient is then no longer at risk of bleeding from their varices; however, this involves an invasive measurement and is therefore not routinely performed in clinical practice. Although most trials have involved propranolol, nadolol, another non-selective beta-blocker, can also be used.

The role of combination propranolol and isosorbide mononitrate therapy has also been explored, as these agents theoretically have a synergistic effect on reducing portal pressure and hence are possibly more effective than monotherapy with a beta-blocker. One study compared combination propranolol and isosorbide mononitrate against propranolol alone, but although combination treatment showed an increased benefit this was not statistically significant. In clinical practice this combination has more side-effects than propranolol alone and is often poorly tolerated, hence monotherapy with propranolol remains the treatment of choice.

What pharmacological treatments can be given to help Mrs CN abstain from alcohol?

A12 Disulfiram, acamprosate or naltrexone.

Abstinence can be achieved by psychological treatments, pharmacological treatments or a combination of both (which tends to be most successful).

Disulfiram is used as an adjunct in the treatment of alcohol dependence. Disulfiram irreversibly inhibits acetaldehyde dehydrogenase, an enzyme involved in the breakdown of alcohol, leading to the accumulation of acetaldehyde. While taking this medication patients are prevented from drinking alcohol by the extremely unpleasant side-effects that occur after the ingestion of even the smallest amounts (including that contained in some oral medicines). These reactions include facial flushing, palpitations, headache, arrhythmias, hypotension and collapse. Because of its powerful interaction with alcohol disulfiram is reserved for patients who have undergone several unsuccessful treatments for alcoholism and have suffered multiple relapses. Trial evidence to support its use is inconclusive, with the quantity of alcohol consumed and the number of drinking days reduced provided the patient adheres to the therapy.

Acamprosate is a gamma-aminobutyric acid receptor antagonist which is used to help maintain abstinence from alcohol by reducing cravings. It should be used in combination with counselling. Several randomised controlled trials and a meta-analysis have shown a reduction in drinking days and an increase in abstinence rates. Treatment should be initiated as soon as possible after the alcohol withdrawal period and maintained if the patient relapses. The recommended treatment period for acamprosate is 1 year, and the most common side-effect is diarrhoea, which occurs in about 10% of patients.

Naltrexone is another agent which has been used to maintain abstinence from alcohol, although it is not licensed for this indication. It is similar to acamprosate in that it has significant anti-craving effects which reduce alcohol consumption. The main side-effects are headache and anxiety, which occur in about 10% of patients. Like acamprosate, naltrexone is also effective in reducing drinking days and increasing abstinence rates.

What are the pharmacological options for treating Mrs CN's ascites, and how should they be monitored?

A13 **Diuretics are the drugs used to treat ascites. Spironolactone in combination with a loop diuretic such as furosemide is first-line treatment, although monotherapy with spironolactone may be used in patients with minimal fluid overload. Amiloride is a suitable alternative for patients who develop gynaecomastia on spironolactone therapy.**

Ascites is the presence of free fluid in the peritoneal cavity. The precise mechanism by which ascites develops is unclear. Contributing factors include portal hypertension, reduced oncotic pressure and activation of the renin–angiotensin–aldosterone system. Spironolactone is a specific antagonist of aldosterone and is the drug of choice for the treatment of ascites. It is initially prescribed at a dose of 100 mg daily, and should be effective after 2 or 3 days. The aim is to induce a negative fluid balance, which can be assessed by daily monitoring of the patient's weight and fluid balance. The rate of fluid loss from the vascular compartment should not exceed the rate at which fluid can be relocated from the ascitic compartment and weight loss should not exceed 0.5 kg/day (1 kg if peripheral oedema is also present). Excessive diuresis may result in hypovolaemia, electrolyte disturbances including hyponatraemia and uraemia, and a risk of precipitating hepatic encephalopathy and renal impairment.

Spironolactone may also cause hyperkalaemia, and close monitoring of serum electrolytes is essential throughout treatment. If necessary, the dose may be increased by increments of 100 mg every 3–5 days to a maximum of 400 mg daily. Dose escalation should be stopped if the serum sodium falls below 130 mmol/L, or if the creatinine level rises to more than 130 micromol/L. Furosemide, at a starting dose of 20–40 mg a day, is used in combination with spironolactone as it has a synergestic diuretic effect. Furosemide may be withheld if the patient has minimal fluid overload or hypokalaemia.

What non-pharmacological options are available if Mrs CN fails to respond to drug treatment?

A14 Paracentesis, a Leveen shunt or TIPS can be used in patients who have diuretic-resistant or tense ascites.

A patient is usually termed 'diuretic resistant' if they have failed to respond to 400 mg of spironolactone a day plus 160 mg of furosemide. Diuretic-resistant ascites has a 1-year mortality of 25–50%. Patients with refractory ascites should be referred for assessment for liver transplant.

Paracentesis (removal of ascites via a cannula inserted into the peritoneal cavity through the abdominal wall) may be indicated if the patient does not respond to diuretics. During paracentesis a large volume of ascites can be drained, and there is a risk of hypovolaemia, renal failure and encephalopathy. These complications can be largely overcome by simultaneously infusing albumin at the time of fluid removal. One bottle of 20% albumin is usually infused for every 2 L of ascites drained. If the volume of fluid removed is <5 L, other colloidal solutions such as HAES-steril can be substituted instead of albumin.

TIPS is the only treatment that relieves portal pressure, and it may be of benefit in selected patients. A Leveen shunt is at least as effective as paracentesis in the control of refractory ascites, but owing to the numerous complications associated with its use it is reserved for patients who are not eligible for transplantation or those who cannot have paracentesis because of surgical scars.

What infection is Mrs CN suffering from, and what treatment should be given?

A15 Mrs CN is suffering from spontaneous bacterial peritonitis (SBP), which is diagnosed by an ascitic polymorphic nuclear count >250/mm^3. A third-generation cephalosporin or agent with a similar spectrum of activity should be initiated and continued for a minimum of 5 days. Mrs CN should then be started on norfloxacin 400 mg daily as prophylaxis against further episodes of SBP.

SBP is an infection of the ascites that occurs in the absence of any clear source of infection. An abdominal paracentesis must be performed, and ascitic fluid analysed to confirm the diagnosis. This fluid should also be sent to microbiology for culture and sensitivity testing. Most cases (70%) of SBP are caused by normal gut flora. *Escherichia coli* accounts for almost half of these. *Klebsiella pneumonia,* and *Enterococcus sp.* are also common. A broad-spectrum antibiotic such as a third-generation cephalosporin, Tazocin or meropenem are effective treatments for SBP. They should be given for at least 5 days, and on average a 7-day course is required for resolution of SBP. It is important to check what the recommended antibiotic is at your hospital. This will be based on local resistance patterns. Long-term prophylaxis with norfloxacin should be initiated as soon as possible after the antibiotic course for the acute event has been completed.

How should Mrs CN's diuretic therapy be adjusted?

A16 Mrs CN should stop her spironolactone until her serum sodium returns to above 130 mmol/L. The spironolactone should then be cautiously recommenced at a dose of 100 mg daily.

Mrs CN's weight has dropped by 5 kg in 2 days, which exceeds the maximum recommended weight loss of 1 kg/day for patients who have ascites plus peripheral oedema. Over-diuresis has also resulted in her serum sodium falling below 130 mmol/L. Her spironolactone dose was increased too quickly from 100 to 300 mg on the first day. Dose increases should be in increments of 100 mg every 3–5 days, with the patient's weight and electrolytes being carefully monitored.

Do you agree with the choice of chlorphenamine for Mrs CN's pruritus? What other agents could be used?

A17 Antihistamines such as chlorphenamine are relatively ineffective (apart from their sedative effect) and should not be used as first-line therapy for pruritus. Colestyramine and colestipol are anion-exchange resins and are the usual first-line therapy.

Bile salts under the skin are one of the factors that cause itching in patients with liver disease. Anion exchange resins are used to bind bile salts in the gut and to help prevent itching by stopping the bile salts being absorbed. It is important to remember that instant relief will not be obtained, and that they usually take at least 7 days to work. Ursodeoxycholic acid is also frequently used in cholestatic liver disease, and its long-term use has been shown to improve pruritus.

Antihistamines such as chlorphenamine can provide symptomatic relief. The older sedating antihistamines are sometimes preferred, especially if given at night. Other drugs, such as low-dose rifampicin, ondansetron and naltrexone, are sometimes used if patients fail to respond to the previous agents. Topical therapy such as aqueous cream with menthol may also give symptomatic relief.

What advice would you give regarding treatment of her acid reflux?

A18 Maalox would be an appropriate first-line agent.

Maalox is a low-sodium antacid containing <1 mmol of sodium per 10 mL dose. For patients with ascites sodium intake should ideally be restricted to approximately 2 g/day (90 mmol). Magnesium trisilicate mixture should be stopped as it contains 3 mmol of sodium per 5 mL dose, and the additional sodium content associated with multiple doses could potentially worsen Mrs CN's ascites. The sodium content of antacids can be found in the *British National Formulary*.

What medication counselling points should be covered with Mrs CN before discharge?

A19 Mrs CN should be told the indication for each of her drugs, how to take them, and any important side-effects. She should be told to use paracetamol for her back pain and not to take NSAIDs.

(a) **Lactulose.** This is a laxative that helps prevent encephalopathy. She needs to take it regularly at the prescribed dose, as it has a delayed action of about 48 hours. Lactulose should be taken at a dose that produces two or three soft stools a day. Care needs to be taken to avoid diarrhoea, as this can cause electrolyte disturbances and precipitate encephalopathy.

(b) **Spironolactone.** This is a diuretic to reduce her ascites which she should take in the morning. If she develops gastrointestinal disturbances the daily dose can be divided. She should be advised to weigh herself regularly (ideally daily), and that if her weight starts to increase significantly she should seek medical advice, as this could be a sign of fluid accumulation.

(c) **Furosemide.** This is a diuretic that works with spironolactone to reduce her ascites. It should ideally be taken in the morning, as if it is taken later in the day it may cause sleep disturbance due to night-time diuresis.

(d) **Norfloxacin.** This is an antibiotic to prevent reinfection of her ascites.

(e) **Colestyramine.** This is an anion-exchange resin used to treat pruritus. To overcome the unpleasant taste it can be incorporated into various foods and drinks to make it more palatable. It can take up to

7 days for colestyramine to take its effect. It must be taken 1 hour before or 4–6 hours after her other tablets. As colestyramine can cause constipation, she must ensure she is taking the appropriate dose of lactulose to counteract this side-effect.

(f) **Propranolol.** This is a beta-blocker to prevent her from having another variceal bleed. Mrs CN should be warned that if she feels faint or dizzy while on this medication she should contact her doctor, as it may be a sign that the dose needs to be reduced.

(g) **Maalox** has been prescribed for her indigestion instead of magnesium trisilicate. This preparation is better for her as it does not contain as much sodium.

(h) Mrs CN should be told not to take any NSAIDs for pain relief but to use paracetamol instead. Finally, she should be advised that it is important with any new medicine (prescribed or purchased) to check that it is safe to take with her liver disease.

Acknowledgements

I would like to thank Gillian Cavell (Deputy Director, Medications Safety, King's College Hospital) for her assistance in preparing this chapter. I would also like to thank Sarah Hulse (nee Stoll), who originally prepared this chapter.

Further reading

Baik SK, Jeong PH, Ji SW *et al.* Acute haemodynamic effects of octreotide and terlipressin in patients with cirrhosis: a randomized comparison. *Am J Gastroenterol* 2005; **100**: 631–635.

Bernard B, Nguyen KE, Opolon P *et al.* Antibiotic prophylaxis for the prevention of bacterial infections in cirrhotic patients with gastrointestinal bleeding: a meta-analysis. *Hepatology* 1999; **29**: 1665–1661.

Chapman R, Gilmore I (eds). Liver disorders – Part 1. *Medicine* 2007; **35**: 1–60.

Chapman R, Gilmore I (eds). Liver disorders – Part 2. *Medicine* 2007; **35**: 61–129.

Cornish JW, O'Brien CP. Pharmacotherapies to prevent relapse: disulfiram, naltrexone and acamprosate. *Medicine* 1999; **27**: 26–28.

Garcia-Tsao G, Sanyal AJ, Grace ND *et al.* Practice Guidelines. Committee of the American Association for the Study of Liver Diseases; Practice Parameters Committee of the American College of Gastroenterology. Prevention and management of gastroesophageal varices and variceal haemorrhage in cirrhosis. *Hepatology* 2007; **46**: 922–938.

Jalan R, Hayes PC. UK guidelines on the management of variceal haemorrhage in cirrhotic patients. British Society of Gastroenterology. *Gut* 2000; **46**: 3–4.

Kennedy PTF, O'Grady J. Diseases of the liver – chronic liver disease. *Hosp Pharm* 2002; **9**: 137–144.

Mason P. Blood tests used to investigate liver, thyroid or kidney function and disease. *Pharm J* 2004; **272**: 446–448.

Mayo-Smith MF. Pharmacological management of alcohol withdrawal. A meta-analysis and evidence-based practice guideline. American Society of Addiction Medicine Working Group on Pharmacological Management of Alcohol Withdrawal. *J Am Med Assoc* 1997; **278**: 144–151.

Mowat C, Stanley A. Review article: spontaneous bacterial peritonitis – diagnosis, treatment and prevention. *Aliment Pharmacol Ther* 2001; **15**: 1851–1859.

North-Lewis P (ed). *Drugs and the Liver – A Guide to Drug Handling in Liver Dysfunction*. Pharmaceutical Press, London, 2008.

Runyon B. Practice Guidelines Committee of the American Association for the Study of Liver Diseases. Management of adult patients with ascites due to cirrhosis. 2003. Accessed via www.aasld.org

Stewart S, Day C. The management of alcoholic liver disease. *J Hepatol* 2003; **38**: S2–S13.

Tome S, Lucey MR. Review Article: Current management of alcoholic liver disease. *Aliment Pharmacol Ther* 2004: **19**: 707–714.

16

Rheumatoid arthritis

Tina Hawkins and David Bryant

Case study and questions

Day 1 A 69-year-old woman, Mrs TD, attended the rheumatology outpatient clinic complaining of increasing pain and stiffness in her hands and knees. The pain was bad all day, but worse in the morning. She had been diagnosed with seropositive rheumatoid arthritis (RA) 4 years earlier. Her other medical history was unremarkable. She had been treated with methotrexate from the date of diagnosis. The dose of methotrexate had been increased in the past, but was not tolerated at doses higher than 10 mg because of gastrointestinal side-effects. Sulfasalazine had been added to her methotrexate in the rheumatology outpatient clinic 6 months earlier, when her Disease Activity Score (DAS28) had been recorded as 5.1.

At this clinic appointment she was taking methotrexate 10 mg orally once a week and sulfasalazine EC 1 g twice a day. Mrs TD was taking both ibuprofen 200 mg and co-codamol 8/500 when required for pain relief. The only other medication she was taking was calcium and vitamin D as prophylaxis against osteoporosis.

On examination Mrs TD was found to have swelling in the joints of both hands, and both her knees were swollen and tender. The swollen joints were warmer than the surrounding areas. Rheumatoid nodules could be felt on her elbows, and she was suffering from dry eyes (Sjögren's syndrome). Her DAS28 score was recorded as 5.8. She had the following blood test results:

- Haemoglobin 10.6 g/dL (reference range 12–16)
- White blood cells (WBC) 12.1×10^9/L ($4–11 \times 10^9$)
- Neutrophils 5.2×10^9/L ($2–7.5 \times 10^9$)
- Platelets 456×10^9/L ($150–400 \times 10^9$)
- Erythrocyte sedimentation rate (ESR) 69 mm/h (0–20)
- C-reactive protein (CRP) 92 mg/L (<10)

- Plasma viscosity (PV) 2.14 mPa/s (1.5–1.72)
- Urea and electrolyte (U&E) levels and liver function tests (LFTs) were unremarkable

A flare of her RA was diagnosed and Mrs TD was admitted. The initial plan was to treat her with drugs and physiotherapy.

Q1 Comment on the previous disease-modifying antirheumatic drug (DMARD) treatment that Mrs TD has received.
Q2 What are the usual signs and symptoms of a flare in RA?
Q3 What initial drug therapy would you advise to treat Mrs TD's symptoms (rather than her underlying disease)?

Day 2 Mrs TD was prescribed the following medication:

- Methotrexate 10 mg orally once a week
- Sulfasalazine EC 1 g orally twice a day
- Folic acid 5 mg orally daily, except on the day of methotrexate
- Calcium 500 mg plus vitamin D 400 units one tablet orally twice a day
- Co-codamol 8/500 orally, two when required for pain
- Ibuprofen 200 mg orally one three times a day when required for pain
- Tramadol 50–100 mg orally four times a day when required for pain

Since admission Mrs TD had taken eight tablets of co-codamol 8/500, three doses of ibuprofen 200 mg and no tramadol. She complained that although the affected joints felt better since she had received intra-articular corticosteroid injections she was still in considerable pain. The Senior House Officer asked for advice on her pain management. He was particularly interested to know whether the addition of a cyclo-oxygenase (COX)-2 inhibitor would be of benefit.

Q4 What advice would you give with respect to the use of non-steroidal anti-inflammatory drugs (NSAIDs)?
Q5 What other advice would you give on her pain medication?
Q6 Is it appropriate for Mrs TD to be taking calcium and vitamin D?
Q7 Outline a pharmaceutical care plan for the initial management of Mrs TD.

Day 4 The long-term management of Mrs TD was discussed on the consultant's ward round. A decision was made to commence the patient on anti-tumour necrosis factor (anti-TNF) therapy and to give her a corticosteroid injection in the interim.

Q8 What is the role of corticosteroids in the management of RA?

Q9 What anti-TNF therapies are currently available for the management of RA?
Q10 What are the criteria for commencing a patient with RA on an anti-TNF?
Q11 What alternative therapeutic options may be considered if treatment with an anti-TNF is contraindicated?

Mrs TD asked if she could talk to the pharmacist about the new medicine the doctor was talking about starting her on. She was concerned about the safety of this new medicine.

Q12 What safety concerns are associated with anti-TNF therapy?
Q13 Which anti-TNF would you recommend for Mrs TD and why?

Day 9 Mrs TD was given an infusion of infliximab. The following day she was discharged from hospital and arrangements were made for her to attend the day unit in 2 weeks' time for her second infusion.

Two weeks later Mrs TD attended the day unit for her second infusion of infliximab. She asked how long she would need to continue this treatment, and what would happen if it did not work. It was explained that treatment is lifelong.

Q14 Are there any subsequent therapeutic options if Mrs TD does not respond to treatment with infliximab?
Q15 What is the long-term prognosis for a patient like Mrs TD?

Answers

Comment on the previous disease-modifying anti-rheumatic drug (DMARD) treatment that Mrs TD has received.

A1 **All patients with a confirmed diagnosis of RA should be commenced on a DMARD. The agent of choice is methotrexate. Sulfasalazine may be added where there is an insufficient response, or may be tried as monotherapy in patients intolerant of methotrexate.**

Several studies have shown that irreversible damage occurs in the first 2 years of this disease. Early therapeutic intervention with DMARDs can improve patient outcomes and reduce disease progression. All patients with a confirmed diagnosis of RA should be commenced on a DMARD.

DMARDs do not provide pain relief but do suppress the disease process. They also have a delayed onset of action: it may take 4–6 weeks before the patient starts to see a response, and up to 4–6 months before a full response is achieved. DMARDs currently used in clinical practice include methotrexate, sulfasalazine, injectable or oral gold, antimalarials, ciclosporin, penicillamine, azathioprine and leflunomide.

The precise mechanism of action of these drugs is unclear. There is good evidence that DMARDs inhibit the activity of inflammatory cytokines. Certain cytokines have been shown to play an important role in the pathogenesis of RA. Activated T cells also play a role in the early induction of RA, and methotrexate, leflunomide and ciclosporin have been shown to inhibit T cells.

Sulfasalazine and methotrexate are generally regarded as first-line therapies owing to their improved efficacy profile (approximately 40% response rates) and high continuation rates compared to other DMARDs.

Methotrexate is generally used in patients with moderate to severe disease, especially those with a poor prognosis. It has an onset of action of approximately 1 month, and can be given either orally or by subcutaneous or intramuscular injection. It tends to be given by injection when patients are unable to tolerate oral doses because of gastric side-effects, or where doses of 25 mg or more are being given. The starting dose tends to be 7.5 mg once a week. The dose is then gradually adjusted according to response and tolerance. Patients should be clearly counselled that the medicine should only be taken once a week. It is recommended that only the 2.5 mg tablets are dispensed to prevent confusion over the dosage. Common side-effects include mouth ulcers (stomatitis) and nausea. Folic acid is commonly prescribed to counteract these. Folic acid tends to be given as a 5 mg once-daily dose, although other regimens are used; however, most regimens omit the dose on the day of methotrexate therapy to avoid any potential impact on the latter's efficacy.

The use of methotrexate has been associated with haematological, hepatic and pulmonary toxicity. Patients should be carefully counselled to watch for signs and symptoms indicating toxicity. Because of methotrexate's potential to suppress bone marrow and cause liver toxicity it is essential that certain blood tests be performed regularly on patients taking methotrexate. All patients should have the following baseline blood tests: full blood count (FBC), urea and electrolytes (U&E) and liver function tests (LFTs). These should then be performed regularly throughout the course of treatment. Both men and women are required to use adequate contraception while taking methotrexate. Also, patients who have not had chicken pox should be advised to contact their general practitioner (GP) immediately if they come into contact with someone who has the disease. A number of commonly prescribed medicines, such as non-steroidal anti-inflammatory drugs (NSAIDs), have the potential to block the excretion of methotrexate, or to increase the risk of methotrexate toxicity, e.g. trimethoprim. Care should be taken when checking for drug interactions with methotrexate, and patients should be advised to check with the pharmacist before buying any medicines over the counter.

Sulfasalazine is indicated in mild to moderate disease. It has an onset of action of 6–12 weeks. In order to reduce nausea, the dose is usually titrated upwards from 500 mg daily, increasing at weekly intervals to 1 g twice daily. Haematological abnormalities have occurred rarely with the use of sulfasalazine, and patients should be counselled to report unexplained bleeding, bruising, purpura, sore throat, fever or malaise. Patients should also be warned that sulfasalazine can colour urine red and stain contact lenses. Baseline FBCs and LFTs should be performed on patients taking sulfasalazine and repeated intermittently throughout the course of treatment.

The use of penicillamine has fallen out of favour owing to its poor side-effect profile and lack of efficacy compared to other agents. The anti-malarials chloroquine and hydroxychloroquine tend to be well tolerated, but are only indicated in mild disease. The agents leflunomide, azathioprine and ciclosporin, or the combination of multiple DMARDs, tend to be reserved for patients in whom the use of biologic therapies is contraindicated (see **A11**).

What are the usual signs and symptoms of a flare in RA?

A2 **Joint pain and loss of function are the most obvious symptoms of a flare in the disease. The peripheral joints of the hands and feet are usually involved first and symmetrically. During a flare there is increased pain and swelling; the affected joints may also feel hot to the touch. There is also morning stiffness that can last for several hours after rising. These factors lead to reduced mobility.**

There are also non-specific indicators of inflammatory processes. The ESR, CRP and PV may be raised. These inflammatory markers can be used as indicators of the success of treatment, but it should be remembered that they are not specific and that normal results do not preclude active disease. There is also often a raised WBC count due to the disease processes, but it may also be high for another reason, such as infection. The count may also be low: an example would be in Felty's syndrome. Rheumatoid factor and antinuclear antibodies (ANA) are often also measured to see if they are raised.

What initial drug therapy would you advise to treat Mrs TD's symptoms (rather than her underlying disease)?

A3 **Pain relief in the form of an NSAID plus simple analgesia, with steroid injection into the worst affected joints.**

Pain relief is important in the early stages of a flare to enable the patient to start to mobilise and be able to receive physiotherapy. Choices of pain relief in RA patients are discussed in greater depth in **A4** and **A5**. An NSAID would be beneficial for this patient. Although there is the potential for NSAIDs to reduce methotrexate excretion and hence predispose Mrs TD to increased toxicity, this should not be a problem as she is being closely monitored.

Intra-articular steroid administration (such as methylprednisolone acetate or triamcinolone acetonide) can effectively relieve pain, increase mobility and reduce deformity in one or more joints. There is no difference in efficacy between different intra-articular corticosteroid preparations and the selection often depends on prescriber preference. The duration of response to intra-articular steroids is variable. The dose used is dependent upon the size of the joint, with methylprednisolone acetate 40–80 mg or triamcinolone acetonide 20–40 mg appropriate for large joints such as knees. The frequency with which injections may be given is controversial, but repeated injections are usually given at intervals of 1–5 weeks or more, depending on the degree of relief obtained after the first one. Patients should be instructed to rest the limb for 24 hours after injection, and that they will start to notice a benefit after 48 hours. The further role of corticosteroids in RA is discussed in **A7**.

What advice would you give with respect to the use of non-steroidal anti-inflammatory drugs (NSAIDs)?

A4 **Because of Mrs TD's age and her concurrent medication, a standard NSAID combined with a proton pump inhibitor (PPI) or a COX-2 selective agent on its own should be used. Ibuprofen, diclofenac and naproxen (in increasing order of relative risk) have the lowest risk of gastrointestinal toxicity of the standard NSAIDs.**

NSAIDs are indicated for short-term use where there are pain and stiffness due to inflammation. NSAIDs suppress inflammation and provide pain relief by preventing the production of prostaglandins through the inhibition of the enzyme COX. This is known to exist in two isoforms, COX-1 and COX-2. Standard NSAIDs block both enzymes, whereas COX-2 inhibitors block only the COX-2 pathway. When only the COX-2 pathway is blocked, the production of prostaglandins responsible for gastric mucosal integrity is retained through the COX-1 pathway.

The differences in anti-inflammatory effects of the various NSAIDs are small, but there is wide variation in the incidence of side-effects. Gastrointestinal bleeding and perforation occur in approximately 1% of patients and result in significant morbidity and mortality. Piroxicam, ketoprofen, indometacin, naproxen and diclofenac are associated with an intermediate risk of gastrointestinal side-effects; azapropazone is associated with the highest risk and ibuprofen the lowest. The COX-2 selective agents etoricoxib and celecoxib are as effective as traditional NSAIDs but produce a lower incidence of gastric side-effects. All NSAIDs, including the COX-2 inhibitors, are contraindicated in the presence of active peptic ulcer disease. Concomitant aspirin therapy greatly increases the gastrointestinal risks of NSAIDs and severely reduces any gastrointestinal safety advantages of COX-2 selective agents. The options for reducing gastric side-effects due to NSAIDs are to avoid the use of NSAIDs and use simple analgesia; to use an NSAID with the fewest associated gastrointestinal side-effects and to use it at the lowest possible dose; to prescribe a gastroprotective agent; or to prescribe a selective COX-2 inhibitor. From studies it would appear that PPIs are most effective for the prevention of gastrointestinal complications associated with NSAID use.

More recent evidence has suggested that patients treated with selective COX-2 inhibitors may be at a slightly increased risk of cardiovascular problems such as myocardial infarction and stroke. Some of the non-selective NSAIDs have also been implicated. Diclofenac has a thrombotic risk similar to that of etoricoxib, whereas naproxen is associated with a lower thrombotic risk than COX-2 inhibitors. COX-2 inhibitors should not be used in patients with a history of ischaemic heart disease, cerebrovascular disease, peripheral arterial disease or moderate to severe heart failure. All NSAIDs are contraindicated in severe heart failure and should be used with caution with patients with renal impairment, as they may cause further deterioration in renal function.

As noted earlier, extra care should be exercised in patients with RA who are co-prescribed an NSAID in conjunction with methotrexate, as there is the potential for interactions which may increase the risks of methotrexate toxicity.

If a patient does not respond to one NSAID they might respond to a different one. It is very important to give a particular NSAID an adequate therapeutic trial before changing to an alternative. Although pain-relieving benefits commence after the first dose, the maximum analgesic benefit takes up to a week to develop and the anti-inflammatory action up to 3 weeks.

Owing to Mrs TD's age and her concurrent medication, it would be reasonable to assume that she will need some sort of protection against gastric ulceration. The options for this would be to use a standard NSAID in combination with a PPI, or to use a COX-2 selective agent. The dose of ibuprofen prescribed is too low, and an 'as required' prescription is inappropriate at this stage of her disease. A higher regular dose of ibuprofen, such as 400 mg three times a day, or diclofenac 50 mg three times a day, would be more appropriate, with co-prescription of a PPI. These drugs have been shown to be efficacious while at the same time having a lesser gastrointestinal side-effect profile than some of the more potent NSAIDs.

What other advice would you give on her pain medication?

A5 **Paracetamol, paracetamol combinations and dihydrocodeine are all useful for simple pain relief. Although they have no anti-inflammatory properties and do not affect the disease process, they do have a place in both early and late stages of the disease. The World Health Organization's analgesic ladder is a good starting point for any decision on analgesia.**

Regular use of paracetamol 1 g four times a day with a weak opioid analgesic either regularly or when required would be a good initial prescription for Mrs TD. There is a need for regular reassessment following review of her pain scores. It is important to avoid co-prescription of analgesia that works on the same receptors. The point of the World Health Organization analgesic ladder is to move up the ladder, not across it. The co-prescription of tramadol with co-codamol will not provide her with additional analgesia and is likely to expose her to unwanted side-effects. This combination requires review with the doctor, and consideration needs to be given to the prescribing of a laxative in conjunction with even a weak opiate.

Is it appropriate for Mrs TD to be taking calcium and vitamin D?

A6 **Calcium and vitamin D supplements are recommended for primary prophylaxis against osteoporosis in frail elderly patients, older people in nursing homes and residential homes, and in patients who are housebound due to illness. Mrs TD should be assessed to see whether she requires bisphosphonate therapy as well as calcium and vitamin D.**

Osteoporosis is characterised by deterioration in bone tissue and low bone mass: the bones become fragile and more likely to fracture. Mrs TD's RA, postmenopausal status and physical disability make her at high risk of developing osteoporosis. The risk of this is further increased by the use of corticosteroids in the management of her RA. In addition to adequate calcium and vitamin D supplementation, the need for an oral bisphosphonate should be considered. Guidance suggests that women aged 65–69 with RA and a T score of –2.5 SD should be treated with an oral bisphosphonate and given adequate calcium and vitamin D supplementation. A T score indicates the number of standard deviations from the mean bone mineral density of young adults and is measured by dual-energy X-ray absorptiometry (DEXA) scanning of the hip. In women of this age group receiving repeated courses of oral corticosteroids, it is suggested that a T score of –1.5 SD indicates the need for osteoporosis prevention with a bisphosphonate.

Outline a pharmaceutical care plan for the initial management of Mrs TD.

A7 The pharmaceutical care plan for Mrs TD should include the following:

(a) Obtain a detailed drug history. Patients often omit to inform medical staff of any eye drops, inhalers or medicines they may buy from their chemist. The pharmacist is in the best possible position to elicit the greatest information.
(b) Contribute to optimising her future treatment according to defined outcomes.
(c) Counsel on all aspects of her treatment.
(d) Monitor all treatment for efficacy and side-effects.
(e) Ensure that all treatment initiated during her hospital stay can be continued and monitored successfully after discharge.
(f) Ensure that she has any aids she might need to manage her medication (such as non-child resistant containers).

What is the role of corticosteroids in the management of RA?

A8 Corticosteroids are used as a bridging therapy to reduce symptoms and disease activity when waiting for the therapeutic onset of a DMARD or when changing from one DMARD to another.

Corticosteroids produce rapid relief of inflammatory symptoms and may have a role in disease modification, but their use is restricted because of their long-term side-effects, such as osteoporosis, peptic ulceration, diabetes mellitus and hypertension.

Low-dose oral prednisolone may be used intermittently if the disease cannot be controlled by other means; however, once oral steroids are started they are often difficult to withdraw, as the patient may flare when the dosage is reduced.

When multiple joints are affected and intra-articular injection would be impracticable, intramuscular depot corticosteroids may be used while awaiting the onset of action of a DMARD. For very severe disease, particularly where there are extra-articular manifestations, pulsed intravenous (IV) infusions of methylprednisolone may be given.

Patients with repeated exposure to corticosteroids are at high risk of glucocorticoid-induced osteoporosis. The risks are highest during the initial stages of treatment. In such patients consideration should be given to the need for bone protection with a bisphosphonate.

What anti-TNF therapies are currently available for the management of RA?

A9 **At the time of writing there are three anti-TNF therapies licensed for the treatment of RA: infliximab, etanercept and adalimumab.**

TNF-α and interleukin (IL)-1 are proinflammatory cytokines present in the synovial fluid and tissue. In RA they are produced in excess. Blocking of TNF-α by anti-TNF agents results in dampening of the inflammatory cascade and blocking of IL-1 activity. Anti-TNF therapy has been shown to reduce the signs and symptoms of RA, improve physical function and slow the progression of joint damage.

Infliximab is a chimeric human–murine monoclonal antibody that binds with high affinity to both soluble and transmembrane forms of TNF-α, leading to inhibition of its functional activity. It is used in combination with methotrexate in patients with active disease who have failed to respond to other DMARDs, including methotrexate. Infliximab is given as a 3 mg/kg IV infusion. The initial infusion is given over a 2-hour period; subsequent infusions are given 2 and 6 weeks after the first. The patient is then maintained on 8-weekly maintenance infusions.

Etanercept is a recombinant human soluble TNF-α receptor. It competitively inhibits the activity of TNF-α by binding to its cell surface receptors. It can be used as monotherapy or in combination with methotrexate for the treatment of moderate to severe active RA. It is given by subcutaneous injection, either 25 mg twice weekly or 50 mg once weekly.

Adalimumab is a recombinant human monoclonal antibody that binds specifically to TNF-α and neutralises its biological function by blocking its interaction with cell surface TNF-α receptors. As the first fully humanised monoclonal antibody against TNF-α, it is less likely to engender an immune response in the recipient than agents that contain non-human or artificial sequences. It is used in combination with methotrexate in patients with moderate to severe active RA who have had an inadequate response to DMARDs, including methotrexate. It can also be used as monotherapy in patients who are intolerant to methotrexate, or where methotrexate is contraindicated. Adalimumab is administered as a 40 mg subcutaneous injection every other week.

There have been no direct comparative trials of anti-TNF agents in patients with RA. Selection is based on prescriber preference, patient factors, the ability to self-inject, and co-prescription with methotrexate. Baseline tests need to be performed prior to therapy initiation to ensure these treatments are not contraindicated (see **A12**).

What are the criteria for starting a patient with RA on an anti-TNF?

A10 **According to NICE guidelines, before patients can be started on an anti-TNF therapy they must have active RA as measured by a disease activity score (DAS28) >5.1. This should be confirmed on at least two occasions, 1 month apart. They should also have undergone trials of at least two DMARDs, including methotrexate (unless contraindicated).**

The DAS28 is a disease activity score based on a 28-joint count and derived from a numerical formula. The value is calculated from the number of tender and swollen joints, the patient's ESR, and a general health status according to a 100 mm visual analogue scale. A score of 5.1 or higher indicates high disease activity; between 5.1 and 3.2 indicates moderate disease activity; and between 3.2 and 2.6 indicates low disease activity. The DAS28 score is also used to evaluate response to treatment. An adequate response to anti-TNF treatment is defined as an improvement in the DAS28 score of 1.2 points or more.

A satisfactory trial of a DMARD is defined as being normally 6 months, with 2 months at standard dose, unless significant toxicity has limited the dose or duration of treatment. Mrs TD has thus fulfilled the NICE criteria for anti-TNF therapy.

What alternative therapeutic options may be considered if anti-TNF therapy is contraindicated?

A11 **For patients where treatment with a biologic is contraindicated, leflunomide monotherapy, or leflunomide in combination with methotrexate, may be given. Where leflunomide is not tolerated, other agents such as azathioprine or ciclosporin, or combination DMARD therapy, could be considered.**

Leflunomide has both immunomodulatory and immunosuppressive characteristics. It inhibits the synthesis of pyrimidine nucleotides in response cells (particularly T cells) and reduces proinflammatory cytokines (TNF and IL6). Studies have shown it to be at least as effective as sulfasalazine and methotrexate, and for quality of life measures some evidence suggests superiority. When given as a loading dose of 100 mg daily for 3 days followed by a maintenance dose of 10–20 mg daily its therapeutic effect starts after 4–6 weeks, and further improvement may be seen for up to 4–6 months. However, many centres do not use this loading dose regimen, as patients are unable to tolerate the gastrointestinal side-effects associated with it. The use of leflunomide has been associated with both haematological and hepatotoxic side-effects. An FBC and LFTs must be performed before therapy is initiated, and then every 2 weeks for the first 6 months, followed by every 8 weeks thereafter. When leflunomide and methotrexate are used in combination extra caution is advised, and patients should be monitored closely because of the increased risk of hepatotoxicity. Leflunomide can also cause hypertension: blood pressure should be checked before commencing leflunomide and periodically thereafter. Both men and women taking leflunomide are required to use adequate contraceptive measures during treatment, and a washout protocol must be followed for any patient considering starting a family.

Azathioprine is an oral purine analogue that inhibits lymphocyte proliferation. It becomes biologically active after metabolism by the liver to 6-mercaptopurine. It is reserved for progressive disease refractory to other DMARDs, as a steroid-sparing agent or where a biologic is contraindicated. Bone marrow suppression and liver toxicity are associated with its use and FBCs and LFTs should be performed during treatment. Renal function should also be monitored as the drug is renally excreted.

Ciclosporin is reserved for severe disease or for use in combination with methotrexate in very active early disease. It works by impairing the function of B and T lymphocytes. Dose-related hypertension and nephrotoxicity are common side-effects. FBCs should be performed during treatment and liver and renal function monitored. Ciclosporin drug levels are not routinely measured when it is used for the management of RA.

Early studies of combination DMARD therapy suggested limited efficacy but excessive toxicity. Recent reviews have shown more positive results. Lower doses of different drugs may reduce the potential for type A adverse drug reactions, and combinations may have synergistic effects owing to their different modes of action. A step-down or step-up approach may be used. The COBRA study involving sulfasalazine, methotrexate and step-down oral prednisolone showed less radiographic damage in patients up to 4 years after the trial. Other combinations include methotrexate, sulfasalazine and hydroxychloroquine; methotrexate and ciclosporin; methotrexate and leflunomide.

What safety concerns are associated with anti-TNF therapy?

A12 **The use of anti-TNF therapy has been associated with an increased incidence of infection and reactivation of latent tuberculosis (TB). Anti-TNFs may also exacerbate heart failure. A small minority of patients have developed lupus-like symptoms or neurological complications as a result of demyelination.**

The use of anti-TNF therapy has been associated with an increased incidence of infection in patients. Therapy should not be started in the presence of serious infection and should be discontinued if the patient develops such an infection. A chest X-ray, tuberculin Mantoux test and hepatitis B+C screen should be performed on all patients being considered for anti-TNF therapy.

Reactivation of latent TB is highest in the first 12 months of treatment, so particular vigilance is required during this time. Active TB must be adequately treated before anti-TNF therapy can be started. Those patients with latent disease may be started on anti-TNF therapy in conjunction with prophylactic anti-TB therapy.

Both infliximab and etanercept have been shown to worsen cardiac failure, so the severity of cardiac failure should be assessed before considering treatment with anti-TNF. Treatment is contraindicated in moderate to severe impairment (NYHA class III/IV) and should be used with caution in patients with mild heart failure (NYHA class I/II). Treatment with anti-TNF should be discontinued in patients who develop new or worsening symptoms of congestive heart failure.

There are a number of reports of demyelination and acute neurological complications associated with anti-TNF therapy: because of this, anti-TNF therapy should not be given to patients with a history of demyelinating disease and is best avoided if there is a strong family history of demyelination. Therapy should be stopped if patients develop signs or symptoms suggestive of demyelination.

Rare cases of systemic lupus erythematosus (SLE) have been reported in association with anti-TNF treatment. SLE symptoms occurred 3–6 months after starting therapy and included fever, malaise, arthritis, discoid lupus rash, erythematous facial rash and hypertension; these resolved 6–14 weeks after stopping therapy. Anti-TNF therapy should be stopped if symptoms of an SLE-like syndrome develop.

Concerns have been raised about the increased risk of cancer associated with anti-TNF therapy. One systematic review has suggested a dose-related increase in cancers, but national registries such as the British Society for Rheumatology (BSR) Biologics Registry have yet to show an increase. In the UK patients started on anti-TNFs are registered in this registry, which tracks the progress of patients with severe RA and other rheumatic conditions who are receiving anti-TNF therapy. The aim of the register is to monitor the long-term safety profile of these agents.

Which anti-TNF would you recommend for Mrs TD and why?

A13 **The choice of anti-TNF is dependent upon both clinician and patient preference. Mrs TD was not keen to self-inject and was already stabilised on methotrexate therapy. She agreed with her clinician that infliximab therapy would be appropriate.**

The three anti-TNFs (infliximab, etanercept and adalimumab) are of equal therapeutic efficacy but differ in their mode of administration and the need for co-prescribing of methotrexate. Infliximab was the first anti-TNF to gain its licence in the management of RA. It has a slightly faster onset of action than the other two and is given by infusion in conjunction with once-weekly methotrexate. As it is an infusion it needs to be given in hospital: this might not suit people who have to work, and it can only be given to patients who are able to tolerate methotrexate. Etanercept and adalimumab are both given by subcutaneous injection. Although these agents are often given in conjunction with weekly methotrexate, co-prescribing of methotrexate is not essential as with infliximab. Patients or their carers are trained to give the injections at home; but some patients are reluctant to self-inject and an alternative person may not be available to administer the medication.

Are there any subsequent therapeutic options if Mrs TD does not respond to treatment with infliximab?

A14 **Patients who have had only a partial or no response to a single anti-TNF agent may respond to an alternative. Patients who fail with anti-TNF may then be considered for treatment with rituximab or abatacept.**

Limited studies have shown that patients who show no response or only a partial response to the first anti-TNF therapy may benefit from an alternative. Infliximab may be considered when etanercept has failed, and vice versa.

Rituximab is a genetically engineered monoclonal antibody which binds to CD20, a protein expressed on B lymphocytes. It is licensed in combination with methotrexate for the treatment of severe active RA in patients who have had an inadequate response or intolerance to other DMARDs, including one or more TNF-inhibitor therapies. It works by killing B cells using CD20 as the target. In RA, B cells can be found in the synovium. They produce antibodies that contribute to the disease and inflammatory cytokines. B cells also affect the function of other cells and cause inflammation. Although rituximab is licensed for both seropositive and seronegative rheumatoid arthritis, only a small group of seronegative patients were studied in the REFLEX trial, and in the DANCER study rituximab was no better than placebo in seronegative patients. Because of this it is used in the management of seropositive patients who have failed with anti-TNF therapy. It is given as two 1 g infusions 2 weeks apart and may be repeated after 6 months if the patient has a detectable B-cell count.

Abatacept is a recombinant human fusion protein that binds to proteins naturally expressed on the surface of activated T cells, causing attenuation of T-cell activity. T cells are central to the immune response and are found in the synovium of patients with RA. In the synovium T cells express activation markers, secrete cytokines and stimulate macrophages, thereby contributing to the development of inflammation and joint destruction. Abatacept in combination with methotrexate is indicated for the treatment of moderate to severe active RA in adults who have had an insufficient response or intolerance to other DMARDs, including at least one TNF inhibitor. In contrast to rituximab, it has been shown to be of benefit in patients with seronegative RA and is given in place of rituximab in such patients who have failed anti-TNF therapy. It is administered as an IV infusion according to weight (<60 kg = 500 mg; ≥ 60 to ≤ 100 kg = 750 mg; >100 kg = 1000 mg). Following the initial infusion it is given 2 and 4 weeks later, then every 4 weeks thereafter.

Anakinra is a naturally occurring IL-1 receptor antagonist licensed for the treatment of RA in combination with methotrexate in patients who have had an inadequate response to methotrexate alone; however, the use of anakinra in the management of RA is no longer recommended by NICE except in the context of a controlled long-term clinical study.

Tocilizumab, an IL-6 receptor antagonist, is, at the time of writing, in phase III trials and is likely to obtain a licence for the treatment of RA. It will be considered as an alternative biologic agent in patients who have failed or are intolerant of anti-TNF.

What is the long-term prognosis for a patient like Mrs TD?

A15 **Anti-TNF therapy can significantly slow disease progression and improve quality of life for patients with RA. It does not, however, reduce existing joint damage, and it takes 3–6 months before patients derive full benefit from treatment. Not all patients respond to the first agent given, and in others therapy may have to be stopped because of adverse side-effects.**

Patients with RA have a shortened life expectancy and an increased risk of cardiovascular disease. A poorer prognosis is associated with a positive rheumatoid factor, raised inflammatory markers, early radiographic joint damage and the presence of tender/swollen joints. It is essential that treatment is commenced with DMARDs as early as possible to prevent joint damage and increase life expectancy.

Acknowledgement

The authors would like to thank Dr Sarah Bingham, Consultant Rheumatologist, Leeds Teaching Hospital NHS Trust, for reviewing and commenting on this chapter.

Further reading

Cohen SB, Emery P, Greenwald MW. Rituximab for rheumatoid arthritis refractory to anti-tumor necrosis factor therapy: results of a multicenter, randomized, double-blind, placebo-controlled, phase III trial evaluating primary efficacy and safety at twenty-four weeks (REFLEX). *Arthritis Rheum* 2006; **54**: 2793–2806.

Emery P. Clinical Review – Treatment of rheumatoid arthritis. *Br Med J* 2006; **332**: 152–155.

Emery P, Fleischmann R, Filipowicz-Sosnowska A *et al.* The efficacy and safety of rituximab in patients with active rheumatoid arthritis despite methotrexate treatment: results of phase IIB randomized, double-blind, placebo-controlled, dose-ranging trial (DANCER). *Arthritis Rheum* 2006; **54**: 1390–1400.

Genovese MC, Becker JC, Schiff M *et al.* Abatacept for rheumatoid arthritis refractory to tumour necrosis factor α inhibition. *N Engl J Med* 2005: **353**; 1114–1123.

Hjardem E, Østergaard M, Pødenphant J *et al.* Do rheumatoid arthritis patients in clinical practice benefit from switching from infliximab to a second tumor necrosis factor alpha inhibitor? *Ann Rheum Dis* 2007; **66**: 1184–1189.

Kremer JM, Genant HK, Moreland LWP *et al.* Effects of abatacept in patients with methotrexate-resistant active rheumatoid arthritis. *Ann Intern Med* 2006; **144**: 865–876.

National Institute for Health and Clinical Excellence. CG79. *Rheumatoid Arthritis: the Management of Rheumatoid Arthritis in Adults*. NICE, London, 2009.

National Institute for Health and Clinical Excellence. TA130. *Adalimumab, Etanercept and Infliximab for the Treatment of Rheumatoid Arthritis*. NICE, London, 2007.

National Institute for Health and Clinical Excellence. TA72 *Anakinra for Rheumatoid Arthritis*. NICE, London, 2003.

National Institute for Health and Clinical Excellence. TA141. *Abatacept for the Treatment of Rheumatoid Arthritis*. NICE, London, 2008.

National Institute for Health and Clinical Excellence. TA160. *Alendronate, Etidronate, Risedronate, Raloxifene and Strontium Ranleate for Primary Pprevention of Osteoporotic Fragility Fracture in Postmenopausal Women*. NICE, London, 2008.

National Institute for Health and Clinical Excellence. TA126. *Rituximab for Treatment of Rheumatoid Arthritis*. NICE, London, 2007 .

Royal College of Physicians. *Glucocorticoid-induced Osteoporosis – Guidance on Prevention and Treatment*. Royal College of Physicians, London, 2002.

Van Vollenhoven R, Harju A, Brannemark S, Klareskog L. Treatment with infliximab (Remicade) when etanercept (Enbrel) has failed or vice versa: data from the STURE registry showing that switching tumour necrosis factor alpha blockers can make sense. *Ann Rheum Dis* 2003; **62**: 1195–1198.

17

Osteoporosis

Jonathan Mason

Case study and questions

Day 1 76-year-old Mrs MG attended A&E following a fall at her care home, where she had been living for the past 2 years. She had a 5-year history of becoming increasingly dependent on others to assist with activities of daily living, and had shown signs of developing dementia, with increasing memory loss and wandering, for which her general practitioner (GP) had prescribed haloperidol 500 micrograms twice daily. Three years earlier, Mrs MG had been diagnosed as suffering from polymyalgia rheumatica (PMR), for which she had been initially prescribed prednisolone orally 10 mg daily. This had been reduced to 5 mg daily after 1 year. She had now been taking this dose for 2 years. She had been a heavy smoker, smoking some 20–30 cigarettes per day, but had stopped completely nearly 10 years ago. She only drank alcohol socially.

Her drug history on admission was as follows:

- Prednisolone 5 mg orally daily
- Nitrazepam 5 mg orally every night
- Haloperidol 500 micrograms orally twice daily

Q1 What is the appropriate dose of prednisolone for the treatment of PMR?

On examination, Mrs MG was found to be small-framed, 1.62 m tall and weighing 49 kg. Blood biochemistry showed that her urea and electrolyte levels were normal. X-ray revealed a fracture to the right radius (Colles' fracture). She was discharged with a plaster cast and a prescription for co-codamol 30/500 capsules one or two to be taken every 4–6 hours. She was referred to the multidisciplinary falls clinic.

Q2 What factors might have contributed to her fall?

Q3 Do you agree with the prescribing of co-codamol 30/500 capsules for analgesia?

Q4 What risk factors does Mrs MG have for osteoporosis?
Q5 How could the diagnosis of osteoporosis be confirmed?

Day 5 Mrs MG attended the multidisciplinary falls clinic at the local hospital outpatient department for a full assessment, which included a review of her medication by a pharmacist. An X-ray was taken of her lower spine, which revealed that she had previously suffered three crush fractures of her lumbar vertebrae.

Q6 What is the purpose of a falls clinic?
Q7 Outline the key points of a pharmaceutical care plan for Mrs MG.
Q8 What changes would you make to her existing therapy?
Q9 What drug treatment options can be considered for her osteoporosis?
Q10 Which would you recommend for this patient and why?
Q11 What non-pharmaceutical interventions should be recommended for Mrs MG?

Mrs MG was started on alendronate 10 mg tablets and Adcal-D3 (calcium and vitamin D tablets). The falls clinic pharmacist stopped the haloperidol and switched the co-codamol to separate paracetamol and codeine tablets. It was agreed that she would be seen at a pharmacist-run sleep clinic in her local surgery. A letter on her proposed management plan was sent to her GP.

Her medication at this time was:

- Prednisolone enteric-coated tablets 5 mg daily
- Nitrazepam tablets 5 mg every night
- Paracetamol tablets 500 mg one or two every 4–6 hours (up to eight tablets in 24 h)
- Codeine tablets 30 mg one every 4 hours if required
- Alendronate tablets 10 mg daily
- Adcal-D3 tablets two daily

Q12 What key points should Mrs MG and her carers be counselled on with regard to her osteoporosis?

Day 14 Mrs MG attended the sleep clinic. The pharmacist stopped the nitrazepam, and provided her carers with advice about sleep hygiene and how to manage her wandering if it became a problem.

A prescription was issued for:

- Temazepam tablets 10 mg one every night if required

Month 3 Mrs MG was seen again in the falls clinic. Her carers reported that she was sleeping well and her wandering was manageable during the day, but that she was experiencing problems swallowing both the alendronate and the calcium tablets.

Q13 What changes would you recommend to her therapy?

Month 6 The community pharmacist from the pharmacy that dispensed medicines for the care home visited the home to conduct medicines use reviews (MURs) for the residents. During the consultation with Mrs MG and her carers, the pharmacist identified that Mrs MG was still experiencing problems swallowing the alendronate tablets.

Her medication at this time was:

- Prednisolone enteric-coated tablets 2.5 mg daily
- Temazepam tablets 10 mg one every night if required
- Paracetamol tablets 500 mg one or two every 4–6 hours (up to eight tablets in 24 h)
- Codeine tablets 30 mg one every 4 hours if required
- Alendronate tablets 70 mg weekly (on the same day each week)
- Calfovit D3 sachets one sachet in water daily

Q14 What is the purpose of an MUR?
Q15 What changes would you recommend to Mrs MG's therapy?
Q16 How long should treatment for osteoporosis be continued?
Q17 How effective is treatment with a bisphosphonate and/or calcium and vitamin D at reducing the risk of fractures?

Answers

What is the appropriate dose of prednisolone for the treatment of PMR?

A1 **Prednisolone should be started at a dose of 15 mg daily. This should then be gradually reduced to the minimum dose that controls symptoms.**

PMR is a chronic inflammatory soft-tissue condition characterised by persistent pain and stiffness of the neck, shoulders and pelvis. It is frequently accompanied by systemic features, and inflammatory markers such as the erythrocyte sedimentation rate (ESR), C-reactive protein (CRP) and plasma viscosity are typically elevated. PMR is rare under the age of 60 (mean age of onset is 70 years) and the condition is three times more common in women than in men.

Corticosteroid therapy is indicated in all cases and should be started as soon as the diagnosis of PMR is suspected. Treatment should be initiated with prednisolone 15 mg/day, as enteric-coated tablets, for at least 1 month. A dramatic symptomatic response would be expected, usually within 2–4 days, whereas inflammatory markers generally normalise over 2 weeks. No advantage has been shown for using starting doses of prednisolone >15 mg daily, and higher doses significantly increase adverse effects.

After 1 month corticosteroid doses should be gradually reduced, taking into account clinical symptoms (pain in shoulders and/or thighs, duration of early morning stiffness, and ability to raise arms) and inflammatory markers (particularly ESR): the patient's symptoms are often a more reliable guide to disease activity than ESR, as it may be normal when the disease is active and raised when the disease is quiescent. If symptoms are controlled, then dosage should be reduced by 2.5 mg every 2–4 weeks until a dose of 10 mg/day is reached; doses should then be reduced by 1 mg every 4–6 weeks until a dose of 5–7 mg/day is reached, and the patient maintained on this dose for the next 12 months. Final reductions from 5–7 mg/day should be at a rate of 1 mg every 6–8 weeks until a dose of 3 mg daily is reached: final reductions should be at a longer interval, for example by 1 mg every 12 weeks.

If symptoms are poorly controlled then the dose of prednisolone should be increased to the lesser of the dose that previously controlled symptoms, or the current dose plus 5 mg. If symptoms relapse fully, then the dose should be increased to the full starting dose.

The patient should be advised that corticosteroid treatment will be required for at least 1 year: the median duration of treatment is approximately 2 years, but may be much longer, with up to 40% of patients still requiring corticosteroid treatment at 4 years. Neither severity of symptoms nor elevation of inflammatory markers at onset can predict the duration of treatment required. Relapse is common after stopping or reducing the dose of prednisolone, occurring in up to 60% of people, but usually responds rapidly to an increase in dose. Relapse is most likely in the first 18 months of treatment and within a year of stopping treatment.

What factors might have contributed to her fall?

A2 **A host of factors might have contributed to Mrs MG's fall, including psychoactive drug therapy (nitrazepam and haloperidol), confusion, problems with balance and environmental factors in the home.**

There are a number of risk factors for falls in older people. These include:

(a) Underlying medical conditions, e.g. transient ischaemic attacks or stroke, heart disease, dementia.
(b) Physical inactivity, which leads to weak muscles and poor balance.
(c) Poor nutritional status.
(d) Medication, e.g. antidepressants, hypnotics, sedatives, diuretics, laxatives.

(e) Sensory disturbance, particularly problems with vision or hearing.
(f) Environmental hazards such as loose carpets, poor lighting, unsafe stairways, rugs on polished floors, ill-fitting shoes or slippers.

Do you agree with the prescribing of co-codamol 30/500 capsules for analgesia?

A3 **No. Fixed combination analgesics are not recommended as they do not provide dose flexibility and can lead to opioid overdosing, particularly in older people such as Mrs MG, who generally require lower doses of opioids.**

Compound analgesic preparations containing a simple analgesic such as paracetamol and an opioid such as codeine are not generally recommended, as there is reduced scope for titrating the individual components to manage pain of varying intensity effectively.

Co-codamol 30/500 is preferable to co-codamol 8/500, because the higher codeine preparation does at least provide a therapeutic dose of the opioid; however, older people are particularly susceptible to opioid side-effects. Using co-codamol 30/500 in an older person may result in the patient receiving either too high a dose of codeine, leading to opioid side-effects, particularly constipation, or too low a dose of paracetamol to provide effective analgesia.

What risk factors does Mrs MG have for osteoporosis?

A4 **Mrs MG has a number of risk factors for osteoporosis, including:**

(a) Chronic corticosteroid use.
(b) Female gender.
(c) Increased age (>60).
(d) White race.
(e) Low weight and body mass index (BMI).
(f) Reduced mobility.
(g) Oestrogen deficiency.
(h) Smoking history.
(i) Being housebound, with a consequent vitamin D deficiency.

Long-term treatment with oral corticosteroids increases the risk of vertebral and hip fractures. Long-term therapy (oral or inhaled) is defined as daily therapy (even at doses <7.5 mg prednisolone or equivalent) for longer than 3 months, or as more than three or four courses of corticosteroid taken in the previous 12 months. The risk of osteoporosis with long-term corticosteroid therapy is increased through a variety of mechanisms:

(a) Reduced gastrointestinal absorption of calcium and increased urinary calcium excretion.

(b) Effects on sex hormones, including reduced adrenal androgens, reduced oestrogen and reduced testosterone, leading to increased osteoclast activity and bone resorption.
(c) Reduced osteoblast activity, leading to reduced bone formation.
(d) Reduced muscle mass.
(e) Effects on growth hormones and growth factors.

The Royal College of Physicians recommends osteoporosis prophylaxis for anyone over the age of 65 taking, or planned to be taking, oral corticosteroids for longer than 3 months. People aged less than 65 with no history of osteoporosis or fragility fracture, but who are likely to remain on corticosteroids for at least 3 months, should have their bone mineral density (BMD) measured using dual-energy X-ray absorptiometry (DEXA) scanning to assess their fracture risk: if their T score is –1.5 or less, or if there is a long wait for DEXA scanning, then prophylaxis for osteoporosis should be initiated.

Female gender, being over 60 years of age (which leads to age-related reduction in vitamin D levels), and a strong family history of osteoporosis, particularly maternal hip fracture, but also a diagnosis of osteoporosis, low-trauma fracture after 50 years of age, and kyphosis (hunched back), are all strong risk factors for osteoporosis. Other patient demographics, such as being of Caucasian or Asian origin, having a low BMI (Mrs MG's BMI is <19 kg/m^2) and reduced mobility (on feet for <4 hours/day) are all predictors of low bone mass and hence increase the risk of osteoporosis. Further risk factors include a personal history of low-impact fractures and height loss, but only as a result of crush fractures of the vertebrae, which may lead to kyphosis.

A number of diseases also predispose to reduced bone mass, as a result of either increased bone turnover or of reduced absorption of calcium and/or vitamin D. These include liver disease, thyroid disease, rheumatoid arthritis and diseases leading to malabsorption.

In women, oestrogen deficiency following the menopause results in the net rate of bone resorption exceeding that of bone formation, which in turn leads to a reduction in bone mass. This effect is heightened in women who have an early (defined as age <45) natural or surgical menopause, women with premenopausal amenorrhoea for more than 1 year which is not due to pregnancy, and women who have had a hysterectomy under the age of 45 with at least one ovary conserved, as this may affect ovarian function.

Smoking is associated with low bone mass, and evidence suggests that patients who smoke have at least double the risk of hip fracture, particularly in postmenopausal women. Smoking may increase the risk for hip fracture through reduced weight, impaired health status and reduced neuromuscular function. It may take up to 10 years after smoking cessation before the excess risks disappear. Other lifestyle/dietary factors, such as alcohol and caffeine intake, are inconsistently associated with low bone mass.

Vitamin D and its major biologically active metabolite 1,25-dihydroxyvitamin D play a central role in maintaining calcium and phosphate homoeostasis. Vitamin D is thus essential for skeletal health. Severe deficiency is associated with defective mineralization, resulting in rickets in children or osteomalacia in adults. Less severe deficiency leads to secondary hyperparathyroidism and increased bone turnover. These effects play an important role in age-related bone loss and osteoporotic fractures. Housebound and institutionalised people are at increased risk of vitamin D insufficiency. Natural dietary sources of vitamin D are limited, and their contribution to vitamin D status assumes importance in individuals with reduced exposure to sunlight. Populations at risk include older people, housebound and institutionalised people, those who avoid exposure to sunlight, and patients with intestinal, liver, renal or cardiopulmonary disease. Low calcium intake is also a significant risk factor.

How could the diagnosis of osteoporosis be confirmed?

A5 **Osteoporosis is diagnosed in terms of bone mineral density (BMD). Dual X-ray absorptiometry (DEXA) scanning of the hip and/or lumbar spine is the gold standard tool for BMD measurement.**

The diagnosis of osteoporosis is confirmed by DEXA scanning demonstrating low BMD. Results are reported as T and Z scores, which indicate the BMD as the number of standard deviations (SD) from the mean BMD for young adults and the patient's age group, respectively. The T score relates to absolute fracture risk, whereas the Z score relates to the individual's risk for their age.

The World Health Organization defines osteoporosis as a BMD of 2.5 SD or more below the young adult mean value, i.e. a T score of ≤ –2.5. For every SD below the mean, the risk of fracture is approximately doubled. A score between –1.5 and –2.5 SD is indicative of osteopenia, i.e. low BMD, which is suggestive of osteoporosis but not diagnostic. DEXA scanning of the hip is generally preferred to that of the spine, particularly in older people, because it is thought to give more information about cortical and trabecular bone and is predictive for fracture risk. DEXA scanning of the spine, albeit easier to perform and probably faster than for the hip, is not suitable for diagnosis in older people because of the high prevalence of arthrosis and arthritis. However, the spine is the preferred scanning site for assessment of response to treatment.

The use of BMD assessment alone has high specificity but low sensitivity. The low sensitivity means that half of all osteoporotic fractures will occur in women said not to have osteoporosis. Screening of individuals without risk factors for osteoporosis is therefore not recommended.

The Royal College of Physicians and NICE recommend that BMD should be measured in people with:

(a) A fragility fracture, except women aged 75 years and older (who should be assumed to have osteoporosis and offered treatment).
(b) Untreated premature menopause.
(c) Prolonged secondary amenorrhoea (for more than 1 year).
(d) Primary hypogonadism.
(e) Chronic disorders associated with osteoporosis (e.g. rheumatoid arthritis, hyperthyroidism, coeliac disease, chronic inflammatory bowel disease, chronic liver disease, hyperparathyroidism).
(f) Family history of maternal hip fracture under the age of 75.
(g) BMI <19 kg/m^2.
(h) Conditions associated with prolonged immobility.
(i) Thoracic kyphosis, and loss of height secondary to vertebral deformity (after radiological confirmation).
(j) X-ray evidence of osteopenia or vertebral deformity.
(k) Those in whom quantitative ultrasound or peripheral DEXA scanning of the wrist or heel suggests osteoporosis (these tests are not recommended for the diagnosis of osteoporosis, but may have been carried out as a screening test).
(l) People under the age of 65 who have been taking oral corticosteroids for 3 months or more.

The National Osteoporosis Society recommends that BMD should also be measured in postmenopausal women who have had two vertebral fractures.

In Mrs MG's case, because she has so many risk factors and has already suffered vertebral crush fractures and a low-impact fracture, DEXA scanning is unnecessary and treatment for osteoporosis should be initiated without delay.

What is the purpose of a falls clinic?

A6 Falls clinics are designed to conduct a comprehensive review of patients with multiple needs who have had a fall (or who are at risk of falling) and who require multiple interventions to reduce their risk of further falls.

Multidisciplinary falls clinics are designed to assess the needs of older people who have had a number of falls (usually three or more), or who are at risk of falling, for example they demonstrate abnormalities of gait and/or balance. Patients are referred following an initial assessment to determine whether they have single or multiple needs. If a faller has single needs then these are more appropriately addressed by the most relevant service, e.g. occupational therapy, district nurses, social services. Fallers with multiple needs are referred to a falls clinic. The multi-disciplinary falls team reviews all aspects of the patient's situation, including medication, vision and hearing, nutrition, walking/gait/balance, environmental hazards, etc. NICE has published clinical guidelines on the management of people at risk of falling.

Outline the key points of a pharmaceutical care plan for Mrs MG.

A7 **The pharmaceutical care plan for Mrs MG should identify and address each of her problems. It should indicate what monitoring is necessary to ensure the desired therapeutic outcomes are achieved with the minimum of adverse effects.**

Mrs MG's identified problems are: cause of fall; pain due to Colles' fracture; PMR; osteoporosis and risk of further fractures. Her care plan should be as follows:

(a) Review her current drug therapy to ensure that any drugs contributing to her risk of falling are discontinued or changed to ones that reduce the risks. Other non-pharmaceutical interventions should also be implemented to reduce her risk of further falls.
(b) Ensure that appropriate analgesia is provided using paracetamol with or without codeine.
(c) Review the need for the continuing use of prednisolone.
(d) Prescribe appropriate therapy for her osteoporosis.
(e) Counsel Mrs MG and her carers on all aspects of her drug therapy, including reasons for changes.
(f) Monitor her treatment for efficacy and side-effects:
    (i) Monitor for insomnia and behavioural problems.
    (ii) Pain relief. Ensure that paracetamol and codeine provide sufficient analgesia. If necessary, increase the dose of codeine or switch to a different opioid. Monitor side-effects of codeine, particularly constipation.
    (iii) Monitor symptoms of PMR and inflammatory markers (ESR, CRP and plasma viscosity).
    (iv) Monitor plasma calcium before treatment and at regular intervals thereafter, and whenever nausea or vomiting occurs.
(g) Ensure she is referred for DEXA scanning of the spine every 2 years.

What changes would you make to her existing therapy?

A8 **The following changes should be made to Mrs MG's medication:**

(a) Switch night sedation from nitrazepam to temazepam.
(b) Stop haloperidol therapy.
(c) Switch co-codamol 30/500 to separate paracetamol 500 mg and codeine 30 mg formulations.
(d) Review the use of prednisolone as Mrs MG is now three years post-diagnosis of PMR.

(a) **Night sedation.** Benzodiazepines increase the risk of falls, particularly in older people, and even more so when used in combination with other psychotropic agents. Benzodiazepines with a longer plasma half-life, such as nitrazepam, are more problematic than those with shorter half-lives such as temazepam. The benzodiazepines with longer half-lives tend to cause a 'hangover' effect, i.e. their sedative effects persist into the following day.

It is advisable to switch patients from longer-acting benzodiazepines to a shorter-acting alternative. A number of studies have shown that it is relatively easy to switch patients from nitrazepam to temazepam. Some have shown that a third of patients taking nitrazepam long term can just stop taking it; a third can be switched directly to temazepam, and the remaining third will need more intensive support.

(b) **Haloperidol.** Antipsychotics such as haloperidol have frequently been used to control behavioural disturbances in patients with dementia even though there is little evidence that they work in such patients. Use of antipsychotics in care home patients with dementia is frequently inappropriate, as some behavioural disturbances occur more frequently in people taking antipsychotics, and <20% of behavioural problems associated with dementia respond to antipsychotics. A number of studies have found an association between the use of psychotropic drugs and falls, restlessness, wandering and urinary incontinence. In addition, the use of antipsychotics in dementia may increase the rate of cognitive decline, reduce inhibitions and increase wandering.

In the USA, the *Nursing Home Reform Amendments* – a component of the *Omnibus Budget Reconciliation Act 1987* (OBRA 87) which came into effect in 1990 – were enacted in an attempt to decrease the unnecessary use of antipsychotics in nursing home residents. The OBRA 87 recommendations specify that antipsychotics should only be used where patients exhibit psychotic symptoms and not for indications such as anxiety, wandering and insomnia. They require documentary evidence that other, non-pharmacological methods have been tried and have failed to control symptoms, and reasons for exceeding recommended doses. Following the implementation of the OBRA 87 guidelines there has been a reduction in the use of antipsychotics of between a quarter and a third in US nursing homes, with no concomitant increase in the prescribing of other psychotropic drugs.

In Mrs MG's case it would be appropriate to just stop the haloperidol and then monitor her behaviour. Withdrawal of antipsychotics has been shown to improve mental state and attention span and is not associated with an increase in problem behaviour. Mrs MG's carers should be given advice on how to cope with problem behaviour. This could include:

(i) Create a calm, predictable environment.
(ii) Take steps to avoid boredom and loneliness.
(iii) Ensure a regular routine, with no unnecessary rules and restrictions.
(iv) Review physical environment, paying attention to room temperature, background noise, lighting etc.
(v) If patients are prone to wandering, ensure they have plenty of opportunity for physical exercise and are encouraged to take walks.
(vi) Warm milky drinks can help induce sleep.

Carers should record details of problem behaviour as follows: date and time of incident; who recorded it; description, including the context of the behaviour; consequences, including how staff responded to the behaviour; and what was thought to trigger the behaviour.

(c) **Analgesia.** As discussed in **A3**, co-codamol 30/500 does not provide flexibility in analgesic dosage and can lead to opioid overdosing. Her prescription should be switched to paracetamol 500-mg tablets one or two up to four times a day, plus codeine 30 mg every 4 hours only if required.

(d) **Corticosteroid.** As Mrs MG has been taking prednisolone for over 3 years it would be worth considering a reduction in dose with a view to stopping corticosteroid therapy completely.

A suitable dose regimen for Mrs MG would be to reduce her dose of prednisolone by 1 mg every 6–8 weeks until a dose of 3 mg daily is reached, and then by 1 mg every 12 weeks. It is important to monitor her condition as the dose is reduced: if she suffers a relapse in symptoms, her dose should be increased again. If she does not, further reduction or complete withdrawal could be considered; however, it should be recognised that it may not be possible to withdraw corticosteroid treatment completely.

What drug treatment options can be considered for her osteoporosis?

A9 **A number of treatment options are available:**

(a) Bisphosphonates, such as alendronate, risedronate, etidronate, ibandronate or zoledronate.
(b) Strontium ranelate.
(c) Teriparatide (parathyroid hormone).
(d) Calcitonin.
(e) Vitamin D derivatives (alfacalcidol and calcitriol).
(f) Calcium and vitamin D supplementation.
(g) Hormone replacement therapy (HRT), either unopposed or with progestogen.
(h) Selective oestrogen receptor modulator (SERM) therapy.

(a) **Bisphosphonates.** The bisphosphonates (alendronate, risedronate, etidronate, ibandronate, zoledronate) are all licensed for the prevention and treatment of osteoporosis. In combination with calcium and vitamin D they prevent bone loss and reduce the risk of osteoporotic fractures; however, the evidence for hip protection is strongest for alendronate and risedronate, particularly in people with established osteoporosis (i.e. T score < –2.5 SD), so these drugs are preferred if hip protection is particularly important. NICE recommends alendronate, risedronate or etidronate as first-line agents for secondary prevention of osteoporotic fragility fractures in postmenopausal women.

Alendronate is licensed at a dose of 10 mg daily. For people who have problems swallowing the tablets, alendronate is also available as a once-weekly formulation at a dose of 70 mg. Risedronate is licensed at a dose of 5 mg daily and is also available as a once-weekly formulation, at a dose of 35 mg. For the treatment for osteoporosis etidronate is taken in 90-day cycles as follows: 400 mg etidronate daily for 14 days followed by 1.25 g calcium carbonate (500 mg elemental calcium) daily for 76 days.

Ibandronate and zoledronic acid are newer and more potent bisphosphonates. Ibandronate is either taken as a 150 mg tablet once a month, or can be given as an intravenous injection (over 15–30 seconds) at a dose of 3 mg once every 3 months. Zoledronate is administered as a 5 mg infusion (50 micrograms/mL in a 100 mL solution, administered over not less than 15 minutes) once yearly. There is limited experience with the use of both ibandronate and zoledronate, so more established bisphosphonates should be used first. However, either agent may be a useful option for people who are unable to swallow any of the oral formulations.

(b) **Strontium ranelate.** Strontium ranelate is licensed for the treatment of postmenopausal osteoporosis. It is taken as a 2 g sachet, dissolved in water, once daily. Strontium ranelate is an option if a bisphosphonate cannot be taken, or for women who have had an unsatisfactory response to a bisphosphonate. Although adverse effects with strontium ranelate are generally mild and transient, the Medicines and Healthcare products Regulatory Agency (MHRA) has recently advised that it may rarely cause severe allergic reactions, including drug rash with eosinophilia systemic symptoms (DRESS): patients should be warned that if a rash develops they should stop taking strontium ranelate and seek urgent medical advice. Strontium ranelate also increases the risk of venous thromboembolism, and should thus be used with caution in people with an increased risk.

(c) **Teriparatide.** Teriparatide is a recombinant human parathyroid hormone that stimulates bone formation. It is given daily by subcutaneous injection at a dose of 20 micrograms and should only be initiated on the recommendation of a specialist. There is evidence that teriparatide reduces both vertebral and non-vertebral fractures. NICE recommends that it should be considered for the secondary prevention of osteoporotic fragility fractures in women aged 65 and over who are intolerant of bisphosphonates, or who have had an unsatisfactory response to bisphosphonates and who have severe osteoporosis. It is only licensed for up to 18 months' treatment.

(d) **Calcitonin.** Calcitonin (salmon) in both injectable form (for subcutaneous or intramuscular injection) and as a nasal spray, is licensed for the treatment of postmenopausal osteoporosis in combination with calcium and vitamin D supplementation. The efficacy of calcitonin for fracture prevention in corticosteroid-induced osteoporosis remains to be established. It appears to preserve bone mass in the first year of corticosteroid therapy at the lumbar spine, but not at the femoral neck. A Cochrane Review suggested that the protective effect on bone mass may be greater for patients who have been taking corticosteroids for more than 3 months. Use of calcitonin should be reserved for people who cannot take either a bisphosphonate or strontium ranelate.

(e) **Vitamin D.** Calcitriol (1,25-dihydroxycholecalciferol), the major active metabolite of vitamin D, is also licensed for the treatment of postmenopausal osteoporosis. Studies of calcitriol on bone loss and fractures have produced conflicting results. It seems to protect against vertebral fracture and is effective in reducing the incidence of vertebral deformity, but it is not known whether it protects against hip fracture. Calcitriol may be useful in younger people, especially women of childbearing age, in whom bisphosphonates should be used with extreme caution, but there is a lack of data in older men and women. Similarly, alfacalcidol (1α-hydroxycholecalciferol) has been shown to prevent corticosteroid-induced bone loss from the lumbar spine but it is not licensed for this indication.

(f) **Calcium supplements.** Used alone, calcium supplements may reduce the rate of bone loss in postmenopausal women with osteoporosis and reduce the risk of vertebral fracture, and there may be some effect on non-vertebral and hip fracture risk; however, calcium supplementation alone is less effective than other agents, and is not generally recommended. Calcium supplements should usually be used in combination with other bone-protective agents.

Historically, calcium and vitamin D supplements have been regarded as adjuncts to treatment; however, recent evidence from large trials indicates that these supplements (providing 800 units vitamin D and 1 g elemental calcium) significantly reduce the risk of both hip and non-vertebral fracture, and may even reduce the risk of falling in older people. It is unclear whether the reduction in risk is due to vitamin D, calcium or the combination of both. Calcium and vitamin D supplementation should be considered as first-line monotherapy prophylaxis for the frail elderly, people in care homes, and those who are housebound. Calcium and vitamin D should also be used as an adjunct to treatment for those with established osteoporosis, unless the clinician is confident that the patient has an adequate dietary calcium intake and is vitamin D replete or is already taking a vitamin D analogue.

(g) **HRT.** HRT with oestrogen prevents bone loss and may increase BMD in postmenopausal women. HRT has been shown to reduce the risk of vertebral fractures. It may also have some effect on reducing the risk of non-vertebral fractures, and observational data support a protective effect against hip fracture. Although there is some evidence that HRT increases BMD in the spine but not the hip in people taking corticosteroids, it is not licensed for the prevention or treatment of corticosteroid-induced osteoporosis. There appears to be no difference in efficacy between the different formulations; however, the bone protective effect is probably dose related. The usual recommended dosages are 0.625 mg oral conjugated oestrogen daily, 2 mg oral estradiol daily or 50 micrograms transdermal estradiol daily.

Lower dosages may also preserve bone mass and may be an option in women intolerant of higher dosages. There is no clear evidence defining either the optimal age for initiation or the duration of therapy. Most evidence suggests that bone-conserving effects are greatest if HRT is initiated at menopause and continued for up to 10 years, but even this may have little residual effect on BMD among women over 75, who have the highest risk of fracture. HRT is no longer recommended as the first-line primary preventative strategy for osteoporosis in postmenopausal women. The results of several long-term studies into the risks and benefits of HRT indicate that for long-term treatment with oestrogen the risks of adverse outcomes such as breast cancer and stroke outweigh the benefits in terms of prevention of bone loss and fractures. Whereas HRT may be appropriate in some older women, the monthly withdrawal bleeds and oestrogenic and/or progestogenic adverse effects generally make it difficult to tolerate in women over the age of 75.

Tibolone, which has both oestrogenic and progestogenic effects, is licensed for prophylaxis of osteoporosis in postmenopausal women; however, its benefits on BMD have not been demonstrated and there is no evidence that it prevents fractures. It is not licensed for corticosteroid-induced osteoporosis.

(h) **SERM.** Raloxifene is a SERM which acts as an oestrogen agonist in bone and in the cardiovascular system and as an oestrogen antagonist in the endometrium and breast. Raloxifene prevents bone loss in postmenopausal women, and is licensed for the treatment and prevention of postmenopausal osteoporosis. It prevents bone loss in the lumbar spine and proximal femur. Although raloxifene in combination with calcium and vitamin D has been shown to reduce the risk of vertebral fracture, it has not been shown to reduce the risk of non-vertebral and hip fractures. Nor has it been evaluated in corticosteroid-induced bone loss. Raloxifene could be considered if a bisphosphonate or strontium ranelate is inappropriate or not tolerated, but its place in the treatment of women more than 10 years postmenopausal is uncertain.

Which would you recommend for this patient and why?

A10 **Mrs MG should be prescribed a bisphosphonate together with calcium and vitamin D supplementation. She has already suffered vertebral crush fractures, a low-impact non-vertebral fracture, and has a number of other factors putting her at high risk of osteoporosis.**

As discussed above, alendronate or risedronate plus calcium and vitamin

D have been shown to prevent bone loss and reduce the risk of osteoporotic fractures at all sites in postmenopausal women. This combination offers the best protection for a woman of Mrs MG's age and fracture history.

What non-pharmaceutical interventions should be recommended for Mrs MG?

A11 **A number of non-pharmaceutical interventions should be recommended. These include the use of external hip protectors, ensuring adequate nutrition (especially with calcium and vitamin D), increased exercise and modifications to the home environment.**

External hip protectors consist of plastic shields or foam pads kept in place by pockets in specially designed underwear. They are designed to divert a direct impact away from the greater trochanter during a fall from standing height. Upon impact the protector transfers released energy to soft tissue and muscles anterior and posterior to the femoral bone. Studies into the effect of such protectors on hip fractures have shown that they significantly reduce the risk. Indeed, in studies in which there were hip fractures in the group wearing protectors, none of those who suffered a hip fracture were wearing their protectors at the time. Other benefits to wearing hip protectors include the fact that they reduce the patient's fear of falling and increase their confidence in participating in exercise and activities of daily living.

The main problem with hip protectors is that their acceptability is generally poor. Studies indicate that only about 50% of patients wear them when they are first issued, and that adherence rates drop to 25–30% within 6 months. Daytime adherence rates are generally better than night-time rates. By their very nature, hip protectors are bulky and many wearers stop using them because they find them uncomfortable, they restrict mobility or they cause practical problems, such as incontinence. Causes of discomfort include warmth, being too tight-fitting, and a feeling that the shells are too hard. Usage can be improved if carers are enthusiastic about the value of hip protectors, and problems with incontinence can easily be overcome by the use of incontinence pads.

At present, hip protectors are not available on NHS prescription, but they can be purchased by the patient or their carers, or may be provided by a hospital or falls clinic.

As discussed earlier, bone loss is influenced by a number of modifiable lifestyle factors, including diet, exercise, smoking and alcohol consumption. Although it is uncertain what benefit people with established osteoporosis gain from lifestyle changes, in Mrs MG's case it would be sensible to encourage an increase in her dietary calcium and vitamin D.

Sources of dietary calcium include milk (200 mL provides approximately 250 mg elemental calcium) and other dairy products (e.g. 30 g Cheddar cheese provides approximately 200 mg calcium); bread; green vegetables, particularly spring greens, broccoli and spinach; nuts, particularly brazil nuts and almonds; and tofu (120 g provides 1776 mg calcium). Dietary sources of vitamin D include margarine, oily fish (herring, sardines), cod liver oil and eggs.

Patients with osteoporosis should also be encouraged to increase their exercise levels. Although exercise has not been consistently shown to improve bone mass, it does improve general wellbeing, muscle strength and postural stability. Physiotherapists working as part of a multidisciplinary falls team can provide a programme of muscle strengthening and balance retraining exercises. Exercise programmes prescribed for fallers generally include elements designed to reduce the risks of injury. So, although such exercises may not prevent the person from falling, the faller knows how to fall more safely.

Finally, Mrs MG's living environment should be assessed to identify potential hazards and to consider measures to reduce the risk of falls. This ideally involves a combined medical and social services assessment. One of the key components of a falls clinic is to assess the patient's home environment, focusing on issues such as provision of nightlights in hallways and bathrooms; provision of footwear with non-slip soles; removal of rugs or the placing of non-slip mats under rugs; the need to ensure that bath, shower and toilet areas are equipped with adequate grab bars, and that stairway railings are sturdy.

What key points should Mrs MG and her carers be counselled on with regard to her osteoporosis?

A12 **Mrs MG and her carers should be counselled on:**

- **(a) The importance of regular treatment.**
- **(b) How to take alendronate.**
- **(c) Diet and exercise.**
- **(d) The need to reduce her night-time sedation regimen.**
- **(e) Coping strategies for wandering.**
- **(f) The benefits of hip protectors.**

Because alendronate can cause oesophageal reactions, the tablets should be taken with a full glass of water on an empty stomach, at least 30 minutes before other drinks and/or breakfast and any other oral medication. Mrs MG should sit upright or stand for at least 30 minutes, and should not lie down until after breakfast. The tablets should not be taken at bedtime or before rising.

What changes would you recommend to her therapy?

A13 Mrs MG's alendronate prescription should be switched to the 70 mg once-weekly formulation and a soluble calcium and vitamin D formulation.

Alendronate may cause oesophageal reactions which include oesophagitis, ulceration, strictures or erosions. These problems can be reduced by using the 70 mg once-a-week formulation, which is licensed for the treatment of postmenopausal osteoporosis and achieves similar increases in bone density to the 10 mg daily formulation. A less frequent dosing schedule will also help Mrs MG cope with her difficulties with taking tablets.

Effervescent granule formulations of calcium and vitamin D are available which provide calcium and the recommended amount of vitamin D per sachet.

What is the purpose of an MUR?

A14 MURs are structured consultations that aim to identify any problems patients may be experiencing taking their medicines as prescribed, and to communicate recommendations to the patient's GP.

MURs were introduced as an advanced service in the English Community Pharmacy Contract in 2005. In order to provide MURs the pharmacist must undertake a training programme and be accredited. MURs are generally provided in the pharmacy in a consultation room/area accredited for the purpose; however pharmacists can apply to their Primary Care Trust for permission to undertake domiciliary MURs. MURs should be undertaken with patients who have been receiving services from the pharmacy for at least 3 months. Patients are asked to bring all of their medicines, both prescribed and non-prescribed, with them to the consultation. During the consultation the pharmacist talks to the patient to ascertain their understanding of each of their medicines and to identify any problems they may be experiencing taking their medicines as prescribed. For each MUR the pharmacist completes either an electronic or a paper-based form, and if they have identified any problems with adherence they send a copy of their recommendations to the patient's GP.

What changes would you recommend to Mrs MG's therapy?

A15 Mrs MG should either be switched to a longer-acting bisphosphonate, or to an alternative second-line drug such as strontium ranelate.

Because Mrs MG is still experiencing difficulty swallowing the weekly alendronate tablets she could either be switched to a longer-acting bisphosphonate such as monthly ibandronate tablets, 3-monthly ibandronate injections, or annual zoledronate infusions, or to an alternative class of drug. In Mrs MG's case it would be reasonable to switch to monthly ibandronate tablets.

How long should treatment for osteoporosis be continued?

A16 **Prophylaxis against corticosteroid-induced osteoporosis should be continued for as long as the patient is taking the corticosteroid. The optimal duration of bisphosphonate therapy for prevention of postmenopausal osteoporosis has not been established. Calcium and vitamin D should be continued long term.**

The optimal duration of bisphosphonate therapy for the prevention of postmenopausal osteoporosis has not been established, because most of the trials have been for less than 4 years. The best approach to long-term management is to perform a DEXA scan on Mrs MG every 2 years (once she has stopped taking prednisolone). If her T score is greater than –2.5 SD (i.e. indicative of osteopenia) it would be reasonable to consider stopping the bisphosphonate therapy, as bisphosphonates are less beneficial in patients with osteopenia. Calcium and vitamin D therapy should, however, be continued.

How effective is treatment with a bisphosphonate and/or calcium and vitamin D at reducing the risk of fractures?

A17 **Both alendronate and risedronate significantly reduce the risk of osteoporotic fractures at all sites in postmenopausal women. Zoledronate has been shown to significantly reduce the risk of osteoporotic vertebral and hip fractures in postmenopausal women. The evidence for efficacy of other bisphosphonates is less substantial. Calcium and vitamin D significantly reduce the risks of osteoporotic fractures at all sites in people over 65. The evidence for fracture risk reduction in people taking long-term corticosteroids is less robust than for interventions used in postmenopausal women with osteoporosis, and has mostly been gained from *post hoc* analysis.**

A number of clinical trials have shown that alendronate prevents osteoporotic fractures in postmenopausal women. For non-vertebral fractures the absolute risk reductions (ARRs) ranged from 1.5% to 6.5%, whereas for vertebral fractures the ARR ranged from 1.6% to 6.8%. However, the trials were of different durations (1–4.25 years) and the rate of fractures in the placebo groups varied between trials (from 3.1% to 4.9% for non-vertebral and from 0.8% to 4.8% for vertebral). Thus the standardised numbers needed to treat (NNTs) for 3 years (adjusted to a baseline risk of 4%) ranged from 17.3 to 75.3 for non-vertebral fractures and from 16.5 to 18.6 for vertebral fractures.

Risedronate has also been shown to prevent osteoporotic fractures in postmenopausal women. For non-vertebral fractures the ARRs ranged from 1.8% to 5.8%, and for vertebral fractures from 3.9% to 8.8%. Again, the trials were of different durations (2.3–3 years) and the rate of fractures in the placebo groups varied between trials (from 2.1% to 7.0% for non-vertebral and from 3.8% to 7.3% for vertebral). For risedronate, the standardised NNTs for 3 years (adjusted to a baseline risk of 4%) ranged from 17.7 to 39.9 for non-vertebral fractures and from 20.6 to 24.2 for vertebral fractures.

There have been two key trials with zoledronate. One involved postmenopausal women with osteoporosis, the other involved both men and women following hip fracture. The trial in postmenopausal women resulted in a significant reduction in vertebral fractures (3.3% compared to 10.9% for the placebo group; $P < 0.001$) and hip fracture (1.4% compared to 2.5% for the placebo group; $P = 0.002$) after 3 years. In the recurrent fracture study there was a significant reduction in new clinical fractures after a median follow-up of 1.9 years (8.6% compared to 13.9% in the placebo group).

A Cochrane Review of the use of etidronate for treating and preventing postmenopausal osteoporosis concluded that although etidronate increases BMD in the lumbar spine and femoral neck, and reduces the risk of vertebral fractures, its effects on non-vertebral and hip fractures are uncertain. However, a recent large observational study suggested that etidronate reduces the risk of fractures at all sites.

There is evidence that oral ibandronate, 150 mg once a month, increases lumbar spine BMD in postmenopausal women, but there is no published evidence that it reduces vertebral or non-vertebral fractures.

In a large trial in relatively healthy mobile older women (mean age 84) living in nursing homes, treatment with calcium and vitamin D resulted in a 4% absolute reduction in hip fracture and a 7% reduction in any fracture over 3 years (NNTs of 25 and 14, respectively). In another trial in community-dwelling older people (both men and women aged over 65) treatment with calcium and vitamin D resulted in a significant reduction in non-vertebral fractures (NNT of 14 over 3 years).

With regard to corticosteroid-induced osteoporosis, the bisphosphonates have been shown to prevent and treat corticosteroid-induced bone loss, and calcium and vitamin D has been shown to prevent bone loss in patients treated with corticosteroids; however, there is a lack of evidence for the efficacy of these agents with respect to fracture prevention.

Further reading

Black DM, Thompson DE, Bauer DC *et al.* Fracture risk reduction with alendronate in women with osteoporosis: the Fracture Intervention Trial. FIT Research Group. *J Clin Endocrinol Metab* 2000; **85**: 4118–4124.

Cranney A, Welch V, Adachi JD *et al.* Calcitonin for preventing and treating corticosteroid-induced osteoporosis (Cochrane Review). In: *The Cochrane Library 2*. Update Software. Oxford, 2003.

Cranney A, Welch V, Adachi JD *et al.* Etidronate for treating and preventing postmenopausal osteoporosis (Cochrane Review). In: *The Cochrane Library 2*. Update Software. Oxford, 2003.

Cryer C, Knox A, Martin D *et al.* Hip protector compliance among older people living in residential care homes. *Injury Prevent* 2002; **8**: 202–206.

Grady D, Cummings SR. Postmenopausal hormone therapy for prevention of fractures. How good is the evidence? *J Am Med Assoc* 2001; **285**: 2909–2910.

Department of Health. *National Service Framework for Older People*. Department of Health, London, 2000.

Gillespie WJ, Avenell A, Henry DA *et al.* Vitamin D and vitamin D analogues for preventing fractures associated with involutional and postmenopausal osteoporosis (Cochrane Review). In: *The Cochrane Library 2*. Update Software. Oxford, 2003.

Homik J, Cranney A, Shea B *et al.* Bisphosphonates for steroid-induced osteoporosis (Cochrane Review). In: *The Cochrane Library 2*. Update Software. Oxford, 2003.

Homik J, Suarez-Almazor ME, Shea B *et al.* Calcium and vitamin D for corticosteroid-induced osteoporosis (Cochrane Review). In: *The Cochrane Library 2*. Update Software. Oxford, 2003.

MHRA. Strontium ranelate (Protelos): risk of severe allergic reactions. *Drug Safety Update* 2007; **1**: 15.

National Institute for Health and Clinical Excellence. CG21. *Falls: the Assessment and Prevention of Falls in Elderly People*. NICE, London, 2004.

National Institute for Health and Clinical Excellence. TA87. *Bisphosphonates (Alendronate, Etidronate, Risedronate), Selective Oestrogen Receptor Modulators (Raloxifene) and Parathyroid Hormone (Teriparatide) for the Secondary Prevention of Osteoporotic Fragility Fractures in Postmenopausal Women*. National Institute for Health and Clinical Excellence 2005.

NIH Consensus Development Panel on Osteoporosis Prevention, Diagnosis and Therapy. Osteoporosis Prevention, Diagnosis and Therapy. *J Am Med Assoc* 2001; **285**: 785–795.

Royal College of Physicians. *Osteoporosis: Clinical Guidelines for Prevention and Treatment*. Royal College of Physicians, London, 1999.

Royal College of Physicians. *Osteoporosis: Clinical Guidelines for Prevention and Treatment. Update on Pharmacological Interventions and an Algorithm for Management*. Royal College of Physicians, London, 2000.

Woolf AD, Akesson K. Preventing fractures in elderly people. *Br Med J* 2003; **327**: 89–95.

18

Epilepsy

Ben Dorward

Case study and questions

Day 1 Miss SL, a 19-year-old student who had recently moved away from home to university, was witnessed 'having a fit' by her friends and was taken to the local A&E department. The fit had stopped by the time she arrived and Miss SL had no recollection of the event. She was sent home from hospital with paracetamol for the resulting headache, and referred to a 'faints and fits' clinic at the local neurology department.

At the neurology clinic she commented that she had been experiencing jerking movements for several years, most notably in the morning, and that these had occasionally led to her dropping her breakfast. Her friends had also commented to her that she was prone to daydreaming. On questioning she stated that initially she had found the transition to university life quite stressful. She admitted to taking full advantage of the social opportunities, and to feeling very tired due to having to get up early for lectures after late nights out.

The neurologist made a diagnosis of juvenile myoclonic epilepsy (JME). Miss SL was prescribed lamotrigine 25 mg once daily, increasing to 50 mg once daily after 14 days, and was referred to an epilepsy nurse specialist.

Q1 What is epilepsy?
Q2 Is the history of stress significant?
Q3 Do you agree with the choice of lamotrigine for Miss SL?
Q4 Is the dose of lamotrigine appropriate?
Q5 Outline a pharmaceutical care plan for Miss SL. What advice would you offer her if she asked about contraception?
Q6 What is the role of the epilepsy nurse specialist?

Month 3 Miss SL presented a prescription for lamotrigine. Her dose was now 50 mg in the morning and 50 mg at night. On receiving the prescription Miss SL commented that the tablets did not look the same as those she was given at the hospital. On further questioning you realise she was previously dispensed a generic brand of lamotrigine and the general practitioner (GP) has prescribed the Lamictal brand.

Q7 Is there a significant difference between the different brands of antiepileptic drugs (AEDs)?

Month 4 Miss SL developed a bad chest infection. As she was known to be allergic to penicillin (previous urticarial rash to amoxicillin) the GP prescribed ciprofloxacin 500 mg twice daily for 7 days.

Q8 Is the choice of ciprofloxacin appropriate?

Month 5 The lamotrigine dose had been slowly titrated up to 150 mg twice daily but Miss SL was not responding to treatment, and now constantly felt quite tired. The myoclonic jerks continued and she had had several further tonic–clonic seizures. The frequency of seizures was increasing, and this was particularly noticeable in the 2–3 days before her period.

Q9 What term is used to describe epilepsy that worsens around the time of menstruation, and how common is it?
Q10 What drug treatments are available for this form of epilepsy?

After discussion with Miss SL and her epilepsy nurse specialist, the neurologist decided to change the lamotrigine to levetiracetam. She was prescribed 250 mg twice daily and instructed to increase the dose to 500 mg twice daily in 2 weeks' time. If she did not experience a reduction in seizure frequency after 2 weeks at 500 mg twice daily, then she was to further increase the dose to 750 mg twice daily. At the same time she was instructed to reduce the morning and evening doses of lamotrigine by 50 mg every 2 weeks.

Q11 Levetiracetam is not licensed as a monotherapy for generalised seizures. What is your opinion of the neurologist's choice?
Q12 Levetiracetam is one of the newer AEDs. What are the advantages of the newer drugs over the older ones?

Month 8 Unfortunately, Miss SL had had to withdraw from her university studies. She had become very low in mood but was not keen to take 'antidepressants'. She had read that St John's wort can be effective for low mood and came to seek your advice.

Q13 What advice can you offer about St John's wort?

Q14 If indicated, what is the appropriate drug treatment for depression in people with epilepsy?

Month 10 Miss SL experienced a particularly bad cluster of seizures and injured herself on falling. She was admitted to a neurological ward for observation and assessment. The consultant neurologist prescribed 10 mg of buccal midazolam to be used when required to terminate tonic–clonic seizures lasting longer than 5 minutes.

Q15 What are the advantages and disadvantages of using buccal midazolam over rectal diazepam?

Month 22 Levetiracetam had been gradually titrated upwards to a dose of 1500 mg twice daily and her seizures had become well controlled. Miss SL had started a career in accounting and met a partner. They had discussed starting a family and wanted to know more about how Miss SL's epilepsy would affect this.

Q16 What are the issues concerning pregnancy in women with epilepsy?
Q17 What drug should epileptic women who wish to become pregnant take, and at what dose?

Answers

What is epilepsy?

A1 **Epilepsy is a neurological disorder characterised by a tendency towards epileptic seizures. An epileptic seizure is the result of abnormal electrical activity in the brain. The manifestation of an epileptic seizure depends on the area of the brain affected by the abnormal electrical activity.**

There are two main seizure types:

(a) Generalised seizures are a result of electrical activity spreading through the entire cerebral cortex. They can be secondary to a focal seizure or idiopathic (see below). Absence, myoclonic and tonic–clonic (grand mal) seizures are forms of generalised seizure.

(b) Partial (focal) seizures are a result of a localised electrical disturbance and are often the result of functional changes caused by brain tumours or congenital structural abnormalities such as focal cortical dysplasia. Partial seizures can be further subdivided into simple–partial and complex–partial, based on whether there is an impairment of consciousness (complex–partial) or not (simple–partial).

There are a large number of epilepsy syndromes that can be characterised by the pattern of seizure type, age of onset and response to drug treatment. Many of the generalised epilepsy syndromes have a genetic basis. The diagnosis of epilepsy is largely a clinical one. An accurate eyewitness account of the seizures is one of the most useful pieces of information in making a diagnosis.

JME is a form of idiopathic generalised epilepsy and is one of the most common epilepsy syndromes. It is characterised by myoclonic jerks and generalised tonic–clonic seizures, often shortly after waking. Many patients also have absence seizures. People with JME can be photosensitive, i.e. myoclonic and tonic–clonic seizures can be precipitated by flashing or flickering light.

Is the history of stress significant?

A2 **Tiredness and a lack of sleep can increase the number of seizures, particularly myoclonic seizures in JME.**

Also, a significant number of people presenting to a neurology clinic with possible epilepsy will be diagnosed with non-epileptic attack disorder (NEAD). Such seizures can be called non-epileptic seizures, pseudoseizures, functional seizures, or non-organic seizures, and although they can look very much like epileptic seizures, during an attack an electroencephalogram (EEG) will show no abnormal electrical brain activity. This is one of the reasons why it is very important that a person with suspected epilepsy should be referred to a suitably trained neurologist.

NEAD can often be a reaction to stress. To complicate matters further, some patients with epilepsy may have non-epileptic as well as epileptic seizures. There is no specific drug treatment for NEAD.

Do you agree with the choice of lamotrigine for Miss SL?

A3 **Sodium valproate and lamotrigine are considered first-line treatments for JME; however, sodium valproate is no longer recommended as a first-line treatment in women of childbearing potential, for a number of reasons:**

(a) Teratogenicity. There is a 2–3% incidence of fetal abnormalities among the general population. The UK Epilepsy and Pregnancy Register (see **A16b**) records a major malformation rate of 5.9% for babies born to mothers treated with sodium valproate during pregnancy.
(b) Side-effects can include weight gain, hair loss and menstrual disturbances, all of which are particularly undesirable in young women.

The SANAD trial was a large-scale practice-based randomised controlled trial comparing the long-term outcomes of the newer antiepileptic drugs (AEDs) against the older ones. One arm of the study compared valproate to lamotrigine in the treatment of generalised epilepsy syndromes and concluded that sodium valproate was more effective but lamotrigine was better tolerated. Overall, sodium valproate was the most cost-effective treatment for generalised epilepsy.

It is generally recommended that preventative drug treatment for epilepsy should only be considered after a person experiences a second seizure, but in certain epilepsy syndromes treatment may be warranted before a second seizure occurs. Miss SL's history indicates she had already experienced absence and myoclonic seizures prior to her presentation at A&E. Many people diagnosed with JME will require lifelong drug treatment.

Is the dose of lamotrigine appropriate?

A4 **Yes. It is very important to adhere to the recommending starting regimen for lamotrigine, which depends on whether it is prescribed as monotherapy or in combination with other antiepileptics. Rapid dose escalation is associated with the development of rash, including cases of toxic epidermal necrolysis and Stevens–Johnson syndrome, which are severe, potentially fatal hypersensitivity reactions. For this reason, people started on lamotrigine should be counselled to seek medical attention immediately if they develop a rash.**

Lamotrigine is metabolised hepatically by glucuronidation. The enzyme-inducing AEDs, which include carbamazepine and phenytoin, can accelerate the metabolism of lamotrigine, whereas sodium valproate inhibits lamotrigine glucuronidation. It is therefore very important to check the patient's concomitant medication to ensure the dose is appropriate, as the starting dose and titration regimen are dependent on whether lamotrigine is prescribed as monotherapy, in combination with sodium valproate, or in combination with enzyme-inducing AEDs.

Outline a pharmaceutical care plan for Miss SL. What advice would you offer her if she asked about contraception?

A5 **The pharmaceutical care plan should ensure that her treatment is prescribed at an appropriate dose, monitored correctly, and that Miss SL receives all the information she needs about her treatment. Checks should be made on whether Miss SL is taking any other medicines, particularly oral contraception.**

Before offering specific counselling to Miss SL it is important to check whether or not she is taking any other medication. Concomitant therapy may affect the starting dose of lamotrigine (see **A4** and below).

(a) **Monitoring.** It is not necessary to monitor serum levels of lamotrigine, and therapeutic dose monitoring generally has limited applications in monitoring AED therapy. Other monitoring includes:

(i) Response to treatment: patients may keep a seizure diary.
(ii) For adverse effects, especially rash.

Women taking oral contraception should be advised to report any breakthrough vaginal bleeding, as this suggests contraception is inadequate.

(b) **Contraception.** Although lamotrigine is not an enzyme-inducing drug, recent evidence suggests it can reduce levels of progestogens and women taking lamotrigine need to be aware that oral contraceptives may not be fully effective. In addition, combined oral contraceptives can reduce lamotrigine levels. Starting or stopping an oral contraceptive may thus require adjustment of the lamotrigine dose. The Summary of Product Characteristics recommends that women's contraceptive needs should be reviewed if lamotrigine is to be prescribed, and they should be advised to use effective alternative non-hormonal contraception.

The efficacy of oral contraceptives is also reduced in women taking the enzyme-inducing antiepileptics phenytoin, carbamazepine, oxcarbazepine, phenobarbital, primidone and topiramate, all of which enhance metabolism of the female sex hormones. The following recommendations are made for oral contraception in women taking enzyme-inducing AEDs:

(i) Enzyme-inducing AEDs are likely to render progesterone-only contraceptives ineffective.
(ii) Women wishing to take combined oral contraceptives should start on a daily ethinylestradiol dosage of at least 50 micrograms. In practice this can be achieved by doubling the dose of preparations containing 30 micrograms of ethinylestradiol
(iii) If breakthrough bleeding occurs then the daily ethinylestradiol dose can be further increased to 75 or 100 micrograms. An alternative option is to consider taking three consecutive pill packets without a break, followed by a 4-day break, rather than the usual 7 ('tri-cycling'). Non-hormonal methods of contraception may also be considered.

(c) General counselling points that should be covered with Miss SL include:

(i) Explaining the name of the drug and the aim of treatment, i.e. to prevent and hopefully stop further seizures. The drug may not have an instant effect, and the dose will be gradually increased to minimise the risk of side-effects.

(ii) Lamotrigine needs to be taken regularly at the same time of the day and evenly spaced out during the day, i.e. take each dose approximately 12 hours apart for a twice-daily regimen. Written information is also beneficial for people with complicated treatment regimens, and for those with epilepsy who have learning difficulties.

(iii) The potential side-effects of lamotrigine should be explained, including the importance of reporting any new rash. Gastrointestinal side-effects such as nausea can occur, as well as tiredness and headache. As with many AEDs, particularly the older drugs, lamotrigine is associated with a risk of haematological toxicity and patients should be advised to seek medical advice if they develop symptoms suggestive of anaemia (fatigue, breathlessness etc); low platelets (bruising or bleeding); or infection (because of potential neutropenia).

(iv) Miss SL needs to ensure her medication does not run out and that doses are not missed, and needs to know where to get further supplies. In some parts of the UK shared care protocols for epilepsy exist where hospitals are responsible for supplying newly prescribed medication until the patient is stabilised on the new treatment. Omission of doses or sudden discontinuation of AEDs can lead to worsening seizures, possibly status epilepticus, and are thought to be a factor associated with sudden unexplained death in epilepsy (SUDEP). This term is used when people with epilepsy die suddenly and no obvious cause is found at *post mortem*. The exact cause of SUDEP is not yet known.

(v) Depending on where they live, people with epilepsy may be entitled to claim exemption from prescription charges.

(vi) If Miss SL has a driving licence then she must be advised that she should contact the Driver & Vehicle Licensing Authority (DVLA). Current UK regulations state that a person can apply for a driving licence when they have been completely free of seizures for 1 year, or have had a pattern of sleep seizures only for 3 years.

(vii) Miss SL could be advised of local and national support groups for patients with epilepsy.

In developed countries with ready access to AEDs the overall prognosis for people with epilepsy is good: up to 70% will have their seizures controlled with drug treatment.

What is the role of the epilepsy nurse specialist?

A6 **Epilepsy clinical nurse specialists perform a vital role in providing practical and emotional support to people with epilepsy and their carers. They may be based in hospital or primary care settings, and can be very useful contacts for patient-specific medication enquiries.**

Is there a significant difference between the different brands of AEDs?

A7 **Generic versions of medicines are often significantly cheaper than branded ones. Although the prescribing of generic medicines is recommended to reduce drug costs, this practice is somewhat controversial in relation to the prescribing of AEDs; however, Miss SL can be reassured if the neurologist and GP feel it is acceptable to switch brands, her response to lamotrigine therapy should not be affected.**

The pharmacist has an important role in listening to patients' concerns about the appearance of their tablets and providing reassurance when appropriate.

Many of the older AEDs, such as carbamazepine and phenobarbital, have narrow therapeutic indices. In the case of phenytoin, its metabolism is saturable. This means that small dose increases, such as those caused by a switch to a slightly more bioavailable formulation, may produce a disproportionate increase in the serum concentration of drug and result in toxicity. There are published case reports and series describing loss of, or worsening, seizure control or side-effects after switching to an alternative brand of AED.

The newer AEDs generally have more predictable pharmacokinetics and broader therapeutic indices. In the case of generic lamotrigine the UK Department of Health has advised that there is no compelling evidence to suggest that swapping to a generic alternative will have an adverse clinical outcome. More research is required into brand switching of AEDs to identify patient groups who may be at risk.

In testing generic medicines, the European Agency for the Evaluation of Medicinal Products (EMEA) stipulates that to prove bioequivalence between a generic and branded medicinal product, the bioavailability must be within 80% and 125%. The pharmacokinetic parameters used for comparison include the maximal concentration (C_{max}) and area under the curve (AUC). A potential variation of up to 25% may seem significant, but the limits of 80% and 125% are statistical ones: they represent the 90% confidence intervals when calculating the ratios of pharmacokinetic parameters between the generic and the branded medicinal product. There are some limitations of bioequivalence studies:

(a) Bioequivalence studies are usually performed in young healthy volunteers who are taking no other, potentially interacting, drugs. Extrapolating results from studies in healthy volunteers to an elderly population with comorbidities and concomitant drug therapy, or to paediatric populations, may not be accurate.
(b) The studies compare generic medicines to their branded equivalent but not against other generic brands.

One AED commonly associated with prescribing and administration errors is modified-release carbamazepine, which is often prescribed for epilepsy and has several advantages over the standard tablet formulations, such as less fluctuation in plasma levels, thereby reducing side-effects and improving seizure control; and twice-daily administration, which may encourage patient adherence. Pharmacists should actively clarify prescriptions for twice-daily regimens of carbamazepine if the modified-release formulation is not prescribed. Occasionally, however, in patients exquisitely sensitive to carbamazepine, the modified-release tablets are prescribed three times a day.

Is the choice of ciprofloxacin appropriate?

A8 **No. Ciprofloxacin is a quinolone antibiotic associated with an approximately 1% risk of seizures. Quinolone antibiotics are thought to inhibit membrane receptor binding of the inhibitory neurotransmitter gamma-amino butyric acid (GABA).**

A macrolide antibiotic such as erythromycin would be appropriate for Miss SL. However, it is important to remember that erythromycin is a strong inhibitor of the cytochrome P450 3A4 isoenzyme and can interact with a number of the older, hepatically metabolised AEDs, notably carbamazepine. Concomitant erythromycin therapy can increase carbamazepine levels resulting in intoxication.

What term is used to describe epilepsy that worsens around the time of menstruation, and how common is it?

A9 **Catamenial epilepsy affects approximately 10% of women of childbearing age.**

The definition of catamenial epilepsy is not an exact one, but around 10% of women with epilepsy experience a worsening of seizures around the time of menstruation. Seizures may also worsen mid-cycle, around the time of ovulation. Catamenial seizures are thought to result from the changing levels of sex hormones that occur throughout the menstrual cycle, in particular the reduction of serum progesterone prior to the onset of menstruation.

What drug treatments are available for this form of epilepsy?

A10 **Clobazam, a benzodiazepine, is often prescribed in short courses for catamenial epilepsy.**

Clobazam at a dose between 5 and 30 mg/day (sometimes higher in refractory cases) may be prescribed to be taken on the days it is anticipated that seizures will be worse. Clobazam is prescribed in addition to the patient's regular AEDs.

Acetazolamide has also been used intermittently for catamenial epilepsy. This is a relatively fast-acting antiepileptic that can be initiated at a therapeutic dose. Its use is based on expert opinion.

Levetiracetam is not licensed as a monotherapy for generalised seizures. What is your opinion of the neurologist's choice?

A11 **AEDs are sometimes prescribed outside of their licence indications, and levetiracetam monotherapy is a reasonable choice for Miss SL.**

The use of leveiracetam as monotherapy is reasonable in this patient. Sodium valproate is not an ideal therapeutic option because of its adverse effect profile and teratogenicity risk. Carbamazapine can exacerbate myoclonic and absence seizures. Topiramate and zomisamide are other therapeutic options for JME.

There are a number of reasons for prescribing outside licensed indications. These include:

(a) Exceeding the maximum dose recommended in the Summary of Product Characteristics. The general principle when prescribing AEDs is to start at a low dose to minimise adverse effects and then increase the dose until seizures are controlled or side-effects become unacceptable. For many AEDs central nervous system (CNS) side-effects such as drowsiness and somnolence are dose related and become the limiting factor in dose escalation. Many of the more severe side-effects of hepatic and haematological toxicity are idiosyncratic reactions, and the incidence is not related to the drug dose; rash from lamotrigine is an exception to this.

(b) Prescribing for an indication not listed in the Summary of Product Characteristics, e.g. for use as monotherapy when it is licensed as an adjunctive therapy only. Most of the newer AEDs gained marketing authorisation as adjunctive therapy in epilepsy. These authorisations were granted based on the results of trials using the drug as adjunctive therapy in refractory epilepsy. It would be ethically very difficult to justify a drug trial in epilepsy where a patient would be given a placebo monotherapy, i.e. no treatment. Given the heterogeneity of epilepsy and the often tight inclusion and exclusion criteria of drug trials, applying results from these trials to every day practice can have limitations.

Specialist epilepsy centres may occasionally use AEDs unlicensed in the UK for refractory cases. One example is felbamate, a drug associated with a risk of hepatic failure and aplastic anaemia. People prescribed felbamate require close monitoring of liver function and full blood count (FBC).

Levetiracetam is one of the newer antiepileptic drugs. What are their advantages over the older drugs?

A12 **The newer AEDs include gabapentin, levetiracetam, oxcarbazepine, pregabalin, topiramate and zonisamide. The properties of each drug should be checked individually, but generally speaking the newer AEDs have advantages over the older AEDs, including:**

- **(a) Linear pharmacokinetics which provide a more predicable dose–response relationship.**
- **(b) Low protein binding, hence less potential to displace and be displaced by other drugs.**
- **(c) Metabolism independent of the cytochrome P450 system, thus reducing drug interactions, particularly with oral contraceptives.**
- **(d) A wider therapeutic index.**
- **(e) More acceptable side-effect profiles.**

Newer AEDs are invariably more expensive than older agents. In the UK newer AEDs can be used in people who have not responded to, or are intolerant of, the older agents, or in those for whom the use of older agents is unsuitable. In women of childbearing potential the older AEDs are usually considered unsuitable because of their teratogenic risk and potential interactions with oral contraceptives.

When taking into account the factors above, and individual patient factors, newer AEDs are sometimes used as first-line therapy.

What advice can you offer about St John's wort?

A13 **In the UK St John's wort is not recommended to be used concomitantly with any AEDs.**

St John's wort is derived from the plant *Hypericum perforatum* and has antidepressant actions that are not fully understood but which may be exerted through the inhibition of neurotransmitter reuptake.

St John's wort has been shown to induce metabolism of cytochrome P450, notably the 3A4 isoenzyme, and thus has the potential to interact with drugs metabolised by this pathway and reduce their effectiveness. Carbamazepine is metabolised by CYP 3A4.

St John's wort can also induce p-glycoprotein, a transport protein implicated in drug resistance in epilepsy by the mechanism of actively expelling drugs from neurons. There are case reports of reduced efficacy when St John's wort has been added to AEDs not metabolised by cytochrome P450. Miss SL should thus be advised to avoid it, even though there is no direct interaction between this product and her prescribed therapy.

If indicated, what is the appropriate drug treatment for depression in people with epilepsy?

A14 **The tricyclic and selective serotonin reuptake inhibitor (SSRI) antidepressants all have potential to lower the seizure threshold and their use in epilepsy is cautioned against. If depression in a person with epilepsy becomes severe enough to warrant drug therapy then the decision to treat with antidepressants is a clinical one, weighing up the risks and benefits of treatment.**

SSRI antidepressants are considered first-line treatment for depression in the general population. Citalopram has been advocated as an appropriate drug to use in people with epilepsy as it is thought to confer a lower risk of inducing seizures.

Recent evidence has shown a small increased risk of suicide with the AEDs. Patients need to be aware of this and know to seek medical advice if they develop mood changes or suicidal thoughts.

What are the advantages and disadvantages of using buccal midazolam over rectal diazepam?

A15 **A number of benzodiazepines are used to terminate epileptic seizures. Rectal diazepam (as a solution, not suppositories) has historically been used, but its use is associated with the stigma and inconvenience of having to remove clothing to enable administration.**

The use of buccal midazolam as an alternative to rectal diazepam is becoming more widespread. Midazolam is sufficiently lipophilic at physiological pH to rapidly cross the buccal mucosa. Controlled trials, mainly in children and adolescents with severe epilepsy, have shown buccal midazolam to be as least as effective as rectal diazepam in terminating epileptic seizures.

Buccal administration represents an unlicensed route of midazolam administration. The injection formulation can be administered buccally or a 10 mg/mL buccal formulation (made as a pharmaceutical special in the UK) can be used. An important counselling point is to administer the drug buccally: oral administration would put a fitting patient at risk of choking. The drug should be given using an oral syringe positioned between the gum and the cheek and by splitting the dose between both sides of the mouth. A usual adult dose would be 5–10 mg, which is 0.5–1 mL of a 10 mg/mL formulation. With such a small volume the risk of accidental swallowing is low.

There are concerns over the risk of respiratory depression when using benzodiazepines outside a hospital setting, but they are relatively safe in carefully selected patients when carers are properly trained in how to administer and when to use them and, importantly, are clear on when to get further help.

What are the issues concerning pregnancy in women with epilepsy?

A16 There are several issues for women with epilepsy wishing to become pregnant.

(a) **Fertility.** Fertility rates are reduced in women with epilepsy compared to age-matched controls. The possible causes of this are multiple and probably not just purely biological.

(b) **Teratogenicity of AEDs.** *In utero* exposure to AEDs is associated with a higher risk of congenital malformations. Accurately assessing the risk of individual drugs is difficult because women are not always treated with monotherapy; however, sodium valproate is associated with the highest risk of congenital malformations. The teratogenic risk of AEDs has to be balanced against the risk to mother and baby from uncontrolled seizures.

The UK Epilepsy and Pregnancy Register was created in 1996 with the aim of collecting data on pregnancy outcomes from women with epilepsy taking AEDs, particularly the newer agents. In 2006 data were published on pregnancy outcomes with *in utero* exposure to levetiracetam. Although no congenital malformations were reported from monotherapy, it is too early to assess accurately the relative safety of levetiracetam in pregnancy.

(c) **Altered pharmacokinetics of AEDs in pregnancy.** In the third trimester the serum levels of a number of AEDs, including lamotrigine, phenytoin, carbamazepine and sodium valproate, can reduce as a result of a variety of pharmacokinetic mechanisms. Regular monitoring of drug levels may be required to guide clinical care.

What drug should women with epilepsy who wish to become pregnant take, and at what dose?

A17 **Ideally pregnancy should be planned and drug therapy reviewed to optimise treatment at the lowest possible doses. Folic acid should be prescribed at a dose of 5 mg/day for women with epilepsy who wish to become pregnant, and should be continued throughout pregnancy.**

Folic acid supplementation has been shown to reduce neural tube defects in the general population. Women with epilepsy may be deficient in folic acid owing to the effects of drug therapy, and so should be prescribed a higher dose than the general population. There are anecdotal reports of folic acid exacerbating seizures, but the benefits of therapy outweigh the risk.

Acknowledgement

The author would like to thank Dr Stephen Howell (Consultant Neurologist, Sheffield Teaching Hospitals NHS Foundation Trust) for reviewing and commenting on this chapter.

Further reading

Crawford P. Best Practice Guidelines for the Management of Women with Epilepsy. *Epilepsia* 2005; **46**: 117–124.

Crawford P, Feely M, Guberman A, Kramer G. Are there potential problems with generic substitution of antiepileptic drugs? A review of issues. *Seizure* 2006; **15**: 165–176.

Duncan JS, Sander JW, Sisodiya SM, Walker MC. Adult epilepsy. *Lancet* 2006; **367**: 1087–1100.

Hunt S, Craig J, Russell A *et al.* Levetiracetam in pregnancy: preliminary experience from the UK Epilepsy and Pregnancy Register. *Neurology* 2006; **67**: 1876–1880.

Mack CJ, Kuc S, Grünewald RA. Errors in prescribing, dispensing and administration of carbamazepine: a case report and analysis. *Pharm J* 2000; **265**: 756–760.

Marson AG, Al-Kharusi AM, Alwaidh M *et al.* The SANAD study of effectiveness of carbamazepine, gabapentin, lamotrigine, oxcarbazepine, or topiramate for treatment of partial epilepsy: an unblinded randomised controlled trial. *Lancet* 2007; **369**: 1000–1015.

Marson AG, Al-Kharusi AM, Alwaidh M *et al.* The SANAD study of effectiveness of valproate, lamotrigine, or topiramate for generalised and unclassifiable epilepsy: an unblinded randomised controlled trial. *Lancet* 2007; **369**: 1016–1026.

MHRA. St John's wort: interactions with all antiepileptics. *Drug Safety Update* 2007; **4**: 7.

National Institute for Health and Clinical Excellence. TA76. *Newer Drugs for Epilepsy in Adults*. NICE, London, 2004.

National Institute for Health and Clinical Excellence. TA79. *Newer Drugs for Epilepsy in Children*. NICE, London, 2004.

National Institute for Health and Clinical Excellence. CG20. *The Epilepsies: The Diagnosis and Management of the Epilepsies in Adults and Children in Primary and Secondary Care*. NICE, London, 2004.

Perucca E. Role of therapeutic drug monitoring in epilepsy. *Hosp Pharm Eur* 2002 (Winter): 37–39.

Shorovan SD. *Handbook of Epilepsy Treatment*, 2nd edn. Blackwell, Oxford, 2005.

Wiznitzer W. Buccal midazolam for seizures. *Lancet* 2005; **366**: 182–183.

19

Parkinson's disease

Stuart Richardson

Case study and questions

Day 1 Mr LN, a 67-year-old retired bookmaker, was admitted to the neurology ward. His presenting complaints included difficulty in getting up from chairs and initiating walking.

Eighteen months earlier he had noticed that his self-winding watch, which he wore on his right wrist, was consistently losing time. When moved to his left wrist, the watch kept perfect time. Friends had pointed out that he had developed a limp, dragging his right foot. These symptoms had worsened over the previous 18 months, and he had also developed a resting tremor in his right hand and leg. He had noticed changes in his bowel habits many years previously.

His general practitioner (GP) suspected Parkinson's disease and referred Mr LN to a neurologist for confirmation of the diagnosis.

Q1 What are the main symptoms of Parkinson's disease?
Q2 Is it possible to make a definitive diagnosis of IPD?
Q3 What biochemical defects are thought to be present in a patient such as Mr LN?
Q4 Outline a pharmaceutical care plan for Mr LN.
Q5 Which drugs are usually considered for the initial treatment of patients with IPD and what are their modes of action?

Day 2 Mr LN was started on ropinirole.

Q6 Do you agree with this choice?
Q7 How should Mr LN's ropinirole therapy be adjusted to optimise his response?

Day 13 Mr LN was discharged on ropinirole 500 micrograms three times daily and instructed to titrate the dose as directed. Mr LN's GP was sent a letter describing his recent admission and advice on how to further titrate the dose of ropinirole.

Month 18 Mr LN was admitted for reassessment. Despite never completely abating, Mr LN's symptoms of bradykinesia and rigidity had temporarily improved following initiation and up-titration of ropinirole; however, recently Mr LN had experienced a worsening of these symptoms, and his wife reported that he had become rather obsessive about cleaning out the garden shed, performing this task on an almost daily basis. On admission he was taking ropinirole 6 mg three times daily.

Q8 What recommendations would you make with regard to Mr LN's drug therapy?

It was decided to start Mr LN on Sinemet Plus 125 mg three times daily and to simultaneously reduce the dose of his dopamine agonist.

Q9 How can the adverse effects of levodopa be minimised?

Month 18, Day 8 Mr LN was discharged. He was now stabilised on Sinemet Plus, two tablets three times daily, and ropinirole 4 mg three times daily and had experienced a significant improvement in his motor function.

Month 66 Mr LN was again admitted for reassessment. His therapy and symptoms had remained stable on the Sinemet and ropinirole until recently, when he had started to notice his arms shaking about 1 hour after each dose of Sinemet Plus. This lasted for about 45 minutes before stopping. Mr LN also complained of painful dystonic cramps at night, which caused him to wake early most mornings. He had attempted to counter this by taking an extra Sinemet Plus tablet shortly before going to bed, which sometimes helped. His wife added that he was becoming profoundly immobile up to 2 hours before his Sinemet doses were due during the day.

On examination he was found to have a mask-like face and a resting tremor in both hands and legs. 'Cog-wheel' rigidity was found in all four limbs. He had difficulty initiating speech and his voice was very quiet. He struggled to rise from his chair, and had a characteristic 'parkinsonian shuffle' when walking. When his shoulders were pulled forward from standing he staggered forward and had to be supported to stop him falling.

Mr LN complained of occasional falls and was not confident to leave the house. He relied on his wife to do everything for him. He admitted to being depressed about his condition.

There was no other medical history of note. All routine laboratory tests were within normal ranges. His drug therapy was ropinirole 4 mg three times daily plus two Sinemet Plus tablets at 8 am, 2 pm and 7 pm and, occasionally, one Sinemet Plus tablet at 11 pm.

Q10 Which of the long-term complications of levodopa therapy is Mr LN suffering from?
Q11 What alterations to Mr LN's drug therapy would you recommend in order to try to minimise these effects?
Q12 How could you monitor and assess Mr LN's response to these changes?
Q13 Can you suggest any non-drug management that might benefit Mr LN?

Mr LN's drug therapy was changed to one Madopar dispersible 62.5 mg tablet on waking around 7 am, and one Sinemet Plus tablet at 10 am, 1 pm, 4 pm and 7 pm. In addition, he was prescribed one Sinemet CR tablet at 10 pm. The nursing staff were asked to complete an hourly 'on–off' chart. Parts of the chart for days 1 and 5 are shown in Table 19.1.

Table 19.1

Time	*Day 1*	*Day 5*
7 am	off	off (dose)
8 am	off (dose)	on (dyskinesia)
9 am	on (dyskinesia)	on
10 am	on (dyskinesia)	off (dose)
11 am	on	on (dyskinesia)
12 noon	off	on
1 pm	off	on (dose)
2 pm	off (dose)	on (dyskinesia)
3 pm	on (dyskinesia)	on

Month 66, Day 6 Mr LN's mobility and dyskinesias were improved; however, he remained depressed about his condition.

Q14 Would Mr LN benefit from an antidepressant?
Q15 If so, which would you choose?

Month 66, Day 8 Mr LN had noticed a significant reduction in the shaking of his arms following his recent regimen change; however, he was still becoming considerably immobile about 1 hour before his dose of

Sinemet. His sleep had improved so that he was getting at least 6 continuous hours' sleep and no longer woke in pain from cramps.

The consultant neurologist recommended commencing entacapone.

Q16 Why has the consultant neurologist recommended entacapone, and does this necessitate the adjustment of Mr LN's other IPD therapy?
Q17 What counselling points would you highlight to a patient commencing entacapone?

Month 66, Day 11 During the ward round, you noted that Mr LN's morning medication was still on his bedside table. His medication now comprised one Madopar dispersible 62.5 mg tablet on waking around 7 am, one Sinemet Plus tablet at 10 am, 1 pm, 4 pm and 7 pm, and a Sinemet CR tablet at 10 pm. In addition, he was taking one entacapone tablet alongside each dose of Sinemet Plus and 3 mg ropinirole three times a day (made up of a 1 mg and a 2 mg tablet for each dose). His regimen thus comprised a total of 16 tablets per day.

On questioning, Mr LN informed you that although he was feeling better, he was concerned at the number of tablets he was taking and feared that he would have problems remembering to take them all when he returned home. He also found the new tablet quite hard to swallow because of its size.

Q18 In view of MR LN's concerns, what options are there for rationalising his medications?

Month 75 Mr LN was admitted as an emergency by his GP, having developed visual and auditory hallucinations over the previous week. He was hearing voices talking about him, threatening to kill him. He was also seeing insects crawling up the walls and burrowing into his skin. On examination he was clearly distressed and very frightened. His medication on admission was one Madopar dispersible tablet on waking, one Stalevo 100/25/200 tablet four times daily, one Sinemet CR tablet at night and one ropinirole XL tablet 8 mg daily.

Q19 Which drugs might have contributed to Mr LN's symptoms?
Q20 What adjustments would you recommend be made to Mr LN's medication?

Month 75, Day 7 The recommendations had been carried out. Mr LN's visual hallucinations had improved, but he was still experiencing distressing auditory hallucinations and the control of his symptoms had deteriorated, such that he was experiencing frequent 'off' periods.

Q21 What course of action would you suggest to improve Mr LN's symptoms?

Mr LN was started on rivastigmine 1.5 mg twice daily. The dose was increased over the next 10 days to 4.5 mg twice daily. His dopaminergic therapy was adjusted to one Stalevo 100/25/200 tablet five times daily, one Sinemet CR tablet at night and one Madopar 62.5 mg dispersible tablet upon waking. His ropinirole XL therapy was discontinued. His hallucinations resolved and acceptable control of his Parkinson's symptoms was achieved. He was discharged on this regimen.

Q22 What is the long-term outlook for Mr LN?

Answers

What are the main symptoms of Parkinson's disease?

A1 **The main symptoms in patients with Parkinson's disease are tremor, rigidity, bradykinesia (slowness of movement), akinesia (loss of movement) and postural abnormalities.**

The onset of Parkinson's disease is usually insidious and progression slow. Many patients first notice a resting tremor. This usually initially affects the hands and may be unilateral. The tremor disappears on movement and during sleep, and may be worse under stress. The patient is usually over 50 years old on presentation.

Rigidity manifests as an increased resistance to passive movement and is classically termed 'cog-wheel' rigidity, with a ratchet-like phenomenon felt at the wrist on passive movement of the hand.

Bradykinesia manifests as a general slowness in movement. Together with the rigidity, it is responsible for the typical abnormalities of gait: difficulty in starting and finishing steps, resulting in shuffling; a stooped head; flexed neck, upper extremities and knees; and a lack of normal arm swing.

A wide range of non-motor symptoms (NMS) have also been described in Parkinson's disease, all of which can have a significant impact on quality of life. These include bowel and bladder problems, fatigue, pain, sleep disorders and autonomic dysfunction, in addition to difficulty in swallowing and speech alteration, drooling of saliva and olfactory disturbance. Loss of postural reflexes leads to postural imbalance and sometimes to frequent falls. NMS are common and can occur at all stages of Parkinson's disease, including long before diagnosis. Symptoms increase in number and severity as the disease progresses.

Until recently, there has been a tendency for healthcare professionals to overlook these features in favour of the more apparent motor symptoms.

Is it possible to make a definitive diagnosis of idiopathic Parkinson's disease (IPD)?

A2 **At present the only way of making a definite diagnosis of IPD is by postmortem study of the brain.**

IPD is the most common cause of parkinsonism, accounting for approximately 75% of cases presenting to neurologists. Other causes include other neurodegenerative diseases such as progressive supranuclear palsy (PSP) and multiple system atrophy (MSA), intoxication with heavy metals, treatment with therapeutic drugs (neuroleptics, metoclopramide), and chronic cerebrovascular disease.

The definitive diagnosis of Parkinson's disease is based on characteristic neuropathological findings of Lewy bodies and neuronal loss in the substantia nigra and other brainstem nuclei. Studies have shown that only 65–75% of patients diagnosed as having early Parkinson's disease had the characteristic findings at postmortem.

Current opinion and guidelines recommend that all patients with a 'suspected' diagnosis of IPD must be referred untreated to a specialist who can reliably differentiate between IPD and other parkinsonian syndromes.

Previously the response to a 'challenge' of levodopa or dopaminergic agents has been used for diagnostic purposes; however the NICE guidance for Parkinson's disease does not advocate that this be performed routinely, although guidelines vary worldwide.

The use of imaging techniques is increasing in this field. Single photon emission computed tomography (SPECT) with DatSCAN, a radiolabelled cocaine derivative, can be used to measure the amount of dopamine-releasing neurons in the brain. This type of imaging can aid differentiation between parkinsonian and non-parkinsonian syndromes, but it is unable to distinguish between IPD, MSA and PSP.

What biochemical defects are thought to be present in a patient such as Mr LN?

A3 **Several biochemical defects are thought to be present in patients with Parkinson's disease.**

A combination of cholinergic (excitatory) and dopaminergic (inhibitory) mechanisms acting in the striatal tracts of the basal ganglia of the brain are thought to be responsible for the smooth control of voluntary movements. Imbalances in the neurotransmitters lead to movement disorders.

In patients with Parkinson's disease, dopamine concentrations in the three major parts of the basal ganglia are reduced to a fraction of normal. Compensatory mechanisms operate and symptoms are not noted until a severe loss (80%) of dopaminergic neurons has occurred. The severity of some symptoms, such as bradykinesia, has been found to correlate with striatal dopamine levels; however, abnormalities of other neurotransmitters, including norepinephrine (noradrenaline), 5-hydroxytryptamine (serotonin) and gamma-aminobutyric acid, have also been reported. The full relevance of these changes is unclear.

Outline a pharmaceutical care plan for Mr LN.

A4 The goals of symptomatic drug treatment are to help the patient function independently for as long as possible, and to achieve this with the minimum of adverse effects.

Patients with Parkinson's disease have a chronic deteriorating condition which will result in lifelong drug therapy of increasing complexity.

A long-term pharmaceutical care plan would include:

(a) Involving Mr LN in the choice of appropriate initial therapy.
(b) Ensuring the development of appropriate treatment outcome measures and a suitable treatment monitoring programme.
(c) Ensuring that the patient understands the role of drugs in the symptomatic treatment of the disease and their possible adverse effects.
(d) Ensuring that the patient and carers understand the importance of adherence and timing of drug doses.
(e) Anticipating problems such as the potential for nausea and vomiting with levodopa preparations, and offering appropriate advice on their prevention.
(f) Counselling the patient and carers about drugs that should be avoided in Parkinson's disease. These include medicines which act as dopamine antagonists, such as metoclopramide and the older antipsychotics (e.g. chlorpromazine, haloperidol).
(g) As the disease progresses and more drugs are added to the regimen, medicine taking may become problematic and advice on methods for improving and maintaining adequate adherence should be given.
(h) As most patients with IPD will be elderly, the general considerations given to elderly patients should also be applied.

As treatment may continue for many years and become increasingly complex, continuity of pharmaceutical care is an issue and consideration should be given to a personal, individualised patient record that can be used by pharmacists at various stages of the disease.

The Parkinson's Disease Society (www.parkinsons.org.uk) publishes a helpful booklet on drug use in IPD which is of value to patients and carers and can be used as a counselling aid. Patients with IPD now have a life expectancy near to normal, so treatment, help and support may be necessary for over 20 years. Non-pharmacological considerations include education on the disease itself, advice on diet, exercise programmes, and other areas such as driving, alcohol intake and recreational activities.

Which drugs are usually considered for the initial treatment of patients with IPD and what are their modes of action?

A5 Initial drug therapy as recommended by NICE guidelines for both early- and late-onset IPD will usually be chosen from the following: levodopa preparations; a dopamine agonist; or a monoamine oxidase B inhibitor (MAOBI).

There is still considerable debate about the best initial choice of therapy for patients with IPD, and also when to start symptomatic treatment. Most experts now advocate early treatment to provide patients with maximal clinical benefit at the start of their illness. Most Parkinson's disease specialists start treatment when a patient's symptoms begin to interfere with their lifestyle. What constitutes this will vary from patient to patient, but may include impairment of activities of daily living, threatened loss of employment, or gait disturbance with a risk of falling.

When a decision is made to initiate treatment the age of the patient, the degree and type of symptoms and the patient's expectations will influence drug choice. Patients should be made aware that drug treatment can provide symptomatic relief, but that there is at present no way of halting the progression of the disease. Levodopa is the most effective drug in the symptomatic management of Parkinson's disease, and virtually all patients will experience meaningful benefit; however, it can cause significant short- and long-term adverse effects, and there is a growing body of evidence and opinion among experts that most patients should initially be started on a dopamine agonist instead.

The rationale for early use of dopamine agonists is that they provide similar benefits to levodopa in early disease, but are significantly less likely to lead to the development of motor complications, particularly dyskinesias. Studies directly comparing levodopa with the dopamine agonists ropinirole, pramipexole and cabergoline as initial therapy for Parkinson's disease have been published and appear to confirm this theory. It is thus generally recommended to begin therapy with a dopamine agonist in patients who require this but who still have relatively mild symptoms. Patients with more severe symptoms, and those over 70 (in whom the development of motor complications is less likely), should probably be started on a levodopa preparation.

Anticholinergic drugs are now rarely used for the treatment of Parkinson's disease. They provide some relief of tremor but are of little value in the treatment of other features, such as rigidity and bradykinesia. In addition, adverse effects are common. These include peripheral effects such as dry mouth, blurred vision and constipation, as well as potentially serious central effects including confusion and hallucinations. Their use is best reserved for younger patients (under 60), in whom resting tremor is the predominant feature. Anticholinergic drugs are thought to act by correcting the relative central cholinergic excess brought about by dopamine deficiency.

The MAOBIs selegiline and rasagiline selectively inhibit monoamine oxidase B, one of the enzyme systems which break down dopamine. The action of endogenous dopamine is thus augmented. Selegiline has a mild anti-parkinsonian effect and is sometimes used either alone in early disease, or later to potentiate the action of levodopa preparations. It is widely believed to possess neuroprotective properties in early disease, but this has yet to be proved. Selegiline is metabolised to amphetamine derivatives, so it may have an alerting effect, especially at night, when it can cause insomnia, vivid dreams and nightmares. Rasagiline, although very similar in chemical structure, is not metabolised to amphetamine derivatives and so is potentially free of alerting side-effects.

Dopamine deficiency cannot be rectified by the administration of dopamine, because dopamine does not cross the blood–brain barrier. Levodopa does cross the blood–brain barrier and is converted to dopamine in the basal ganglia. Levodopa is thus thought to act primarily by increasing brain dopamine concentrations. If levodopa is administered alone, over 95% of a dose is decarboxylated to dopamine peripherally, which results in reduced amounts being available to cross the blood–brain barrier and problematic peripheral side-effects such as nausea, vomiting, and postural hypotension. Levodopa is therefore now almost always administered with a dopa-decarboxylase inhibitor, either carbidopa or benserazide. These dopa-decarboxylase inhibitors do not cross the blood–brain barrier and so smaller daily doses of levodopa can be administered, thereby reducing the incidence of peripheral side-effects. Levodopa therapy is particularly helpful in controlling symptoms of bradykinesia or akinesia.

Do you agree with this choice?

A6 **Yes. The choice of initial therapy is based on many different factors that will vary from patient to patient. The use of a dopamine agonist is indeed appropriate in this situation, as would be the use of levodopa.**

The dopamine agonists can be split into two different categories: ergot and non-ergot. Ergot-derived dopamine agonists include the older generation products bromocriptine, lisuride, pergolide and cabergoline. Non-ergot-derived agonists include the newer agents pramipexole, ropinirole, and rotigotine.

Use of the ergot-derived agonists has declined considerably over the last few years as a result of increased concerns about long-term side-effects, specifically cardiac fibrosis. There are clear monitoring guidelines for patients who remain on these agents.

Critical appraisal of the literature evaluating the two non-ergot-derived oral agonists provides no evidence to prefer one over the other. Rotigotine, the transdermal patch formulation, although considered less potent than the other non-ergot-derived dopamine agonists, provides continuous dopaminergic stimulation (CDS) over a 24-hour period. Although it is suggested that 24-hour continuous drug release more closely resembles endogenous dopamine release and may reduce the risk of motor fluctuations and dyskinesias developing, there are at present no firm clinical data to support this. Ropinirole XL is also available as a once-daily preparation, but requires patients to be previously stablised on the three times a day preparation before switching.

How should Mr LN's ropinirole therapy be adjusted to optimise his response?

A7 **Like any dopaminergic therapy, ropinirole must be started at a low dose and increased gradually in order to reduce the incidence of side-effects and to establish the lowest effective dose.**

In order to facilitate gradual up-titration, ropinirole is available as a 'starter pack' that contains all the medication required for a stepwise dose titration over a 4-week period. A 'follow-on' pack allows further stepwise titration over a similar period to a therapeutic dose. This dose can then be further increased as required and tolerated by the patient.

Rotigotine patches are also available in a starter pack format. Pramipexole doses are often referred to in both the salt and the base form. It is important to be aware of this when referring to doses with patients and other healthcare professionals; however, there are a number of information materials available to aid patients and reduce confusion.

What recommendations would you make with regard to Mr LN's drug therapy?

A8 **Mr LN should at this stage be commenced on a low dose of levodopa as an adjunct to the dopamine agonist. The dopamine agonist dose should be reduced in view of his history of punding (the obsessive and repetitive perfomance of a useless task). The levodopa dose should be gradually increased, with decisions based on symptom relief and adverse effects.**

Levodopa and dopa-decarboxylase inhibitors are marketed in the UK as Sinemet (levodopa plus carbidopa: co-careldopa) and Madopar (levodopa plus benserazide: co-beneldopa). There are six Madopar preparations and six Sinemet preparations available in a variety of levodopa strengths and formulations (standard, dispersible and controlled release). The potential for confusion among clinicians and pharmacists is considerable, and care must be taken to ensure that the patient receives the intended preparation.

At the start of levodopa therapy the effects of a dose usually last for 4–8 hours, so the tablets may be prescribed three times daily. The dose should be increased by one tablet every 2–3 days until optimum effects are seen or adverse effects occur. If daily doses of <70 mg carbidopa are used, the peripheral decarboxylase will not be saturated and Mr LN will be more likely to suffer from nausea and vomiting. For this reason there are low levodopa Sinemet preparations containing 25 mg carbidopa plus 100 mg levodopa. There are also preparations containing 10 mg carbidopa plus 100 mg levodopa that are suitable when higher levodopa doses are needed. This is not a problem with benserazide preparations. Most patients are initially controlled on 400–800 mg levodopa daily.

Mr LN is beginning to display symptoms of 'punding'. This is characterised by repetitive pointless behaviours carried out for long periods of time at the expense of all other activities, and is associated with excessive dopaminergic stimulation. Although it has a relatively low incidence (5%) it can cause considerable distress to the patient, their family and friends, and should be carefully monitored.

Punding is managed by reducing and discontinuing dopaminergic stimulatory agents, predominantly dopamine agonists, although levodopa is also implicated. In view of Mr LN's worsening motor function it is reasonable to reduce his dopamine agonist to manage the side-effect of punding, and to supplement this with (initially) low doses of levodopa in view of its superiority in improving motor function. Abrupt withdrawal of dopamine agonists has been associated with neuroleptic malignant syndrome and should therefore be avoided. As there are no defined reduction regimens for these agents, the rate of withdrawal can vary. In the case of Mr LN, complete withdrawal may not be necessary and so slow reduction would be appropriate, depending on symptom control. Reducing the daily dose by 3 mg at 5-day intervals would be a reasonable regimen.

How can the adverse effects of levodopa be minimised?

A9 **The peripheral side-effects of levodopa are significantly reduced by combining it with a dopa-decarboxylase inhibitor (see A5); however, peripheral side-effects may still occur.**

Levodopa therapy is therefore best started at a low dose and increased gradually. In addition, ensuring that the drug is taken with or after food can reduce the incidence of nausea and vomiting still further. Using domperidone, a dopamine antagonist that does not cross the blood–brain barrier, can also reduce nausea and vomiting. Doses of 10–20 mg domperidone 1 hour before levodopa preparations are effective.

Which of the long-term complications of levodopa therapy is Mr LN suffering from?

A10 **End-of-dose akinesia and dyskinesias.**

Initial treatment with levodopa leads to sustained improvement throughout the day. Most patients will show a slow improvement in response during the first 18–24 months of treatment. Symptoms are then adequately controlled for 3–5 years. Unfortunately, after long-term treatment (>5 years) only about 25% of patients continue to have a good, smooth response. The main complications that develop are fluctuations in response, dyskinesias, psychiatric side-effects and partial or substantial loss of efficacy.

Fluctuations in response initially consist of end-of-dose deterioration or end-of-dose akinesia. End-of-dose akinesia is the term used when the therapeutic effects of a dose of levodopa are lost. This commonly occurs first thing in the morning (after the longest dosage interval) or just before or after a dose during the day, when the effect of the previous dose wears off and before the next one is taken or becomes effective. Patients may become immobilised and unable to do anything except wait for the next dose. After prolonged treatment, gradual deterioration in symptoms may begin between 1 and 3 hours after a dose.

Long-term levodopa therapy is also associated with the 'on–off' phenomenon. The patient develops a sudden loss of effectiveness (off), when 'freezing' occurs, which may last for only a minute or for up to several hours before normal function returns (on).

Dyskinesias (abnormal movements) can occur in 60–90% of patients and are usually dose related. They are generally worse when the response to a dose is maximal, and have been correlated with high levodopa plasma levels. They are therefore commonly seen after a dose has been taken. Symptoms include grimacing, gnawing and involuntary rhythmic jerking movements.

What alterations to Mr LN's therapy would you recommend in order to try to minimise these effects?

A11 Increase the frequency of levodopa administration to 3-hourly and reduce the amount given with each dose.

The most common approach to response fluctuation is to reduce each individual dose of levodopa and to increase the frequency of administration. This can reduce end-of-dose akinesia, but care must be taken to ensure a clinical response is maintained.

End-of-dose bradykinesia or akinesia is thought to be caused by a progression of the underlying disease or an unexplained occurrence of symptoms of dopamine deficiency after an initial response to each dose. Although there is no change in the plasma half-life of levodopa, it appears that the pharmacological half-life is reduced. End-of-dose akinesia has been shown to be corrected by levodopa infusion; however, this is not a genuine therapeutic option, as levodopa must be infused in large volumes, owing to its acidity, and it also commonly causes thrombophlebitis. The initial approach taken to minimise the end-of-dose effect is therefore to try to reduce the dosage interval.

Modified-release versions of co-careldopa (Sinemet) and co-beneldopa (Madopar) are available which result in a more prolonged and constant plasma level of levodopa. Both preparations lead to delayed action and lower peak concentrations than standard levodopa, but the risk of dose failure may be higher. Patients may still need to take controlled-release preparations every 3 or 4 hours, and may need doses of standard preparations to produce optimal clinical effects, especially with the first dose of the day.

Dyskinesias may occur at the time of peak benefit, at the beginning or end of a dose, or both (diphasic), or during 'off' periods. A reduction in levodopa dose may reduce peak dose dyskinesias, as may the partial replacement of levodopa with a dopamine agonist. Diphasic dyskinesias may also be helped by partially replacing levodopa with dopamine agonists. 'Off' period dyskinesia may be improved by administering a fast-acting (e.g. dispersible) preparation or, for those occurring in the early morning, a controlled-release preparation last thing at night.

How could you monitor and assess Mr LN's response to these changes?

A12 By charting his mobility regularly.

Some neurology wards use mobility charts on which an indication of a patient's mobility can be recorded at suitable intervals. Such charts can be a valuable aid to the manipulation of drug administration in order to optimise therapy. One version of a scoring system is described in Table 19.2. In addition to a score, a brief description of the patient's condition may be added.

Table 19.2

State	*Description*
On	No rigidity, mobilising
Off	Rigid, with or without tremor Unable to mobilise or only with assistance
On with dyskinesia	No rigidity, mobilising but with involuntary movements

Can you suggest any non-drug management that might benefit Mr LN?

A13 Mr LN may benefit from some remedial therapy, such as speech and language therapy, physiotherapy or occupational therapy. This should be available to patients with IPD and has been endorsed in NICE guidance for IPD.

The role of these therapies is to maintain the maximum level of functional mobility and capacity to perform activities of daily living (ADL). Early therapeutic intervention cannot reverse the course of Parkinson's disease, but it can delay potential deformity and functional decline.

Physiotherapy for Parkinson's disease patients addresses the functional limitations caused by rigidity and bradykinesia. It may include an exercise programme that focuses on maintaining flexibility, balance and strength.

Occupational therapy focuses on finding solutions to difficulties patients encounter with ADLs. Specialist adaptive equipment may be provided if necessary.

Mr LN and his relatives should also be made aware of the existence of the Parkinson's Disease Society, which can provide education and general advice.

Would Mr LN benefit from an antidepressant?

A14 Probably.

Depression is very common in Parkinson's disease, approximately 40–50% of patients suffer from depression at least once during the course of their disease. Depression in Parkinson's disease is characterised by feelings of guilt, helplessness, remorse and sadness. It is independent of age, disease duration, severity of symptoms or cognitive impairment.

Ensuring adequate treatment for Parkinson's disease should be the first step before considering more specific antidepressant therapy. This has been achieved in Mr LN, so a trial of an antidepressant would be reasonable.

If so, which would you choose?

A15 A tricyclic antidepressant (TCA) or selective serotonin reuptake inhibitor (SSRI) could be prescribed for Mr LN.

At present, there is insufficient evidence to recommend one antidepressant/antidepressant class over another. This lack of data is also highlighted in the NICE guidance. Clinical practice, as well as trial data, supports the use of some TCAs (e.g. amitriptyline, nortriptyline) in Parkinson's disease; however, they are often associated with anticholinergic effects and orthostatic hypotension, which may limit their usefulness.

The SSRIs (e.g. fluoxetine, sertraline, citalopram) have also been shown to be effective in Parkinson's disease. They are free of the anticholinergic effects associated with the tricyclics, and theoretical concerns that they may worsen parkinsonian symptoms have not been borne out by recent studies.

Why has the consultant neurologist recommended entacapone, and does this necessitate the adjustment of Mr LN's other IPD therapy?

A16 Mr LN is still displaying signs of end-of-dose akinesia, despite appropriate adjustment to his levodopa therapy. Entacapone therapy may improve these symptoms, but his other IPD therapies will need to be adjusted as the drug is introduced.

Entacapone is a catechol-*O*-methyltransferase (COMT) inhibitor and works in synergy with Sinemet and Madopar preparations, resulting in a 30–50% increase in levodopa half-life.

Entacapone works by inhibiting the peripheral metabolism of levodopa by the enzyme COMT, thereby increasing its availability to the brain. Entacapone is licensed for use as an adjunct to levodopa in

Parkinson's disease. Studies have shown that its use can significantly reduce 'off' time and increase 'on' time in patients with 'wearing-off' episodes. It should be given at a dose of 200 mg with each dose of levodopa, up to 10 times daily. The introduction of entacapone to a regimen can cause a new-onset or worsening of existing dyskinesias. In order to minimise this, the daily dose of levodopa should be reduced by about 10–30% by extending the dosing intervals and/or by reducing the amount of levodopa per dose. In practice, the choice varies from patient to patient.

Tolcapone, the only other commercially available COMT inhibitor, differs from entacapone in that it also blocks central COMT. Tolcapone was withdrawn in 1998 after a number of cases of hepatitis, but has since been relaunched with strict monitoring parameters and guidance on use.

What counselling points would you highlight to a patient commencing entacapone?

A17 **Entacapone can discolour the urine reddish brown. Patients should also be advised that nausea and vomiting can occur due to augmentation of levodopa, and that diarrhoea is a common adverse effect.**

The large size of the tablets may cause problems for patients with swallowing difficulties.

In view of Mr LN's concerns, what options are there for rationalising his medications?

A18 **The use of combination products and alternative formulations could be considered.**

In the literature it has been noted that approximately 20% of patients with IPD are non-adherent with their medication. Younger patients and those with complex regimens are associated with the highest levels of non-adherence.

A number of pharmaceutical companies have recently developed combined preparations and modified-release preparations in an attempt to reduce the patient's 'pill burden'.

Stalevo is a combined preparation of levodopa, carbidopa and entacapone formulated into one tablet. A Stalevo tablet is smaller than a tablet of entacapone alone and is thus also helpful in patients with swallowing difficulties who require therapy. Stalevo is available in a number of strengths, although dose titration is more limited than with the individual components. Mr LN could be started on Stalevo in place of Sinemet and entacapone.

The transdermal patch rotigotine and the oral formulation ropinirole XL are both designed for once-daily administration. At the time of writing, pramipexole, the remaining non-ergot dopamine agonist is in the process of being developed as a once-daily formulation that is expected to come to market.

There are therefore a number of options for the rationalisation of Mr LN's medication regimen. A reasonable option would be to convert each dose of levodopa/carbidopa and entacapone to one tablet of Stalevo 100/25/200. Ropinirole could also be converted to the XL preparation, as recommended in the Summary of Product Characteristics (SPC) to one 8 mg tablet daily. These changes would more than halve the number of tablets taken by Mr LN from 16 per day to seven.

Which drugs might have contributed to Mr LN's symptoms?

A19 All the drugs prescribed for Mr LN can cause the psychiatric complications described.

Levodopa causes a variety of psychiatric symptoms, including hallucinations. Dopamine agonists such as ropinirole can cause central nervous system effects such as hallucinations and confusion. These psychiatric complications are especially common in elderly patients. In addition, progression of the disease itself may contribute to these symptoms.

What adjustments would you recommend be made to Mr LN's medication?

A20 Gradually reduce his dose of ropinirole XL and stop if necessary.

The psychiatric complications of most anti-parkinsonian drugs are dose related and often respond to a reduction in dosage.

It is generally recommended to reduce or eliminate anti-parkinsonian drugs in the following order, corresponding to their relative propensity to cause psychiatric problems versus degree of anti-parkinsonian activity: anticholinergics, amantadine, MAOBI, dopamine agonist, levodopa.

Mr LN's dose of ropinirole should be reduced to the point of improving his hallucinations without drastically worsening his parkinsonism, if possible. It should be reduced gradually, as sudden withdrawal of dopaminergic agents may precipitate a neuroleptic malignant syndrome. The levodopa dose should only be reduced if hallucinations persist after elimination of all other anti-parkinsonian agents.

What course of action would you suggest to improve Mr LN's symptoms?

A21 Add a low dose of an 'atypical' antipsychotic drug, or consider a cholinesterase inhibitor.

Haloperidol and chlorpromazine are effective antipsychotics but are not recommended for Parkinson's patients because of their capacity to block striatal dopamine D_2 receptors and exacerbate parkinsonism.

The newer 'atypical' antipsychotics (e.g. clozapine, olanzapine, risperidone, quetiapine) are relatively free of D_2-receptor-blocking potential, and in principle should improve psychotic features without worsening parkinsonism. The best-studied of these is clozapine, which has been shown to reduce hallucinations without worsening parkinsonism. However, the potential for clozapine to cause agranulocytosis (1–2% of patients) and the consequent rigorous monitoring requirements often deter its use. Olanzapine and risperidone have proved less effective than clozapine in comparative studies, and have also worsened parkinsonism.

The early work with quetiapine was more hopeful; however, more recent controlled studies have been negative. When quetiapine is considered, a starting dose of 12.5 mg at bedtime is recommended and the dose should be titrated upwards at 3–5-day intervals until the desired effect is achieved.

The cholinesterase inhibitors rivastigmine, galantamine and donepezil, which were developed primarily for Alzheimer's disease, have been shown to reduce psychotic features and improve cognition in some patients with Parkinson's disease dementias. Rivastigmine is the only agent licensed for use in Parkinson's disease dementias. A relative cholinergic excess is already present in the striatum of Parkinson's disease patients, and thus the use of an agent likely to further support this imbalance should only be undertaken under specialist supervision.

What is the long-term outlook for Mr LN?

A22 It is likely that Mr LN's condition will continue to deteriorate with time, and that he will experience more 'off' time and increasing dyskinesias. His cognitive function may also decline further.

Amantadine has been used for the management of dyskinesias based on its antiglutamate activity; however, its side-effects (confusion, hallucinations) would preclude its use in Mr LN. Other side-effects of amantadine include ankle swelling and livedo reticularis.

A small number of other therapies can be used at this stage in patients with Parkinson's disease, but their risks and financial implications are considerable.

The use of apomorphine, a potent dopamine agonist licensed for the treatment of refractory motor fluctuations ('off' periods) in IPD, is a possibility in patients who deteriorate despite maximum tolerated oral therapy. The drug cannot be given orally and must be administered subcutaneously. It may be given as a continuous subcutaneous infusion or as single injections. It causes severe nausea and vomiting, so 3 days' pretreatment with domperidone (20 mg three times daily) is used to minimise this. Domperidone therapy may be continued until tolerance to this side-effect develops. Apomorphine is effective within 5–10 minutes, and patients may remain in the 'on' state for up to 60 minutes. During this time an oral dose of medication should have taken effect. Many patients are helped by up to five injections a day, although up to 10 may be needed in some patients. If the number of injections needed is high, then continuous infusions of apomorphine should be considered. If the nausea and vomiting can be overcome, apomorphine therapy is generally well tolerated. Bruising, nodules or abscesses may form at the site of an infusion, so the site should be changed daily. As Mr LN has had psychotic features in the past that resolved following discontinuation of his dopamine agonist, the use of apomorphine may not be appropriate and may further exacerbate this symptom.

The use of surgical techniques such as subthalamic deep brain stimulation (STN-DBS) may also be precluded in Mr LN by his previous psychotic symptomatology. The relatively high morbidity and mortality rate associated with lesioning operations such as thalamotomy and pallidotomy has recently made STN-DBS more favourable. STN-DBS involves the placement of tiny wires into the subthalamic nucleus (STN). These emit continuous electrical impulses from a neurostimulator, which is similar to a heart pacemaker. This stimulation can have a positive effect on the brain activity involved in controlling movement, and can improve tremor, stiffness, slowness and dyskinesia. In addition, with improvement in these symptoms medication can be reduced, thereby further reducing dyskinesias.

Mr LN may, however, be an appropriate candidate for Duodopa, a gel formulation of levodopa/carbidopa that is infused directly into the duodenum. Duodopa is designed to mimic the pharmacokinetic profile of endogenous dopamine release. The technique, albeit initiated using a nasogastric tube, requires a percutaneous gastrostomy tube for long-term administration. Such a procedure in patients with advanced Parkinson's disease can be hazardous.

It is estimated that the cost of intraduodenal levodopa therapy is in the region of £30,000 per patient per annum, which compares with around £10,000 for apomorphine and £6000 for STN-DBS.

Although there have been many recent advances in the management of IPD, there is still no cure. Ongoing research is targeted at neuroprotection strategies: interventions to protect or rescue vulnerable dopaminergic neurons, and to slow down or stop disease progression. Gene therapy trials are also currently under way.

Acknowledgement

This revision is based on a case originally written by Robert C Hirst.

Further reading

Antonini A, Isaias I, Canesi M *et al.* Duodenal levodopa infusion for advanced Parkinson's disease: 12-month treatment outcome. *Mov Disord* 2007: **22**; 1145–1149.

Chaudhuri KR, Healy D, Schapira AHV. The non-motor symptoms of Parkinson's disease. Diagnosis and management. *Lancet Neurol* 2006; **5**: 235–245.

Clarke CE, Guttman M. Dopamine agonist monotherapy in Parkinson's disease. *Lancet* 2002; **360**: 1767–9.

Deane KHO, Spieker S, Clarke CE. *Catechol-O-methyltransferase Inhibitors Versus Active Comparators for Levodopa-induced Complications in Parkinson's Disease.* Cochrane Database of Systematic Reviews 2004, Issue 4.

Emre M, Aarsland D, Albanese A. Rivastigmine for dementia associated with Parkinson's disease. *N Engl J Med* 2004; **351**: 2509–2518.

Fernandez HH, Friedman JH, Jacques CC *et al.* Quetiapine for the treatment of drug-induced psychosis in Parkinson's disease. *Mov Disord* 1999; **14**: 484–487.

Friedman JH, Factor SA. Atypical antipsychotics in the treatment of drug-induced psychosis in Parkinson's disease. *Mov Disord* 2000; **15**: 201–211.

Ghazi-Noori S, Chung TH, Deane KHO *et al. Therapies for Depression in Parkinson's Disease.* Cochrane Database of Systematic Reviews 2003, Issue 3.

Grosset KA, Bone I, Grosset DG. Suboptimal medication adherence in Parkinson's disease. *Mov Disord* 2005; .**20**: 1502–1507.

Hibble JP. Long-term studies of dopamine agonists. *Neurology* 2002; **58**: S42–S50.

National Institute for Health and Clinical Excellence. CG35. *Parkinson's Disease – Diagnosis and Management in Primary and Secondary Care.* NICE, London, 2006.

Nutt JG. Continuous dopaminergic stimulation: is it the answer to the motor complications of levodopa? *Mov Disord* 2007: **22**; 1–9.

Nutt JG, Wooten GF. Diagnosis and initial management of Parkinson's disease *N Engl J Med* 2005; **353**: 1021–7.

Olanow CW, Obeso JA, Stocchi F. Continuous dopamine receptor treatment of Parkinson's disease: scientific rationale and clinical implications. *Lancet Neurol* 2006; **5**: 677–687.

O'Sullivan SS, Evans AH, Lees AJ. Punding in Parkinson's disease. *Prac Neurol* 2007; **7**: 397–399.

Schapira AHV. Present and future drug treatment for Parkinson's disease. *J Neurol Neurosurg Psychiatr* 2005; **76**: 1472–1478.

Scherfler C, Schwarz J, Antonini A *et al*. Role of DAT-SPECT in the diagnostic work up of Parkinsonism. *Mov Disord* 2007: **22**; 1229–1238.

Shade R, Andersohn F, Suissa S *et al*. Dopamine agonists and the risk of cardiac valve regurgitation. *N Engl J Med* 2007; **356**: 29–38.

Singh N, Pillay, Choonara Y. Advances in the treatment of Parkinson's disease. *Prog Neurobiol* 2007; **81**: 29–44.

Thanvi B, Lo N, Robinson T. Levodopa-induced dyskinesia in Parkinson's disease: clinical features, pathogenesis, prevention and treatment *Postgrad Med J* 2007; **83**: 384–388.

Walter BL, Vitek JL. Surgical treatment for Parkinson's disease. *Lancet Neurol* 2004; 3: 719–728.

Zanettini R, Antonini A, Gatto G *et al*. Valvular heart disease and the use of dopamine agonists for Parkinson's disease. *N Engl J Med* 2007; **356**: 39–46.

20

Depression

Stuart Gill-Banham

Case study and questions

Day 1 35-year-old Miss CT made an appointment to see her general practitioner (GP) because she felt run-down and generally unable to cope. She said she felt tired all day long, yet at night she could not sleep. Concentrating on any task had become difficult, and she felt everything was getting on top of her. Frequently she would be reduced to tears when faced with a task and she dreaded having to go out, as she felt quite panicky when she left the house. She had not felt 100% for the last few months, since she had split up with her partner. She denied ever having felt like this in the past, although she had been extremely saddened by the sudden death of her mother when she was 14 years old. The GP prescribed fluoxetine 20 mg daily plus diazepam 2 mg twice daily for just 2 weeks.

Q1 Are Miss CT's presenting symptoms typical of depression?
Q2 Is this depressive episode purely a reaction to the end of her relationship, or could it be due to other factors?
Q3 In what ways can depression be treated?
Q4 Is the combination of fluoxetine and diazepam appropriate?

Week 3 Miss CT had been concerned that she would become addicted to the medication, so after 2 weeks she had stopped both the fluoxetine and the diazepam as she was feeling slightly better. However, her mood had quickly deteriorated and so she returned to her GP.

Q5 Are antidepressants addictive, and how long should they be prescribed for?

The GP persuaded Miss CT that antidepressants are not addictive and she restarted the fluoxetine plus a further 2-week course of diazepam.

Q6 Outline a pharmaceutical care plan for Miss CT.

Week 12 Miss CT was still experiencing poor concentration and feeling unable to cope with daily activities. When her GP saw her he noticed that she had lost a considerable amount of weight and had an unkempt appearance. Miss CT was adamant that she has been taking the fluoxetine regularly every day.

Q7 What treatment options are available to the GP now?

The GP decided to try Miss CT on venlafaxine 37.5 mg twice daily.

Q8 Was the starting dose of venlafaxine appropriate?
Q9 How should venlafaxine therapy be monitored?

Week 20 The dose of venlafaxine had reached 225 mg daily. It had been higher than this, but Miss CT could not tolerate the associated severe nausea, so the dose had had to be reduced. Miss CT described herself as 50% better. She was now able to leave her house without feeling panicky, and she no longer felt like crying as much as before. However, she still lacked motivation and her appetite remained poor.

Q10 What options are there to improve Miss CT's mood further?

The GP decided to try to augment her antidepressant therapy with lithium.

Q11 Is augmentation with lithium appropriate?
Q12 What baseline checks need to be performed before lithium is started, and how frequently should lithium levels be monitored?
Q13 What points should be covered when counselling Miss CT about her lithium therapy?
Q14 How long should treatment with lithium and venlafaxine be continued?
Q15 What other treatment options could be considered if Miss CT fails to respond to this therapy?

Answers

Are Miss CT's presenting symptoms typical of depression?

A1 **It is difficult to say exactly which symptoms of depression are typical because of the varied ways in which the illness can present; however, Miss CT does display some key symptoms of a depressive illness.**

Depression is a syndrome characterised by persistent low mood, anhedonia, a lack of interest in usual daily activities and a lack of energy. In addition to these key symptoms a wide range of accompanying symptoms can be present. Accompanying symptoms can be psychological (e.g. anxiety, increased sense of guilt, pessimism or suicidal thoughts and plans), physical (e.g. disturbed sleep, early morning wakening, tiredness, lack of energy, loss of appetite and increased sensitivity to pain), cognitive (e.g. impaired concentration and memory) and psychomotor (e.g. agitation, physical slowing or refusal of food and drink). In order to make a diagnosis of mild depression at least four symptoms, two of which need to be key, need to have been present for at least the preceding 2 weeks. Moderate depression is diagnosed when six symptoms are present, two of which must again be key. Severe depression is diagnosed when eight symptoms are present, at least three of which must be key symptoms.

Depressive symptoms are more common than most people realise. Up to 10% of the population will experience some form of depressive illness at some time in their life. Women are more than twice as likely as men to develop depression, partly as a result of an increased readiness to admit what their true feelings are.

The key symptoms displayed by Miss CT were low mood and lack of energy accompanied by poor sleep, pessimism, lack of concentration and severe anxiety, which together were impairing her daily routine. Frequently depression is not diagnosed when patients seek medical help, especially when they present with predominantly physical complaints. Depression ratings scales, which are formal sets of questions that can be used to give a numerical score to symptom severity, can be helpful in the diagnosis. However, such scales should not be seen as providing a black and white answer to the question of whether somebody is depressed: rather, they serve as a guide to indicate when an individual's underlying problem might be depressed mood.

Is this depressive episode purely a reaction to the end of Miss CT's relationship, or could it be due to other factors?

A2 **Although a depressive episode is frequently triggered by a stressful life event, it is not possible to say that one event is solely responsible. Several factors, such as genetic predisposition, previous experiences and childhood upbringing, can influence how an individual handles life events, and in turn the likelihood of a stressful event leading to an episode of depression.**

The degree to which somebody has a predisposition to depression is determined by a combination of genetic factors along with their upbringing and previous life experiences. Studies comparing rates of depression in identical and non-identical twins have found depression to be almost twice as likely in the brother or sister of an identical twin with depression as in a non-identical twin. Genetic predisposition could exert its influence on the biochemical structure of the brain, or its influence could be subtler, by altering individual character traits. Along with genetic factors, early life experiences, particularly parental discord or abuse, can influence the degree of predisposition faced by an individual.

Regardless of an individual's predisposition to depression, some life events may be more likely than others to cause depression. Events that lead to feelings of entrapment or humiliation are thought to be particularly important.

For Miss CT the break-up of her relationship was a significant factor, but it may not have been the cause of her depression. In her personal history she had coped with the loss of her mother at an early age. It is impossible to say how this influenced her upbringing, but it could have affected the way she coped with stressful events. Although the relationship ended about the same time as the depressive episode started, it might have been the emerging depressive illness that caused the relationship to end.

In what ways can depression be treated?

A3 **A range of options are available to treat depression, including psychological therapy, drug therapy and electroconvulsive therapy (ECT).**

Deciding which treatment option is the most appropriate depends on the severity of the depressive episode, and the preferences of both the doctor and the patient. Drug therapy is not necessarily the best option for mild depressive episodes.

The NICE clinical guideline No. 23 (*Depression: Management of Depression in Primary and Secondary Care*) introduces the concept of stepped care for the management of depression. This highlights the different needs of depressed individuals, depending on the characteristics of their depression and their personal and social circumstances. The steps range from 1, with a focus on recognition and assessment, to 5, which focuses on the most severe presentations where the individual requires complex inpatient treatment in order to minimise risk to life or self-neglect.

Studies of mild depression frequently fail to demonstrate that antidepressants have a significant effect, largely as a result of high placebo response rates. Many patients prefer non-drug approaches: they particularly value practical support and problem-solving approaches. Additional non-drug therapies may include dynamic psychotherapy, which examines interpersonal dynamics and how these may contribute to an individual's predisposition to experiencing depression; or cognitive therapy, which examines how an individual interprets adverse events and how this may make depression more likely. Cognitive behavioural therapy (CBT) links the way individuals think about themselves, others and the world around them with the impact that this has on thoughts, feelings and behaviours. Unlike some other psychotherapies, the focus is on present difficulties rather than past events that might have caused current problems. Like other psychotherapies, CBT can be particularly difficult if the underlying disorder impairs concentration. When combined with medication the effects of CBT are thought to be more durable than the effects of medication alone. The availability of non-drug therapies can be limited, as they require a greater level of support than can sometimes be offered.

A wide range of antidepressant drugs are available, classified according to either their mechanism of action, e.g. selective serotonin reuptake inhibitors (SSRIs) or monoamine oxidase inhibitors (MAOIs), or their chemical structure, e.g. tricyclic antidepressants (TCAs). Many of the more recently introduced antidepressants cannot be classified into any of these groups and are placed in groups of their own, e.g. venlafaxine, a selective norepinephrine (noradrenaline) and serotonin reuptake inhibitor, or reboxetine, a selective norepinephrine reuptake inhibitor. Classifying antidepressants in this way causes confusion, as it implies that some have a unique mechanism of action when this is not the case. For example, venlafaxine is not the only antidepressant to block the reuptake of both norepinephrine and serotonin, as several TCAs have an effect on both of these neurotransmitters.

Antidepressants from different therapeutic classes differ little in their overall effectiveness. Studies that have directly compared different antidepressants have found the response rates achieved to be comparable; however, individual patient response to antidepressants and tolerance of side-effects can vary considerably. Different classes of antidepressants have quite distinct side-effect profiles. The TCAs predominantly cause sedation, dry mouth, blurred vision, constipation and weight gain. SSRIs predominantly cause headaches, nausea, diarrhoea and initial weight loss, although when patients start to respond to the antidepressant effect, weight gain occurs. Selecting the most appropriate antidepressant for an individual is largely based on a consideration of the likely response and the side-effects that may be seen.

ECT has been found to be effective in cases of severe depression, especially when psychotic symptoms are present. Owing to its rapid onset of action patients can improve after just one session. ECT is a treatment option when the patient is refusing fluids and so is in grave danger of harm.

Is the combination of fluoxetine and diazepam appropriate?

A4 **Fluoxetine is a reasonable first-line choice of antidepressant, and combining it with a short course of benzodiazepine therapy could have many advantages. Care is needed to ensure that any potential benefits of this combination are not outweighed by the risks of addiction or tolerance to the benzodiazepine.**

All antidepressants are equally effective in treating depression. The choice therefore relies on considering response to previous treatment, potential side-effects, the likelihood of an intentional overdose, the age and physical condition of the patient, whether there are any other concurrent drug therapies, and the personal preferences of the prescriber. Miss CT is young, fit and healthy, and has never been treated with an antidepressant before, so the choice will be based largely on the potential side-effects.

It is widely believed that SSRIs are better tolerated than TCAs, although evidence from clinical trials is not necessarily as conclusive as popular belief. Another potential benefit of prescribing an SSRI as first-line therapy is their safety in overdose. It is estimated that the average number of deaths from overdose with TCAs is 34 per million prescriptions, whereas for SSRIs the figure is two per million prescriptions.

These potential benefits of SSRIs need to be considered against potential risks, namely the risk of gastric bleeding and the risk of suicide.

SSRIs have been associated with an increased risk of gastric bleeding, which is brought about by reduced platelet aggregation. This mechanism differs from the way in which other drugs cause gastric bleeding. For example, non-steroidal anti-inflammatory drugs (NSAIDs) cause direct damage to the gastric mucosa. The absolute risk of an SSRI inducing a gastric bleed serious enough to require hospital admission is quite low, but is increased by co-administration of aspirin and further increased by co-administration of NSAIDs. It is not thought necessary to routinely prescribe a gastric protectant to patients prescribed an SSRI, but those who are also prescribed aspirin or an NSAID are at increased risk. The risk of SSRI-induced gastric bleeding is also increased by old age and a previous history of gastric bleeds.

Concerns have been raised as to the potential of antidepressants in general, and SSRIs in particular, to increase the risk of suicide or self-harm. The relationship between antidepressants and suicidal behaviour is complex, not least because individuals prescribed antidepressants are already at a higher risk of suicide, and when treatment is started not all symptoms improve at the same time. This can result in an individual whose mood is low gaining more energy and motivation after starting antidepressant therapy. Antidepressants that cause initial agitation, including SSRIs, can heighten the risk of suicide at the start of therapy. The NICE clinical guideline makes several recommendations about managing the risk of suicide in depression, including close monitoring of patients at increased risk, especially those under 30 years of age; supplying limited quantities of medication for those at increased risk; and stopping therapy if marked agitation or akathisia (restlessness) is seen in the first few weeks.

In deciding which SSRI to use it needs to be remembered that studies have failed to demonstrate any single agent to be more effective than another. As the main SSRIs have similar side-effect profiles, the choice is based on the individual prescriber's experience and preferences or on cost considerations.

The addition of a benzodiazepine to antidepressant therapy has numerous potential benefits, particularly when anxiety symptoms predominate. It is likely that Miss CT's anxiety is a symptom of her depression, so if the depression is treated then the anxiety will resolve. However, depression can take between 2 and 4 weeks to respond to an antidepressant, and during this time the anxiety may become worse, particularly as fluoxetine, like other SSRIs, can cause an initial increase in anxiety. A Cochrane Collaboration Review found that adding a benzodiazepine to an antidepressant improved the initial antidepressant response and reduced the likelihood of therapy being discontinued. A benzodiazepine such as diazepam will quickly reduce anxiety symptoms, and by the end of the 2-week course there will hopefully be some response to the antidepressant. The duration of use of the benzodiazepine should be restricted to less than 4 weeks to minimise the risk of tolerance and addiction.

Are antidepressants addictive, and how long should they be prescribed for?

A5 **Contrary to popular belief, antidepressants are not addictive but sudden discontinuation can produce a withdrawal reaction. The minimum length of time they should be prescribed for is 6 months after all symptoms have been resolved. Continuous therapy may need to be considered for patients who have had multiple episodes of depression.**

One of the major concerns that patients have when prescribed an antidepressant is that they are addictive, and by taking them they may become dependent on them for life. This simply is not true. Antidepressants are not addictive, and needing to take them for long periods should not be confused with being dependent on them. A useful analogy is to compare treatment of depression with the treatment of any physical illness. For many patients with a physical condition medication is needed to control symptoms of that disease. When the medication is stopped the symptoms may return, but this is not the same as dependence. It is true that many antidepressants, if stopped abruptly, will produce withdrawal symptoms such as anxiety, flu-like aches and pains or irritability, but this should not be seen as evidence of addiction because there is no physical craving for the drug. Withdrawal symptoms can be avoided by gradually reducing doses before the drug is stopped. For Miss CT the risk of any withdrawal reaction is minimal, as fluoxetine has one of the longest half-lives of any antidepressant and so hardly ever causes a withdrawal reaction.

Despite this, patients tend to only be prescribed antidepressants for a short period. It is widely accepted that the minimum they should be prescribed for is 6 months after all symptoms have disappeared. This figure comes from studies which found that in patients who had responded to antidepressant therapy, those who were switched to placebo were more than twice as likely to relapse in the following 6 months as those who remained on antidepressant therapy. Allowing between 2 and 3 months for all symptoms to respond to therapy means that most patients will need to take an antidepressant for around 9 months for any single episode of depression. Individuals who have experienced one episode of depression are at an increased risk of further episodes. For those patients who have had two or more episodes, 75% will remain well for 5 years if they continue to take their medication, whereas only 10% of those who stop their medication will remain well for the same period. Patients who have had multiple episodes of depression may therefore benefit from long-term therapy with an antidepressant.

Outline a pharmaceutical care plan for Miss CT.

A6 The pharmaceutical care plan for Miss CT should include the following:

(a) Ensure that the antidepressant and benzodiazepine are restarted at a dose appropriate for the presenting symptoms.
(b) Ensure that the benzodiazepine is prescribed for as long as anxiety remains a problem, but stopped before addiction occurs.
(c) Counsel Miss CT about the potential side-effects of both agents, and also how they will be of benefit.
(d) Explain how long it will take before any antidepressant response is seen.
(e) Reassure Miss CT that antidepressants are not addictive.
(f) Monitor her for signs of side-effects.

What treatment options are available to the GP now?

A7 Change to a different antidepressant. Other options could include non-drug strategies or ECT.

If the first-line antidepressant fails to produce a therapeutic response despite being prescribed for an adequate length of time at an adequate dose, then an alternative will need to be considered. An adequate length of time is usually defined as being at least 4 weeks, but if some response is seen then there is benefit in continuing with the antidepressant for longer.

Defining what constitutes an adequate dose can be more difficult. Most SSRIs are effective at their initial starting dose, although there is some debate as to whether sertraline is effective at 50 mg daily, so doses of at least 100 mg/day are sometimes preferred.

It has been previously recommended that doses of TCAs need to be at least 100 mg/day of amitriptyline or equivalent. These recommendations were not supported by the NICE clinical guidelines, which took a more pragmatic approach to TCA dosing levels, recommending that patients starting on low doses of TCAs should be carefully monitored for side-effects and efficacy, and the dose gradually increased if there is a lack of efficacy and no major side-effects.

The choice of an alternative antidepressant will again depend on the potential side-effects, as well as which antidepressant was used initially. The Sequenced Treatment Alternatives to Relieve Depression (STAR*D) was a large multicentre trial that looked at the outcomes of different sequential treatment strategies in the outpatient management of depression. The study found that individuals who did not obtain full remission from depression symptoms after initial treatment with citalopram could go on to achieve remission if they were switched to either a different antidepressant class or to a different antidepressant within the same class. There was no evidence of a significant difference in response rate between the two strategies. TCAs have potentially greater differences in response, as they are less homogeneous in their specific mechanisms of action; however, despite these factors it is still usual to select a second choice antidepressant from a different class to the first choice.

Other treatment options at this point may include non-drug therapies, although if the depression is severe it may impair the patient's ability to engage with such therapies. If the symptoms are particularly severe then ECT may be indicated, although as Miss CT is remaining under the care of her GP it is unlikely that her depression is severe enough to warrant ECT.

In summary, Miss CT has failed to respond adequately to the first antidepressant that was prescribed. She should be switched to another antidepressant, and typically this will be an agent from a different class. This could be either a TCA or one of the newer agents such as venlafaxine or mirtazapine. There is no evidence to suggest one would be more effective than another, so the choice would be based on likely side-effect profiles and overall tolerability.

Was the starting dose of venlafaxine appropriate?

A8 **It is recommended that therapy with venlafaxine be initiated at 75 mg/day. As venlafaxine has a wide dose range Miss CT will gain more benefit from a higher dose, especially as the drug's noradrenergic effect is only seen at higher doses.**

The major benefit of choosing venlafaxine for Miss CT is that it has a different mechanism of action from the SSRIs. In addition to blocking the reuptake of serotonin by presynaptic neurons, venlafaxine also blocks the reuptake of norepinephrine. This dual effect may be advantageous, as Miss CT failed to respond to an SSRI. As many of its side-effects are dose related, especially nausea, sedation and postural hypotension, a low starting dose is used; however, at these low doses venlafaxine has an effect predominantly on serotonin pathways, so has a mechanism of action similar to an SSRI. It is only after the dose is increased beyond 112.5 mg/day that any activity on norepinephrine reuptake is seen. In order to gain maximum benefit from prescribing venlafaxine the dose will therefore need to be increased to 150 mg/day after a couple of weeks.

How should venlafaxine therapy be monitored?

A9 **Response to therapy can be monitored subjectively or objectively using an appropriate rating scale. Particular side-effects that need to be monitored for are sedation, nausea and (possibly) changes in blood pressure.**

Therapeutic response can be measured subjectively by assessing the patient to see whether key depressive symptoms have resolved. For Miss CT this will be to see whether her mood improves, if she takes more pride in her appearance and if any weight is gained. If necessary, an objective assessment of her mental state can be made by using a standard depression rating scale.

Venlafaxine causes a considerable number of side-effects, including constipation, nausea, dizziness, headache and dry mouth. NICE Clinical Guidelines (CG23) warn prescribers that there is an increased likelihood of patients stopping venlafaxine therapy because of its side-effects. Dose-related hypertension is seen with venlafaxine, and in patients with existing hypertension this needs to be controlled before commencing the drug, and blood pressure should be regularly monitored while they are taking it. Venlafaxine can also cause increases in serum cholesterol, particularly following prolonged use. Again, in susceptible patients routine monitoring may be advisable.

What options are there to improve Miss CT's mood further?

A10 **If only a partial response is seen then the dose of antidepressant can be increased further, a new antidepressant can be prescribed, or an augmenting strategy can be considered.**

Miss CT is already taking the maximum dose of venlafaxine that she can tolerate, so a further increase in dose would seem inappropriate. Using a sustained-release formulation can help reduce the incidence of nausea, but the maximum licensed dose for this formulation is 225 mg/day. If another antidepressant were to be considered then either a TCA, mirtazapine or possibly even a MAOI might be appropriate. MAOIs are infrequently used in clinical practice because of their adverse effects and their interactions with other medicines and foods; however, they are still indicated for atypical depression, where symptoms include pronounced phobic anxiety. Moclobemide differs from other MAOIs in that it reversibly inhibits monoamine oxidase type A enzyme. This gives an antidepressant effect without any interaction with foodstuffs, plus a quicker offset of action.

The main disadvantage of switching to an MAOI at this stage would be the time that a switch would take. In order to minimise any withdrawal symptoms it would be necessary to gradually reduce the dose of venlafaxine over 2 weeks, then have a washout period of 7–14 days before initiating the MAOI; however, a specific washout period would not be required if either a TCA or mirtazapine were prescribed for Miss SL.

As there has been some response to venlafaxine it may be possible to augment its effect by adding another agent to the regimen. Several agents have been suggested for possible augmentation, including levothyroxine, liothyronine, tryptophan, anticonvulsants and lithium. Another means of augmenting antidepressant therapy might be to add a second antidepressant into the regimen. Generally this approach is only recommended as a last resort, and should be undertaken by somebody experienced in using antidepressant combinations because of the potential of many antidepressants for interacting with others.

Is augmentation with lithium appropriate?

A11 **Lithium is a recognised augmentation option for patients who fail to respond or respond only partially to antidepressant therapy.**

Several studies have shown that the addition of lithium to antidepressant therapy is beneficial in reducing symptoms in patients who are not suffering from a bipolar illness. Antidepressants studied in combination with lithium include lofepramine, fluoxetine, sertraline, citalopram and venlafaxine. When using lithium as an augmentation agent the same plasma level should be aimed for as when it is used to treat bipolar disorder, i.e. at least 0.4 mmol/L. Part of the STAR*D trial assessed the impact of lithium augmentation on remission rates in patients who had failed to respond adequately after two optimally delivered trials of antidepressants. Modest remission rates were seen when lithium was added to antidepressant therapy, but it would appear that tolerance of lithium side-effects was low. Significantly greater numbers of lithium-treated patients left the study compared to those receiving alternative augmentation strategies such as liothyronine (T_3).

What baseline checks need to be performed before lithium is started, and how frequently should lithium levels be monitored?

A12 Before lithium therapy is started the following baseline checks are needed: renal function, thyroid function and general health, including cardiac function. Once an appropriate plasma level has been reached lithium levels should be checked monthly for the first 3 months, then every 3–6 months thereafter.

It is essential to check renal function before starting lithium therapy, as lithium is excreted predominantly unchanged by the kidneys. If renal function is reduced, especially if glomerular filtration rate is <50 mL/min, then lithium clearance will be correspondingly reduced and a lower starting dose may be required.

An assessment of thyroid function is necessary because lithium therapy can cause changes in thyroid function in 5–20% of patients. Lithium-induced hypothyroidism can be managed by administering replacement levothyroxine, and is reversible when lithium therapy is withdrawn.

There is some debate about the clinical significance of the electrocardiogram (ECG) changes lithium therapy can produce. They are thought to be largely benign, but initial assessment can be useful in determining whether any subsequent ECG abnormalities are due to lithium treatment.

Lithium therapy should be started at a dose of 400 mg lithium carbonate each night (200 mg in the elderly or those who are physically frail). Four to 5 days after the first dose the lithium level should be measured 12 hours after the last dose and the dose adjusted to a range of 0.4–1.0 mmol/L. Once a stable plasma level has been reached it should be rechecked every month for the first 3 months, then every 3–6 months after that.

What points should be covered when counselling Miss CT about her lithium therapy?

A13 **Before lithium is started Miss CT needs to be told that it will be a long-term treatment; that regular blood tests will be required, and why; what the side-effects of lithium are; how to recognise toxicity; the dangers of dehydration or low-salt diets; and which over-the-counter medicines should be avoided.**

The common side-effects of lithium include fine tremor, polyuria (passing a lot of urine), polydipsia (increased thirst), nausea and diarrhoea. These are usually mild and transient. Other side-effects can also be a sign of lithium toxicity. These include blurred vision, confusion, drowsiness or palpitations, and if any of these are experienced then the patient needs to have an urgent lithium level measurement.

As the body handles lithium in the same way as sodium ions, so altered sodium levels in the body can affect lithium levels. Thus, if sodium levels fall, due to either dehydration or reduced dietary intake, to compensate the body will reduce the amount of sodium excreted by the kidneys and, as a consequence, will also reduce lithium excretion. This in turn will lead to lithium toxicity. Patients taking lithium need to know how dangerous dehydration or low-salt (sodium) diets can be.

Several medicines can potentially interact with lithium, including angiotensin-converting enzyme (ACE) inhibitors, diuretics and NSAIDs. Patients need to be warned about avoiding aspirin or aspirin-like painkillers if they self-medicate, and they need to tell any doctor who prescribes medicines for them that they are taking lithium.

How long should treatment with lithium and venlafaxine be continued?

A14 **If a response is seen with this combination then therapy may need to be continued for a considerable time, well beyond the 6 months recommended for uncomplicated cases of depression.**

The prognosis for Miss CT is not good, as her depressive episode failed to respond to the first two antidepressants prescribed. This may mean that therapy should be continued for longer than the 6 months after the resolution of symptoms recommended in straightforward cases. Antidepressant therapy for up to 5 years, and possibly longer, will continue to prevent the return of symptoms. If there was a desire to withdraw therapy, then each agent should be gradually withdrawn one after the other, starting with lithium first. It should be remembered that even if gradually withdrawn, the risk of relapse would be high.

What other treatment options could be considered if Miss CT fails to respond to this therapy?

A15 **Other treatment options might be augmentation with a different agent, prescribing two antidepressants together, or ECT.**

Alternatives to lithium augmentation might include sodium valproate, tryptophan or a thyroid hormone. The use of tryptophan or a thyroid hormone to treat depression requires specialist knowledge and experience, and would best be undertaken by a consultant psychiatrist. Tryptophan, an amino acid precursor of the neurotransmitter serotonin, is sometimes used to treat resistant depression. Owing to an association with eosinophilia myalgia syndrome (EMS), it can only be prescribed on a named-patient basis by hospital specialists. Patients receiving tryptophan require routine blood monitoring to prevent the development of EMS.

ECT would be indicated for Miss CT if she continued to lose weight or started to refuse fluids. Her care would need to be referred to a consultant psychiatrist in order for ECT to be used.

Further reading

Cipriani A, Pretty H, Hawton K *et a*l. Lithium in the prevention of suicidal behaviour and all-cause mortality in patients with mood disorders: a systematic review of randomised trials. *Am J Psychiatr* 2005; **162**: 1805–1819.

Furukawa T, Streiner D, Young L. Antidepressant plus benzodiazepine for major depression (Cochrane Review). In: *The Cochrane Library 2*. Update Software, Oxford, 2003.

Geddes JR, Carney SM, Davies C *et al*. Relapse prevention with antidepressant drug treatment in depressive disorders: a systematic review. *Lancet* 2003; **361**: 653–661.

Gelder M, Harrison P, Cowen P. *Shorter Oxford Textbook of Psychiatry*. Oxford University Press, Oxford, 2006.

Gilbody S, House A, Sheldon T. Routinely administered questionnaires for depression and anxiety: systematic review. *Br Med J* 2001; **322**: 406–409.

National Institute for Health and Clinical Excellence. CG23 (amended). *Depression: Management of Depression in Primary and Secondary Care*. NICE, London, 2007.

National Prescribing Centre. Management of depression in primary care. MeReC Briefing No. 31. Liverpool, 2005/2006.

Nirenberg AA, Fava M, Trivedi MH *et al*. A comparison of lithium and T_3 augmentation following two failed medication treatments for depression: a STAR*D report. *Am J Psychiatr* 2006; **163**: 1519–1530.

Peveler R, Carson A, Rodin G. ABC of psychological medicine: depression in medical patients. *Br Med J* 2002; **325**: 149–152.

Rush AJ, Trivedi MH, Wisniewski SR *et al.* Acute and longer-term outcomes in depressed outpatients requiring one or several treatment steps: a STAR*D report. *Am J Psychiatr* 2006; **163**: 1905–1917.

Timonen M, Liukkonen T. Management of depression in adults. *Br Med J* 2008; **336**: 435–439.

Williams JW, Mulrow CD, Chiquette E *et al.* A systematic review of newer pharmacotherapies for depression in adults: evidence report summary: clinical guideline, part 2. *Ann Intern Med* 2000; **132**: 743–756.

21

Schizophrenia

Stuart Gill-Banham and Carol Paton

Case study and questions

Day 1 Mr MB, a 22-year-old man, was visited at home by a psychiatrist at the request of his general practitioner (GP). Mr MB's mother had become increasingly concerned about his isolating himself in his room. He only ever went out to visit the library, where he selected books on various religious and philosophical themes. Mr MB no longer watched television with his family, as he said that it 'wound him up', and he had not been out with his friends for several months. He had not been to work for 2 weeks. He told his mother that there was no longer a job for him, but she later discovered that his attendance and timekeeping had been deteriorating over a period of weeks and that he had then failed to attend at all. She said that he 'refused to discuss the matter sensibly with her'. As Mr MB had always been a reasonably outgoing and sociable young man, this behaviour was very out of character.

Mr MB's mental state examination revealed that he was unkempt, wearing his pyjamas under his trousers. He appeared slightly over-aroused. His speech was at a normal rate, but very disjointed, e.g. 'I have books in my room – it's special, the moon – God controls it – do you know him – he controls life – the forces can win'. The content of his speech mainly concerned religion and philosophy, and how they affect us all. His mood was euthymic and somewhat incongruous. Mr MB said that he could feel something was going on 'out there'. He also said that he had heard people talking about him in the street, and occasionally he heard a single male voice saying 'Go to your room, it is safe there'. He said that he had seen cosmic rays. His orientation and cognition were grossly intact.

After some discussion, Mr MB accepted the offer of a few days in hospital 'for a rest'. On admission his routine physical examination and baseline bloods were unremarkable. His urine screen was positive for nicotine and cannabis.

Q1 Which of Mr MB's symptoms are consistent with a psychotic illness?
Q2 What is the significance of Mr MB's positive urine screen for cannabis?
Q3 Outline a pharmaceutical care plan for Mr MB.
Q4 Would you recommend treatment with an antipsychotic at this time, and if so, which one would you recommend?

Mr MB was prescribed risperidone. The dose was titrated against response up to 4 mg taken as a single dose at bedtime.

Q5 Was this dose appropriate?
Q6 What is meant by 'response', and over what time course does this usually occur?

Week 4 Mr MB's symptoms had improved. He still felt that spiritual matters were important, but he was less preoccupied by them. He refused to stay in hospital any longer, and as he was not 'sectionable' he was discharged home. He was given a supply of risperidone 4 mg tablets and was noted to be ambivalent about taking medication.

He did not attend for outpatient follow-up. His mother said that he was living at home and 'doing OK'.

Month 7 Mr MB was brought to the ward by his brother. He had developed an interest in martial arts and had punched a hole in his bedroom wall 'in order to defend himself'. A mental state examination revealed systematised paranoid delusions surrounding a plot to steal his soul. He also admitted to his thoughts being interfered with by an outside agent that removed thoughts from his head and inserted its own.

Mr MB refused to stay in hospital and punched out at a nurse who tried to prevent him from running off. It was decided to place him under Section 2 of the Mental Health Act.

Q7 What is the scope and purpose of Section 2 of the Mental Health Act 2007?
Q8 How should Mr MB's acutely disturbed behaviour be dealt with?
Q9 What medication would you recommend for Mr MB and why?

Mr MB was given haloperidol 5 mg and lorazepam 2 mg intramuscularly. Fifteen minutes later his head was tipped to the side and his eyes fixed upwards towards the ceiling.

Q10 What is happening to Mr MB, and what would you recommend should be done?

Mr MB was sensitive to extrapyramidal side-effects (EPSEs) with typical antipsychotics and refused to take risperidone again as he said it 'didn't agree' with him. He was therefore prescribed olanzapine Velotabs 10 mg at night, increased to 20 mg over the next 5 weeks. His urine screen was negative for drugs of abuse.

Mr MB remained very symptomatic albeit no longer aggressive. He still believed that someone was out to get him, and his thinking continued to be muddled. Nursing staff suspected that Mr MB was not taking his medication (by taking a sip of water and spitting the Velotab back into the cup). The consultant decided to prescribe a depot antipsychotic.

Q11 What is the main advantage of administering a depot antipsychotic to Mr MB?

Q12 Which depot antipsychotic would you recommend and why?

Mr MB's Section 2 was converted to a Section 3, which is a treatment order lasting a maximum of 6 months in the first instance. Mr MB accepted risperidone depot, but over the next 2 months his mental state remained virtually unchanged. He was then prescribed zuclopenthixol depot 200 mg every 2 weeks. Again, little response was apparent. Trifluoperazine 10 mg daily was added to his prescription. Mr MB protested by refusing his injection. A second-opinion doctor was requested to visit Mr MB for the purposes of the Mental Health Act.

Q13 Why has a second opinion been requested?

Q14 What role can the pharmacist play in this process?

Q15 Can anything be done to change Mr MB's attitude towards antipsychotic drugs?

The trifluoperazine was discontinued. Over the next 2 months the zuclopenthixol dose was increased to 600 mg/week. Mr MB became slightly less suspicious, but was still very unwell. Sulpiride 600 mg/day was added to his prescription.

Q16 What are the risks associated with high-dose and combination antipsychotics?

After a lengthy discussion with Mr MB and his family it was agreed that there was little point in pursuing the above prescription and that Mr MB should be offered treatment with clozapine.

Q17 Why has clozapine been prescribed for Mr MB, and is its use appropriate at this time?

Q18 How should treatment with clozapine be initiated and monitored?

Q19 How should treatment with clozapine be optimised?

Q20 What side-effects might you anticipate, and how would you deal with them?

Q21 What further options are available if Mr MB fails to respond to clozapine?

Answers

Which of Mr MB's symptoms are consistent with a psychotic illness?

A1 **Formal thought disorder, probable delusional ideas, auditory and visual hallucinations, and poor self care and social isolation.**

(a) **Formal thought disorder.** This is the term used to describe the abnormal construction (form) of speech that occurs in psychotic illness. In milder forms occasional derailment may be all that is seen. This is when the line of thought jumps from one topic (rail) to another and the connection is not easily understood by the listener. Other terms commonly used to describe this phenomenon include loosening of associations, tangential thinking and 'knight's move' thinking (as in a game of chess). In more severe cases, such as Mr MB's, the conversation may change themes several times within the same sentence and eventually the speech becomes completely incomprehensible. This is sometimes described as schizophrenic word salad. Formal thought disorder occurs in various forms in many psychiatric syndromes and its presence is by no means diagnostic of schizophrenia.

(b) **Delusions.** A delusion is a culturally inappropriate belief that is firmly held despite any logical argument to the contrary. Delusions can take many forms. There are three pieces of evidence in Mr MB's presentation that are suggestive of delusional ideas:

(i) He no longer watches television. This may be due to *delusions of reference*: Mr MB may interpret the content of a television programme as being directly related to himself, e.g. the presenter may be speaking directly to him or making comments about him. Many people with schizophrenia are unable to watch television or listen to the radio because they are troubled by delusions of reference (also called ideas of reference).

(ii) The content of Mr MB's speech is concerned entirely with religion and philosophy. Although there is insufficient evidence to be sure, Mr MB may think that his presence is central to the situation that he is describing. This is an example of a *grandiose delusion*.

(iii) Mr MB says that he can 'feel something going on out there'. This phenomenon can be described as both an abnormal perception and a delusional idea. It is usually called a *delusional perception*.

(c) **Hallucinations.** An hallucination is a perception for which no stimulus exists. Any of the senses can be affected, although auditory hallucinations are the most common. Mr MB describes three types of hallucination:

(i) *Second-person auditory hallucinations*, where he hears a single voice speaking directly to him. The particular voice that Mr MB is hearing is giving him an instruction. This is called a command hallucination. People with schizophrenia may find it difficult to resist these 'commands', and acting upon them is not uncommon.

(ii) *Third-person auditory hallucinations*, where he hears other people talking about him. These are also called commentary hallucinations, and of all the abnormal perceptions they are the most predictive of schizophrenia.

(iii) *Visual hallucinations*. Mr MB says that he has seen cosmic rays.

(d) **Poor self-care and social isolation.** In schizophrenia, symptoms abnormal by their presence, such as hallucinations and delusions, are referred to as positive symptoms. Symptoms abnormal by their absence, such as lack of self-care, poverty of speech, social isolation or blunting of emotional response, are referred to as negative symptoms (and sometimes, where their presence dominates the clinical picture, as the defect state). Mr MB has negative symptoms in that his self-care is poor and his social interactions limited.

The above description has only touched the surface of abnormalities that can be found in the mental state. Each case of psychotic illness is different, and many phenomena not described above can be present. No individual symptom described above is diagnostic of schizophrenia. For a more complete understanding of psychopathology, terminology and the way in which symptoms are grouped together to reach a diagnosis, further reading is strongly recommended. The *Oxford Textbook of Psychiatry* gives an excellent account of psychopathology. The diagnosis of schizophrenia is described in the *International Classification of Diseases (ICD–10)* and the *Diagnostic and Statistical Manual of Mental Disorders (DSM-IV)*.

What is the significance of Mr MB's positive urine screen for cannabis?

A2 **Acute psychotic episodes can be precipitated by cannabis. Cannabis can also exacerbate symptoms in patients with schizophrenia. Mr MB should be discouraged from using cannabis in the future.**

Although there is good evidence that cannabis may contribute to the presentation of psychotic illness, the relationship is complex. People with schizophrenia are six times more likely to develop a problem with substance misuse than the general population. The most frequently misused drug is cannabis. This may cause an acute toxic psychosis characterised by euphoria, fragmented thoughts, paranoia, hyperacusia, depersonalisation, derealisation, and auditory and visual hallucinations, particularly if large quantities are consumed. Symptoms usually resolve within a week of abstinence. The literature in this area consists mainly of uncontrolled studies and case reports, although some population-based longitudinal studies have been undertaken. A systematic review of published studies identified an increased risk of any psychotic outcome in individuals who had ever used cannabis. The risk was greatest in those who used it frequently. The overarching conclusion of this review was that cannabis increases the risk of psychotic outcomes regardless of confounding effects. Although it is not possible to state that cannabis directly causes psychosis, it is thought best to warn individuals that its use could increase the risk of developing psychosis later in life.

Cannabis has a very long half-life, and in chronic users can be detected in the urine for 4 weeks or more after consumption. A positive urine screen (which is usually qualitative) cannot confirm acute intoxication. The situation is further complicated by the fact that cannabis may ameliorate the negative symptoms of schizophrenia as well as some of the side-effects of antipsychotic drugs, and may be used as 'self-medication' for these purposes. Cannabis use in some patients may post-date rather than pre-date the emergence of psychotic symptoms.

Although the use of cannabis in those with psychotic illness should be discouraged, the exact role that it plays in each clinical presentation must be determined from the individual circumstances of that case.

Mr MB's symptoms are of at least several weeks' duration and his presentation is suggestive of a primary psychotic illness, but as this is his first episode the possible role of cannabis should not be excluded. Mr MB should be discouraged from using cannabis in the future as it may predispose him to further episodes and/or exacerbate his psychotic symptoms.

Outline a pharmaceutical care plan for Mr MB.

A3 The pharmaceutical care plan for Mr MB should include the following:

(a) The decision to administer any drugs at all should be discussed with the multidisciplinary team.
(b) The anticipated effects and side-effects of antipsychotics should be discussed with Mr MB. This must be done sensitively, with regard to his mental state and level of insight.
(c) Mr MB's views about drug choice should be respected if possible.
(d) The antipsychotic dose should be titrated against both clinical symptoms and side-effects. The aim is to prescribe one antipsychotic at a therapeutic (not high) dose.
(e) Physical health parameters such as weight, blood pressure, blood glucose and blood lipid profile should be monitored periodically (every 6–12 months) while Mr MB remains on antipsychotic therapy.
(f) The effect of Mr MB's Mental Health Act status on the multidisciplinary team's ability to medicate him should be constantly reviewed.

Would you recommend treatment with an antipsychotic at this time, and if so, which one would you recommend?

A4 Yes, treatment with an antipsychotic is appropriate at this time, but the choice of drug is a matter for negotiation with the patient and should be determined by consideration of a number of factors. For Mr MB a typical or atypical antipsychotic would be appropriate, depending on his views and the views of his psychiatrist. In the absence of any previous drug history or physical pathology, risperidone is a reasonable first choice.

Mr MB has well-documented psychotic symptoms which are sufficiently severe to interfere markedly with his ability to function normally. The potential benefits of antipsychotics therefore outweigh the risks in his case.

Three main factors influence the choice of antipsychotic drug:

(a) **Previous response to treatment**. If there is a history of a previous good response to any individual antipsychotic it is logical to use the same drug again. Similarly, a previous poor response or a history of adverse reactions would militate against the use of an individual drug. For Mr MB this is the index episode, so no useful information is available in this respect.
(b) **The clinical presentation**. This requires consideration of both the severity of the illness and the predominant symptoms. Mr MB is a

young man with a florid psychotic illness. However, he has come into hospital voluntarily and is not an immediate danger to himself or others. There is no need to select a drug that is available in a parenteral form.

(c) **Physical pathology and anticipated side-effect profile**. All antipsychotics have in common the ability to block dopamine receptors, but they vary in the degree to which they block other central neurotransmitter pathways. Sometimes this difference can be clinically relevant. For example, cholinergic blockade is associated with dry mouth, blurred vision, constipation and urinary retention. It is obviously unwise to administer antipsychotics which have significant anticholinergic effects to patients who have narrow-angle glaucoma or prostatism. Alpha-adrenergic blockade is associated with postural hypotension: the elderly are particularly at risk. Blockade of histamine receptors is associated with sedation: sometimes this can be desirable, sometimes not. The relevant potencies of antipsychotics at dopamine, serotonin, Alpha-adrenergic, histaminergic and cholinergic receptors is well documented and can be found in several standard texts. Extrapyramidal side-effects (EPSEs) are a major problem with typical antipsychotics. Acute dystonias are painful and frightening. Akathisia (inner restlessness) is felt by many patients to be intolerable. Pseudo-parkinsonism can interfere with activities of daily living, and tardive dyskinesia (which can be irreversible) is very stigmatising. Atypical antipsychotics are relatively free from these motor side-effects but tend to cause more weight gain than the older drugs. Clozapine and olanzapine may also cause impaired glucose tolerance, frank diabetes and unfavourable lipid profiles. The distinction between typical and atypical drugs is not clear: the original definition of atypicality was a lack of potential to cause EPSEs or raise serum prolactin, yet the atypical antipsychotics risperidone and amisulpride cause prolactin-related side-effects and risperidone causes EPSEs in doses >6 mg/day. It is more useful clinically to think of all antipsychotic drugs as being on several spectra: those that can produce severe EPSEs to those that cause none; those that can lead to enormous weight gain to those that cause less; and those that are very sedative to those that are not, etc.

Drug choice should be negotiated between Mr MB, his psychiatrist and the pharmacist. NICE clinical guidelines on schizophrenia (CG01) emphasise a joint decision regarding the choice of antipsychotic therapy between the patient, the clinician responsible for prescribing and, when possible, the patient's advocate or carer. For patients with diagnosed schizophrenia it is also recommended that advanced directives be drawn up for use in times of acute illness. These are written documents that outline the treatment preferences an individual wishes to be considered at times when they are unable to communicate those preferences themselves.

Was the dose appropriate?

A5 **The optimal dose for many antipsychotic drugs has been determined in randomised controlled trials. Often this is considerably less than the licensed maximum dose for the drug. It is important to be aware of these optimal doses and not titrate the dose too rapidly, as this will only lead to an increased side-effect burden.**

For example, the majority of patients respond to risperidone 6 mg/day or less, or haloperidol 10 mg/day or less. Higher doses have not been shown to confer any benefit in either the speed or magnitude of response. Mr MB has been prescribed risperidone 4 mg, an 'optimal dose'.

What is meant by 'response', and over what time course does this usually occur?

A6 **The aims of antipsychotic treatment are to treat positive and negative symptoms and normalise social functioning. The time course of response to antipsychotics is poorly documented, although most therapeutic gain tends to be seen in the first 6 weeks.**

(a) **Positive symptoms.** Antipsychotics are most effective at treating positive symptoms such as delusions and hallucinations, both of which are present in Mr MB. The onset of this effect is variable. Improvements can sometimes be seen after 4 or 5 days' treatment, but can take much longer. Psychotic symptoms should not be expected to disappear suddenly, but rather to 'melt away'. Delusions often change in quality from being overvalued ideas to being of no importance at all, although they may be remembered as having been true in the past.

As a general rule of thumb, the longer a delusion has been held, the longer it will take to go. Untreated psychotic symptoms of many months' or sometimes years' duration can be very difficult to treat in clinical practice. This is the most powerful argument for early intervention with antipsychotics. In addition, approximately one-third of patients with schizophrenia will have repeated episodes of acute illness. These can be progressively more difficult to treat, with a worsening post-treatment baseline after each episode. This is a powerful argument for maintenance treatment. Unfortunately, there is no way of identifying those who are at risk of having subsequent episodes.

(b) **Negative symptoms**. Negative symptoms such as poverty of speech, emotional blunting, lack of volition etc. are less successfully treated by antipsychotics. Primary enduring negative symptoms are particularly difficult to treat. By virtue of their side-effects, typical antipsychotics can produce secondary negative symptoms such as akinesia and an expressionless face. It is important not to confuse the lack of EPSEs seen with atypical antipsychotics with their ability to treat negative symptoms.

(c) **Social functioning**. Improved socialisation can take many months and may never be completely achieved.

A 'response' to antipsychotics in clinical trials can be as little as a 20% reduction in the Brief Psychiatric Rating Scale, a scale used to quantify psychotic symptoms. By definition, many patients who are classified as 'responders' have residual symptoms.

Approximately 30% of patients will fail to 'respond' to typical or atypical antipsychotics. The management of these patients is discussed in more detail in **A17**.

What is the scope and purpose of Section 2 of the Mental Health Act 2007?

A7 **Section 2 of the Mental Health Act 2007 involves a compulsory admission to hospital for a maximum of 28 days for the purpose of assessment and treatment of mental disorder.**

Section 2 is used when an individual who is thought to suffer from mental disorder refuses to come into hospital voluntarily and admission is considered to be in the best interests of the patient or the public. An application to invoke Section 2 can be made by the patient's nearest relative or a social worker. Two independent medical recommendations are required, one of which must be by a psychiatrist who has been approved for the purpose. The patient has the right of appeal, when he can present his case to the Mental Health Review Tribunal.

How should Mr MB's acutely disturbed behaviour be dealt with?

A8 **De-escalation strategies should be tried first. These include 'talking down' and offering Mr MB voluntary 'time out' in a room on his own with an open door and staff nearby. This may be followed by voluntary oral, then enforced parenteral medication. In extreme cases seclusion may be used.**

Acute behavioural disturbance can occur in the context of psychiatric illness, physical illness, substance abuse or personality disorder. Psychotic symptoms are common and the patient may be aggressive towards others secondary to persecutory delusions or auditory, visual or tactile hallucinations.

With skilled handling, only a small proportion of 'incidents' require enforced parenteral medication. A balance must be drawn between building a trusting relationship with the patient and maintaining the safety of the ward environment. All psychiatric inpatient units should have guidelines for the treatment of behavioural emergencies as they will otherwise be dealt with by junior (inexperienced) doctors on call. This is at best unfair and at worst potentially dangerous. Pharmacists have a key role to play in developing local guidelines and reinforcing their content.

What medication would you recommend for Mr MB, and why?

A9 **The principal objective is to calm Mr MB, which will be best achieved by the combination of a parenteral antipsychotic and a benzodiazepine. Haloperidol 5 mg intramuscularly or olanzapine 10 mg intramuscularly plus lorazepam 2 mg intramuscularly would be a suitable choice.**

Rapid tranquillisation (RT), defined as the use of drugs to rapidly control disturbed behaviour, is required at this point. The common clinical practice of RT is not underpinned by a strong evidence base. Patients who require RT are usually too disturbed to give informed consent and therefore cannot be included in randomised controlled trials. The largest randomised controlled trials to date were the licensing studies conducted with intramuscular olanzapine, although a series of recent studies conducted around the world by the TREC Collaboration has examined a range of other agents. However, no single drug therapy has been found to be best overall for the management of acute agitation or aggression. The best approach would appear to be the use of either a benzodiazepine, particularly lorazepam, or an antipsychotic such as haloperidol or olanzapine. These specific agents are favoured because of considerable experience of their use and their availability as intramuscular injections, although oral therapy should always be offered prior to forced injections.

If olanzapine injection is given then it is recommended that lorazepam injection is not given within 1 hour either side of the olanzapine dose. Oral olanzapine can, however, be given at the same time as oral lorazepam. Diazepam is not recommended as an intramuscular injection because of the erratic absorption from this route of administration.

Parenteral chlorpromazine is best avoided for RT because of the association between low-potency phenothiazines, QTc prolongation and sudden cardiac death. It must be remembered that all antipsychotics have the potential to prolong the QTc interval in vulnerable patients, and that QTc prolongation is a risk factor for *torsades de pointes*, a potentially fatal cardiac arrhythmia. Risk factors for developing QTc prolongation include genetic vulnerability, ischaemic heart disease, hypokalaemia, autonomic arousal and co-prescribing of metabolic inhibitors of antipsychotics.

The slow onset of action of Clopixol Acuphase makes it unsuitable for use in RT, and its long duration of action (72 hours) raises ethical questions about its enforced administration to informal patients. This is not an issue for Mr MB.

Care should always be taken when administering intramuscular injections to a struggling patient, as vasodilation secondary to autonomic arousal may lead to inadvertent bolus intravenous administration.

It is essential to perform regular physical observations in all patients following RT. As a minimum, temperature and blood pressure should be recorded. Patients who are asleep should be subject to 'constant observation' until they are ambulatory again.

What is happening to Mr MB, and what would you recommend should be done?

A10 **Mr MB is experiencing a type of acute dystonic reaction called an oculogyric crisis. This is both painful and frightening, and should be dealt with by the immediate administration of intramuscular or intravenous procyclidine. One 10 mg dose is usually sufficient, although it can be repeated if required.**

What is the main advantage of administering a depot antipsychotic to Mr MB?

A11 **Adherence can be assured.**

Non-adherence and partial adherence with antipsychotic drugs is common in inpatient settings. One study found that 10% of inpatients had no trace of prescribed medication in their blood despite the existence of signed administration records.

Which depot antipsychotic would you recommend, and why?

A12 **Mr MB experienced an acute dystonic reaction with haloperidol. Ideally he should receive risperidone depot for its reduced propensity to cause motor side-effects. If Mr MB refuses risperidone depot, any of the others could be used; however, if this is the case, a test dose would be essential.**

The nature of Mr MB's objections to oral risperidone are unclear. It is important to clarify whether he experienced intolerable side-effects or just objected to taking any medication at all.

If the latter is found to be the case (as is likely), risperidone depot should be prescribed at a dose of 25 mg every 2 weeks. A test dose is not required as Mr MB has tolerated oral risperidone. He should also be prescribed oral risperidone in liquid form for the first 3 weeks of treatment, although he may refuse to take it.

The pharmacokinetics of risperidone depot are very different from those of conventional depots. The risperidone is contained in microspheres which need to be suspended in diluent immediately prior to administration. The microspheres slowly dissolve, releasing the active drug into the intramuscular site over a period of weeks. The first injection does not give therapeutic plasma levels until 3 weeks after administration. Thereafter the drug has to be administered every 2 weeks to maintain therapeutic levels.

If Mr MB had experienced side-effects with oral risperidone, such as headaches or nausea, a typical antipsychotic in depot form could be used as an alternative. Conventional depot antipsychotics are virtually indistinguishable with respect to efficacy or side-effects. Whichever one is chosen, a 'test dose' should be administered. This allows Mr MB to be observed for EPSEs and any allergic (local) reaction to the depot oil. Systemic (anaphylactic) reactions to depot antipsychotics have not been documented.

Why has a second opinion been requested?

A13 **Mr MB is refusing his injection and more than 3 months of his Section 3 have elapsed.**

When patients are detained under Section 3 of the Mental Health Act medication can be administered against their will for the first 3 months only. After this time, medication can only be enforced if a second-opinion doctor, who is a representative of the Mental Health Act Commission, has reviewed the patient and the proposed care plan. Any drugs that are prescribed should be strictly in accordance with those stated on the form completed by the second-opinion doctor. Future changes in drug therapy may require a further visit from the second-opinion doctor.

What role can the pharmacist play in this process?

A14 **In order to comply with the Mental Health Act legislation the second-opinion doctor must consult with two professionals involved in the clinical care of the patient. The first is usually the key nurse. The Mental Health Act states that the second person should be 'neither a doctor nor a nurse'. As an understanding of drug therapy is required, pharmacists are in an ideal position to fulfil this role.**

Can anything be done to change Mr MB's attitude towards antipsychotic drugs?

A15 **Mr MB is not accepting of the need to take medication. There is much to be gained from trying to work with him on this issue. Psychoeducation to address the nature of his illness and the likely effects and side-effects of medication is a priority. His views should be listened to and accommodated if at all possible. This approach, which has been called 'compliance therapy', has been shown to improve attitudes towards medication, increase adherence and delay readmission to hospital.**

What are the risks associated with high-dose and combination antipsychotics?

A16 **High-dose antipsychotics may be associated with sudden cardiac death and carry a high risk of motor side-effects. Combinations of typical and atypical antipsychotics are particularly illogical, as the patient may experience two different sets of side-effects simultaneously.**

It is unlikely that high-dose and combination antipsychotics confer significant therapeutic benefit to the majority of patients who receive them, although the evidence from studies examining this issue is not incompatible with individual patients deriving benefit occasionally. This is where the problem lies in clinical practice: the majority of psychiatrists claim to treat many such patients.

An audit conducted by the Royal College of Psychiatrists Research Unit found that 20% of all inpatients who were prescribed antipsychotics could potentially receive a high (i.e. greater than the *British National Formulary* maximum) dose. 'As-required' prescribing was a major source of 'high-dose' prescriptions, and in the majority of cases there was no record in the patient's notes that a high dose had been prescribed. Monitoring for physical side-effects, particularly QTc prolongation, in these patients was poor. Antipsychotic polypharmacy was found in 48% of patients, and 60% of those who were prescribed an atypical drug were prescribed a typical one in addition.

Patients receiving high-dose and combination antipsychotics are invariably disabled by a plethora of side-effects, including EPSEs, sedation, anticholinergic side-effects, postural hypotension and potential QTc prolongation leading to life-threatening cardiac arrhythmias. As can be seen from the above audit, these side-effects often go unnoticed.

An excellent review of the evidence for the efficacy of high-dose antipsychotics and the risks associated with their use is to be found in the Royal College of Psychiatrists consensus statement. This statement also gives good practical guidelines on how to review treatment and document the clinical decision to use high-dose antipsychotics. It is both essential reading and a good audit tool for examining local practice.

Why has clozapine been prescribed for Mr MB, and is its use appropriate at this time?

A17 **Mr MB has treatment-resistant schizophrenia. Clozapine is the only antipsychotic that has superior therapeutic efficacy in this situation, and its use is thus indicated for Mr MB at this time.**

Mr MB's symptoms have failed to respond to three different antipsychotics given in adequate doses for adequate periods of time. His symptoms are disabling and his quality of life poor. His illness can therefore be described as treatment-resistant schizophrenia. The excellent study by Kane *et al*. demonstrated the superior efficacy of clozapine in otherwise treatment-resistant schizophrenia, with 30% of patients responding after 6 weeks of treatment. Follow-up studies have shown that double this number will show worthwhile therapeutic benefit if treatment is continued for 6 months to 1 year. These findings have been replicated by several groups. Clozapine therefore offers Mr MB the best chance of relief from his symptoms.

How should treatment with clozapine be initiated and monitored?

A18 **Clozapine is associated with a 3% risk of neutropenia, and haematological monitoring is a mandatory condition of treatment. This is coordinated by the individual monitoring schemes provided by the manufacturers of the available clozapine brands. Mr MB should be registered with the monitoring scheme, as should the prescriber and the pharmacist responsible for making the supply. Depot antipsychotics should be discontinued and oral antipsychotics used during the changeover period. Treatment with clozapine can be initiated once the monitoring service receives satisfactory haematological results. The dosage should be titrated gradually upwards as described in the product data sheet, and Mr MB should be observed for side-effects.**

Mr MB is currently receiving zuclopenthixol depot 600 mg/week and sulpiride 600 mg/day. It is routine clinical practice to omit the depot for one dosage interval before starting clozapine. In Mr MB's case this would mean starting clozapine 12.5 mg at night 7 days after his last depot injection was administered, and reducing the dose of sulpiride over the next few weeks as the clozapine dose is increased. There are no set rules for the duration of this crossover period, as it will be determined by Mr MB's mental state and ability to tolerate increasing doses of clozapine. Most patients can be successfully switched to clozapine monotherapy within 4 weeks.

When treatment is initiated, patients should be monitored for postural hypotension (due to alpha-adrenergic block), sedation (due to histaminergic block), tachycardia (due to cholinergic block) and fever (can be due to agranulocytosis, but is usually unexplained and benign and settles despite continued treatment). Weekly blood counts, to monitor white cells, neutrophils and platelets, are performed for the first 18 weeks of treatment as this is the period of maximum haematological risk. Thereafter, fortnightly monitoring is required. If the haematological profile remains stable throughout the first year, the patient can move on to monthly monitoring.

For patients who are clinically stable – defined as stable mental state plus monthly monitoring – the option exists for shared care protocols, when GPs can prescribe continuing treatment and community pharmacies supply the clozapine.

Whichever system is used, clozapine can only be dispensed on receipt of satisfactory haematological results: i.e. no blood, no drug.

How should treatment with clozapine be optimised?

A19 **The dose should be titrated up to 300–400 mg/day unless limited by side-effects. If there is no response after several weeks, a trough serum level should be measured. If the serum concentration is <350 micrograms/L, the dose should be increased to achieve a level over this threshold. If there is still no response, the dose should be increased to the maximum tolerated (up to 900 mg/day).**

It is important to remember that only 50% of eventual responders show therapeutic gains in the first 6 weeks. Clozapine should be prescribed for 6 months to 1 year before concluding that Mr MB has not responded.

What side-effects might you anticipate, and how would you deal with them?

A20 **Excess sedation, hypersalivation, postural hypotension, hypertension, tachycardia, nausea, constipation, nocturnal enuresis, weight gain, impaired glucose tolerance, diabetes and seizures can all occur. Myocarditis and cardiomyopathy have also been reported. EPSEs are extremely rare.**

Some of these side-effects are dose related, others are idiosyncratic. Dose-related side-effects are obviously best dealt with by slowing the rate of dosage titration or by reducing the dose. If this is not clinically possible or the problematic side-effect is not dose related, the following approaches can be useful:

(a) **Excess sedation**. This sometimes responds to alterations in the timing and distribution of the daily dose, e.g. early-morning hangover may be reduced by giving the last dose of the day at 8 pm. Care must be taken to distinguish true drug-induced sedation from the lack of volition often seen in schizophrenia, or simple inactivity due to boredom.

(b) **Hypersalivation**. Simple measures such as propping up the pillows at night can sometimes resolve the problem. Hyoscine (Kwells) or pirenzepine often help. Pirenzepine is widely prescribed for hypersalivation as it does not cross the blood–brain barrier and cause central side-effects; however, it must be imported for use in the UK as it has been discontinued.

(c) **Tachycardia**. If persistent, beta-blockers may help. This is also a useful strategy in clozapine-induced hypertension.

(d) **Nausea**. The aetiology of clozapine-induced nausea is poorly understood. Pragmatically, domperidone, ranitidine or a proton pump inhibitor often help.

(e) **Nocturnal enuresis**. If restricting evening fluids fails to correct the problem and nocturnal seizures are not implicated, oxybutynin often helps. In severe cases desmopressin may be used.

(f) **Weight gain**. This should be anticipated and steps taken to prevent it. The mechanisms of antipsychotic weight gain are poorly understood, and once the weight has been gained it is very difficult to lose. Obesity increases the risk of cardiovascular disease, some cancers, diabetes and osteoarthritis.

(g) **Diabetes**. This requires evaluation of risk versus benefit in each case. There is no guarantee that the diabetes will resolve if clozapine is discontinued.

(h) **Seizures**. These occur in 5% of patients who receive doses of clozapine in excess of 600 mg/day. Sodium valproate is effective. A dose of at least 1000 mg/day is usually required.

(i) **Sensitivity myocarditis and cardiomyopathy**. It is important to be aware of these very rare side-effects. A high degree of vigilance should be shown if the patient displays any symptoms or signs suggestive of new-onset cardiovascular disease.

What further options are available if Mr MB fails to respond to clozapine?

A21 **There are no other antipsychotics either currently available or in development that are as effective overall as clozapine. Various strategies have been used to augment response to clozapine. These include the addition of sulpiride, lamotrigine, valproate and benzodiazepines. It is essential to consult the primary literature before embarking upon any of these options.**

Further reading

Adams CE, Fenton MKP, Quraishi S *et al.* Systematic meta-review of depot antipsychotic drugs for people with schizophrenia. *Br J Psychiatr* 2001; **179**: 290–299.

Alexander J, Tharyan P, Adams C. Rapid tranquillisation of violent or agitated patients in a psychiatric emergency setting. *Br J Psychiatr* 2004; **185**: 63–69.

Allison DB, Mentore JL, Heo M *et al.* Anti-psychotic-induced weight gain: a comprehensive research synthesis. *Am J Psychiatr* 1999; **156**: 1686–1696.

Chong SA, Remmington G. Clozapine augmentation: safety and efficacy. *Schizophrenia Bull* 2000; **26**: 421–440.

Correll CU, Schenk EM. Tardive dyskinesia and new antipsychotics. *Curr Opin Psychiatr* 2008; **21**: 151–156.

Cree A, Mir S, Fahy T. A review of the treatment options for clozapine-induced hypersalivation. *Psychiatr Bull* 2001; **25**: 114–116.

Geddes J, Freemantle N, Harrison P *et al.* Atypical anti-psychotics in the treatment of schizophrenia: systematic overview and meta-regression analysis. *Br Med J* 2000; **321**: 1371–1376.

Gelder M, Harrison P, Cowen P. *Shorter Oxford Textbook of Psychiatry.* Oxford University Press, Oxford, 2006.

Harrington M, Lelliott P, Paton C *et al.* The results of a multi-centre audit of the prescribing of anti-psychotic drugs for in-patients in the United Kingdom. *Psychiatr Bull* 2002; **26**: 414–418.

Johns A. Psychiatric effects of cannabis. *Br J Psychiatr* 2001; **178**: 116–122.

Kane J, Honigfeld G, Singer J *et al.* Clozapine for the treatment resistant schizophrenic. *Arch Gen Psychiatr* 1988; **45**: 789–796.

Keck P, Cohen B, Baldessarini R *et al.* Time course of anti-psychotic effects of neuroleptic drugs. *Am J Psychiatry* 1989; **146**: 1289–1299.

Kemp R, Kirov G, Everitt B *et al.* Randomised controlled trial of compliance therapy. *Br J Psychiatr* 1998; **172**: 413–419.

Mir S, Taylor D. Atypical anti-psychotics and hyperglycaemia. *Int Clin Psychopharmacol* 2001; **16**: 63–73.

Moore THM, Zammit S, Lingford-Hughes A *et al.* Cannabis use and risk of psychotic or affective mental health outcomes: a systematic review. *Lancet* 2007; **370**: 319–328.

National Institute for Health and Clinical Excellence. TA43. *The Clinical Effectiveness and Cost Effectiveness of Newer Atypical Antipsychotic Drugs for Schizophrenia.* NICE, London, 2002.

National Institute for Health and Clinical Excellence. CG1: *Schizophrenia.* NICE, London, 2002.

Overall JE, Gorham DR. The Brief Psychiatric Rating Scale. *Psychol Rep* 1962; **10**: 799–812.

Paton C, Okocha C. Anti-psychotic drugs: old and new. *New Med* 2001; **1**: 45–50.

Paton C, Lelliott P, Harrington M *et al*. Patterns of antipsychotic and anticholinergic drug prescribing for hospital inpatients. *J Psychopharmacol* 2003; **17**: 223–229.

Reilly J, Ayis S, Ferrier IN *et al*. QTc interval abnormalities and psychotropic drug therapy in psychiatric patients. *Lancet* 2000, **355**: 1048–1052.

Reilly JG, Thomas SHL, Ferrier IN. Recent studies on ECG changes, antipsychotic use and sudden death in psychiatric patients. *Psychiatr Bull* 2002; **26**: 110–112.

Rifkin A, Doddi S, Karajgi B *et al*. Dosage of haloperidol for schizophrenia. *Arch Gen Psychiatry* 1991; **48**: 166–170.

Taylor D, Paton C. *Case Studies in Psychopharmacology*, 2nd edn. Martin Dunitz, London, 2002.

Thompson C for the Royal College of Psychiatrists Consensus Panel. Consensus statement on the use of high dose anti-psychotic medication. *Br J Psychiatry* 1994; **164**: 448–458.

World Health Organization. *The ICD–10 Classification of Mental and Behavioural Disorders – Clinical Descriptions and Diagnostic Guidelines*. WHO, Geneva, 1992.

Wright P, Birkett M, David SR *et al*. Double-blind, placebo controlled comparison of intramuscular olanzapine and intramuscular haloperidol in the treatment of acute agitation in schizophrenia. *Am J Psychiatry* 2001; **158**: 1149–1151.

22

Dementia

Denise Taylor

Case study and questions

Day 1 Mr LD, a 76-year-old retired sales manager, attended a memory clinic at his local district general hospital with his wife. He had a 2-year history of aphasia, mild memory difficulties and problems with activities of daily living. His wife reported that he needed help in dressing appropriately, often putting on pyjamas or suits at the wrong time of day unless she laid out his outfits each morning and evening. She said that he also used to be the one who looked after all the household bills, but now he just ignored bank statements and had also misplaced his chequebook and wallet.

His Mini Mental State Examination (MMSE Folstein) score was 24/30 and the Activities of Daily Living (ADL) score was 16/20. He exhibited no extrapyramidal signs, had no medical history of note and scored 12 on the Hamilton Depression (HAMD) rating scale. His blood pressure was 135/75 mmHg, pulse 75 beats per minute (bpm), capillary blood sugar 4.6, and his urea and electrolyte levels were all within normal ranges. Tests for folate, B_{12}, haemoglobin, thyroid and liver function were also all within normal ranges.

Q1 Briefly describe the purpose and function of the MMSE, ADL and HAMD rating scores.
Q2 What is the purpose of the other baseline measures assessed for Mr LD?

Mr LD agreed to start an antidepressant and attend the memory clinic once a month for review. He was given information on ways in which he could improve his memory and a prescription for fluoxetine 20 mg each morning.

Q3 What is the purpose of trying to improve Mr LD's memory?
Q4 Was fluoxetine therapy appropriate for Mr LD?

Month 3 Mr LD arrived for the day dressed in his pyjama bottoms, and a shirt and tie. He was adamant that he had been brought against his will and that there was nothing wrong with him, and he accused the ambulance driver of stealing his wallet. He became very agitated and displayed mild symptoms of aggression (shouting and pacing up and down) until one of the nurses distracted him with a photo-album depicting London in wartime. Eventually he agreed to see the doctor. His MMSE score was now 20/30, the HAMD score 4, ADL rated 12/20 and his ADAS-cog score was 22.

A computed tomography (CT) scan showed enlarged lateral ventricles, widening of the sulci and atrophy of the medial structures in keeping with a neurodegenerative disorder. No space-occupying lesions or cerebral ischaemia were seen.

Q5 What is an 'ADAS-cog' score, how is it calculated, and what is the relevance of the final score?
Q6 What is the relevance of the CT results?
Q7 What is the probable diagnosis for Mr LD and how can it be confirmed?

Mr LD's wife was contacted and asked if she could accompany her husband to his next memory clinic appointment. At this appointment, they were both informed that Mr LD probably had Alzheimer's disease (AD).

Q8 Why is an early diagnosis of AD better for the individual and their family?
Q9 What are the pharmacological treatment options for Mr LD?
Q10 What therapy would you recommend? Outline a dosing and monitoring schedule.
Q11 Outline a pharmaceutical care plan for Mr LD.

Month 7 Mr LD had his 3-monthly assessment after starting rivastigmine. He had complained of feeling nauseous and dizzy when the rivastigmine was initially started, but he had eventually tolerated the dose increases until the last increase to 4.5 mg twice daily, when he had begun to vomit and feel unwell. On observation he was lethargic and pale and reluctant to speak. He refused to complete any of the assessment scales because he was feeling so poorly.

Q12 What is the possible cause of these side-effects and how might they be treated?

Mrs LD asked whether her husband should take any herbal remedies, as she had heard at the Alzheimer's Society carer support group that they could help.

Q13 What is the role of ginkgo biloba and other dietary supplements in the symptomatic treatment of AD?

Month 8 Mr LD was looking much brighter and was telling the nursing staff about his day out to the zoo with his great-grandchildren at the weekend. His MMSE score was now 24/30, ADL rated 16/20 and the ADAS-cog score was 18. His wife thought that he 'was doing brilliantly', and that he seemed much happier and contented in himself.

Month 12 Mr LD was admitted to a general medical ward with deteriorating cognitive function and increasing confusion. That morning Mrs LD had woken up to find her husband was missing from their bedroom. She could not find him downstairs, then had heard 'banging noises' coming from the upstairs bedroom. She found Mr LD in the front bedroom wardrobe 'hiding from the b..... Germans'. Mr LD's general practitioner (GP) arranged his admission to hospital for further investigation.

On examination Mr LD was increasingly confused and would not settle for a full physical examination. Observations noted were: a temperature of 39°C, an empty bladder and no signs of constipation. He had an increased respiratory rate, with a 'chesty' cough and crepitations at the left base.

He then became extremely anxious and 'escaped' from behind the curtains to the safety of the corridor near the nurses' station. He now believed that he was back in the army and had to 'take control of the lake' to protect everybody. He would not allow anyone to come near him, and was having conversations with an imaginary person he referred to as 'Captain'.

Q14 What is the likely diagnosis for Mr LD?
Q15 Would you recommend antipsychotic therapy for Mr LD at this point?

Two days later Mr LD's cognitive symptoms had resolved and his temperature was now normal. Antibiotics had controlled his chest infection and he now wanted to go home to be with his wife. He complained that the ward was 'full of old people.'

Month 24 Mr LD's dose of rivastigmine had been increased 3 months earlier to the maximum licensed dose of 6 mg twice daily. This was in response to a fall in his MMSE, ADAS-cog and ADL scores. Since then there had been no improvement in the scores (MMSE 14/30, ADAS-cog 38 and ADL 8/20), but no further fall in scores. His wife was distressed because Mr LD was now very agitated and shouted at her for bringing 'strangers into the house'. (The strangers were his grandchild and great-grandchildren). He had started to wander aimlessly from room to room and seemed unable to settle. He had also been having increasingly frequent episodes of urinary incontinence, and Mrs LD was feeling 'at the end of my tether'.

Q16 What are the next therapeutic options?
Q17 What care issues are necessary for Mrs LD?

Month 40 Mr LD was now very frail (he had lost 8 kg since the first diagnosis of probable AD). He had been admitted to a nursing home 3 months earlier when Mrs LD no longer felt able to cope. Although his medication of memantine 10 mg twice daily had been continued after admission, he now no longer seemed to be aware of his surroundings. He no longer recognised his wife or any of his family. Increasingly he had been calling for his mother, getting very agitated in the evenings, and had difficulty sleeping. He was often observed 'talking' to an imaginary person who sat at the end of his bed. His speech was rambling and confused, and mainly incoherent. He was also now doubly incontinent and unable to feed himself successfully.

Q18 How might Mr LD's increasing agitation and hallucinations be controlled?
Q19 Outline a pharmaceutical care plan for the treatment of double incontinence.
Q20 When might pharmacological treatment for Mr LD be withdrawn?

Answers

Briefly describe the purpose and function of the MMSE, ADL and HAMD rating scores.

A1 **These provide a baseline measurement of a patient's cognitive function, orientation in time, space and place, and ability to carry out activities of daily living. They also ascertain whether clinical depression is present.**

(a) **MMSE.** The Folstein MMSE tests eight domains of cognitive function, including orientation, memory, recall, language and attention. It takes 10–15 minutes to complete. It is scored from 0 (lowest) to 30. A score of 27–30 = normal cognitive function, 21–26 = mild dementia, 10–20 = moderate dementia (10–14 = moderately severe dementia) and <10 = severe dementia.

In September 2006 the MMSE scoring outlined was proposed by a NICE health technology assessment as an indicator of when to start or to stop a person on a cholinesterase inhibitor (ChEI). Prior to this updated guidance, ChEIs were recommended for use for people with mild to moderate Alzheimer's disease (AD). In the updated guidance this was changed to use in moderately severe disease only. In October 2006 the Royal College of Psychiatrists published guidance on behalf of several parties reminding prescribers that MMSE scores can fluctuate from day to day, and that prescribing decisions should be made in 'the light of the individual patient's circumstances'. Subsequently, the decision by NICE has been criticised by the Health Select Committee for restricting access to beneficial medicines, and the Court of Appeal ruled that the economic modelling used in these decisions was less than transparent.

Other tests with similar function include the Abbreviated Mental Test Score (AMTS), e.g. Hodkin's, which takes less than 4 minutes to complete. It is scored from 0 (lowest) to 10, with 7 or less indicating cognitive impairment.

The results of these tests help to establish the level of a person's cognitive impairment. Where a shortfall in performance is seen within a particular domain, the effect on day-to-day activities such as following commands, orientation to time, person and place or the ability to remember new concepts, can be determined.

These tests are not without drawbacks. For example, English needs to be the patient's first language. Also, if the patient being tested has learning difficulties or a poor educational background, they may have never have known the answers to some of the questions. The tests are also relatively insensitive to change; however, there is proven sensitivity to the effects of ChEI therapy compared to placebo in mild to moderate AD. There is also a proven statistically significant inverse correlation between the MMSE score and the ADAS-cog score (see **A5**). This means that as the MMSE score decreases (reflecting increasing severity of cognitive impairment and/or dementia), there is an increase in the ADAS-cog score (reflecting an increasing severity in the AD). However, a significant point is that people with dementia experience wide fluctuations in their day-to-day behaviour and cognitive function. Therefore, decision making purely on the results of a single test should be undertaken with great caution.

(b) **ADL.** In a clinical setting the Barthel Assessment scale rates the patient's ability to complete basic ADL. These include dressing, –continence, grooming, eating, bathing and walking. It is scored out of a total of 20 (best outcome). A score <16 is associated with the need for care services or carer support. It must be remembered that as cognitive function declines, the ability of the patient to perform physical tasks will also decline because the memory is no longer present for that particular task.

Complicated ADL can also be rated, and include shopping, cooking, finances and keeping appointments.

(c) **HAMD.** Severe depression may present with the same symptomatology as a dementia (e.g. slowing down, memory loss, social withdrawal, low mood or personality change). These symptoms may also be reflected in low MMSE and/or ADL scores. When depression presents in this fashion it is often termed a 'pseudo-dementia'. However, because depression is eminently treatable and effective treatment reduces the associated morbidity and mortality, every patient suspected of having cognitive dysfunction, including dementia, should be assessed for depression. The HAMD scale rates a series of 17 domains ranging from mood to insomnia to anxiety and somatic symptoms. These are then attributed a score. A score of 0–7 = absence of depression, 8–17 = mild depression, 18–25 = moderate depression and >26 is associated with a severe depressive episode.

What is the purpose of the other baseline measures assessed for Mr LD?

A2 **These results (if normal) rule out the presence of a treatable cause for the cognitive disturbance.**

Cardiovascular assessment should include blood pressure monitoring, heart rate (undiagnosed arrhythmia), heart failure (possible hypoxia) and history of stroke or ischaemic disease (cause of cerebral ischaemic lesions).

Biochemical monitoring should include blood glucose (to detect hypoglycaemia or untreated diabetes), serum urea and creatinine (renal failure is a rare cause of cognitive decline), serum electrolytes (hyponatraemia and hypercalcaemia are a common cause of cognitive dysfunction, including delirium in the elderly, and are often medication related), and haematological indices such as haemoglobin, folate and B_{12} levels (severe anaemias of any type may produce cognitive impairment in the elderly, and these should be treated if detected). Thyroid function should also be assessed, as hypo- and hyperthyroidism can be associated with cognitive abnormalities. Liver function tests are generally done to complete the work-up and to establish baseline levels when starting certain pharmacological treatments.

A full physical and medical examination is also necessary, as making a diagnosis of probable AD is one of exclusion. All other possible causes for the symptoms observed should be eliminated. Common causes of cognitive dysfunction (especially delirium) in the elderly include infection (urinary, chest or skin); less common causes are HIV or syphilis and concomitant medication (especially on initiation or withdrawal of an agent).

What is the purpose of trying to improve Mr LD's memory?

A3 Memory dysfunction is a common complaint in ageing. This dysfunction may not be related to a neurodegenerative process.

Often older people complain about changes in their memory. This may or may not be associated with changes after formal cognitive assessment. If minor changes are found but nothing else of note, the person is said to have age-related cognitive decline (ARCD). If slightly more abnormalities are found but insufficient to make a diagnosis of probable dementia, then the person is said to have mild cognitive impairment (MCI). It is thought that about 15% of people presenting with MCI will go on to develop dementia; generally those whose symptoms are predominantly memory impairment.

Giving people with ARCD or MCI guidance on how to remember things and/or improve memory allows them some control over their symptoms, but also these skills may normalise the initial symptoms. Such guidance includes:

(a) The use of diaries or notebooks to act as memory aids.
(b) Repeatedly practising a task.
(c) Using alarm clocks or mobile phone alarms to remember appointments (with a note by the clock of the reason for the alarm).
(d) Using strategies such as mnemonics to remember an action plan (although sometimes only the mnemonic can be remembered, and not the reason why it is remembered).
(e) When being introduced to new people, to repeat their name immediately once or twice to ensure that it enters the memory. Then when speaking to the person, to use their name in the sentence.
(f) To concentrate on things that are important to remember and ignore the less important, e.g. keep telephone numbers in a telephone book for referral.
(g) Establish routines for placing frequently 'lost' items, e.g. always place car keys in a specific place, or carry spectacles on a neck-chain so they cannot be lost.
(h) There is increasing evidence that keeping the brain active by memory-enhancing activities such as crosswords and/or Sudoku

type puzzles, 'brain teasers' (computerised or written) and other activities can enhance cognitive function and improve memory.

(i) Keeping physically active helps to restore cerebrovascular circulation.

(j) To admit to others that there is a problem with short-term memory and ask for assistance and prompting.

Was fluoxetine therapy appropriate for Mr LD?

A4 **Yes. An antidepressant is indicated. Mr LD had a HAMD score that indicated mild depression. The choice of an antidepressant in an elderly patient is dependent on comorbidity and concomitant medication. In patients with cognitive impairment it is best to select an agent with fewer anticholinergic side-effects, as these may enhance the impairment. Fluoxetine is thus an appropriate choice.**

Mr LD's HAMD score of 12 indicates a mild depression, therefore it would be reasonable to initiate effective treatment to achieve resolution of his depressive symptoms.

There is little therapeutic difference in terms of efficacy between any group of antidepressants, especially between the tricyclic antidepressants (TCAs) and the selective serotonin reuptake inhibitors (SSRIs). Treatment decisions are dependent on patient acceptability, tolerability, toxicity, suicide risk and cost. Owing to age-related changes in pharmacokinetic and pharmacodynamic parameters, the elderly are most susceptible to the adverse effects of any medication. These may also be exacerbated by concomitant medication and/or pathology.

In the elderly, pharmacokinetic changes markedly reduce clearance and the elimination half-life of TCAs. These changes can lead to increased plasma concentrations and an increased risk of dose-related toxicity. Pharmacodynamic changes in the elderly mean that organ sensitivity is increased to the adverse effects associated with these pharmacokinetic changes. The adverse effects of TCAs are well known, and the cognitive impairment resulting from their anticholinergic activity precludes their use in patients with dementia.

Owing to the heterogeneity of the elderly and often the concurrent pathology and associated polypharmacy, it is appropriate to use an SSRI first, with the particular choice of agent governed by patient factors such as anticipated pharmacokinetic changes and tolerability. Mr LD has no cardiovascular disease, no history of movement disorders (which may preclude treatment with fluoxetine or paroxetine), and his renal and hepatic function (which may affect the clearance of citalopram, paroxetine and fluoxetine) is unremarkable. He is not on any other medication that might lead to the drug–drug interactions seen with many of the SSRIs. SSRIs have a selective effect on CYP isoenzymes, leading to many pharmacokinetic interactions with other medicines. Paroxetine and fluoxetine are potent inhibitors of CYP2D6, whereas fluvoxamine mainly affects CYP1A2 and CYP2C19 activity, so it is safer to avoid these agents in older people taking concomitant medications that are substrates of these isoforms. The safest agents for older people with concomitant medications are those with a low propensity for drug interactions: citalopram and sertraline. Common side-effects on starting SSRIs are increased anxiety and/or nausea. These can be reduced by starting at half the recommended dose for the first 2 weeks (i.e. 10 mg citalopram) and then increasing to a maximum of 20 mg.

Fluoxetine is thus a reasonable choice for Mr LD; however, the time to therapeutic effect may be delayed because of the long half-life of the drug and its active metabolite norfluoxetine in the elderly. Therefore, the full therapeutic effect may not be attained for 1–3 months. Conversely, once stable plasma levels are reached a missed dose will have less of an effect than an agent with a shorter half-life.

What is an 'ADAS-cog' score, how is it calculated, and what is the relevance of the final score?

A5 **ADAS-cog (the Alzheimer's Disease Assessment Scale – cognitive subscale) is a tool designed for research and clinical purposes to monitor the progression of disease, and also the response to pharmacological treatment.**

The ADAS-cog (there is also a non-cognitive subscale, which is used less frequently) was developed to measure all the major symptoms of AD and the severity and progression of the symptoms in a variety of settings and languages. It is a performance-based test that assesses 11 domains of cognitive function, including word recall, naming, orientation, commands, praxis, word recognition, spoken language and comprehension, word-finding, and recall. It takes about 1 hour to complete and is scored from 0 (no errors) to 70 (profoundly demented). Patients with moderate dementia (untreated) show an annual rate of change of about 13 points. In comparison, those who are mildly or severely affected have a point change of about 6 or 7, respectively. There are many other similar scales. Some centres use the Cambridge Mental Disorders of the Elderly Examination (Camdex), others the Clinician's Interview-based Impression of Change (CIBIC); the CIBIC-plus for global outcomes; or the Progressive Deterioration Scale (PDS) for functional/quality of life measures. All scales have their limitations and some have wide inter-rater variability.

What is the relevance of the CT results?

A6 **A CT scan is used to eliminate reversible causes of dementia and to act as a baseline measurement for disease progression.**

The first purpose of a magnetic resonance imaging (MRI) or CT scan in AD is to rule out reversible causes such as tumours, strokes, haemorrhages, hydrocephalus, ischaemia and other lesions. The findings on CT of enlargement of lateral ventricles and sulci, and the appearance of cerebral atrophy are only supportive diagnostic indicators of dementia. In normal ageing, brain volume reduction is estimated at 5–10% at 80 years, with enlargement of the lateral and third ventricles and cortical cerebral sulci. False positives (apparent cerebral atrophy in normal subjects) and false negatives (appearances within the normal range in definite dementia) are frequently seen. MRI scanning can help to distinguish between the various dementias and normal ageing. It is increasingly used for people with a history of cerebrovascular ischaemic disease (i.e. stroke or transient ischaemic attacks) and early dementia (MCI) and is an important investigation to facilitate choice of appropriate therapeutic options. The use of follow-up rescanning and identification of progressive changes makes for a more accurate diagnosis.

What is the probable diagnosis for Mr LD, and how can it be confirmed?

A7 **The diagnosis is probable Alzheimer's disease (AD). Confirmation is only possible via postmortem necropsy.**

Dementia has been defined as a syndrome consisting of progressive impairment in two or more areas of cognition (memory, language, visuospatial and perceptual ability, thinking and problem-solving, and personality) which is sufficient to interfere with work, social function or relationships and represents a significant change from the previous level of function. It generally occurs in the absence of delirium or major nonorganic psychiatric disorders such as depression or schizophrenia, or impaired consciousness. The *Diagnostic and Statistical Manual of Mental Disorders (DSM)-IV* diagnostic criteria, which are American, or the International Classification of Disease (ICD-10) criteria, which is the WHO classification system, should be referred to before a diagnosis of probable dementia is made.

The histopathological indicators of AD found at necropsy include significant loss of neurons and synapses and resultant neurochemical changes; intracellular neurofibrillary tangles; extracellular neuritic amyloid plaques; and, in some cases, the presence of Lewy bodies. These findings cannot at present be detected by any visualisation techniques while the patient is still alive. Research is currently underway to determine a less invasive screening tool, such as urinary analysis; however, the specificity of such tests remains as yet unproven.

Why is an early diagnosis of AD better for the individual and their family?

A8 **It allows them the opportunity to arrange things such as wills, Advance Decisions, power of attorney and long-term care arrangements while the patient has insight and can make informed choices.**

An early definitive diagnosis is becoming more important, both for the patient, their carers and loved ones and the patient's physician and multidisciplinary team. The Mental Capacity Act 2005 set out for the first time the legal rights of people with dementia to make decisions for themselves. The Act assumes that people have the capacity to make decisions for themselves unless otherwise proved. For people with dementia this capacity may fluctuate on a day-to-day or moment-to-moment basis, so it is a reminder for all those involved in their care that capacity to consent (or incapacity) needs to be reassessed with each decision. An Advance Decision is also legally recognised and allows people with dementia to specify what types of treatment they do NOT want in the future. These Advance Decisions need to conform to the specifications of the Act, but are legally binding documents and must be followed by health professionals. The Act also allows people with early dementia to decide on up to two people with Lasting Power of Attorney: the first for property and financial decisions and the second for personal welfare (health, day-to-day care etc.). The Act applies to England and Wales; Scotland has its own legislation. The British Medical Association has published guidance for healthcare professionals on assessing capacity for consent to treatment (including taking medication).

Other benefits of early diagnosis are:

(a) Reversible conditions can be excluded.
(b) It allows early access by the patient and their family to support groups (e.g. the Alzheimer's Society) for further information and planning purposes.
(c) It helps to determine the prevalence of the disease.
(d) It permits future research into treatments that may slow or halt the progression of the disease to be more effectively targeted to the right stage of the disease.
(e) It enables the appropriate medical treatment to be started at the most beneficial time for the patient.

What are the pharmacological treatment options for Mr LD?

A9 **There are currently three licensed ChEIs for the symptomatic treatment of mild to moderate AD in the UK.**

ChEIs increase the bioavailability of acetylcholine, a neurotransmitter which is depleted in AD, by reducing its hydrolysis. All have shown statistically significant improvement in randomised controlled trials against placebo in patients with mild to moderate AD. However, not all patients will show a response to treatment, and some will have only a partial response. It is estimated that approximately 25% of patients show a definite response, and some 40–50% of all patients are likely to show some benefit. The reason for these findings is unclear, but is perhaps due to the heterogeneity of the dementias as diseases. Patients with the apolipoprotein allele-4 (a genetic risk factor for AD) seem to have a different response rate from those patients without; however, this finding is inconsistent across studies.

The numbers needed to treat (NNT) with reference to a significant improvement in cognition, ADL or global functioning are relatively low (ranging from three to seven for a low dose of any ChEI), indicating that this is a clinically significant treatment. A higher NNT would also be acceptable in view of the chronic nature of the disorder.

Each of the agents available has a different side-effect profile and different cautions and contraindications to use. The choice of pharmacological agent is therefore dependent on the patient's concomitant pathology and medication.

Other agents have also been investigated. Long-term studies of patients taking non-steroidal anti-inflammatory drugs have shown a reduced incidence of dementia compared to normal population groups; however, there is currently no evidence for their use in established dementia, and the risk of adverse effects outweighs possible benefit.

What therapy would you recommend? Outline a dosing and monitoring schedule.

A10 **A ChEI is justified. The choice and dose regimen is dependent on patient comorbidity and local prescribing guidance. For Mr LD, rivastigmine is an appropriate choice.**

Mr LD is suitable for treatment with an ChEI because he has been diagnosed by a specialist physician as having probable moderate AD. The choice of ChEI depends on the patient's concomitant disease factors. The presence of severe hepatic or renal disease precludes the use of galantamine, and the presence of respiratory and cardiovascular disease is a caution against the use of ChEIs in general. Another consideration is that of adherence: once-daily dosing is often preferred by both the carer and the patient.

Rivastigmine is a reasonable choice for Mr LD. It is generally well tolerated, the most common side-effects being drowsiness, nausea, vomiting and diarrhoea, which occur most commonly with upward dose titration. Rivastigmine has a short half-life of about 2 hours but a prolonged action, as acetylcholinesterase is inhibited for up to 10 hours after the parent drug has been eliminated from the plasma. Excretion of inactive metabolites is via the kidney. There is no hepatic metabolism and little protein binding.

The starting dose is generally 1.5 mg twice daily, increasing slowly by steps of 1.5 mg twice daily at monthly intervals to a maximum of 6 mg twice daily. This is in an attempt to increase the tolerability to rivastigmine and to determine the most effective response to a particular dosage. Rivastigmine is marketed in 1.5, 3, 4.5 and 6 mg strengths to aid flexibility in titration. Some patients may need a longer titration interval, e.g. by increments of 1.5 mg daily at monthly intervals.

In some centres the propensity of rivastigmine to cause severe vomiting and diarrhoea, plus its twice-daily dosing regimen which means its use requires greater input from carers to ensure the medication is taken and not forgotten, has however made this a second- or third-line agent.

The monitoring requirements of the ChEI selected will be guided by local policy, but will generally include a barrage of cognitive, physical and psychological assessments to assess continuing efficacy and guide the need for continued treatment.

In 2001, NICE suggested that prior to initiation of therapy a mutually agreeable endpoint for withdrawal of therapy be agreed with the individual and their carer. With emerging evidence of rapid deterioration on withdrawal, this is increasingly hard to establish. Therapy is usually reassessed during titration of dosing every 2–4 months until an appropriate maintenance dose is achieved. Often it takes longer than 3 months to achieve a therapeutically effective maintenance dose owing to the patient's inability to tolerate dose increments. Once reached, assessment can be made every 6 months and the agent continued if the MMSE remains >10; however, overall benefit is still judged in terms of behaviour, global functioning and ADL in patients with MMSE scores <10.

In those who demonstrate no therapeutic response, or who cannot tolerate the adverse effects of a first-line agent, evidence shows that they may respond to an alternative ChEI. If ChEIs are contraindicated then memantine is now licensed for moderate to severe dementia. NICE guidance does not recommend memantine for the treatment of moderately severe to severe dementia except as part of well-designed clinical studies;

however, it says that 100% of people with moderate illness should be offered suitable treatment. NICE did not comment on the suitability of memantine in moderate dementia.

There is no currently available guidance on when to withdraw treatment in patients who have previously demonstrated a therapeutic response but have since shown no improvement. One could argue that if the disease progression itself is being held static and no deterioration is shown, then the treatment should continue. Recent evidence demonstrates that stopping ChEIs can result in a dramatic decline in individual functioning and behaviour. In practice, if the decision is made to withdraw the ChEI then the person is carefully monitored over a 2-week period, and if there is a substantial decline in behaviour or symptoms, or if a previously unappreciated benefit emerges, then treatment is reinstated. NICE's decision in the UK to treat only people with moderate illness is based primarily on the observation that those in this stage of the disease generally have a greater measurable response to treatment than those in the mild stages. It is not clear whether similar concepts of treatment have been incorporated into other NICE guidance.

In 2007 Ballard *et al.* found that in postmortem tests on the brains of people prescribed ChEIs there was a dramatic (70%) fall in the levels of the β-amyloid and τ proteins associated with the cause and progression of AD. This evidence supports the hypothesis that ChEIs slow progression of the illness at a cellular level.

Outline a pharmaceutical care plan for Mr LD.

A11 The pharmaceutical care plan for Mr LD should include the following:

(a) The patient's and, with the patient's consent, the carer's understanding of the illness and its treatment should be fully assessed with reference to local support services.
(b) All members of the team providing healthcare to the patient should be identified within the pharmaceutical care plan.
(c) Prior to starting the ChEI a full medication history should be taken, and if possible all medicines with highly anticholinergic side-effects withdrawn/changed to agents with lesser effects. This is because dementia is associated with reduced levels of cerebral acetylcholine, so that medicines with anticholinergic side-effects will make this imbalance worse.
(d) Pharmaceutical needs may include the need for concomitant medication, advice and treatment about adverse effects, titration schedule, medicine reminder devices, patient and carer information,

medication reminder aids, patient and carer agreement with the treatment plan, and monitoring of efficacy.

(e) At each dose titration a medication review may aid the early detection of intolerable adverse effects which could lead to the suggestion of treatment options for adverse effects or a switch to an alternative ChEI.

(f) Identification of main carer and relevant carer needs. (The National Dementia Strategy (2009) provides further information.)

(g) Generally the aim of a pharmaceutical care plan is to achieve concordance. It must be taken into account that people with dementia will probably not remember what is said, or even that anything has been said. There should therefore be written supporting information at each consultation, even if the carer is present. A difficult thing to take on board for many pharmacists is that true concordance may never be achieved between the person with dementia and their health professionals. The best to aim for is adherence, and to achieve this the pharmacist needs to involve the main carer in charge of medication and explore medication issues in general. Once-daily dosing regimens are often preferred, and donepezil and long-acting galantamine preparations may be beneficial if there are issues regarding multiple dosing regimens. Liquid formulations should be considered if there are swallowing difficulties, which are common in advancing illness.

What is the possible cause of these side-effects, and how might they be treated?

A12 They are probably due to the cholinergic side-effects of the increasing rivastigmine dose.

Susceptible patients may find it increasingly difficult to tolerate dose increases because of increased vomiting and nausea, which may be so severe that the patient loses a clinically significant amount of weight. If there is no evidence of a movement disorder such as Parkinson's disease or Lewy body dementia, then prescribing a long-acting form of metoclopramide for 2 days prior to the dose increase and the first week of the increased dose may help. Staggering the upward titration over a longer period may also help (e.g. 4.5 mg each morning and 6 mg each evening for 4 weeks prior to a final increase to 6 mg twice daily). In patients with movement disorders domperidone 10 mg four times daily as a regular medication, again starting 2 days prior to dose increases and continuing until tolerance is achieved, may help. If diarrhoea is a problem then loperamide can be used.

What is the role of ginkgo biloba and other herbal agents in the symptomatic treatment of AD?

A13 There is some evidence to support their efficacy but few robust data are available.

(a) ***Ginkgo biloba.*** The *Ginkgo* (sometimes spelled *Gingko*) *biloba*, or maidenhair tree, dates back some 200 million years. Its leaves have been used in the treatment of asthma and as a memory enhancer for perhaps 5000 years in Chinese medicine. It is licensed in Germany for the symptomatic treatment of cognitive disorders, intermittent claudication and vertigo of vascular origin. It is becoming increasingly popular in the USA and UK as a dietary supplement to enhance memory.

The active ingredients are unknown and may include one or all of the following: flavonoids, terpenoids, organic acids. This means that there is no product standardization, and different formulations have different ingredients and dosage specifications. This factor contributes to the inconsistency of results in clinical trials.

Ginkgo biloba is thought to produce a vasoregulatory effect on arteries, capillaries and veins, which improves blood flow, and to antagonise platelet-activating factor. There is a theoretical increased risk of adverse bleeding events if it is taken by patients on either aspirin or warfarin; however, there are only isolated case reports in the literature. A Cochrane Review updated in February 2007 suggests that overall the evidence for the use of ginkgo for people with dementia is inconsistent and unconvincing. The SIGN guidelines in 2006 suggested that people wanting to use ginkgo should consult a qualified herbalist and be made aware of possible interactions with other prescribed medicines.

(b) **Lecithin supplementation.** A Cochrane Review found no evidence to support the use of lecithin in the treatment of people with dementia.

(c) **Vitamin E supplementation.** Although one large randomized controlled trial of vitamin E supplementation demonstrated a slowing in the decline of cognitive function associated with a reduction in numbers of patients reaching an endpoint of severe dementia in the active supplementation arm, an increased number of falls was also noted in the active group of the study. Subsequently a Cochrane Review in 2006 stated there was no evidence for the use of vitamin E in people with MCI or dementia.

(d) **Other supplements or interventions.** The NICE Dementia Guidelines published in 2007 outlined a number of non-pharmacological interventions to help in the treatment and/or support of cognitive or behavioural problems in dementia. Cochrane have also completed a number of reviews in this area. There has been increasing evidence for the use of bright light therapy (>1000 lux) to help improve some cognitive and non-cognitive symptoms of dementia. This has been shown to be especially beneficial in the winter months. Lemon balm (*Melissa officinalis*) or lavender are used in aromatherapy interventions to induce sleep or to calm behaviour.

It is also pertinent to remember that the environment in which the person is cared for contributes a great deal to mood and behaviour. Cochrane and the Dementia guidelines both uphold the importance of the environment, including its design, content, accessibility, the use of colour, and access to garden and walking areas.

What is the likely diagnosis for Mr LD?

A14 **Infection-induced delirium superimposed on a background of dementia. Supporting factors include signs of infection, sudden onset, and both visual and auditory hallucinations.**

Delirium is extremely common in this age group, affecting as many as 24% of all hospital admissions. There are many triggers for delirium and the reader is referred to the DSM-IV criteria, which aid in the final diagnosis by outlining the exclusions and investigations that need to be made. The most common triggers for delirium are:

(a) Infection, especially of the urinary or lower respiratory tract (the elderly have a delayed immune response to infection and can become systemically very unwell before changes in X-rays, temperature or blood cultures are seen), but also skin infections and more rarely neurosyphilis or HIV.
(b) Metabolic and endocrine disorders, especially thyroid disorders and electrolyte disturbances.
(c) Neurological disorders, especially stroke and transient ischaemic attacks.
(d) Cardiovascular disease, especially heart failure (poor cerebral perfusion) and arrhythmias.
(e) Medication toxicity, including intoxication, withdrawal effects and side-effects of certain pharmacological classes. Alcohol or nicotine withdrawal should be considered, as well as the starting and stopping of any pharmacological agent.
(f) Other medical conditions, such as chronic constipation, chronic pain or urinary retention.

Impairment of consciousness is defined in DSM-IV terminology as 'reduced awareness of the environment'. In delirium this fluctuates throughout the day, with the intensity of the impairment generally greater at night. This can often present as a disturbance in the sleep–wake cycle, where the patient experiences daytime sleepiness and night-time agitation. Sometimes complete reversal of the sleep–wake cycle can occur. The patient's behaviour and thought processes are often slow and muddled, visual perception is distorted, and hallucinations are frequently noted. The patient can present with mood changes, disorientation for time and place and memory disturbance. Emotional disturbances such as anxiety, fear, depression, irritability, anger, euphoria and apathy may also be demonstrated, with a rapid and unpredictable shift from one emotional state to another. Fear may distress the patient to such an extent that they try to climb out of bed while still attached to medical equipment such as intravenous lines and urinary catheter bags. They may also attack those who are falsely perceived to be threatening, e.g. the nurse trying to get them back into bed.

Would you recommend antipsychotic therapy for Mr LD at this point?

A15 No. Antipsychotic therapy is only indicated if Mr LD's behaviour puts either himself or others at risk of physical harm.

The underlying principle for the successful treatment of delirium is to treat the physical condition or the underlying cause. During the acute phases of cognitive impairment it is important to relieve the distress of the patient and to prevent behaviour that may result in an injury to themselves or others.

Where possible, non-pharmacological methods should be employed to treat behavioural disturbances in this age group. Patients who have poor concentration are often easily distracted, and behavioural intervention methods are recommended. These include:

(a) Creating a calming environment.
(b) Providing activities to reduce boredom and loneliness.
(c) Providing a regular routine.
(d) Providing proactive non-confrontational care.
(e) Ensuring the physical environment is optimal, i.e. temperature control, space to walk, good lighting.

Other psychological strategies include the ABC analysis, where the patient is carefully observed over a 2-week period for:

(a) Antecedents (television programme, meal times, nurse of the opposite sex involved in bathing routine).
(b) Behaviour (clear description of behaviour exhibited).
(c) Consequences (if the consequence is unimportant, does the behaviour require treatment?).
(d) The next step is to record what stops the behaviour (so that it can be used again if necessary).

Recent research has demonstrated a statistically significant association between the rate of cognitive decline, pneumonia and/or death from cerebrovascular or cardiovascular disease and the prescribing of antipsychotics. Current advice is not to use antipsychotic medication unless the behavioural symptom places the individual and/or others at risk of injury.

The Omnibus Budget Reconciliation Act (OBRA) legislated in the US in 1998 recommends that behaviour be observed for up to 1 month in patients with neurodegenerative disease before any pharmacological treatment is initiated. This is to ensure that the behaviour is not just a short-term manifestation of disease progression. Unnecessary medication puts the elderly person at risk of increased morbidity and mortality from iatrogenic illness.

Behavioural problems can include restlessness, irritability, nocturnal wakening, aggressive behaviour and resistive behaviour. The first course of action is to attempt to identify any underlying treatable cause. The following questions should be considered:

(a) Is the patient in pain? (Remember, these patients have reduced visuospatial awareness and are often confused, and therefore at greater risk of falls or walking into things.)
(b) Is there an underlying depression causing the apathy and lethargy?
(c) Is there a superimposed delirium due to infection or some other cause?
(d) Is the patient's communication hampered by visual or hearing or speech difficulties? Always remember to check for glasses, hearing-aids or false teeth when communicating with an elderly patient.
(e) Has the patient recently moved from another care environment? Changes in environment can greatly distress patients with dementia as they no longer have familiar items by which to reorientate themselves.
(f) Does the patient become more distressed in certain situations, such as when being bathed by a member of the opposite sex, mealtimes etc.? If so, try to establish the causative factor.

(g) Ask yourself 'is the patient really wandering or actually just walking?' People need exercise and mental stimulation. Medication should not be a substitute for inappropriate staffing levels or lack of activities.

Each problem should be analysed to identify causality if possible, and specific procedures for assessment and treatment should be agreed so that all members of the multidisciplinary team and any visitors can handle the problem in the same manner.

In 1998, the *Expert Consensus Guidelines for the Treatment of Agitation in Older Persons with Dementia* (updated annually) were first published, giving guidance on two treatment strategies: environmental intervention and the use of medication. The guidelines describe mild agitation as behaviour which is somewhat disruptive but not aggressive, such as moaning, pacing, crying or arguing. They describe severe agitation as behaviour that is aggressive or endangers others (or the patient), e.g. screaming, kicking, throwing objects, scratching others or self-injury. Their first recommendation is that the family and/or carer(s) should be educated about dementia and agitation and encouraged to join a support group. The most important aim is to identify the trigger for any problem behaviour.

Efforts should be made to reduce disorientation, e.g. at night try using low lights so that the patient can orientate to place, and to avoid sensory over- and under-stimulation. It may be easier to care for restless agitated patients in a side room where there is less disturbance from noise and other patients.

Carer (and healthcare professional) education groups on dementia are often provided by the Alzheimer's Society or the local memory clinic. These groups can help carers to understand changing/challenging behaviour and learn how to cope with it. This greatly increases the support mechanism for the caring process, and also ensures people with dementia are cared for appropriately.

What are the next therapeutic options?

A16 Memantine, a novel *N*-methyl-D-aspartate (NMDA) antagonist, is licensed for the symptomatic treatment of moderate to severe AD.

Transfer to an alternative ChEI may be tried at this point, but it would seem more logical to initiate (or co-prescribe, depending on local policy) the non-competitive NMDA receptor antagonist memantine. Memantine is licensed in the UK for the symptomatic treatment of moderate and moderately severe to severe AD. When a patient is classified as having a moderate to moderately severe dementia it is often difficult to assess their cognitive function owing to reduced attention span and poor memory. Therefore, the burden on the carer is also measured in relation to assisting the patient with ADL.

Double-blind placebo-controlled studies have demonstrated significant improvements in cognitive impairment, lack of drive, motor dysfunction, ADL and elevation of mood, with reduced lability of affect also reported. In two double-blind placebo-controlled randomised trials, memantine demonstrated statistically significant improvement in the following domains of ADL as measured by the Global Deterioration Scale: overall behaviour, ability to move, to wash and to dress.

Memantine targets excitatory amino acids such as glutamate. A chronically released high level of glutamate is associated with the pathomechanism of neurodegenerative dementia. An excess of glutamate causes over-stimulation of NMDA receptors, which allows the free flow of calcium into the cell. Sustained elevation of glutamate leads to a chronic overexposure to calcium, which in turn leads to cell degeneration and ultimately neuronal cell death. Memantine is thought to bind to NMDA receptor sites, thereby reducing this overexposure to calcium. However, although memantine blocks the glutamate-gated receptor channels allowing the physiological activation of the receptors (involved in memory formation), it blocks the pathological activation. Owing to the pharmacological effects and mechanism of action of memantine, there are several drug–drug interactions and the reader is advised to refer to the agent's latest Summary of Product Characteristics for further information.

The initial dose is 5 mg once daily, increasing to twice daily, then 10 mg each morning and 5 mg in the evening, eventually leading to the maximum dose of 10 mg twice daily. Dose increments should be made at weekly intervals. Memantine is available as 5 mg tablets or a solution to aid dosing regimens. This slow upward titration is to reduce the incidence of side-effects. The most common side-effects are hallucinations (5% versus 2.1% in placebo); confusion (1.3% versus 0.3%); dizziness (5% versus 2.8%); headache (5% versus 3.1%) and tiredness (1% versus 0.3%). Uncommon adverse reactions include anxiety, hypertonia (increased muscle tone), vomiting, cystitis and increased libido.

Anecdotal evidence shows that some people respond extremely well to memantine, often those with driven and agitated behaviours. A Cochrane Review highlighted its possible usefulness in treating vascular and mixed dementias as well as AD. Increased efficacy and safety have also been demonstrated when this drug is used concomitantly with ChEIs.

What care issues are necessary for Mrs LD?

A17 Mrs LD requires a personal care plan that meets her emotional, physical and psychological needs.

Carers of people with AD need a great deal of support to ensure that their own physical, mental and social needs are met. The institutionalisation of patients with AD is generally dependent on when the carer feels unable to cope with the demands of a 24-hour, 7-day week regimen of caring (consult the National Dementia Strategy (2009) for further detail).

Early intervention for carer needs is vital, as many will suffer from depression, and many will be frail and elderly themselves, with concomitant healthcare needs. Frequently the stress associated with caring can lead to physical and mental ill health. Healthcare professionals need to be aware that many people are completely unaware of any services and appreciate actually knowing that they are a carer. The Carer Rights Act aims to support all carers appropriately; however, many healthcare trusts and organisations suggest that there is insufficient funding to support its recommendations, and this is why support is often not proactively offered.

It is advised that each carer has a care plan agreement which outlines respite care needs, additional service needs, community psychiatric nurse monitoring, psychiatric care support programme, carer and patient counselling/support/stimulation activities, and local day hospital services. There should also be a social worker assessment. The Alzheimer's Society and the local memory clinic are useful first contacts for any carer.

How might Mr LD's increasing agitation and hallucinations be controlled?

A18 The treatment of agitation and hallucinations should be by non-pharmacological methods if possible; however, if these fail, an atypical antipsychotic may be warranted.

Patients with AD are often reported to have associated psychotic presentations such as persecutory delusions and hallucinations. When these occur with behavioural changes (agitation, aggression etc.) they are termed behavioural and psychological symptoms in dementia (BPSD). A recent study demonstrated that the incidence of visual hallucinations in dementia was actually 3%, compared to the more accepted 40%. Researchers found that poor lighting combined with ageing eyesight, onset of cataracts, glaucoma and/or macular degeneration resulted in an interaction where the person made mistakes in seeing what was there, and also had errors in their perception of what was there. For example, seeing little people in the corner of the room was actually linked to the television being on at the other end of a room!

Historically such symptoms were often treated first by the use of antipsychotic medication. We now need to be more circumspect about prescribing, and determine whether the patient is actually distressed by these hallucinations or whether they can be distracted from them or they can be ignored. All antipsychotics are known to increase morbidity and mortality in older people. Stroke is increased more than threefold with risperidone or olanzapine, and more than doubled with any other atypical antipsychotic agent. This does not mean that typical (conventional) antipsychotics should be used indiscriminately. Two large epidemiological studies have demonstrated that the safety profiles of typical and atypical antipsychotics are similar. The consensus on safe prescribing in older people with dementia is that any antipsychotic should be used with caution under specialist supervision and for a short period of time, with regular review. The decision to prescribe should be documented in the patient's notes and state clearly all factors that were considered in the decision-making process.

An added concern is that people who have Lewy body dementia or Parkinson's disease dementia show an exaggerated sensitivity to the extrapyramidal side-effects (EPSE) of antipsychotics and an increased risk of morbidity and mortality. Conventional antipsychotics should not be used in these people (because of the increased risk of EPSE), and atypical antipsychotics should be used with extreme caution. Finally, two recent studies have shown that when antipsychotics are withdrawn there is no change in the amount of behavioural disturbances in individuals, illustrating that generally they seem to be ineffective.

In June 2008 the FDA alerted prescribers to the increased risk of mortality in people treated for dementia-related psychosis with both conventional and atypical agents, and that this increased risk of mortality should be discussed with their patient, the patient's family and carers prior to commencing treatment.

Alternative approaches may instead be more appropriate. Increasingly studies in the treatment of BPSD are showing a statistically significant reduction in behavioural problems following treatment with a ChEI or memantine. Another agent used for restlessness and agitation is trazodone (dose 50–150 mg at night).

Despite these concerns, in some situations an antipsychotic may be warranted. If the decision is taken to prescribe, the following factors need to be taken into account. Pharmacokinetic changes in the elderly lead to higher plasma concentrations at low doses of antipsychotics, thereby increasing susceptibility to side-effects, which will occur at much lower doses than in younger patients. The elderly have reduced lean body mass, with a corresponding increased lipophilic store and decreased serum albumin, all of which affect the distribution and transportation of a pharmacological agent. Clinically this means that when dosing with a lipophilic agent it may seem to take an unexpectedly long time before therapeutic effect is reached. Ageing also results in decreased renal and hepatic mass (indeed, all organ mass is reduced), which affects the body's ability to metabolise and then excrete medicines. A corresponding reduction in hepatic and renal blood flow also exacerbates this delay in clearance.

At the time of writing low-dose quetiapine is the antipsychotic drug of choice; however, quetiapine clearance rates are reduced by 30–50% in the elderly, so it is recommended that dosing is started at 12.5–25 mg once daily, increasing by 12.5–25 mg increments every 1–3 days until a therapeutic effect is reached. Quetiapine is well tolerated in the elderly, has a low incidence of seizures, no anticholinergic activity, and sedative effects similar to those of chlorpromazine; however, postural hypotension can be a problem if titration is too rapid. Amisulpride or aripiprazole are other alternatives.

If absolutely necessary, risperidone starting at a dose of 250–500 micrograms at night (and increasing in 250–500 microgram increments) can lead to symptom control. Increasing side-effects (EPSEs and postural hypotension) are seen at doses >2 mg daily. Risperidone does not reduce the seizure threshold or block histamine receptors, and has no anticholinergic side-effects. However, the cerebrovascular and cardiovascular risks need to be discussed with the patient's carer and the agent withdrawn as soon as possible.

Olanzapine has been used extensively for the treatment of psychoses in the elderly. Fewer EPSEs have been reported than with risperidone, but there is a 10% incidence of drowsiness, anticholinergic effects and weight gain. Therefore, it is less useful in elderly patients with worsening cognitive dysfunction. Olanzapine is also associated with cerebrovascular and cardiovascular risks.

The efficacy of clozapine is well documented in this age group but its use is associated with many side-effects, including sedation, hypersalivation, tachycardia, hypotension, hypertension, constipation and urinary incontinence. Its propensity to cause fever and agranulocytosis also necessitates mandatory monitoring of blood cell counts on a regular basis. It also has high anticholinergic activity and will therefore adversely affect cognitive function. It is generally only considered as a last resort.

Low-dose haloperidol (250–500 micrograms once daily, adjusting the dose accordingly), seems to be used increasingly for agitation and rapid tranquillisation with or without lorazepam (500 micrograms to 1 mg). An alternative is promazine. In 2005 Schneider *et al.* demonstrated an increased risk of mortality of 107% with the use of haloperidol in particular.

Whatever agent is chosen, if an antipsychotic is being prescribed, its dose, frequency and continued use should be reviewed daily. As the patient responds to the treatment of the behavioural disturbance, antipsychotic therapy should be reduced and withdrawn as soon as possible. It is also prudent to remember that the neurodegenerative process will be ongoing, and that as this progresses the observed behaviour will change in response.

Outline a pharmaceutical care plan for the treatment of double incontinence.

A19 **Double incontinence puts the patient at risk of infection and skin problems. It is often a leading reason for institutionalisation of the patient by carers.**

As social awareness declines and the patient no longer remembers how to find the toilet, or that they actually physically need to go to the toilet, alternative measures are needed. Behavioural treatment suggests a toilet training regimen, e.g. taking the patient to the toilet at regular intervals during the day, such as on waking, after breakfast, lunch and dinner, and then again before going to bed. The co-prescription of agents such as oxybutynin is not to be recommended as they have anticholinergic side-effects and may exacerbate confusion and cognitive functioning. Continence pads are also an option. Catheterisation is generally not acceptable because of problems with bladder infections and the distress associated with changing the catheter; however, it may be an option if the patient is bed-bound and has no bladder control and/or a permanent catheter *in situ*.

If the patient is doubly incontinent a 'constipating and laxative' regimen is often employed. This is where the patient is kept deliberately constipated using codeine or loperamide, and then has a stimulant laxative or enema once or twice weekly so that bowel actions can be controlled. Toilet training options involve less medication and less distress and discomfort for the patient. Dietary interventions are often less effective owing to the reduced appetite of the patient. High-fibre products should be avoided in people with poor mobility and poor fluid intake, as they can lead to bowel obstruction.

It is also important to be aware of the risk of the skin breaking down and leading to chafing or pressure areas. The use of a good barrier preparation, such as Morhulin, Calendula or Drapolene, will help to protect vulnerable areas.

When might pharmacological treatment for Mr LD be withdrawn?

A20 When there is no halt in progression of baseline disease monitoring scales for at least 3 months.

There is no current guidance for the withdrawal of memantine or ChEIs from patients with end-stage AD. However, it would seem obvious that if there is no halt in the progression of the disease, and if the patient is requiring full nursing care and is unaware of their surroundings, a full review of all pharmacological agents should be completed with a view to stopping all except those that are essential. Death is commonly due to bronchopneumonia or embolism (as a result of reduced mobility). Also, loss of awareness of hunger and thirst often results in profound weight loss and/or dehydration. At this stage of the illness the principles of palliative medicine should apply.

Further reading

Alexopoulous GS, Silver JM, Kahn DA *et al.* (eds) Expert Consensus Guideline Series. *Treatment of Agitation in Older Persons with Dementia.* 1998. Updated annually.

Ancelin MI, Artero S, Portet F *et al.* Non-degenerative mild cognitive impairment in elderly people and use of anticholinergic drugs: longitudinal study. *Br Med J* 2006; **332**: 455–459.

Ballard C, Fossey J. Clinical management of dementia. *Psychiatry* 2008: **7**: 88–93.

Department of Health. *Living Well With Dementia: A National Dementia Strategy*. London, February 2009.

Drugs and Therapeutics Bulletin Review. Safety of Antipsychotics in Dementia. *Drug Ther Bull* 2007; **45**: 81–85.

Fossey J, Ballard C, Juszczak E *et al.* Effect of enhanced psychological care on antipsychotic use in nursing home residents with severe dementia: cluster randomised trial. *Br Med J* 2006; **332**; 756–761.

Gauthier S, Emre M, Farlow MR *et al.* Strategies for continued successful treatment of AD: switching cholinesterase inhibitors. *Curr Med Res Opin* 2003; **19**: 707–714.

Lee PE, Gill SS, Freedman M *et al.* Atypical antipsychotic drugs in the treatment of behavioural and psychological symptoms of dementia: systematic review. *Br Med J* 2004; **329**: 75.

Maidment I, Fox CG, Boustani M *et al.* Efficacy of memantine on behavioural and psychological symptoms related to dementia: a systematic meta-analysis. *Ann Pharmacother* 2008; **42**: 32–38.

Masand PS. Side effects of anti-psychotics in elderly. *J Clin Psychiatr* 2000; **61**: 43–49.

Mental Capacity Act 2005 Summary. Department of Health, London, 2005.

National Institute for Health and Clinical Excellence. CG42. *Dementia: Supporting People with Dementia and their Carers in Health and Social Care.* NICE, London, 2006.

National Institute for Health and Clinical Excellence. TA111. *Donepezil, Galantamine, Rivastigmine and Memantine for the Treatment of Alzheimer's Disease (amended).* NICE, London, 2007.

Overshott R, Burns A. Treatment of dementia. *J Neurol Neurosurg Psychiatry* 2005; **76**: 53–59.

Riemersma-can der Lek RF, Swaab DF, Twisk J *et al.* Effect of bright light and melatonin on cognitive and noncognitive function in elderly residents of Group Care facilities. *J Am Med Assoc* 2008; **299**: 2642–2655.

Royal College of Psychiatrists Faculty for the Psychiatry of Old Age. *Atypical Antipsychotics and Behavioural and Psychiatric Symptoms of Dementia.* Prescribing Update for Old Age Psychiatrists. Royal College of Psychiatrists, London, 2008.

Royal College of Psychiatrists. Implementation of the NICE guidance on donepezil, galantamine, rivastigmine and memantine for the treatment of Alzheimer's disease: Position statement by the Royal College of Psychiatrists Faculty of Old Age Psychiatry, Royal College of Psychiatrists Faculty of Learning Disability and the British Geriatrics Society, London, 2006.

Schneider LS, Dagerman KS, Insel P. Risk of death with atypical antipsychotic drug treatment for dementia: meta-analysis of randomized placebo-controlled trials. *J Am Med Assoc* 2005; **294**: 1934–1943.

Sink KM, Holden KF, Yaffe K *et al.* Pharmacological treatment of neuropsychiatric symptoms of dementia: a review of the evidence. *J Am Med Assoc* 2005; **293**: 596–608.

Wang PS, Schneeweiss S, Avorn J *et al.* Risk of death in elderly users of conventional vs atypical antipsychotic medications. *N Engl J Med* 2005; **353**: 2335–2341.

23

Substance misuse

Rosemary Blackie

Case study and questions

Day 1 29-year-old Mr SM asked the assistant who was manning the needle exchange facility in the community pharmacy for injecting materials for heroin/crack use.

The needle exchange facility in this pharmacy had been set up not only to provide needles, syringes and condoms, but also to provide safer injecting advice. This includes ensuring that the message about safe needle disposal is given; encouraging referral to treatment services; checking that the client knows what they are doing; passing on information about current problems with drug batches; and referring injecting and any other problems to the pharmacist, who can deal with them more appropriately.

Mr SM mentioned that he had a wound and asked the assistant what would be best for it. The pharmacy assistant referred him to the pharmacist on duty.

Q1 What general advice about injecting can be given to Mr SM? What are the risks of injecting?
Q2 What are the typical signs of injection wounds, and what should the pharmacist suggest he does?

Week 3 Mr SM presented at the needle exchange again, but this time he was being supported by two friends and was looking much the worse for wear. On questioning it was clear Mr SM had overdosed. It was known he had been using heroin and crack, but his friends were not sure whether or not he had taken anything else. They had brought him to the pharmacy partly because it was the closest place, but also because they did not want to call the emergency services for fear of the police becoming involved.

Q3 What are the signs and symptoms of heroin overdose?
Q4 What should the pharmacist do?

Week 7 Mr SM returned to the needle exchange and asked to see the pharmacist. He had clearly recovered and wanted to thank the pharmacist for the help that had been given to him. He admitted that the experience had been a shock and had made him realise what a problem his drug use had become. He wondered if there was anything the pharmacist could do to help him get some sort of help.

Q5 How could you describe which stage in the Cycle of Change Mr SM has reached?
Q6 What could the pharmacist do to help him?

The relevant referral forms were completed and sent off.

Week 8 Mr SM received an appointment for an initial assessment. At this appointment a comprehensive range of issues were covered, including drug use (both past and present); employment; health (mental and physical); and social history.

Q7 What factors can precipitate drug use?

Mr SM's drug use and social history were recorded as follows during the assessment:

Mr SM is aged 29 years. He comes from a middle-class family where his parents remained married throughout his childhood. He has one brother, aged 24, who is currently abroad in Africa helping at an orphanage. His sister is 21 and at university. He went to the local comprehensive where he achieved good GCSEs and three A levels and attended university.

He began drug use as teenager, starting with cannabis aged 14 then LSD, amphetamines and ecstasy aged 15, but did not try heroin until age 21 following peer pressure. Since then he has been using heroin on and off, but with substantial periods of abstinence. He does not enjoy the feeling that alcohol offers, especially the hangovers, as he always likes to be out and about.

Mr SM was not really sure what triggered his drug use and says that it just seemed the thing to do, as his friends at school at the time were taking drugs. He says that he did feel pressurised to do well and that he was constantly seeming to fight a feeling of failure. Drugs helped with this. His drug use increased at university when he was encouraged to try heroin, which he smoked, but this remained controllable until about two years ago, when he found that it started to increase. The company he worked for collapsed and he became unemployed.

Mr SM found that he could not get another job and his drug use increased to the stage where he could no longer fund it from his savings and so he turned to shop-lifting. This subsequently landed him in prison. His parents' divorce occurred at the same time.

After 4–5 months' abstinence he had recently relapsed, a few weeks after his prison release. Mr SM stated that he had come to the stage where he really needed to do something, and not only because of the probation service! He lives with his supportive girlfriend, a non-drug user.

Once the assessment had been completed, it was decided which services would be of best help to Mr SM at this stage and he received an appointment with a doctor.

Q8 What would the main aims of treatment be?
Q9 What are the prescribing options for the treatment of heroin addiction?
Q10 How do they work, and what are the advantages and disadvantages of each?

Week 9 Having undergone assessment and urine tests to ensure that opioids had been used, a treatment plan was decided upon. Mr SM was started on methadone mixture 1 mg/mL at a dose of 30 mg daily by supervised consumption, to be titrated upwards over the next few days to 50 mg daily for 1 week. His urine test had also shown benzodiazepines, but it was decided at this stage not to provide a prescription for them.

Mr SM came from his appointment and handed in a green FP10 prescription completed as follows:

Methadone mixture 1 mg/mL
Mitte 30 mL daily supervised
Total quantity 210 mL

Q11 What is your response to this prescription? What issues need resolving?
Q12 What practical issues do you need to discuss with Mr SM about the supply of his medication?
Q13 What advice should be given to Mr SM regarding starting methadone treatment?

Mr SM had been collecting his prescription each day during the course of the first week, as well as continuing to collect needles from the needle exchange unit. During the week his doctor contacted the pharmacy to find out whether Mr SM had been collecting his medication and whether he had been requesting needles.

Q14 What are you able to tell the doctor?

Week 10 At his next doctor's appointment Mr SM reported that he had been using extra heroin on top of his methadone prescription. The doctor was able to convert the amount Mr SM reported spending (£10 daily) into the dose of heroin he had been injecting, and increased his methadone dose to 60 mg daily by supervised consumption.

Q15 Why can the dose of methadone be increased now, but cannot be higher at the start of treatment?
Q16 What other issues should be addressed as well as the provision of methadone for Mr SM?

Protection against hepatitis infection was discussed with Mr SM and he was offered vaccinations for hepatitis A and B.

Q17 There are a number of strains of hepatitis. What are they, and how are they transmitted? Which is the main one to affect intravenous drug users (IDUs) and should Mr SM be offered vaccinations against this infection?
Q18 Is Mr SM likely to be infected, and should he be screened for this strain?

Week 13 Mr SM was looking and feeling much better, having stopped using extra heroin and cocaine; however, his urine still tested positive for benzodiazepines. His doctor decided to provide him with a prescription for benzodiazepines.

Q19 What are the advantages and disadvantages associated with prescribing benzodiazepines for a patient like Mr SM?

Mr SM was started on diazepam 5 mg tablets, 30 mg daily, with a view to starting to reduce them within the next 6 months if he remained stable, and eventually stopping them completely. He was advised that he should take the dose spread throughout the day, which would also help with his reported insomnia at night.

Week 14 At his next appointment Mr SM reported that he was buying an extra 20 mg diazepam daily on top of his prescription. This issue was addressed but no increase in diazepam was prescribed, as this was against the treatment centre's prescribing protocol and the available evidence for the use of prescribed benzodiazepines. Mr SM received counselling support to help him overcome this extra use, and over the next 4 weeks he was able to stop it.

Weeks 15–30 During this 4-month period Mr SM was able to obtain employment as a farm labourer. He also produced his first urine sample that was clean for illicit drugs: two major achievements in the progress of a recovering drug addict. As a result, his daily supervised methadone consumption was able to be reduced to three times weekly, with supervised consumption on the day of each pick-up to help ensure that he was still able to tolerate the dose and was not diverting some or all of his methadone.

As part of the interview process, his employer had carried out a urine screen for drugs and during his employment random urine samples were collected.

Q20 How long do common drugs of abuse remain in the urine?

Week 31 Unfortunately a chance encounter with an old friend caused him to start using heroin again, initially smoking but then progressing to injecting.

Q21 What other events can lead to relapse in patients like Mr SM?
Q22 What stage has Mr SM now reached in the Cycle of Change? Is this a common occurrence?

As a result of this relapse his methadone dose was increased to 100 mg daily of supervised consumption. He received a lot of support from his key workers to help him address the issues that had led to this relapse, and to help him to recognise trigger factors and learn how to deal with them to avoid being led back into illicit drug use and relapse.

Week 50 Mr SM had again managed to become stable and he had decided that, after a lengthy period of stabilisation, now was the right time to start reducing his methadone dose. He had moved on to collecting his methadone fewer times each week and had a very good collection history. However, one week he came in on a Tuesday having missed his collection on the Monday.

Q23 Can you supply his prescription?
Q24 Could this problem have been avoided?
Q25 What are the advantages and disadvantages of maintenance and reduction treatment strategies?
Q26 What are the options for treatment reduction?

Mr SM decided to remain on methadone and to reduce at a slightly slower rate of 2 mg every 2 weeks until he reached a dose of 10 mg each day, when he would then reduce by 1 mg every 2 weeks.

At one pick-up he told the pharmacist that he was really struggling with diarrhoea, as it made him feel tired and irritated, and he also could not sleep properly.

Q27 What advice can you offer, including self-help techniques and medication?

A couple of weeks later Mr SM came into the pharmacy with a prescription for loperamide, diazepam, lofexidine and Buscopan.

Q28 What are these for, and how are they used in the detoxification process?

Mr SM did not attend the pharmacy for a further 2 weeks, then came in and presented a prescription for naltrexone.

Q29 What is the place of naltrexone in treatment? Is there anything that you should check with Mr SM at the time of dispensing?

Answers

What general advice about injecting can be given to Mr SM? What are the risks of injecting?

A1 **Mr SM can be advised on safe injecting techniques. It can also be ensured, by asking simple questions, that the right equipment is being provided. Advice on safe disposal of equipment is also vital.**

It is important that anyone working in this setting is aware of the terms used by drug users. Table 23.1 includes some, but there are many others. There will also be local slang, so it is worth finding out about some of this so that you have a better understanding of what is being talked about.

Although Mr SM may know how to inject heroin and crack ('speedballing') it is worth a brief question such as: 'Where are you planning to inject?' This will help to establish that the right equipment and techniques are being used. Ideally, it should be checked that Mr SM knows how to inject and how to prepare his 'works' correctly. Leaflets are available that cover needles, sites and preparation, among many other issues.

The right sized needles are vital: brown needles are required for 'skin popping', whereas orange needles are for surface veins such as in the arms and long blue and green needles for muscles or deeper veins. If the needle is too short there is a very high risk of it snapping while in the body.

When injecting into blood vessels it is vital not to hit any surrounding arteries or nerves, as this can lead to severe consequences (further guidance can be found in *The Safer Injecting Handbook*). It should be ensured that Mr SM has something to dispose his used 'works' into. Small black 'sin bins' are ideal to supply as they are fairly discreet and, once used, can be returned to the pharmacy for safe disposal. Other clients will have big bins at home, which can be obtained from certain centres.

Table 23.1 Slang terms used by the drug user population

Term	*Definition*
User	Person who uses heroin – smokes, injects
Speedballing	Injecting both heroin and crack cocaine
Gouch	Makes the person sleepy (usually had too high a dose of the opiate: the term is also used in reference to methadone)
'Benzo'	One of the benzodiazepine drugs: diazepam, temazepam are most commonly found on the street
OD or 'She OD'd'	Overdose, which may or may not be as a result of heroin use
'Skin-popping'/ popping	Injecting just below the skin
'Having a dig'	Injecting
'Dirty hit'	An injection which was contaminated or the person missed the vein
'Rattle'	Withdrawing from opiates
Gear	Heroin

Under no circumstances should used works be left lying around or thrown into the nearest bin. They carry huge risks of harm and other infection if discovered by unsuspecting people.

Safer injecting advice includes:

(a) Do not use lemon juice (carries bacterial infection risks especially to the eyes).
(b) Use the smallest amount of citric acid needed to dissolve the heroin.
(c) NEVER EVER share any works (carries bacterial, viral and other infection risks).
(d) ALWAYS dispose of the sharps into a sharps bin.
(e) Avoid using on your own.
(f) Avoid using in unfamiliar environments.
(g) Avoid using with people you do not know – you never know whether they will look after you should you overdose.
(h) Don't used bottled or tap water (contains bacteria): if you can't get ampoules, boil and cool your water (some needle exchange units provide sterile water ampoules).
(i) Wash the area using soap and water before injecting.
(j) If you hit an artery (pressure will be felt forcing back the plunger) remove the needle straight away and apply lots of pressure.

(k) Do not use the mixture if it looks unusual: it is the contaminants that are causing this. Try to stick to the same supplier, as they are more likely to tell you if the strength is much different from usual.
(l) Avoid the femoral vein ('fem'), as this is one of the most risky sites, and use the forearm instead.
(m) Give the veins a rest by using different sites.
(n) Don't double up: allow time to assess the strength of the first hit.
(o) Smoke heroin if at all possible: you may waste more, but the effects come on faster and there is much less risk involved.

Citric and other acids are harmful to the site of injection, but should be used in preference to lemon juice, vinegar or any other acid. Lemon juice carries the risk of contracting bacterial infection. Advice on use of citric acid can be found in the *Harm Reduction Works* DVD.

The team manning the needle exchange facility should be aware of any current alerts about the purity of local heroin supplies. This information can be obtained from a number of sources, such as the users themselves, alerts from the Drug And Alcohol Team (DAAT) and other agencies, both local and national. There are also numerous resources which can be used for training staff and to help increase awareness in the users themselves of overdose. See Resources at the end of this chapter for places to obtain materials.

What are the typical signs of injecting wounds, and what should the pharmacist suggest he does?

A2 **The typical signs are of swelling, pain, redness, and the area weeping or turning black, pale or discoloured. The pharmacist should refer Mr SM to his general practitioner (GP) or the nearest walk-in centre.**

Anything that looks untoward near the injecting site or that the patient feels is very different from usual should be checked out, and the sooner this is done the less long-term damage there is likely to be. It is a good idea to watch out for any reactions occurring specifically in your area: the HPA (Health Protection Agency) releases alerts and information, as well as local DAATs.

The patient should be referred to the GP or a walk-in centre. A&E may be required, and referral here can also be advised if needed. Some areas may have centres with nurse-led clinics where there is a drop-in service for this type of problem.

This may also be an opportunity to briefly broach the subject of use and suggest a treatment referral. This could plant the seed of contemplation into the patient's mind (as part of the Cycle of Change, see **A5**).

What are the signs and symptoms of heroin overdose?

A3 **The signs and symptoms range from moderate to severe and may not always occur straight after a hit:**

- (a) **Moderate: slurred speech, nodding head, pinpoint pupils, unable to focus, slowing pulse.**
- (b) **Serious: unable to talk, shallow breathing, vomiting, making choking sounds.**
- (c) **Severe: unconscious, unable to breathe, blue skin.**

The risks of overdose (OD) are much greater when the following occur:

- (a) More than one substance is being used (prescribed or illicit). This could include alcohol, benzodiazepines, other prescription and non-prescription medications. One of the most common combinations seen in OD is a mixture of alcohol, benzodiazepines and heroin.
- (b) The person is newly out of prison.
- (c) Injecting.

What should the pharmacist do?

A4 **The main thing is not to panic! Mr SM should be laid on the floor in the recovery position, basic first aid principles (ABC) followed and an ambulance called.**

It will be important to convince his friends that you really must call for help, as otherwise it is very likely that Mr SM will die. You can reassure them that you will not be calling the police and that the police will not turn up at the pharmacy or at the hospital (unless there are other reasons about which you have not been informed). Finally, it is important to try to elicit what has been injected or otherwise used.

How could you describe which stage in the Cycle of Change Mr SM has reached?

A5 **Mr SM is following the Cycle of Change as described by Prochasaka and DiClemente, and has reached the Action stage.**

The cycle can be represented as shown in Figure 23.1. It can be used to help with understanding how a person feels about their attitude to their drug use and treatment. At different stages, different methods and approaches are employed to help further the person in the treatment process. For example, at the pre-contemplative and contemplative stages (which are likely to be at the time of the first request for help) and at assessment, motivational interviewing and advice is helpful; relapse prevention is best given at the maintenance stage of treatment.

Mr SM has now reached the Action stage, probably as a result of the combination of the information provided at needle exchange and

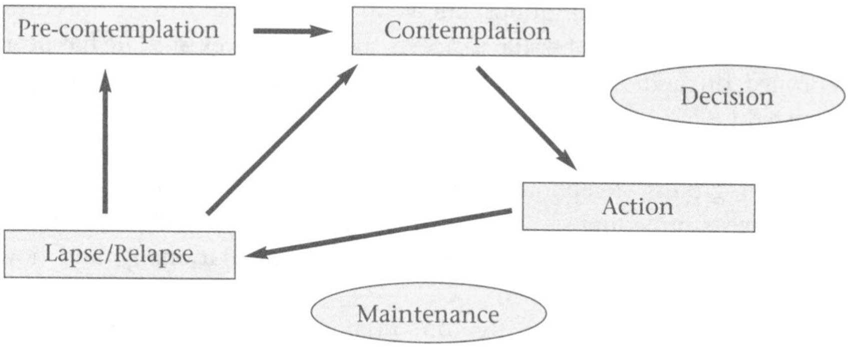

Figure 23.1 The cycle of change.

following his OD, as well as possibly because of a lack of money and some other personal factors.

What could the pharmacist do to help him?

A6 **This will depend on local policies and available services, but the pharmacist should be able to refer Mr SM into a local drug treatment programme.**

Treatment of substance misusers requires a multidisciplinary team approach involving 'drugs at sufficient doses, supported by ongoing psychosocial interventions'. Substance misusers can consume vast resources in a wide range of areas, including medical services and the criminal justice system. For example, in 1996 in the UK half of all crime was drug related, costing about £1 billion in associated costs to the Criminal Justice System. Half to two-thirds of prisoners were reported to be problem drug users. Mortality rates in this group are 12 times higher than in the general population, and in 2003 there were over 1400 drug-related deaths, 55% of these being associated with heroin or morphine.

Data for 2004–5 showed that 1% of 15–64-year-olds in the UK used illicit drugs in a chronic and potentially damaging way; 64% of those accessing treatment had been using heroin and 43% inject heroin. Sharing equipment vastly increases the risks of spreading all manner of infections, including hepatitis C and HIV, with all the long-term medical and social cost implications: 28% of those injecting reported sharing needles and syringes, and 48% shared other injecting paraphernalia.

It has been shown that treatment works. For example, opiate use decreases from 62% to 20% in patients treated in the community with methadone; injecting decreases from 60% to 37%. Criminal involvement reduces from 61% to 20–28% at 4–5 years (NTORS data 1995).

Each area of the UK will have a service to support substance misusers. There may be a referral system into specialist treatment centres as well as to various other groups, but as Mr SM is still an intravenous drug user (IDU) he may not be able to access specific services until he has been enrolled on a drug treatment programme where he can be formally assessed.

There are also many other support services available in the form of self-help groups, telephone services, private and charitable services. Pharmacists providing services for drug misusers should find out what is available, both in the area where they work and nationally, and how these services can be accessed.

As well as organising any appropriate referral, or directing him to other services, motivational comments will greatly help Mr SM to try and reduce his drug use in preparation for structured treatment.

What factors can precipitate drug use?

A7 **Many factors can precipitate drug use, and many people who take illicit drugs come from supportive and stable backgrounds and lead very successful lives.**

Key factors include:

(a) Social deprivation/background.
(b) Bereavement.
(c) Stress.
(d) Family problems, such as marriage break-up, parents splitting up.
(e) Being brought up in a drug-using environment.
(f) Curiosity.
(g) Peer pressure.
(h) Abuse (sexual, physical, mental), either when younger or currently.

These are just a few of the many potential factors involved. Many patients come from very supportive and stable families and may just have fallen in with the 'wrong crowd', or simply found that what was a weekend or occasional drug use has escalated to levels that have resulted in addiction.

What would the main aims of treatment be?

A8 **When providing treatment for addiction it is very important that all aspects of the patient's life are addressed, as it is rarely just drugs that are the issue; however, at the beginning the first aim is to control drug use with substitute prescribing and support, which will then provide a more stable lifestyle which enables other issues such as housing, childcare, triggers and mental health issues to be considered.**

It is vital to take into account the aims and expectations of the patient at this stage, as if these are not listened to and addressed there is very little likelihood that the patient will take a full part in their treatment.

There are four main areas to be addressed:

(a) Drug and alcohol use.
(b) Physical and psychological healthcare.
(c) Criminal activity and offending.
(d) Social functioning.

Each patient will have their own aims and expectations, but the overall aims for all patients should be to reduce and stop illicit drug use; commence substitution treatment; and allow stability which will enable other areas of the patients' life to be successfully addressed.

What are the prescribing options available for the treatment of heroin addiction?

A9 **There are four opioid replacement options in the community setting: methadone 1 mg/mL mixture (or other variations); buprenorphine sublingual tablets; buprenorphine/naloxone (Suboxone) sublingual tablets; diamorphine injections.**

How do they work, and what are the advantages and disadvantages of each?

A10 **Each provides a substitute for the illicit drug use, preventing the symptoms of withdrawal but not providing the 'highs' associated with illicit drug use. Each has different properties, and the choice of product depends largely on patient factors and their level of illicit drug use.**

(a) **Methadone.** Methadone is a synthetic opioid agonist that acts with greater affinity for the μ receptors than does heroin. It has a half-life of 24–36 hours once steady state is reached and is lipid soluble, so it is well absorbed. As with all opioid substitutes it does not give the peak highs characteristic of heroin, but at sufficient doses of between 60–120 mg (although more or less may be required) it will block the opioid receptors to stop the feelings of withdrawal and craving. Missing a dose causes a drop in blood levels, so if constant daily consumption is not achieved, receptor saturation is not reached or maintained and a patient will still experience the need to use heroin as well as methadone (although some will continue to use heroin as well as take methadone).

Methadone causes broadly the same effects and side-effects as all opioids. Some of these will subside with time, but tolerance to constipation usually does not develop. There are many interactions, as methadone is metabolised through the liver by the cytochrome p450 enzyme system, which can result in potentially serious interactions if it is given in combination with either inducers or inhibitors of this system. This can often be overcome by taking into account other medication being taken and adjusting doses as necessary. If this is the case, it is vital that all prescribers (GPs, substance misuse specialists etc.) are aware of the patient's full medical and medication history. It is more likely to be an issue if medication has been commenced at different times. Often patients will have other mental health issues, such as depression, or infections and deep-vein thromboses, therefore it is important that the patient is asked in the pharmacy when the methadone is supplied or supervised if they are taking other medication. Patients should be asked this on a regular basis and not just at the start of treatment, as they may not tell you that they have been prescribed any new medication when further into methadone treatment.

Methadone increases the effects of alcohol and other central nervous system (CNS) depressants. Indeed, a significant cause of death in methadone patients is consumption of a cocktail of methadone, alcohol and benzodiazepines. There is increasing evidence that methadone, especially at doses >100 mg daily, increases the QT interval, therefore patients with other risk factors such as heart or liver disease and those taking >100 mg daily should be monitored.

There are several strengths of methadone solution available at the time of writing: 1 mg/mL methadone oral solution (and a sugar-free version) which is green; 10 mg/mL oral solution which is blue; 20 mg/mL oral solution which is brown. In addition there are tablet and injectable versions. It is vital that any concern regarding the strength or form of preparation prescribed is addressed before it is dispensed, to avoid the serious consequences of a possible overdose.

(b) **Buprenorphine.** Buprenorphine is a semi-synthetic opioid with a duration of action of up to 72 hours. It is a partial opioid agonist/antagonist which gives it unique properties. It must be administered sublingually as it has poor oral bioavailability. It differs from methadone in that it has partial opiate agonist activity at the μ receptors, and antagonist activity at the κ receptors, thus resulting in less euphoria and sedation than full agonists. However, it binds with a greater affinity than heroin, methadone and morphine, and exerts enough activity to prevent withdrawal symptoms. It differs from methadone and heroin in that binding to the κ receptors results in antagonist activity. It also differs from methadone and heroin in that it has a ceiling effect, whereby above 32 mg no further opioid effects or respiratory depression occur. This also makes it safer in overdose. Full receptor blockade occurs between 8 and 16 mg daily, although a dose of up to 32 mg is licensed.

Buprenorphine comes in three different strengths: 8 mg, 2 mg and 0.4 mg. Subutex is the branded version licensed for treatment of opioid addiction, whereas Temgesic is licensed for pain relief. There are now generic versions available for treatment of substance misuse. At doses of between 8 and 16 mg daily it blocks all receptors to prevent withdrawal and craving. As a result of its greater affinity and efficacy for opioid receptors than heroin, it should not be first administered until 6–8 hours after the last heroin dose, and preferably only once withdrawal effects have been observed. This will help to ensure that a forced heroin withdrawal is avoided (and means the patient is more likely to continue with the treatment!). If a patient is transferring to Subutex from methadone, the methadone dose should be 30 mg daily or less, and a window period of 24–36 hours left between the last dose of methadone and the first dose of the buprenorphine (methadone has a much longer half-life than heroin). A dose of 8–16 mg Subutex is approximately equivalent to 60–70 mg methadone daily, therefore it is less suitable for patients with the larger heroin habits. However, as increased experience and evidence are obtained there are some practitioners who will transfer patients from methadone to Subutex at doses >30 mg methadone.

Buprenorphine is metabolised by cytochrome P3A4 (part of the cytochrome P450 system) in the liver, therefore care is needed with potential interactions. Titration to full dose can be carried out over 2–3 days, also as a result of its partial agonist activity. Best practice for induction regimens is constantly changing, therefore current manufacturer information and guidance should be consulted. Different doctors and centres also have differing and preferred regimens.

(c) **Suboxone.** These sublingual tablets are the newest opioid addiction treatment available, launched in 2008 in England. They differ from Subutex in that they also contain naloxone. They come in 8 mg/2 mg and 2 mg/0.5 mg strengths. When taken sublingually the naloxone is unable to pass through into the bloodstream in an active form and the patient will feel no adverse effects; however, if the tablets are injected the naloxone exerts its activity, causing immediate withdrawal effects. Naloxone was added in order to prevent the diversion of Subutex onto the illicit market.

Table 23.2 The advantages and disadvantages of opioid substitution therapies

Methadone mixture 1 mg/mL		*Buprenorphine sublingual tablets*		*Suboxone tablets*	
Advantages	*Disadvantages*	*Advantages*	*Disadvantages*	*Advantages*	*Disadvantages*
Easy to administer in a supervised environment	Takes 7–10 days to reach steady state	Takes less room to store	Takes time to dissolve	Prevents diversion and misuse	Lack of information on use in practice
	Higher risk of overdose	Safer in overdose	More easily diverted	Gives a feeling of clear-headedness	
	Acidic nature increases risk of tooth decay, which is often already an issue in this group		Tablets can be crushed and injected as they are soluble	More pleasant taste	Can cause mouth irritation
	Gives more of a 'foggy' feeling		Less suitable for the higher opioid-using patients	Safer in overdose	Harder to start due to the 'window period' needed to avoid precipitated withdrawal
	Larger volumes can be harder to take, making some patients feel nauseous		Harder to start due to the 'window period' required to avoid precipitated withdrawal		

The advantages and disadvantages of the three products are summarised in Table 23.2.

Current evidence demonstrates that both methadone and buprenorphine are suitable for prescribing in this situation, but that methadone retains more patients in treatment. At the time of writing, no comparisons or NICE appraisals for Suboxone use have been made. As always, prescribing should take into account experience, history and risks and benefits, but where both methadone and buprenorphine are suitable, methadone should be prescribed first.

Because of the nature of the condition and the treatment being issued, supervised consumption is recommended for at least the first 3 months of treatment. This is to help support the patient by giving them: daily contact with a healthcare professional; avoiding diversion of a controlled drug into the community; reducing the risks of overdose; and reducing the risks of death to other people (10 mg methadone can kill a child).

Methadone mixture 1 mg/mL would be an appropriate opioid replacement therapy for Mr SM. The main reason for this is that at his reported level of heroin use, which is equivalent to 80–90 mg methadone, buprenorphine has been found to be unsuitable. Mr SM will need to choose a pharmacy to dispense his prescription, and the pharmacist should enter into an agreement to take him on.

What is your response to this prescription? What issues need resolving?

A11 **Methadone is prescribable on a daily instalment basis, but should be prescribed on a blue FP10 (MDA) form which complies with all current controlled drugs legislation. Methadone can also be prescribed on green FP10 prescriptions, but these are used for single supplies only, again complying with all controlled drugs legislation. Mr SM is being supplied on a daily basis, therefore the prescription he has presented you with is incorrect. The prescriber needs to be contacted to obtain the correct prescription.**

The correct prescription can be faxed through to the pharmacy, but only to confirm that the prescription exists. Mr SM must return to the surgery in order to pick up the original and bring it back to you in order to receive his medication.

A blue FP10 (MDA) form, as well as the usual prescription requirements, states the amount of methadone (or other instalment medication) to be prescribed and on what day. On days when the pharmacy is closed, a supply will need to be made the previous day to be taken away for consumption on the day that the pharmacy is shut. This should be made clear on the prescription.

Although Mr SM will be initially presenting to the pharmacy on a daily basis, there will be a time when he starts to collect on fewer occasions. The prescription should then state what should be supplied on each day, and care should be taken to ensure that the amount supplied correlates with the daily dose.

Methadone, buprenorphine, Suboxone, diamorphine and diazepam are the most common products supplied on an instalment basis. The right-hand side of the FP10 (MDA) is divided into sections to allow a record to be kept of the medication supplied. It is vitally important that this section and the controlled drugs register are completed once the methadone has been collected (and not just when it is dispensed). If the supply is not collected, this must be recorded. If 3 consecutive collection days are missed, the prescription should be put on hold and the prescriber contacted. The patient will then need to contact the prescriber to assess whether it is safe to restart treatment at the current dose, or at a lower dose and titrate upwards again. It is not safe to restart at the previously prescribed dose of methadone if 3 days have been missed without first assessing the opiate intake of the patient during the time missed. Tolerance to methadone is lost and there is a great risk of overdose, especially at the higher doses. Although this risk is less with buprenorphine, owing to its longer half-life, it is usual to follow the same procedure.

There is insufficient space in this chapter to cover all the scenarios that could occur, so interested pharmacists are directed to the resources listed at the end of the chapter.

What practical issues do you need to discuss with Mr SM about the supply of his medication?

A12 **When Mr SM first presents with his prescription there are several practical issues that should be covered with him:**

(a) Behaviour in the pharmacy: waiting patiently for his turn, not shoplifting etc.
(b) Times to collect his medication. Some pharmacies state certain times between which prescriptions can be collected.
(c) What supervised consumption entails: confidentiality and supervision in the consultation area.
(d) Clarity about the '3-day rule' and what will happen should 3 days be missed.
(e) The need to present himself in a non-intoxicated state.
(f) The shared care arrangements and on what basis you will speak to the prescriber.
(g) Safe storage of any take-home supplies. It should be checked that he has a lockable box, kept away from anyone else.

(h) Clarity about any discovered diversion or 'spitting' of methadone.

It is very good practice to obtain identification from any new substance misuse patient and to verify the validity of the prescription and signature (especially if it not recognised) of the prescriber. You can also contact the prescriber and ask for a description of the patient. Some centres will phone ahead of a patient arriving to ask if you are able to accept a new patient, and will also provide details of the patient and prescription. You should be especially careful when receiving prescriptions and patients who present 'out of area'. You should also not hesitate to take the time to ensure that all is as it should be. The patient may well be withdrawing, agitated, and just want to get the methadone and go; however, if you explain the reasons for any delays, potential arguments and incidents can be avoided.

You must be sure that the full methadone dose is consumed before the patient leaves the pharmacy. This can be done by insisting that they have a drink of water afterwards, and by making sure they respond fully to a question.

Although Mr SM will be only taking away one day of methadone (to cover the dose on Sunday), it is vitally important that he stores it safely, preferably in a locked box. Just 10 mg can kill an opioid-naive child, and its colour makes it look exciting for someone to try if it is left lying around.

Some pharmacies create patient files with photographic identification onto which details of any of the above agreements are recorded and signed. The patient can be issued with a pharmacy card, which must be presented each time supplies are collected,

There are numerous variations in how supply and supervised consumption are managed, so interested pharmacists should find out about local processes as well as consult the resources at the end of the chapter.

What advice should be given to Mr SM regarding starting methadone treatment?

A13 **Mr SM should be told that the starting dose of 30 mg daily of methadone he has been prescribed is very unlikely to 'hold' him in terms of blocking effects to withdrawal symptoms, but that it will reduce them. He should also be advised not to 'top up' his dose with heroin.**

This is because of the pharmacokinetics of methadone as well as the amount of heroin Mr SM has been using. Ideally, Mr SM should not use any heroin on top of the methadone at this time, and should be advised to that effect, owing to the risks of overdose, which can increase, as often a patient will use the same amount of heroin as used previously. Any withdrawal symptoms will get better with time: the best option is to ride them through. However, it should be recognised that it is very unlikely that a patient will just stop their drug use straight away, as this also requires a change in lifestyle to avoid the triggers for use: something very hard to achieve when suffering withdrawal! Therefore, if Mr SM does use heroin on top of his methadone it would be better if he smoked it (less risk of overdose) and used much less than usual.

In order to aid adherence it is a good idea to explain how methadone works in terms of how it builds up in the system, and why a low dose is started as a result of this; and the fact that the purity of the street heroin consumed by Mr SM is unknown. Mr SM could be totally uninterested in this at the first instalment, as it is likely he will just want the methadone and to go, but this can be covered over the next 2–3 days when he comes in for his next doses.

It is likely that, subject to successful initiation and titration, Mr SM will continue to collect his methadone on a daily supervised basis for at least 3 months; however, this period is variable and depends on his progress during this time.

What are you able to tell the doctor?

A14 **This depends on the local shared care policy. As part of most shared care arrangements you would be able to confirm that Mr SM has been collecting his prescription. In addition, you could inform the prescriber of any concerns you may have regarding his appearance or behaviour in the pharmacy; however, you could not disclose that he is continuing to collect needles.**

Each area will have its own shared care polices. Shared care arrangements are set up between the prescriber, patient and pharmacist to help ensure effective communication between all involved in the prescribing and supply of medication and other treatment interventions. The policy should also enable the pharmacist to have named contacts with others caring for the patient, which makes it much easier to sort out any problems as they occur.

The shared care policy would thus clearly state what should be communicated between the prescriber and the pharmacist. If, for example, Mr SM had been presenting to the pharmacy in an intoxicated state, causing a disturbance which you have been unable to resolve with him, shoplifting, or if he seems to be deteriorating either physically or mentally, then you can discuss your concerns with his prescriber; however, you should be aware that you are not at liberty to disclose whether or not a patient is continuing to request needles. One of the cornerstones of needle exchange provision is that supply is confidential for all parties. Data that may be collected from needle exchange units for analysis is anonymised, and hence not traceable to a particular client.

If you have concerns about the request for needles you can discuss them with the patient and encourage him to speak to his GP/treatment centre. Other behavioural issues, such as presenting consistently late or causing disturbances, are best dealt with in the first instance by speaking directly to the patient in order to resolve them. However, if problems continue or become more serious (such as shoplifting or diversion), it may be appropriate to contact the prescriber to discuss this as soon as you are able (this may be later, when the patient is not in the pharmacy).

Why can the dose of methadone be increased now, but cannot be higher at the start of treatment?

A15 **Methadone reaches a steady-state blood level after about 7–10 days. After this, it is safe to increase the dose by larger amounts than at the beginning. Tolerance will have been established but not all receptors blocked, therefore where a patient is still using on top of the methadone dose it is shown that they have tolerance to extra opiate. The aim is therefore to reach a dose whereby all receptors are blocked as soon as possible, to reduce the risk of harm.**

At the time of writing, £10 of injected street heroin is equivalent to about 20 mg methadone, so a 70 mg daily dose of methadone could be enough for Mr SM. However, the aim is to stop his extra use as soon as possible, so increasing his dose to 80 mg daily will help this as all receptors will be blocked. As a result, cravings and withdrawal symptoms will be prevented, resulting in avoidance of the physical and psychological need to use; however, work may be needed on how to overcome his routines and times of using. This is often dealt with by key workers either in group or one-to-one sessions.

If Mr SM was not using extra heroin on top of the methadone, but was still feeling withdrawal symptoms, the methadone dose would need to be increased at a slower rate, such as 10–30 mg per increase, with between 4 and 10 days between increases to allow the full effects of each increase to be assessed; however, it is possible to increase the dose between 60 and 120 mg each time for people using on top after the first week, but there is still the need to leave time between increases to assess the affects.

Optimum dosing has been achieved when: Mr SM is not using illicit opioids; not experiencing sedation or euphoria after doses; and is suffering no signs and symptoms of withdrawal.

What other issues should be addressed as well as the provision of methadone for Mr SM?

A16 **Once Mr SM has started treatment it is important to start addressing other issues that will have an effect on the overall outcome.**

These include: counselling and other psychological support; support with housing; help finding employment or educational opportunities; and provision of information to relatives. A care plan will have been drawn up by either the key worker or the prescriber. Key workers play a very important part in patient care, in terms of both coordination and referral to the relevant agencies and delivering interventions themselves. In some treatment centres every patient will have a key worker; others will only use key working as required by the patient.

A care plan in the context of substance misuse treatment is 'a collaborative venture' and is a written agreement between patient and key worker (or other main contact in the drug treatment programme, such as a doctor). It outlines the goals that should be achieved during treatment, who will do what towards achieving them, and by when. The care plan will include details of all the different types of drug treatment a client needs, including substitute prescribing, and it will cover the patient's journey through all stages of treatment, helping to ensure that all areas of the patient's life are addressed. The care plan should be reviewed regularly to ensure that all aspects are still relevant.

There are a number of strains of hepatitis. What are they and how are they transmitted? Which is the main one to affect intravenous drug users (IDUs), and should Mr SM be offered any vaccinations against this infection?

A17 **There are five main strains of hepatitis: A, B, C, D and E. The main one to affect IDUs is hepatitis C. If he is not yet infected and has not already had full courses of vaccinations, Mr SM should be offered vaccinations against hepatitis A and hepatitis B. There are no vaccinations against the other strains of hepatitis.**

(a) **Hepatitis A.** Hepatitis A is spread by consuming food or drinks that have been contaminated by the virus, which is passed out of the body in the faeces. It is common in areas where sanitation and hygiene are poor, such as parts of Africa and the Far East. Symptoms are often confused with influenza; jaundice can also be a symptom.

There is a vaccination which is recommended for those travelling to high-risk areas, and vaccination is recommended for IDUs.

Infection confers lifelong immunity. Hepatitis A does not usually cause long-term liver damage.

(b) **Hepatitis B.** This is spread by cross-contamination of body fluids as it is carried in blood, saliva, semen and vaginal fluids. Transmission can therefore be through sharing injecting equipment, via unprotected sex, and from mother to baby during pregnancy, birth and breastfeeding.

Most people experience no symptoms once infected, although mild influenza-like symptoms can occur, but this is unlikely to be for at least 1–6 months after infection. Hepatitis B can develop in one of two ways: acute and chronic. The acute form will resolve within a few weeks, whereas the chronic form lasts for more than 6 months. The person can remain infected without ever knowing it. In about 25% of cases more serious liver disease, such as cirrhosis, occurs following infection and it is possible that this will lead to cancer. If diagnosed, chronic hepatitis B can be treated with antivirals such as interferon and lamivudine.

There is a vaccination which is routinely offered to those at risk, such as healthcare workers and those travelling to high-risk areas. It is a course of three injections, which must all be given if full immunity is to be achieved. A blood test is needed to check that immunity has been acquired. Many treatment clinics will vaccinate those who come for addiction treatment, and it is recommended for all users regardless of injecting status.

(c) **Hepatitis C**. Hepatitis C is carried in the blood and spread mainly through contact with the blood of an infected person. Other ways of spread are less common but include an infected mother to her baby before or during birth; unprotected sex; having tattoos, piercings or acupuncture with unsterile equipment; and sharing razors or toothbrushes which have been contaminated with infected blood.

Hepatitis C is the most common form of the virus contracted by drug users and is acquired through sharing equipment. The greatest risk is through shared injecting equipment, but anything causing cross-contamination of blood could result in infection. It is also spread through sexual contact, as it is found in semen and vaginal fluids. The only way to prevent spread is by not sharing or reusing any equipment, or making sure that any equipment is fully disinfected if reused. Practising protected sex is also vital.

IDUs are at great risk of contracting hepatitis C, but it can also be spread by snorting and smoking drugs if there is blood transfer as a result of the presence of open sores in the nose or mouth. The virus is able to survive for up to 1 week inside a syringe: this is much shorter than for HIV, but hepatitis C is much more infectious in that there could be up to one million viral particles per millilitre of blood, compared to HIV at about 10 000 per millilitre.

One of the main problems with hepatitis C is that there are often no signs or symptoms for years, so the infection can unknowingly be passed on with great ease. There is currently no vaccination against hepatitis C.

(d) **Hepatitis D.** Hepatitis D strain is more complex in that it requires co-infection with hepatitis B in order to reproduce, and the combination can be more serious than hepatitis B on its own; however, it has a low rate of infection in Europe.

Spread is by infected blood and unprotected sex. Incubation is between 3 and 12 weeks and symptoms are similar to those of hepatitis B. There is no vaccine, and it is treatable at the same time as chronic hepatitis B.

(e) **Hepatitis E.** This is spread in a similar way to hepatitis A; epidemics occur when water supplies are contaminated with infected sewage.

Incubation time is 2–12 weeks and the infection can be spread for up to 2 weeks after symptoms appear. Symptoms are general and non-specific. The main concern is in pregnant women in the third trimester, when it can be fatal in one-fifth of cases.

There is no vaccination available and treatment is based on symptom control.

Is Mr SM likely to be infected, and should he be screened for this strain?

A18 There is a strong possibility that Mr SM might be infected with hepatitis C, but the decision to test for infection is not one to be undertaken lightly, as the consequences are wide ranging.

Hepatitis C is a RNA virus of the Flaviviridae family. There are several genotypes, with the most common, 1a and 1b, accounting for approximately 60% of worldwide infection. As Mr SM injected he is at much greater risk of contracting bloodborne or other infections for a number of reasons: injecting allows pathogens directly past the skin barrier; possible transfer of infection from other people from using the same equipment; unclean environments etc. Therefore, it is likely that Mr SM will have contracted hepatitis C, although a test will be required for confirmation.

In 1997, data showed that almost half of IDUs in the UK had been infected with hepatitis C and one-fifth had become infected within 3 years of becoming IDUs. Also, about half of all IDUs who had accessed treatment services did not know that they had hepatitis C.

It takes about 3 months after infection for the virus to show in the blood. About 20% of those infected will clear the virus at the acute stage, but the rest will progress to chronic (>6 months) infection. Once infection has occurred, it often takes many years to destroy the liver to an extent where the person experiences symptoms, but the rate of liver damage varies greatly from person to person.

There are several places where tests can be carried out: through some treatment services; through sexual health clinics; through GUM (genitourinary medicine) clinics. Following a positive result, further tests are required to establish viral load, progression and strain. Not all genotypes respond to treatment to the same extent. For example, genotypes 2 and 3 achieve an 80% treatment success rate, in contrast to genotype 1 at 50%. Progression varies from person to person, with some living for many years after infection until a stage is reached where liver function is severely affected.

Once infection has been identified, the decision of when and whether to treat is complex, involving many factors, all of which need to be discussed extensively with the patient. One of the most important issues is whether the patient is in a physical, mental and social situation that will enable the vigorous and demanding treatment to be completed. Treatment lasts either 24 or 48 weeks, depending on the genotype.

Many factors can affect the success of treatment. Those that reduce the rates of successful eradication include: increased age; male gender; high level of liver damage already present; present and past high alcohol intake; smoking; infection with genotypes other than 1, 2 or 3; high viral load.

What are the advantages and disadvantages associated with prescribing benzodiazepines for a patient like Mr SM?

A19 **The main reason for prescribing benzodiazepines for Mr SM would be that he showed the signs and symptoms of anxiety, for which it has been shown that up to 30 mg daily diazepam is effective. Unlike sleeping, tolerance does not appear to develop to the anxiety-attenuating effects of benzodiazepines at such doses. Diazepam can also help to reduce alcohol intake, another major concern, both in the general population and especially so where other CNS depressant drugs are being prescribed; however, in Mr SM's case alcohol use is not an issue.**

It is dangerous to stop benzodiazepine use abruptly, and not prescribing would very likely mean that Mr SM would continue to go out and buy his daily diazepam, thereby keeping himself in contact with other drug users and suppliers, factors that will greatly increase the likelihood that he will continue using other substances such as heroin or crack on top of his prescription. This would completely counteract one of the main aims of providing treatment, which is to reduce the patient's risk-taking behaviour.

One of the disadvantages of benzodiazepines is that they are used illicitly in this population, and providing them on prescription could result in Mr SM selling them for other drugs. He could also crush the tablets and inject them. He may also use them to aid a suicide, accidental or otherwise, or in an overdose. He may also continue to buy extra supplies even if he does have a prescription. One option is therefore to provide the diazepam in daily instalments, along with his methadone prescription. This would also mean that, should Mr SM comply fully, a managed reduction and withdrawal could be more safely carried out through prescribing, rather than expecting Mr SM to do this by controlling his buying habits.

Other disadvantages include the fact that drug users take benzodiazepines to enhance or counteract the effects of other drugs and for their intrinsic intoxification effects, whereas for methadone users benzodiazepines can be used to give the 'high' that is lost with methadone use.

It is recommended that benzodiazepines should not be prescribed on a long-term basis. Starting a prescription for these should be with the agreement that reduction in about 6 months or so should be part of the plan. The benefits of prescribing bezodiazepines long term have not been fully established, but the benefits of short-term prescribing are that it can help to stabilise their use and the patient's life in general. Prescribing also means that benzodiazepine use has been acknowledged, and therefore support can be given to help reduce use in a constructive and safe manner.

How long do common drugs of abuse remain in the urine?

A20 Table 23.3 indicates the time that drugs remain detectable in urine.

It is important to note that drug retention times will vary between patients as well as be related to which urine drug test is used, but Table 23.3 provides a good guideline.

Factors that affect drug retention times include the amount used, bodyweight, and the combination of drugs used. Some patients become 'fast metabolisers' as a result of high drug use as the liver adapts to the demands placed on it for metabolism by producing more enzyme, with the result that the drug is metabolised at a faster rate.

Self-test kits are available for drugs of abuse, and guidance is given with each product as to the substances detectable and how long after

Table 23.3 Urine detection times of common drugs of abuse

Drug	*Urine detection time*
Amfetamine	1–4 days
Benzodiazepines	Very short acting (such as midazolam) 12 hours Intermediate acting (such as temazepam) 2–5 days Long acting (such as diazepam and nitrazepam) 7 days or longer
Barbiturates	3–8 days, depending on the type
Cannabis	3–45 days. Single use will be the shortest time and chronic heavy use much longer
Methadone	1–7 days. After regular dosing, detectable time increases to 7 days
Metamfetamine	1–4 days
Heroin	Up to 2 days. Heroin is detected in the urine as the morphine metabolite. (Urine tests will detect other opiates too, such as morphine, codeine and dihydrocodeine. Laboratory testing is needed to determine which opiate is present)
Phencyclidine (PCP)	2–6 days
Buprenorphine	8 days
Cocaine	2–3 days

consumption they can be detected. The legal implications surrounding the use of these tests are beyond the scope of this chapter.

What other events can lead to a relapse in patients like Mr SM?

A21 **There are many causes for relapse back to using illicit drugs. They include:**

(a) Meeting up with old contacts who are still using and being unable to 'get out of' the situation
(b) Difficult events in family life, such as relationship break-up, bereavement
(c) Other stressful situations, such as debt, housing problems
(d) Parties/gatherings where drugs are available and there is pressure to use

(e) An urge just to try it again, having convinced themselves that it will be 'just this once'
(f) A need to relax or 'get out of a situation' because in the past using drugs has worked and may still be the only real way a patient has ever been able to achieve relaxation
(g) A feeling of frustration/fed-up with being on substitution and wishing to use illicit medication again
(h) Having money in the pocket
(i) Loss of employment
(j) A previous conviction resulting in some sort of penalty, such as a fine, prison, community service and the resulting change to the person's outlook.

Part of the support and key work will be to cover with the patient how to deal with these types of more stressful event, but the advice can be much harder to actually apply when such a situation first presents itself.

What stage has Mr SM now reached in the Cycle of Change? Is this a common occurrence?

A22 **Mr SM has reached the lapse/relapse stage, which is a well-recognised part of the cycle in the progression towards full recovery. It can be reached many, many times before a person reaches the stage of full recovery, and it can occur at any time, from shortly after treatment initiation to after many years of stability.**

Can you supply his prescription?

A23 **No. As the prescription stands, you are legally unable to supply the medication because it is stated that none should be supplied on the day Mr SM has presented.**

The prescriber will need to be contacted and a new prescription issued in order for you to be able to supply legally.

Could this problem have been avoided?

A24 **Yes. With future prescriptions this problem could be avoided by making sure that the following wording, or very similar, is written on them: 'Instalment prescriptions covering more than one day should be collected on the specified day. If this collection is missed, the remainder of the instalments (i.e. the instalment, less the amount prescribed for the day(s) missed) may be supplied.'**

This advice was correct at the time of writing. Current legislation should be checked to ensure that it is still appropriate.

What are the advantages and disadvantages of maintenance and reduction treatment strategies?

A25 **Although the advantages and disadvantages can be described, every patient is different in terms of how they see their treatment progressing, and that view can change over time. It is thus important to fully consider a patient's wishes in order to get the best for, and from, them over the course of their treatment programme.**

There can be pressure from external sources such as the government, national guidelines or new research, as well as from other people around the person being treated (employers, family, friends, prescriber) to pursue a certain path of treatment.

At the beginning the overall aim is to achieve stability, which then gives a platform from which to look at the issues surrounding drug use as well as the other issues covered earlier. Some patients will not want to reduce medication at all, therefore maintenance is the best strategy to avoid relapse into illicit drug use. Pressure from external sources should not be the reason why a particular plan is decided upon.

(a) Maintenance treatment (Table 23.4)

Table 23.4 The advantages and disadvantages of maintenance treatment

Advantages	*Disadvantages*
Gives long-term stability in a mental state where a feeling of being in control prevails	Can develop a 'habit' for both methadone and heroin
Reduces crime	Cost of prescribing, consultation etc
Reduces risk-taking behaviour	No reduction in risk of diversion
Enables the patient to be able to return to some form of education or employment	
Enables the patient to stop using illicit opioids where they feel that they are unable to abstain from all opioids at that time	

(b) Reduction treatment (Table 23.5)

Table 23.5 The advantages and disadvantages of reduction treatment

Advantages	*Disadvantages*
Enables a patient the freedom to pursue all interests and employment options by stopping medication	Withdrawal effects can destabilise the patient and cause them to relapse
Reduces the amount of controlled medication being released from the pharmacy with potential for diversion	Enforced reduction can result in reversion to illicit drug use

What are the options for treatment reduction?

A26 **First, it is important to establish that it is the right time to attempt reduction and that the patient is ready. Withdrawal effects such as sweating, insomnia and shivers can be experienced, but these reduce once stable blood levels are reached. Options for reduction would be:**

(a) Reduction using only methadone
(b) Reduction using only buprenorphine/Suboxone
(c) Reduction to 20–30 mg methadone and transfer to buprenorphine/Suboxone for the rest of the process
(d) Reduction to 20–30 mg methadone or lower followed by an inpatient detoxification in a specialist clinic.

There are also other options that individual patients will come up with through their own research, and these wishes should be discussed and a plan decided upon. Inpatient detoxification is beyond the scope of this chapter, but would be governed by local guidelines. If this is the route chosen it is vital to ensure there are appropriate aftercare arrangements in place and support from the community team.

The withdrawal effects are usually more pronounced once lower doses (<20–30 mg methadone) are reached, but every patient is different. Some will state that withdrawal from methadone is the worst thing ever, whereas others will have very little difficulty.

As the body gets used to the reduced dose, the effects subside and symptomatic treatment can be provided as necessary. There are many different options in the reduction and cessation of substitute medication. Much support will be needed, especially in the later stages when the patient comes closer to stopping completely. There is no 'best way' to stop substitute medication, other than gradually.

Generally speaking, reducing methadone at a rate of 5 mg every 2–4 weeks or so down to about 30 mg is good, as it gives the patient the time to get used to it and become stable again. At every stage it should be emphasised that, should the patient fail to cope, or if there is a change in circumstances which means that further reduction at that particular time is not such a good idea, this is not a problem and that indeed it would be much better to stay on the dose that has been achieved until such a time as the reduction can be continued.

Many patients express the desire just to stop medication as they are 'fed up with it', or find it a drag and a tie to keep having to come back to the pharmacy to collect it, and also always having to think further ahead to organise holidays, prescribing and appointments. It is, however, not recommended to stop substitute medication abruptly, as the chances of relapse into previous drug-using behaviour are extremely high as the patient seeks to stop the withdrawal effects that will be experienced.

Although each patient is different, a general plan for reduction for Mr SM would be at a rate of 5 mg methadone every 4 weeks, with a reduction in dose 1–2 weeks before an appointment with the doctor. This would allow him to get used to any effects felt as a result of the reduction, but also enable frequent review of the situation to ensure that the reduction is going smoothly, which will reduce the risk of destabilisation.

It should be emphasised that, much as Mr SM may want to stop methadone as soon as possible, it would be best to stick to the plan, which can be reviewed. Also, that it is not a problem or a failure if at any stage he should want to maintain again or even increase the dose. This is far preferable to reverting to illicit drug use, with all its risks. A good relationship with the doctor, key worker and pharmacist will help to ensure that Mr SM feels able to communicate any problems he may be having at an early stage.

Once 30 mg methadone has been reached, there are two options that can be discussed with him: carry on reducing with methadone or transfer to buprenorphine or Suboxone.

What advice can you offer, including self-help techniques and medication?

A27 **It is first important to reassure him that these symptoms will get better with time, but meanwhile there is much that he can do to help make things easier by using over-the-counter medication such as paracetamol and loperamide for symptom relief.**

Some form of relaxation or other distraction activity can help. Ideas include sport or participating in another interest that he may have: generally keeping occupied helps. He should avoid alcohol, as this will not help in the long run, especially with the risk of developing an alcohol habit. Speaking to his girlfriend, prescriber and key worker will also enable him to overcome some of the anxiety. Relaxation music and other therapies are available. Some people also find that ear acupuncture and other complementary therapies can help. Herbal preparations containing valerian and other 'anxiety-reducing' extracts can be purchased which may be of help. It is also important to ensure that he eats a healthy diet, which includes the recommended levels of nutrients. Eating regularly throughout the day and avoiding too many sweets and other 'junk food', which can bring 'sugar highs' but then leave the person feeling worse later on, will all help. He could also be offered sleep advice, such as not eating too late at night; use of lavender products which have good sleep and relaxing properties; and having a hot milky drink before bed.

What are these for, and how are they used in the detoxification process?

A28 **These products have been prescribed to counter the side-effects of withdrawal, which comprise a number of physical and psychological symptoms.**

The final stage of reduction and cessation can for some patients be the hardest, because at this stage a number of physical and psychological issues can appear. These include anxiety, diarrhoea, insomnia, aches and pains, which can all be helped with prescribed medication on a short-term basis. Not all of the following will be used for every patient, and each clinic and doctor will have their own preference, but all are commonly used:

(a) **Loperamide** is an opiate antimotility agent, but safe to use in this patient group as it has its effects on the gut and does not penetrate the blood–brain barrier. It is used for diarrhoea, a common symptom of withdrawal. It can be given at a dose of 2–4 mg immediately, then up to 16 mg daily.

(b) **Diazepam** is a short-acting benzodiazepine which can be used to help with anxiety. The dose will be different for every patient, and it is only prescribed in very small amounts in order to control its use and prevent the risk of overdose and misuse.

(c) **Lofexidine** is an alpha$_2$-adrenergic agonist which helps with the epinephrine/norepinephrine (or 'adrenergic storm') effects of withdrawal from opiates, such as piloerection, runny nose and sweating. It is started at 0.8 mg daily in divided doses and gradually increased until symptom relief is obtained, up to a maximum of 2.4 mg daily, with a maximum single dose of 0.8 mg (four tablets). It is then gradually reduced over 7–10 days, if there is no opioid use, but longer may be required. Each clinic or doctor may have their own protocol, so you can check with them and also with Mr SM that he is clear about what he is to do with the tablets. Care should be taken, as lofexidine can cause hypotension and bradycardia, so blood pressure should be monitored, especially during dose titration.

(d) **Buscopan** (hyoscine butylbromide) is a muscarinic antagonist used for stomach cramps at a dose of 2 mg, four times daily before food.

Further commonly used products are shown in Table 23.6.

Table 23.6 Preparations used to ameliorate the side-effects of opiate withdrawal

Drug	*Indication*	*Typical dose*
Paracetamol 500 mg	Aches and pains	Two, four times daily when required
NSAIDs	Aches and pains	As per drug
Dicycloverine 10 mg	Stomach cramps	One to two, three times daily before food
Zopiclone	Insomnia	3.75–7.5 mg at night
Promethazine	Insomnia	25 mg at night

At this stage Mr SM may well receive daily visits from his key worker and be presenting frequently at the pharmacy. Again, this will help to ensure that cessation goes as smoothly as possible: lots of support and encouragement can be given, and any medical complications can be dealt with at a very early stage.

Another useful resource which can be given to Mr SM is *The Detox Handbook,* which gives other practical advice.

What is the place of naltrexone in treatment? Is there anything that you should check with Mr SM at the time of dispensing?

A29 **Naltrexone is an opiate antagonist which can be used after the final cessation of opiates to help prevent relapse. It is very important that it is not started until Mr SM has had no methadone (or other opiates) for at least 7–10 days. Naltrexone is hepatotoxic, so you should check that Mr SM has had a liver function test before starting therapy. You should also double check that he has remained opiate-free since you last saw him.**

Naltrexone is initiated at a dose of 25 mg and increased to 50 mg daily. It is very important that Mr SM carries the naltrexone warning card in case of an emergency.

Further reading

British Liver Trust. Various leaflets on adult liver disease. www.britishliver trust.org.uk

CPPE. An Open learning programme for Pharmacists. *Substance Use and Misuse.* University of Manchester, Manchester, 2006.

Department of Health (England) and the devolved administrations. *Drug Misuse and Dependence: UK guidelines on clinical management.* London: Department of Health (England), the Scottish Government, Welsh Assembly Government and Northern Ireland Executive, 2007.

Exchange Supplies: Tools for harm reduction. Exchange Supplies, 1 Great Western Industrial Centre, Dorchester, Dorset DT1 1RD. www.exchange supplies.org.

Ford C, Roberts K, Barjolin JC. *Guidance on Prescribing Benzodiazepines to Drug Users in Primary Care.* Updated 2005. Published by Substance Misuse Management in General Practice (SMMGP).

Harm Reduction Campaign: various resources, see website/address for latest products and information. www.harmreductionworks.org.uk.

National Treatment Agency for Substance Misuse. www.nta.nhs.uk.

RCGP Substance Misuse Unit. *Guidance for the Use of Methadone for the Treatment of Opioid Dependence in Primary Care.* Royal College of General Physicians, London, 2005.

RCGP. *Guidance for the Use of Buprenorphine for the Treatment of Opioid Dependence in Primary Care.* RCGP Drug and Alcohol Misuse training programme 2nd Edition, Royal College of General Physicians, London, 2004.

24

Human immunodeficiency virus (HIV) disease: opportunistic infections and antiretroviral therapy

Elizabeth Davies

Case study and questions

Day 1 A 34-year-old man, Mr IH, presented to A&E with a 10-day history of increasing shortness of breath. He also complained of a non-productive cough, with fevers and night sweats, but had had no haemoptysis. His appetite had decreased over the last few days and his weight had fallen from 73 to 64 kg during the last month.

On examination he was pyrexial, with a temperature of 39.5°C, and tachycardic with a pulse of 125 beats per minute (bpm). He was also tachypnoeic with a respiratory rate of 30 breaths per minute. He had poor lung expansion on both sides; however, his breath sounds were clear, with no bronchial breathing or crepitations. His blood pressure was 120/80 mmHg. He had white plaques with surrounding areas of inflammation on his tongue suggestive of *Candida albicans* infection. The rest of his examination was unremarkable.

A chest X-ray was requested which showed diffuse bilateral shadowing with no signs of consolidation. Pulse oximetry without supplementary oxygen showed an oxygen saturation (O_2 sat) of 82% at rest.

His arterial blood gases on admission (on 40% oxygen) were:

- PaO_2 7.2 kPa (reference range 11.9–13.2)
- $PaCO_2$ 4.1 kPa (4.8–6.3)
- HCO_3 21 mmol/L (22–30)
- pH 7.42 (7.35–7.45)

From his presentation, a clinical diagnosis of either *Pneumocystis jirovecii* (formerly *carinii)* pneumonia (commonly referred to as PCP) or another atypical pneumonia was made. Mr IH was admitted to hospital and nursed in a negative-pressure isolation room until a diagnosis of tuberculosis could be excluded.

Mr IH's serum biochemistry and haematology on admission were:

- Sodium 138 mmol/L (135–144)
- Potassium 3.9 mmol/L (3.1–4.4)
- Calcium 2.2 mmol/L (2.15–2.55)
- Albumin 35 g/L (30–42)
- Urea 4.9 mmol/L (2.2–7.4)
- Creatinine 91 micromol/L (60–115)

His liver function tests were within normal ranges.

- White blood cells (WBC) 2.3×10^9/L ($4–11 \times 10^9$)
- Neutrophils 1.5×10^9/L ($2.0–7.5 \times 10^9$)
- Lymphocytes 0.7×10^9/L ($1.5–4.0 \times 10^9$)
- Monocytes 0.1×10^9/L ($0.2–0.8 \times 10^9$)
- Haemoglobin 11 g/dL (13–18)
- Mean cell volume 108 fL (85–95)
- Platelets 238×10^9/L ($150–400 \times 10^9$)

Q1 How should Mr IH be treated to cover for PCP and atypical pneumonias?
Q2 Would you recommend the use of steroids to help manage Mr IH's hypoxia?

Day 2 An induced sputum test was performed for further respiratory microbiological examination. His arterial blood gases (on 60% oxygen) were:

- PaO_2 11.6 kPa (11.9–13.2)
- $PaCO_2$ 3.28 kPa (4.8–6.3)
- HCO_3 30.3 mmol/L (22–30)
- pH 7.46 (7.35–7.45)
- O_2 sat 90% at rest

Mr IH had been started on high-dose intravenous (IV) co-trimoxazole and IV steroid therapy the previous evening. His current drug therapy was:

- Co-trimoxazole 3840 mg (40 mL strong co-trimoxazole ampoules) IV twice daily
- Methylprednisolone 40 mg IV four times daily
- Metoclopramide 10 mg IV three times daily (for prevention of co-trimoxazole-induced nausea)
- Fluconazole 200 mg orally once daily
- Clarithromycin 500 mg orally twice daily

A full medical and social history was taken. Following this, HIV testing was discussed, and after Mr IH had consented, a blood sample was taken. Mr IH was subsequently found to be positive for HIV antibody and his CD4 lymphocyte count was found to be very low, at 33/microlitre.

Q3 Is a systemic agent appropriate for treating Mr IH's oral *Candida* infection?

Day 4 Results of the induced sputum test confirmed the diagnosis of PCP. Mr IH was now apyrexial with a temperature of 37°C and was feeling better, although he was still short of breath and tired. His nausea was controlled with regular metoclopramide.

Day 7 As Mr IH had improved it was decided on the ward round to change his co-trimoxazole therapy from IV to oral administration. His IV steroids were changed to oral prednisolone. A dose of 40 mg prednisolone twice daily was prescribed with a reducing regimen to follow, which reduced the dose to zero over the next 10 days.

Q4 What oral dose of co-trimoxazole would you recommend?

Day 9 Mr IH's respiratory symptoms were improving. However, he complained of painless blurred vision, which had worsened over the last few days. Examination revealed retinal haemorrhage with exudates in the right eye, characteristic of cytomegalovirus (CMV) retinitis.

Q5 What agents are available for the treatment of CMV infection? What are their advantages and disadvantages?

His haematology, urea and electrolytes were all within normal ranges. The consultant decided to commence treatment with IV ganciclovir at a dose of 5 mg/kg twice daily.

Q6 What monitoring is necessary throughout treatment with IV ganciclovir?
Q7 Would you now consider any adjustment to his PCP treatment, in view of the need to commence ganciclovir?

Day 14 Mr IH was feeling much better. The PCP treatment course was due to be completed and the CMV retinitis was being treated. Mr IH's drug therapy was as follows:

- Clindamycin 600 mg orally four times daily
- Primaquine 30 mg orally once daily
- Prednisolone 40 mg orally once daily
- Metoclopramide 10 mg orally three times daily
- Fluconazole 50 mg orally once daily
- Ganciclovir 320 mg IV twice daily

Q8 What PCP prophylaxis would you recommend for Mr IH?
Q9 In view of his low CD4 cell count, is there any other antibacterial therapy that Mr IH ought to be prescribed?

Mr IH was to complete a 3-week induction course as treatment for his CMV retinitis, at which point he would then continue on maintenance therapy with oral valganciclovir 900 mg once daily.

In view of his low CD4 count and diagnoses of PCP and CMV retinitis, Mr IH needed to start antiretroviral therapy (to fight the virus itself and promote immune system recovery).

Q10 When should antiretroviral therapy usually be commenced to treat established HIV infection? When specifically should Mr IH start treatment?

Q11 What factors ought to be considered when choosing an antiretroviral regimen? Are any specific tests required before treatment is commenced?

It was agreed that Mr IH would start antiretroviral treatment during his hospital admission. Following discussion, Mr IH felt that he required a simple regimen, which he could take once daily if possible.

Q12 Which regimen would you recommend for Mr IH?

Day 20 Mr IH was commenced on triple antiretroviral therapy with tenofovir plus emtricitabine (Truvada) and efavirenz.

Q13 Which classes of pharmacological agents would you advise Mr IH to avoid while on his chosen antiretroviral regimen?

Day 27 Mr IH was due to be discharged from hospital following completion of his PCP and CMV treatment, and having been stable on his new antiretroviral therapy for 1 week.

Q14 Outline a pharmaceutical care plan for Mr IH.

Day 60 Mr IH returned to the outpatient clinic for follow-up. He was taking the following medication:

- Co-trimoxazole 960 mg once daily
- Valganciclovir 900 mg once daily
- Azithromycin 1250 mg once weekly
- Truvada one tablet once daily at night
- Efavirenz 600 mg once daily at night

Blood was taken to check his CD4 lymphocyte count and viral load.

One week later Mr IH returned to clinic to obtain his results. His CD4 count had risen to 150 cells/microlitre and his viral load was now 5000 copies/mL, indicating that the antiretroviral therapy was working.

Mr IH was given a prescription for more medicines and advised to return to clinic 2 months later for these tests to be repeated, then every 3 months.

Month 6 Mr IH was now taking the following medication:

- Co-trimoxazole 960 mg once daily
- Valganciclovir 900 mg once daily
- Azithromycin 1250 mg once weekly
- Atripla one tablet once daily

His CD4 lymphocyte count was 280 cells/microlitre and his viral load was undetectable (<50 copies/mL).

Q15 Is it safe for Mr IH to discontinue his prophylactic medication for PCP, CMV and *Mycobacterium avium* complex (MAC)?

Q16 If Mr IH's viral load result not been undetectable, what tests should have been carried out?

Answers

How should Mr IH be treated to cover for PCP and atypical pneumonias?

A1 **Co-trimoxazole at a dose of 120 mg/kg/day intravenously (IV) in two divided doses (usual dose 3840 mg IV twice daily unless under 60 kg) plus a macrolide antibiotic.**

Co-trimoxazole is highly effective for the treatment of HIV-associated PCP. Treatment should be continued for 14–21 days, depending on the severity of infection. As Mr IH has presented with severe disease, a 3-week course is indicated. Although co-trimoxazole is well absorbed from the gastrointestinal tract, in severe disease it should initially be administered IV, switching to oral therapy as the patient improves. Local practice often deviates from the administration guidelines recommended by the manufacturers. Practice also varies between hospitals, although a common regimen is to infuse IV co-trimoxazole 3840 mg in 500 mL 5% glucose over a 2-hour period. Higher concentrations have been used, e.g. in patients in whom fluid restriction is necessary. In practice, if large doses are given quickly the patient is at greater risk of developing nausea and vomiting. Patients receiving high-dose co-trimoxazole should always be co-prescribed an antiemetic. An appropriate choice is IV metoclopramide, which is effective at controlling drug-induced nausea and vomiting through its action on D_2 receptors in the chemoreceptor trigger zone area of the brain. At higher doses metoclopramide also acts as a 5-hydroxytryptamine (5-HT_3) receptor antagonist. Unfortunately, HIV-positive patients appear to be more susceptible to extrapyramidal side-effects of metoclopramide at high doses. If these occur, domperidone is a suitable alternative, although there is no IV preparation. As Mr IH's HIV status on admission was unknown it is important to consider other possible causes of his chest infection, such as *Legionella* or *Mycoplasma*. Co-trimoxazole is a suitable choice of antibiotic for most bacterial chest infections, but the addition of an oral macrolide antibiotic will cover atypical pneumonias. Once a diagnosis of PCP is confirmed this can be discontinued. While Mr IH is on high-dose co-trimoxazole his renal, liver function and full blood count should be monitored twice each week.

Would you recommend the use of steroids to help manage Mr IH's hypoxia?

A2 **Yes. In patients with moderate to severe PCP and hypoxia there is evidence that by reducing inflammation in the alveoli, gaseous exchange is improved, hypoxia is reduced and the need for mechanical ventilation is prevented.**

It is common practice for patients presenting with a PaO_2 <8 kPa to be prescribed steroids, but many hospitals use a lower PaO_2 threshold. Various regimens have been described (different regimens are used in different treatment centres). One suggested regimen is 40 mg IV methylprednisolone four times daily until the PaO_2 is >10 and there is clinical improvement. This should be followed by a switch to a reducing dose of oral prednisolone, starting with 40 mg twice daily for 5 days then once daily for 5 days.

There are risks associated with prescribing steroids for patients with HIV infection, particularly if establishing a definitive diagnosis of PCP is difficult. Patients with tuberculosis or disseminated fungal infections may present with clinical and radiological features similar to those of PCP. For this reason steroids should be tailed off at the earliest opportunity. In addition, a long-term complication of steroid treatment in HIV infection is osteonecrosis. Finally, it should always be ensured that the steroid courses are completed before the patient finishes the course of co-trimoxazole, otherwise there is risk of reactivation of PCP.

Is a systemic agent appropriate for treating Mr IH's oral *Candida* infection?

A3 **Yes. Patients with early HIV infection can often be managed with topical agents such as nystatin suspension and amphotericin lozenges. However, as they become more immunosuppressed it becomes necessary to use systemic therapy. As Mr IH is acutely unwell and receiving large doses of antibiotics and steroids, it is unlikely that topical treatment will clear his oral *Candida* infection.**

There are five oral azole antifungal agents that can be used for the treatment of oral *Candida*: ketoconazole, fluconazole, itraconazole, voriconazole and posaconazole. The choice will vary between centres. Ketoconazole is nowadays used to a lesser extent than fluconazole because it is metabolised in the liver via the cytochrome P450 microsomal enzyme system, and therefore has the potential to interact with drugs metabolised via the same route, many of which are used in HIV infection. Fluconazole is predominantly excreted unchanged in the urine, so drug interactions are less common. Itraconazole is another option, more often used in its liquid formulation than capsule form owing to the more favourable bioavailability of the liquid, although some centres prefer to reserve the use of itraconazole to treat refractory *Candida* or dermatophyte infections. Voriconazole and posaconazole should be reserved for more serious fungal infections such as aspergillosis or for proven resistant *Candida* infection.

For uncomplicated oral *Candida* a suitable choice is a single dose of fluconazole 400 mg orally. Therapy should be confined to single doses where possible, with courses of treatment reserved for more severe infections in order to minimise the risk of resistance. Mr IH is on steroids, and so the *Candida* infection is likely to persist. For this reason it is sensible to prescribe fluconazole as a course until the oral steroids have been discontinued. A suitable dose would be 200 mg daily until the infection has resolved, then 50 mg daily until the steroids have been discontinued.

As all the above agents have been associated with hepatotoxicity, baseline and then regular liver function tests should be carried out on patients prescribed azole antifungals.

What oral dose of co-trimoxazole would you recommend?

A4 Dosage adjustment is not required when changing from IV to oral co-trimoxazole. Mr IH's IV dose of 3840 mg twice daily can be converted to four 960 mg tablets twice daily, or more commonly two 960 mg tablets four times daily.

Co-trimoxazole is rapidly and well absorbed from the gastrointestinal tract. Patients should be counselled to take the tablets after meals to reduce the probability of gastrointestinal side-effects.

What agents are available for the treatment of CMV infection? What are their advantages and disadvantages?

A5 There are four agents available for the treatment of CMV retinitis: IV ganciclovir, foscarnet, cidofovir and the oral preparation valganciclovir.

Ganciclovir is a nucleoside analogue closely related in structure and mode of action to aciclovir, but with activity against additional members of the herpes group of viruses, including CMV. The treatment dose is 5 mg/kg IV twice daily for 3 weeks. Its main disadvantage is bone marrow suppression. Foscarnet is a pyrophosphate analogue which inhibits the replication of herpes viruses. The treatment dose is 90 mg/kg IV twice daily for 3 weeks. Its main disadvantages are nephrotoxicity, electrolyte disturbances, and the fact that there is no oral preparation available. Cidofovir is a nucleotide analogue which is administered once weekly for 2 weeks during induction therapy and then once every 2 weeks as maintenance therapy, each dose being 5 mg/kg. The main advantage of treatment with cidofovir is the convenient dosing schedule. The main drawback is its renal toxicity. Patients must receive concomitant IV hydration and oral probenecid, which protects the kidneys by blocking secretion of the drug into the renal tubules. Co-administration of other nephrotoxic drugs is absolutely contraindicated, which can often lead to treatment management problems.

Most centres will use ganciclovir as first-choice treatment, reserving cidofovir and foscarnet for patients with bone marrow suppression or those who have relapsed on ganciclovir.

Valganciclovir is an oral prodrug of ganciclovir. It is administered at a dose of 900 mg twice daily as induction treatment, and 900 mg once daily as maintenance thereafter. Its main advantage is that is allows treatment as an outpatient, but many ophthalmologists may be hesitant about using this for sight-threatening CMV retinitis, as success relies on patient adherence to therapy. Its main disadvantage is its high cost, and it shares all the same toxicities as ganciclovir.

Mr IH has no specific contraindications to any of the above treatment options. Although his WBC count and haemoglobin levels seem low, these are relatively normal for someone with advanced HIV disease and do not contraindicate the use of ganciclovir/valganciclovir.

What monitoring is necessary throughout treatment with IV ganciclovir?

A6 **All patients should have a full blood count and urea and electrolyte monitoring twice weekly during induction therapy.**

The major side-effect of ganciclovir is bone marrow suppression. If neutropenia occurs patients may require treatment with colony-stimulating factor, or a switch to alternative therapy. Ganciclovir is excreted renally, and dose adjustment is required as renal function declines. Electrolyte results should be monitored twice weekly and the patient's calculated creatinine clearance should be checked to ensure the dose prescribed is still appropriate.

Would you now consider any adjustment to his PCP treatment in view of the need to commence ganciclovir?

A7 **One option is to switch to clindamycin and primaquine as alternative treatment for his PCP.**

As previously discussed, the major toxicity of ganciclovir is bone marrow suppression. Co-trimoxazole can also cause haematological changes, mainly leukopenia, neutropenia, thrombocytopenia and, to a lesser extent, agranulocytosis. There is a high risk of neutropenia if the two drugs are co-prescribed. Different centres will have different treatment protocols, but one option is to consider an alternative form of PCP treatment, particularly now that clinical improvement has been made. Second-line treatment for PCP is clindamycin 600 mg orally or IV four times daily combined with primaquine 30 mg orally once daily. The other option is to continue with the co-trimoxazole and monitor for haematological toxicity, and use colony-stimulating factors when necessary.

What PCP prophylaxis would you recommend for Mr IH?

A8 Oral co-trimoxazole 960 mg once daily or three times a week.

HIV-positive patients are at risk of PCP infection once their CD4 lymphocyte count falls below 200 cells/microlitre. It is recommended practice to prescribe primary prophylaxis for all such patients. Secondary prophylaxis should be given to all patients following an acute episode of PCP. Mr IH should continue with PCP prophylaxis until his immune system function has been restored sufficiently by the use of antiretroviral medication. Co-trimoxazole has been shown in large clinical trials to be the most effective agent for both primary and secondary PCP prophylaxis. Common dose regimens are 960 mg daily, 480 mg daily and 960 mg three times a week. A thrice-weekly dosage of 960 mg, usually taken on Monday, Wednesday and Friday, appears to be as effective as 960 mg daily and is accompanied by a lower incidence of side-effects. In addition, co-trimoxazole will offer patients some protection against infection with *Toxoplasma gondii*, a protozoon that affects the brain, as well as some other bacterial infections.

Other agents that can be used for PCP prophylaxis in the presence of co-trimoxazole allergy include dapsone (100 mg daily), nebulised pentamidine isetionate (300 mg every 2–4 weeks) or atovaquone (750 mg twice daily).

Up to 20% of patients develop a skin rash while taking co-trimoxazole. Such patients can be changed to one of the alternative agents described above, or a desensitisation regimen can be tried. This involves minute doses being given initially, increasing gradually over a 10-day period to the therapeutic dose of 960 mg. If patients have previously had a co-trimoxazole-associated rash there is an increased risk of a rash in patients treated with dapsone, owing to its sulphonamide moiety.

In view of his low CD4 cell count, is there any other antibacterial therapy that Mr IH ought to be prescribed?

A9 Mr IH should be started on azithromycin 1250 mg once a week as prophylaxis against MAC (*Mycobacterium avium* complex).

Mr IH has a CD4 lymphocyte count of only 33 cells/microlitre. The Centres for Disease Control (CDC) and other guidelines indicate that patients with CD4 counts <50 cells/microlitre should receive prophylaxis for MAC. Clarithromycin or azithromycin are the preferred prophylactic agents for MAC, but if they cannot be tolerated rifabutin is an alternative, although rifabutin-associated drug interactions can make this agent difficult to use. A suitable prophylactic regimen for Mr IH would be azithromycin 1250 mg orally once weekly.

When should antiretroviral therapy usually be commenced to treat HIV infection? When specifically should Mr IH start treatment?

A10 The 2008 British HIV Association (BHIVA) guidelines advise that initiation of therapy should be recommended for all patients with a confirmed CD4 cell count of <350 cells/microlitre (confirmed in at least one consecutive blood sample). In addition, it has been clearly shown that starting therapy with a CD4 cell count <200 cells/microlitre is associated with a substantially greater risk of disease progression and death. Every effort should therefore be made to start treatment before the CD4 cell count has fallen to <200 cells/microlitre.

Given that adherence is vital for treatment success, and that this may be based to some extent on patient perception of the need for treatment, it is advisable to begin discussions about the relative advantages and disadvantages of starting treatment at an earlier stage, for example when the CD4 count drops to just below 500 cells/microlitre.

In a small number of patients, treatment may be started or considered before the CD4 count is <350. They include the following:

(a) Aquired immunodeficiency syndrome (AIDS) diagnosis (e.g. Kaposi's sarcoma).
(b) Hepatitis B infection where treatment of hepatitis B is indicated.
(c) Low CD4%. The CD4% is the percentage of functional lymphocytes that are CD4 cells and is thus a measurement that takes into account the total lymphocyte count when assessing immune system health. It is felt by many to be a more reliable indicator of immune system health than the CD4 count. Typically, HIV-negative people will have a CD4% of about 40%, but an HIV-positive person would have a

CD4% of 25% or less. In this situation, a CD4% <14%, at which PCP prophylaxis would be indicated, may be a factor prompting early antiretroviral therapy.

Mr IH has a diagnosis of PCP and CMV retinitis – both classified as AIDS-defining diagnoses – and a CD4 count of only 33 cells/microlitre. He should therefore start antiretroviral therapy. A decision has to be made as to whether treatment is urgent, or whether it is better to wait until the acute infections have been treated. Mr IH is severely immunocompromised, and therefore there is some urgency to start therapy. Early initiation needs to be balanced against the risks of drug interactions, overlapping toxicities and the risk of immune reconstitution disease/syndrome (IRS). IRS manifests as acute respiratory failure following initiation of antiretroviral therapy soon after treatment for PCP, and is thought to be the immune system reacting in an exaggerated fashion to microbial antigens. Despite these potential disadvantages, a recent study has suggested that in the majority of patients presenting with opportunistic disease, antiretroviral therapy should be started early.

What factors ought to be considered when choosing an antiretroviral regimen? Are any specific tests required before treatment is commenced?

A11 Factors such as number of tablets, side-effects, resistance patterns, drug interactions, comorbid conditions and viral load need to be considered before deciding on a regimen.

Before any antiretroviral treatment is begun, all patients require a resistance test. If abacavir is being considered as part of the regimen, the patient will require an HLA-B*5701 test to detect genetic predisposition to abacavir hypersensitivity. Only patients who are HLA-B*5701-negative should receive abacavir.

Patients co-infected with hepatitis B require a regimen that will treat both infections. The patient's drug history must be taken into account when deciding on a regimen, as numerous drug interactions can occur with antiretroviral agents owing to their metabolism via the cytochrome P450 microsomal enzyme system. Some antiretroviral regimens are considered more potent than others and therefore safer to use in patients with high viral loads. Certain regimens have been shown to increase the long-term risks of cardiovascular disease: this should be particularly borne in mind in patients already at increased risk (smoking, obesity, family history). Certain antiretroviral combinations have been shown to be safe and effective at reducing vertical transmission, and so are recommended for pregnant women.

Which regimen would you recommend for Mr IH?

A12 A suitable option for Mr IH is a three-drug combination of tenofovir, emtricitabine and efavirenz.

There are three classes of antiretroviral drug that have so far been used routinely as first-line therapy for treatment-naive patients: nucleoside/tide reverse transcriptase inhibitors (NRTIs), non-nucleoside reverse transcriptase inhibitors (NNRTIs), and protease inhibitors (PIs). Other classes exist but are usually reserved for later in treatment, when patients are resistant to the groups named above. It is common practice to use an NNRTI or PI in combination with two NRTIs. This is commonly referred to as the nucleotide backbone. A combination of three or more effective drugs is termed highly active antiretroviral therapy (HAART) and is the standard of care in the developed world.

The 2008 BHIVA guidelines recommend efavirenz (an NNRTI) as standard first-line therapy for all patients, reserving boosted PIs inhibitors for certain groups, e.g. those with primary NNRTI resistance, pregnant women or patients with a history of certain psychiatric illness. Nevirapine (another NNRTI) should be reserved for women wishing to become pregnant or for patients with mental health problems, but must be used within the set CD4 cell count criteria (consult product literature).

Truvada (tenofovir/emtricitabine) and Kivexa (abacavir/lamivudine) are both available as once-daily preparations of co-formulated tablets containing two NRTIs and are therefore the preferred options for the nucleotide backbone. However, Kivexa should be reserved for those patients who are HLA-B*5701 negative and used with caution in those with high viral loads (>100 000 copies/mL) or where there is significant risk of cardiovascular disease. ACTG study 5202 demonstrated that patients started on Kivexa with a viral load >100 000 copies/mL were significantly less likely to achieve an undetectable viral load than those started on Truvada, and the D:A:D study revealed a correlation between the incidence of myocardial infarction and abacavir therapy. Given these findings, at the time of writing the BHIVA guidelines suggest that Kivexa should be reserved for patients in whom Truvada is contraindicated.

Atripla is a co-formulated product containing all three drugs that are recommended for Mr IH: tenofovir, emtricitabine and efavirenz. The Summary of Product Characteristics for Atripla specifies that it should be used in patients already stable on antiretroviral therapy with a viral load <50 copies/mL; however, in clinical practice in the UK it is now routinely used in some centres for patients commencing HAART for the first time, because of its convenience and patient preference.

Which classes of pharmacological agent would you advise the patient to avoid while on his chosen antiretroviral regimen?

A13 Mr IH should be advised to avoid medicines capable of inducing liver enzymes, e.g. phenytoin, carbamazepine and St John's wort.

Efavirenz is metabolised primarily in the liver via the cytochrome P450 microsomal enzyme system. The primary enzyme responsible for its metabolism is CYP4503A4. This is responsible for the metabolism of many other drugs, and is also subject to potential enzyme induction or inhibition. Enzyme induction would lead to a reduction in plasma efavirenz drug levels, thereby increasing the development of drug resistance and virological failure. Mr IH should be advised to consult a specialist HIV pharmacist or HIV physician before receiving any prescribed medicines from a general practitioner (GP). Rifampicin is another enzyme inducer that interacts with efavirenz; however, this may be prescribed with careful dose adjustment by a physician specialising in both HIV and tuberculosis.

Efavirenz itself acts as a mixed enzyme inducer/inhibitor. It has been shown to lower plasma methadone levels and induce withdrawal in patients stabilised on methadone maintenance. An increase in the patient's methadone maintenance dose may sometimes be required.

Tenofovir and emtricitabine are renally excreted and therefore do not exhibit metabolic drug–drug interactions.

Outline a pharmaceutical care plan for Mr IH.

A14 The pharmaceutical care plan for Mr IH should include the following:

(a) Ensure that PCP prophylaxis is prescribed in the form of co-trimoxazole 960 mg once daily or three times each week.
(b) Ensure that the steroid course is reduced to zero prior to discharge, as remaining on steroids after completion of the PCP treatment course is not recommended.
(c) Ensure the patient is prescribed the correct dose of oral valganciclovir as maintenance treatment for his CMV retinitis following completion of the 3-week treatment with IV ganciclovir.
(d) Ensure that arrangements have been made for the patient to have blood monitoring performed at least every 2 weeks while he is taking valganciclovir.
(e) Counsel Mr IH on his new antiretroviral medication, paying particular attention to the importance of adherence to maintain viral control and prevent the development of resistance. Side-effects of efavirenz include drowsiness, dizziness, sleep disturbance and

hallucinations. The patient should be advised to return to clinic if these become troublesome.

(f) Counsel Mr IH on the remainder of his discharge medication.

Is it safe for Mr IH to discontinue his prophylactic medication for PCP, CMV and *Mycobacterium avium* complex (MAC)?

A15 It is safe for him to stop his PCP prophylaxis and MAC prophylaxis. His CMV retinitis maintenance therapy may be stopped provided his CMV infection is quiescent.

PCP prophylaxis may be safely discontinued if the CD4 count is maintained >200 cells/microlitre for 3 months. If the CD4 count falls below this, prophylaxis should be recommenced.

The Centers for Disease Control and Prevention (CDC) guidelines indicate that patients with CD4 lymphocyte counts <50 cells/microlitre should receive prophylaxis for MAC. Primary prophylaxis can be discontinued with minimal risk of developing MAC in patients who have responded to HAART, with an increase in the CD4 count >100 cells/microlitre for at least 3 months. Secondary prophylaxis or maintenance therapy is lifelong, unless immune reconstitution occurs as a consequence of HAART. There are few firm recommendations on when to discontinue secondary prophylaxis, but patients appear to have a low risk of recurrence if they have completed a course of at least 12 months of MAC treatment, are clinically well, and have a sustained increase over 3–6 months in their CD4 count to >100 cells/microlitre with HAART. Prophylaxis should be reintroduced if the CD4 count falls to <100 cells/microlitre (although some physicians use a lower cut-off of 50 cells/microlitre for primary prophylaxis).

In CMV retinitis infection a maintenance regimen must be chosen for the patient in order to prevent reactivation of disease and risk of blindness. The maintenance phase for CMV retinitis is indefinite, or until an adequate CD4 count rise has been achieved with HAART. Maintenance treatment can often be safely discontinued once the CD4 count has risen above 100 cells/microlitre. As some patients will not receive specific CMV immunity despite an increase in CD4 lymphocyte cells, these patients require regular ophthalmological follow-up. In addition, the CD4 count needs to be monitored as patients may relapse if it falls below 50 cells/microlitre. There are no definitive guidelines for when to stop CMV maintenance therapy, but generally patients are treated until the CD4 count rises to >100 cells/microlitre. Therapy is then continued for 3 months, at which point it may be stopped if the CMV is inactive, the CD4 remains >100 cells/microlitre and the patient's HIV viral load is undetectable.

If Mr IH's viral load result had not been undetectable, what tests should be carried out?

A16 **A repeat viral load test should always be performed. Following this, a resistance test is required. Therapeutic drug monitoring may also be useful. If the patient needs to change therapy and did not have this test prior to commencing HAART, an HLA*5701 genetic test should be performed to detect for genetic predisposition to abacavir hypersensitivity.**

When a patient has previously had a stable undetectable viral load which then becomes detectable, a repeat test should always be performed to check that the result is not just a 'blip'. The two tests should normally be performed a month apart. Often at times of acute illness a patient's viral load can become detectable and later return to undetectable levels without further intervention.

If a detectable viral load is confirmed then a resistance test should be performed on a sample of blood taken from the patient, during his current drug therapy. Genotypic tests are widely available and represent the most cost-effective approach for resistance testing in both treatment-naive and experienced patients. The genotypic test is used to identify specific mutations in the viral genome (compared to wild-type virus). Certain mutations are known to convey resistance to specific drugs. The interpretation of resistance test results is complex, and especially difficult with new drugs, and expert advice should be sought with complex or unusual resistance profiles. It is now common for laboratories performing resistance testing to also provide expert support for their service.

Therapeutic drug monitoring for some antiretroviral drugs is available and can provide a useful tool to monitor patient adherence to therapy. In the case of Mr IH, therapeutic drug monitoring of efavirenz is readily available. It is also available for PIs, but less established for the NRTI drugs, as with this group it is the intracellular triphosphate levels of the drug that are important, rather than the plasma levels.

If drugs levels are adequate it is likely that resistance to some or all of the therapy will have developed, and the exact extent of this will be demonstrated by the resistance test results. If the drug levels are inadequate and the patient is still sensitive to the same therapy according to the resistance profile, a dose increase may be an option, assuming the patient is adhering to treatment.

Acknowledgements

The author wishes to thank Dr Mark Nelson MA MBBS FRCP, HIV Consultant at Chelsea and Westminster Hospital, London, and Ms Leoni

Swaden MRPharmS, Consultant HIV Pharmacist at The Royal Free Hospital, London, for their assistance.

Further reading

Gazzard B (ed.). *AIDS Care Handbook*. Mediscript, London, 2002.

Gazzard BG on behalf of the BHIVA Treatment Guidelines Writing Group. British HIV Association (BHIVA) Guidelines for the treatment of HIV-1-infected adults with antiretroviral therapy 2008. www.bhiva.org.

Medical Management of HIV. www.Hopkins-HIVGuide.org.

Oxford Handbook of Genitourinary Medicine, HIV and AIDS. Oxford Medical Publications, Oxford, 2007.

Recommendations from Centres for Disease Control, the National Institutes of Health, the HIV Medicine Association of the Infectious Diseases Society of America and the Paediatric Infectious Diseases Society. Guidelines for Prevention and Treatment of Opportunistic Infections in HIV-Infected Adults and Adolescents – June 18, 2008. www.aidsinfo.nih.gov.

Useful websites

www.i-base.info
www.hiv-druginteractions.org

25

Oncology

Nicola Stoner

Case study and questions

Day 1 Mrs DC, a 49-year-old woman, was referred to the breast clinic at the hospital by her general practitioner (GP) after presenting with a self-detected lump in her left breast. Following an ultrasound, fine needle biopsy and mammogram she underwent a lumpectomy and wide local excision. She was diagnosed with breast cancer (stage T2N1 (1/9) M0). Her tumour was found to be 26 mm, grade 3, mixed invasive ductal and infiltrating lobular carcinoma which was oestrogen-receptor and progestogen-receptor positive, and also HER2 positive.

There was no family history of breast cancer. Mrs DC's father had been diagnosed with prostate cancer aged 72, but was still alive and well. Mrs DC had two children, a daughter aged 21 who was away at university and a son aged 15 who was still at home. She had never smoked, and drank approximately four units of alcohol per week.

Mrs DC was taking hormone replacement therapy, as she was post-menopausal. She had no known drug allergies.

Q1 What advice should be given to Mrs DC about her current medication?

Her treatment plan was to receive adjuvant FEC75 (5-fluorouracil, epirubicin, cyclophosphamide) chemotherapy for four cycles, followed by four cycles of adjuvant docetaxel chemotherapy. Adjuvant trastuzumab chemotherapy was to be given concurrently with the docetaxel chemotherapy. The chemotherapy treatment was to be followed by local radiotherapy and hormonal therapy with anastrozole 1 mg orally daily.

Based on Adjuvant On Line, adjuvant chemotherapy with FEC followed by docetaxel would offer a 12.7 % improvement in survival at 10 years in addition to an 11.5% survival improvement from the adjuvant anastrazole.

Day 30 Mrs DC attended the chemotherapy day unit for cycle 1 of FEC75 chemotherapy. Her weight was 79 kg, her height 1.72 m, and her body surface area 1.94 m². Her chemotherapy was prescribed as follows:

- FEC75 chemotherapy every 3 weeks:
  - 5-fluorouracil 600 mg/m² = 1164 mg intravenous bolus (IVb) day 1
  - Epirubicin 75 mg/m² = 146 mg IVb day 1
  - Cyclophosphamide 600 mg/m² = 1164 mg IVb day 1

Mrs DC was prescribed antiemetics with her chemotherapy according to the local hospital policy:

- Granisetron 2 mg once daily orally 1 hour prior to FEC75 chemotherapy, and a second dose 24 hours later
- Dexamethasone 8 mg twice daily orally for three doses, starting the morning of chemotherapy
- Metoclopramide 10 mg four times daily orally starting the morning of chemotherapy for 3 days regularly, then if required

Her biochemistry and haematology results prior to cycle 1 were as follows:

Biochemistry results:

- Sodium 139 mmol/L (reference range 135–145)
- Potassium 4.2 mmol/L (3.5–5.0)
- Urea 5.7 mmol/L (2.5–6.7)
- Creatinine 95 micromol/L (70–150)
- Bilirubin 4 micromol/L (3–17
- Alanine aminotransferase (ALT) 16 IU/L (10–45)
- Alkaline phosphatase (ALP) 150 IU/L (95–320)
- Gamma-glutamyltransferase (GGT) 25 IU/L (15–40)
- Phosphate 1.12 mmol/L (0.8–1.45)
- Magnesium 0.81 mmol/L (0.75–1.05)
- Lactate dehydrogenase (LDH) 208 IU/L (110–250)

Her calculated creatinine clearance was 79 mL/min using the Cockcroft–Gault formula.

Haematology results were:

- Haemoglobin 14 g/dL (13–17)
- White cells 8.63 × 10⁹/L (4–11)
- Platelets 204 × 10⁹/L (150–400)
- Neutrophils 6.10 × 10⁹/L (2–7)

Q2 Outline a pharmaceutical care plan for Mrs DC.
Q3 Describe how you would screen this chemotherapy prescription for Mrs DC clinically.
Q4 Is the combination of antiemetics prescribed for Mrs DC appropriate? Why?

Q5 Which order should the chemotherapy drugs be administered in, and why?

Q6 How would you recommend the nursing staff manage an extravasation of each of the chemotherapy drugs administered?

Day 52 Mrs DC attended for assessment prior to cycle 2 of FEC75 chemotherapy. She complained of suffering from grade 2 nausea and vomiting after her first cycle. She had experienced moderate nausea starting the evening of treatment, and her oral intake had decreased without significant weight loss, dehydration or malnutrition. This continued for 3–4 days. The vomiting had started at bedtime the night of the chemotherapy. She had vomited twice overnight and once the following morning. She had taken her antiemetics as prescribed.

Q7 How would you advise Mrs DC's antiemetic regimen be adjusted?

Mrs DC's neutrophil count was 0.9×10^9/L (2–7). The consultant decided to go ahead with chemotherapy on time at the full dose, but to add in a granulocyte colony-stimulating factor (G-CSF) to the regimen.

Q8 Is this an appropriate course of action? Discuss your answer.

Day 73 Mrs DC attended for cycle 3 of FEC75 chemotherapy. She complained of experiencing stomach discomfort in the 3 weeks between treatments, which had been relieved in the last week by lactulose and opening her bowels.

Q9 What was the most likely cause of Mrs DC's stomach discomfort? What prophylactic treatment would you recommend be prescribed with her third cycle of chemotherapy?

Day 84 Mrs DC attended for cycle 4 FEC75 chemotherapy.

Q10 What should Mrs DC be prescribed in preparation for starting docetaxel and trastuzumab chemotherapy in 3 weeks' time? What tests must be undertaken prior to this regimen?

Q11 How would you counsel Mrs DC?

Day 105 An 8 mg/kg loading dose of trastuzumab (632 mg) was prescribed with the first cycle of docetaxel 100 mg/m^2 (194 mg), then a maintenance dose of traztuzmab 6 mg/kg (474 mg) every 3 weeks thereafter.

Q12 What should the duration of the trastuzumab treatment be?

Q13 If Mrs DC has a delay in her trastuzumab treatment at any stage, how should this be managed?

At the end of the docetaxel chemotherapy regimen Mrs DC was prescribed anastrozole 1 mg daily and AdCal one daily. She was referred for a dual-energy X-ray absorptiometry (DEXA) bone density scan at the same time as starting her anastrozole therapy.

Q14 How would you counsel this patient with respect to the anastrozole? Why was the AdCal prescribed?
Q15 How long should anastrazole treatment be continued for?

Mrs DC completed her planned treatment and was followed up at the hospital regularly.

Year 3 During a routine blood test her biochemistry results were reported as follows:

- Sodium 142 mmol/L (135–145)
- Potassium 3.9 mmol/L (3.5–5.0)
- Urea 6.0 mmol/L (2.5–6.7)
- Creatinine 97 micromol/L (70–150)
- Bilirubin 22 micromol/L (3–17)
- ALT 60 IU/L (10–45)
- ALP 418 IU/L (95–320)
- GGT 72 IU/L (15–40)
- Phosphate 1.12 mmol/L (0.8–1.45)
- Magnesium 0.81 mmol/L (0.75–1.05)
- LDH 681 IU/L (110–250)

Her calculated creatinine clearance using the Cockcroft–Gault formula was 77 mL/min. Her height was recorded as 1.72 m, weight 82 kg, and body surface area 1.98 m^2.

She complained of pain over her left upper ribs. An ultrasound scan, bone scan, computed tomography (CT) scan and magnetic resonance imaging (MRI) showed that her disease had metastasised to her liver and bones. Mrs DC was advised of her metastatic disease and the need for further treatment. Her anastrozole therapy was stopped and she was prescribed docetaxel and trastuzumab, plus bisphosphonate therapy.

Q16 Why was bisphosphonate therapy started? Which bisphosphonate should be prescribed?
Q17 What information should be given to Mrs DC about her bisphosphonate treatment?
Q18 Is it appropriate to restart trastuzumab? What dose should be prescribed?
Q19 Is it appropriate to restart docetaxel? What dose should be prescribed?

Following six cycles of docetaxel a CT scan confirmed a marked response in the liver and sclerosis of the bone metastases, which may imply a degree of healing. Mrs DC had a repeat cardiac echogram which was normal. An MRI scan showed no impingement of disease on the spinal cord and confirmed healing of the bony metastases, some of which were appearing more sclerotic. She had thus had an excellent response to docetaxel therapy and it was decided to continue treatment with pamidronate and trastuzumab.

Q20 Is it appropriate to continue pamidronate and trastuzumab treatment? How long should they be continued for?
Q21 What monitoring is required?

Year 4 A year after being diagnosed with metastatic disease, Mrs DC had a repeat MRI scan which showed stable disease in her bones. A CT scan showed fewer and smaller liver metastases. Therefore, she continued to have responding disease and it was decided to continue with pamidronate and trastuzumab treatment. A repeat cardiac echogram showed good systolic function, with an ejection fraction of 55%.

Year 5 Mrs DC had started to complain of headaches, initially in the morning, then lasting all day (and for the last 5 days). She also had mild nausea and general lethargy. She had a feeling of pressure in her head. An MRI scan of the brain showed multiple brain metastases, including one near the fourth ventricle. The metastases were mainly in the cerebellum. The plan was to start dexamethasone 8 mg twice daily orally for 1 week, then reduce the dose weekly over the following few weeks to the lowest effective dose. Radiotherapy to the brain was to be administered daily for five sessions at 20 Gy. Mrs DC was told she was no longer able to drive.

Q22 How would you counsel Mrs DC on her dexamethasone treatment?

Mrs DC was prescribed capecitabine and lapatinib every 3 weeks.

Q23 What should happen with Mrs DC's pamidronate and trastuzumab treatment?
Q24 What considerations need to be taken into account when prescribing oral chemotherapy?
Q25 How should Mrs DC be counselled on her oral chemotherapy?
Q26 What side-effects should she be warned about?
Q27 What supportive treatment should be prescribed concurrently?

A CT scan was performed after three courses of lapatinib and capecitabine and showed a reduction in one of the cerebellar lesions, which had reduced in size from 16 mm at the start of treatment to 10 mm. The right parietal lobe lesion was unchanged at 7 mm. There was no significant change to the left-sided cerebellar lesions. No liver metastases were identified on the scan. It was agreed that Mrs DC was to proceed with a further three cycles of lapatinib and capecitabine.

Q28 How long should lapatinib and capecitabine treatment be continued for?

A CT scan at the end of six cycles of lapatinib and capecitabine showed no significant change from the scan that had been performed at the end of three cycles of treatment.

Mrs DC was advised to discontinue her capecitabine treatment and continue with the lapatinib. She was able to maintain a relatively normal quality of life for a further 6 months before her disease progressed further. Mrs DC then refused any further chemotherapy and her symptoms were controlled by the palliative care team until her death 3 months later.

Answers

What advice should be given to Mrs DC about her current medication?

A1 Mrs DC must be advised to stop her hormone replacement therapy.

As Mrs DC has oestrogen-receptor and progestogen-receptor positive breast cancer, the hormone replacement therapy could stimulate the growth of any remaining cancer cells in the body. Hormone replacement therapy is contraindicated in breast cancer. She could be advised of alternative treatments to manage her menopausal symptoms if necessary.

Outline a pharmaceutical care plan for Mrs DC.

A2 A pharmaceutical care plan for Mrs DC should include the following:

(a) Advise on the choice and dose of any supportive drug therapy required with Mrs DC's chemotherapy regimen.
(b) Ensure that all the medication is prescribed and administered correctly, through both verbal and written communication with the nursing and medical staff.
(c) Ensure that Mrs DC's prescribed treatment is made available in a timely manner.
(d) Counsel Mrs DC on her prescribed medication to ensure she is aware of how to take it appropriately, to ensure adherence.

(e) Counsel Mrs DC on the possible side-effects of her treatment, and how to manage them if they occur.
(f) Counsel Mrs DC on 24-hour contact numbers if she should have any problems and need to contact the hospital.
(g) Mrs DC must be monitored for the side-effects of her chemotherapy treatment. These need to be assessed and her treatment adjusted accordingly at the second cycle of treatment.

Describe how you would screen this chemotherapy prescription for Mrs DC clinically.

A3 All chemotherapy prescriptions for both oral and intravenous (IV) chemotherapy must be clinically screened by a pharmacist. The items that should be checked are as follows:

(a) The patient's name, date of birth, and hospital number on the prescription must be checked against the notes, to ensure that the prescription matches the patient.
(b) The pharmacist must check that the correct chemotherapy regimen has been prescribed.
(c) The patient's height and weight must be checked as to their accuracy with the patient records.
(d) The patient's surface area calculation must be checked either with a nomogram or with the following calculation:

$$\text{Surface area (m}^2\text{)} = \sqrt{\text{height (cm)} \times \text{weight (kg)} / 3600}$$

(e) Surface area is often capped at 2 or 2.2 m^2. Local policy on this should be checked.
(f) Check the patient's ideal body weight. If they are significantly more or less than the ideal, discuss with doctor:

$$\text{Ideal body weight (IBW) kg} = (\text{height (m)} \times \text{height (m)} \times 25)$$

(g) The chemotherapy drug doses must be checked against the chemotherapy protocol. Check the correct drugs have been prescribed. Check maximum doses according to the protocol.
(h) Check the frequency of intended cycles and appropriate interval since any previous chemotherapy.
(i) Check patient's age, as some doses/protocols are age related.
(j) Check cumulative lifetime doses, i.e. for anthracyclines (e.g. doxorubicin maximum cumulative dose 550 mg/m^2 and bleomycin maximum cumulative dose 500 000 units).
(k) The chemotherapy dose calculations must be checked. Check whether any patient-specific modifications are required.

(l) The biochemistry must be checked to see whether any dose reduction is required, e.g. impaired renal function, clotting disorders, liver function tests (when appropriate for drug). Doses may need to be adjusted according to renal and liver function. Cyclophosphamide is excreted renally and can be nephrotoxic, although usually at higher doses. 5-Fluorouracil is mainly eliminated by the liver. Etoposide is metabolised in the liver. The patient's creatinine clearance should be calculated using the Cockcroft–Gault equation as an estimation.

Cockroft–Gault equation in adults:

$$\text{Creatinine clearance (mL/min)} = \frac{F\,(140 - \text{age}) \times \text{weight (kg)}}{\text{Serum creatinine (micromol/L)}}$$

where F = 1.04 in females and 1.23 in males.

(m) Haematology must be checked. The full blood count must be acceptable before chemotherapy is administered. The neutrophil count should be $>1.5 \times 10^9$/L and the platelets $>100 \times 10^9$/L. However, as this chemotherapy is curative in intent, treatment may be able to proceed with a lower blood count than for palliative chemotherapy, so local policies should be checked.

(n) Check whether there are any drug interactions between the chemotherapy and the patient's regular medication, and whether there are any drugs that are contraindicated with the chemotherapy.

Is the combination of antiemetics prescribed for Mrs DC appropriate? Why?

A4 **Yes, the combination of antiemetics prescribed for Mrs DC is appropriate because she has been prescribed emetogenic chemotherapy.**

FEC75 chemotherapy is moderately emetogenic. It is essential that a combination of antiemetics is prescribed to prevent nausea and vomiting. If patients experience nausea and vomiting with chemotherapy they are at higher risk of developing anticipatory nausea and vomiting prior to their next cycle of treatment.

Chemotherapy causes acute nausea and vomiting through the release of serotonin from the enterochromaffin cells of the gut mucosa. This stimulates vagal afferents in the gut mucosa, which send stimuli to the chemotherapy receptor trigger zone in the fourth ventricle of the brain stem. This then stimulates the vomiting centre to cause nausea and vomiting. It is therefore essential that a 5-HT_3 receptor antagonist antiemetic is prescribed acutely. As cyclophosphamide can have a delayed onset of acute nausea and vomiting, it is also essential to ensure that a 5-HT_3 receptor antagonist is continued for at least 36 hours.

Dexamethasone increases the efficacy of the 5-HT_3 receptor antagonists by 20–30%, and is a useful adjunct to chemotherapy antiemetic therapy. It is also an effective treatment for delayed nausea and vomiting, which occurs after the first 24 hours. The mechanism of delayed nausea and vomiting has not been established.

Metoclopramide is a dopamine receptor antagonist, which blocks both central and peripheral receptors that are involved in the vomiting process. Patients should be advised to take this regularly for at least 3 days after chemotherapy, then if required.

Which order should the chemotherapy drugs be administered in, and why?

A5 The chemotherapy with the greatest risk of extravasation should be administered first, followed by the next most irritant and finally the least irritant. Epirubicin is a vesicant, cyclophosphamide is neutral and 5-fluorouracil is an inflammatory agent.

Vesicant drugs can cause pain, inflammation, and blistering of the skin and underlying tissue, which can cause tissue death and necrosis. Inflammatory agents can cause mild to moderate inflammation in the local tissues. Neutral agents do not cause inflammation or damage. The most vesicant drug should be administered first while the access site is most patent. In this case, the order of chemotherapy administration should be as follows:

1. Epirubicin.
2. 5-Fluorouracil.
3. Cyclophosphamide.

How would you recommend the nursing staff manage an extravasation of each of the chemotherapy drugs administered?

A6 The extravasation of each of the chemotherapy drugs must be managed according to the extravasation risk of each and the local extravasation policy, using the extravasation kit, which must be available in areas where chemotherapy is administered.

Extravasation is the inappropriate or accidental administration of drug into the subcutaneous or subdermal tissues, instead of into the intended IV compartment. A number of agents used in cancer chemotherapy are extremely damaging if they extravasate or infiltrate into the tissues rather than remain within the vasculature. Extravasation may have occurred if there is evidence of:

(a) Pain on administration, either at the cannulation site or around the area.
(b) Swelling around or above the cannulation site.
(c) Redness or heat at or around the area.

If left undiagnosed or inappropriately treated, extravasation can cause necrosis and functional loss of the tissue and limb concerned. Extravasation can occur with any IV injection, but is only considered to be a problem with compounds known to be vesicant or irritant. Appropriately treated extravasation which is dealt with within 24 hours should ensure that the patient has no further problems.

The risk factors associated with extravasation include:

(a) Administration technique: risk is increased if staff are inadequately trained.
(b) Administration device: the use of unsuitable cannulae, e.g. >24 hours old.
(c) Location of cannulation site: the forearm is the favoured site.
(d) Patient factors. These include:
    (i) Underlying conditions such as lymphoedema, diabetes, and peripheral circulatory diseases.
    (ii) Patient age: additional precautions are required for paediatric and elderly patients.
(e) Concurrent medication such as steroids, anticoagulants
(f) The physical properties of the drugs concerned

Prevention of extravasation is best, using one or more of the following techniques:

(a) Use of a central line for slow infusions of high-risk drugs.
(b) Administer cytotoxic drugs through a recently sited cannula.
(c) Ensure the cannula cannot be dislodged during drug administration.
(d) Ensure the cannula is patent prior to administration.
(e) Administer vesicants by slow IV push into the side arm of a fast-running IV infusion of a compatible solution.
(f) Administer the most vesicant drug first (as discussed in A5).
(g) Assess the site continuously for any signs of redness or swelling.
(h) Ensure the patient is aware of extravasation risks and reports any burning or pain on administration of the drug.
(i) Take time and do not rush drug administration.

If extravasation is thought to have occurred, the local extravasation policy must be followed. Administration of the infusion or injection should be stopped immediately, and the site checked. Extravasations are usually managed as follows:

(a) The administration of infusion/ injection must be stopped and the cannula left in place.
(b) The healthcare professional administering the treatment should remain with the patient and ask a colleague to summon a doctor to examine and prescribe the appropriate treatment, according to the local extravasation policy.
(c) If a vesicant drug has been extravasated, the plastic surgical specialist registrar on call 24 hours may need to be contacted as per the local policy. Emergency intervention/antidote may be required as per the local policy.
(d) 3–5 mL of fluid should be aspirated from the extravasation site through the cannula if possible.
(e) The area should be marked and the cannula removed.
(f) 100 mg hydrocortisone should be administered IV via a new cannula that is re-sited remotely from the extravasation area.
(g) 100 mg hydrocortisone (2 mL) can be administered subcutaneously or intradermally in 0.2 mL aliquots in a 'pincushion' fashion at six to eight points of the compass around and in the extravasated area. Omit this step if the extravasation is around a central line.
(h) Hydrocortisone cream 1% should be applied topically to the extravasated site three times a day, as long as redness persists.
(i) The extravasated area should be covered with sterile gauze. Heat can be applied to disperse the extravasated drug, or the area can be cooled to localise the extravasation, depending upon the drug extravasated and the local policy.
(j) The site should be elevated while swelling persists.
(k) Antihistamine cover should be given (e.g. chlorphenamine 4 mg orally).
(l) Analgesia should be provided if required.
(m) For the management of each individual drug refer to management plans in the local policy.
(n) The following documents should be completed within 4 hours according to local policy: standard local documentation for extravasation that should be filed in the patient's notes: a local incident form.
(0) The patient's consultant should be informed within 24 hours (at the discretion of the specialist registrar on call).
(p) If IV chemotherapy is to be continued on the same day as an extravasation incident, where possible avoid using the limb where the extravasation has occurred. Review the extravasation site (suggested at approx. 24 hours and at 7 days). If it is not ulcerated, advise a gradual return to normal use. For subsequent cycles of

chemotherapy a surgical opinion should be considered if there is persistent pain, or swelling or delayed ulceration occurs.

How would you advise Mrs DC's antiemetic regimen be adjusted?

A7 **Mrs DC had experienced grade 2 acute vomiting and delayed nausea with her first cycle of FEC75 chemotherapy. Her antiemetic treatment needs to be adjusted to prevent chemotherapy-induced nausea and vomiting during cycle 2.**

Mrs DC should be advised to adjust her antiemetic medication as follows:

(a) To take the dexamethasone as for cycle 1, but to continue at a dose of 4 mg twice daily orally for a further 2 days. Dexamethasone tablets can be dissolved in water if the patient finds that swallowing them initiates an episode of vomiting. Dexamethasone is one of the best agents for delayed chemotherapy-induced nausea and vomiting, and should be the first line of treatment in refractory cases. If dexamethasone is not effective for the delayed phase, then aprepitant can be considered for addition to the antiemetic regimen.

(b) Aprepitant is a neurokinin-1 receptor antagonist and is licensed to be administered with dexamethasone and a 5-HT_3 receptor antagonist antiemetic to prevent moderately and highly emetogenic chemotherapy-induced nausea and vomiting. It is administered as a 125 mg dose orally 1 hour before chemotherapy, then 80 mg daily for the next 2 days.

(c) To take one additional dose of granisetron 2 mg once daily orally, that is, a total of 3 days' treatment. Mrs DC must be warned of the additional risk of constipation that may result from prolonging the duration of the 5-HT_3 receptor antagonist antiemetic.

(d) Prochlorperazine tablets 5–10 mg four times daily should be prescribed instead of the metoclopramide, starting the day of chemotherapy and continuing for 5 days. Prochlorperazine is a broad-spectrum phenothiazine antiemetic which is a dopamine-2 antagonist, antihistamine, antimuscarinic, and 5-HT_2 receptor antagonist. It can cause drowsiness, so Mrs DC must be warned that if she has that symptom she cannot drive or operate machinery.

(e) In addition to the antiemetic medication above, lorazepam 1 mg at night can be prescribed orally or sublingually, to start the night of chemotherapy for up to 3 nights. Lorazepam is a benzodiazepine that acts centrally on the cerebral cortex. It is useful in anticipatory emesis and as an adjunct to other antiemetics in refractory emesis. It causes sedation and amnesia.

Is this an appropriate course of action? Discuss your answer.

A8 **Yes, this is the appropriate course of action as it will help to ensure that Mrs DC's therapy, which is potentially curative, can be administered on time.**

Pegfilgrastim is a pegylated human granulocyte colony-stimulating factor (G-CSF), which is indicated to reduce the duration of neutropenia and the incidence of neutropenic sepsis in patients with a malignancy treated with cytotoxic chemotherapy. Pegfilgrastim is only prescribed prophylactically for patients who are at high risk of a neutropenic episode, who have had to have treatment delayed on a previous cycle due to low neutrophil count, or those who have been admitted with a neutropenic episode following a previous cycle of chemotherapy. Pegfilgrastim is prescribed to ensure that the patient can receive their treatment on time, as the regimen is prescribed with curative intent. There is no evidence that G-CSF therapy improves survival.

Pegfilgrastim is administered as one 6 mg dose by subcutaneous injection 24 hours after cytotoxic chemotherapy. Its main side-effects include bone pain and allergic-type reactions. G-CSF is a glycoprotein which regulates the production and release of neutrophils from the bone marrow. Pegfilgrastim is a sustained-duration G-CSF, and its elimination is mediated by neutrophil clearance in a self-regulating manner.

What was the most likely cause of Mrs DC's stomach discomfort? What prophylactic treatment would you recommend be prescribed with her third cycle of chemotherapy?

A9 **Mrs DC's stomach discomfort was most likely to be caused by constipation, as it was relieved by lactulose.**

The main side-effects with 5-HT_3 receptor antagonist antiemetics are constipation and headache. If these occur, patients should be advised to use a prophylactic laxative following the next cycle of chemotherapy. Mrs DC should be advised to take lactulose 10–15 mL twice daily regularly prophylactically, starting at the commencement of granisetron therapy and for at least 3 days after discontinuation. If lactulose alone is not effective, senna in a dose of one to two tablets at night could be added to the regimen.

What should Mrs DC be prescribed in preparation for starting docetaxel and trastuzumab chemotherapy in 3 weeks' time? What tests must be undertaken prior to this regimen?

A10 **Mrs DC must be prescribed dexamethasone premedication prior to starting docetaxel. Her cardiac function must be assessed prior to the trastuzumab therapy.**

The dexamethasone should start the morning of the day prior to docetaxel chemotherapy and continue for 3 days at a dose of 8 mg twice daily orally. This is to prevent any hypersensitivity reactions and fluid retention. The G-CSF should be continued with the docetaxel, and administered 24 hours after docetaxel chemotherapy.

Trastuzumab should be administered the day before docetaxel chemotherapy for the first cycle of treatment. If there are no adverse reactions, both drugs can be administered on the same day on subsequent cycles. Trastuzumab should always be administered prior to chemotherapy, as there may be a synergistic effect.

Mrs DC should also have baseline cardiac assessment and cardiac function tests prior to starting on trastuzumab. These include an echocardiogram, electrocardiogram (ECG), or magnetic resonance imaging (MRI). Patients with symptomatic heart failure, a history of hypertension or coronary artery disease, or with a left ventricular ejection fraction (LVEF) of 55% or less must be treated with caution. If the LVEF drops by 10% from baseline and to below 50%, trastuzumab treatment must be stopped and a repeat LVEF assessment undertaken. If there is no improvement or further deterioration of LVEF, trastuzumab treatment should be discontinued.

How would you counsel Mrs DC?

A11 Mrs DC must be counselled on her dexamethasone premedication treatment and on possible side-effects associated with her new chemotherapy regimen.

Mrs DC must be informed that it is essential for her to start the dexamethasone in the morning of the day before her docetaxel treatment. Her dose of dexamethasone is 8 mg twice daily, which will be four 2 mg tablets each morning and lunchtime/early afternoon for a total of 3 days. Mrs DC must be informed of the possible side-effects of the dexamethasone. She must be advised not to take her second dose too late in the day, as it may keep her awake at night. She must be informed of the possible increase in appetite, mood swings or mood changes, and the risk of inducing diabetes (rare).

She must be informed that the dexamethasone premedication is to try to prevent any hypersensitivity reaction and to reduce the risk of fluid retention with docetaxel treatment. Mrs DC must have the possible nature of a hypersensitivity reaction explained to her. If a reaction were to occur, it would most likely be during the first or second dose of docetaxel. A hypersensitivity reaction can occur within a few minutes of starting the infusion. Symptoms can be minor, including flushing or localised cutaneous reactions; or severe, including hypotension, bronchospasm or generalised rash/erythema. Severe reactions require discontinuation of the docetaxel infusion, and these patients should not be rechallenged.

What should the duration of the trastuzumab treatment be?

A12 The duration of adjuvant trastuzumab is 1 year.

Trastuzumab was approved by NICE for the adjuvant treatment of early stage HER2-positive breast cancer in the UK. It should be administered every 3 weeks for 1 year, or until disease recurrence, whichever is the shorter period, after surgery, chemotherapy and radiotherapy. Cardiac function tests need to be performed prior to trastuzumab treatment and repeated every 3 months during treatment. Some local protocols may recommend cardiac assessment at intervals following completion of treatment.

Trastuzumab is a recombinant humanised IgG1 monoclonal antibody which targets the human epidermal growth factor receptor 2 (HER2). HER2 is overexpressed in 20–30% of primary breast cancers. Patients with HER2 overexpression have a shortened disease-free survival compared to patients who do not overexpress HER2. HER2 is measured in the serum, and detected using an immunohistochemistry-based assessment. It is detected using fluorescence *in situ* hybridisation (FISH) or chromogenic *in situ* hybridisation (CISH) of fixed tumour blocks in a specialised laboratory. Trastuzumab inhibits the proliferation of human tumour cells overexpressing HER2. It is also a potent mediator of antibody-dependent cell-mediated cytotoxicity in cancer cells overexpressing HER2. Trastuzumab is only indicated in patients whose breast cancer overexpresses HER2 by a score of 3+.

If Mrs DC has a delay in her trastuzumab treatment at any stage, how should this be managed?

A13 If trastuzumab treatment is delayed by more than 7 days, then on recommencement of treatment a loading dose should be re-administered, followed by the maintenance dose 3 weeks later (for a 3-weekly schedule).

For adjuvant treatment trastuzumab is administered as a loading dose of 8 mg/kg, followed by 6 mg/kg every 3 weeks for 1 year. The half-life of trastuzumab is approximately 28.5 days, and it takes up to 24 weeks for the washout period. It would thus take approximately 20 weeks to reach steady state; however, if a loading dose is given followed by a maintenance dose, steady state is reached within 13 weeks.

How would you counsel this patient with respect to the anastrozole? Why was the AdCal prescribed?

A14 Mrs DC must be informed when to take the drug, what side-effects may occur, and that she is taking AdCal as prophylaxis against anastrazole-induced osteoporosis.

Anastrozole is a potent and highly selective non-steroidal aromatase inhibitor. Oestradiol is produced mainly from the conversion of androstenedione to oestrone in peripheral tissues through the aromatase enzyme complex in postmenopausal women. Oestrone is converted to oestradiol, and the reduction in circulating oestradiol levels is beneficial in women with breast cancer. The 1 mg daily dose of anastrozole in postmenopausal women produces oestradiol suppression >80%. Mrs DC must also be told that she should avoid all oestrogen-containing therapies, as they will counteract the effect of the anastrozole.

Anastrozole lowers circulating levels of oestrogen and hence may cause a reduction in bone mineral density, thereby increasing the risk of fractures. The incidence of osteoporosis with anastrozole is 10.5%. Mrs DC must be informed that she needs to have her bone density assessed with a DEXA scan when she starts her anastrozole treatment and at regular intervals thereafter. She has been prescribed AdCal one tablet daily as prophylaxis against osteoporosis.

Mrs DC must also be informed of the other possible side-effects of her treatment. The most common are hot flushes, asthenia, joint pain or stiffness, vaginal dryness, hair thinning, rash, nausea, diarrhoea and headache, all of which are mild or moderate. Some of the more uncommon side-effects that can occur include vaginal bleeding, anorexia, vomiting, somnolence and allergic reactions. If Mrs DC has the symptoms of asthenia and somnolence she must be careful about driving or operating machinery.

Anastrozole is rapidly absorbed with a maximum plasma concentration approximately 2 hours after dosing on an empty stomach. It has a plasma elimination half-life of 40–50 hours. Food does not affect its absorption. Steady-state concentrations are reached after 7 days of daily dosing; therefore, if Mrs DC misses a tablet one day, she can be reassured that it will not adversely affect her overall treatment.

How long should anastrazole treatment be continued for?

A15 Anastrozole therapy should be continued for a total of 5 years.

Anastrozole is one of the treatment options for adjuvant treatment of postmenopausal women with hormone receptor-positive early invasive breast cancer. It has been shown to be statistically superior to tamoxifen in disease-free survival, following a phase 3 study of 9366 postmenopausal women treated for 5 years. It was especially effective for hormone-receptor positive patients. Anastrozole is also statistically superior to tamoxifen in time to recurrence and distant recurrence, with a reduced incidence of contralateral breast cancer. Therefore, anastrozole is at least as effective as tamoxifen with respect to overall survival.

Why was bisphosphonate therapy started? Which bisphosphonate should be prescribed?

A16 **Bisphosphonates are indicated in patients with metastatic breast cancer as they may prevent the skeletal complications of bone metastases. The bisphosphonate chosen would depend on the local hospital formulary. Options include IV disodium pamidronate, oral ibandronic acid, oral sodium clodronate, and IV zoledronic acid.**

There is a choice of bisphosphonates indicated for metastatic breast cancer with bony metastases, some of which are administered orally and some IV. Some cancer centres/units prefer to use IV formulations to avoid adherence issues, an option that can be convenient for the patient if they are receiving concurrent chemotherapy. Some hospitals choose to prescribe oral treatments via shared care protocols with primary care. Oral treatment is more convenient for the patient if they are not receiving concurrent chemotherapy, as it avoids repeated visits to the hospital. The doses and administration details for each individual agent at the time of writing are as follows:

(a) **Disodium pamidronate**. For osteolytic lesions and bone pain due to bone metastases with metastatic breast cancer: 90 mg in 500–1000 mL sodium chloride 0.9% over 90 minutes IV every 3–4 weeks. The rate may need to be adjusted if there is renal impairment.

(b) **Ibandronic acid**. For reduction of bone damage in patients with breast cancer and bone metastases: 50 mg orally daily or 6 mg by IV infusion every 3–4 weeks. Tablets must be swallowed whole and with plenty of water while sitting or standing. They must be taken on an empty stomach at least 30 minutes or 1 hour before breakfast or other oral medicine, and the patient must continue to fast and stand or sit upright for at least another 30 minutes to an hour after taking the tablet: the length of time depends on the tablet strength (30 minutes for the 50 mg tablets and one hour for the 150 mg tablets).

(c) **Sodium clodronate**. For osteolytic lesions and bone pain in patients with metastatic breast cancer and skeletal metastases: 1.6–3.2 g orally daily in a single or two divided doses. Patients must be counselled to avoid food for 1 hour before and after treatment, especially calcium-containing products such as milk. Patients must also avoid iron, mineral supplements and antacids. Patients must maintain an adequate fluid intake.

(d) **Zoledronic acid**. For reducing bone damage in advanced breast cancer with bone metastases: 4 mg as an IV infusion in 100 mL sodium chloride 0.9% over 15 minutes every 3–4 weeks.

Mrs DC has pain with her bony metastases, so she should be prescribed a bisphosphonate that is indicated to treat bone pain, which would be either sodium clodronate or disodium pamidronate. As Mrs DC has to attend the hospital day unit every 3 weeks for her chemotherapy and trastuzumab treatment, IV disodium pamidronate would be a suitable option. This is also available generically, so may be the more cost-effective option.

What information should be given to Mrs DC about her bisphosphonate treatment?

A17 Counselling should include the duration of treatment, the rationale, and how it is to be administered. She must also be informed of any possible side-effects and how to manage them.

Mrs DC was prescribed disodium pamidronate as discussed in **A16**. It must be explained to her that this is for her bony metastases, to prevent skeletal problems in the future, and also to treat her bone pain.

She must be informed that her treatment will be administered IV over 90 minutes every 3 weeks when she is attending the unit for her trastuzumab and docetaxel treatments. If she suffers any deterioration in her renal function, the disodium pamidronate infusion would have to be administered over 4 hours. The treatment will continue until disease progression.

The side-effects of disodium pamidronate include fever and flu-like symptoms which can be accompanied by malaise, rigors, fatigue and flushes, bone and musculoskeletal pain, nausea, vomiting, diarrhoea or constipation, anorexia, headache, insomnia, drowsiness, hypertension, rash, anaemia, thrombocytopenia, lymphocytopenia, and abdominal pain. Paracetamol can be used to relieve some of these symptoms. Disodium pamidronate can also cause hypophosphataemia, hypomagnesaemia and hypocalcaemia, so these biochemical parameters need to be monitored. Rarely it can cause muscle cramps, dyspepsia, agitation, confusion, dizziness, lethargy and pruritus. One of the very rare side-effects of IV bisphosphonates in cancer patients is osteonecrosis of the jaw, and this has been reported with disodium pamidronate. Patients must be advised to maintain good oral hygiene and to avoid invasive dental procedures while on treatment. Mrs DC should be advised to have any dental work carried out prior to starting bisphosphonate treatment.

Is it appropriate to restart trastuzumab? What dose should be prescribed?

A18 It is appropriate to restart the trastuzumab at the same dose as used for adjuvant therapy.

Trastuzumab is indicated for the treatment of both metastatic and early breast cancer. It is licensed to be administered to patients overexpressing HER2 in combination with docetaxel in patients who have not received chemotherapy for metastatic disease, or in combination with paclitaxel in patients who have not received chemotherapy for metastatic disease and for whom an anthracycline is not suitable. Trastuzumab can be administered as monotherapy in patients who have received at least two cycles of chemotherapy for metastatic breast cancer, including a taxane and hormonal therapy (for hormone-receptor positive patients).

There are two possible dosing schedules for trastuzumab in metastatic breast cancer:

(a) The licensed loading dose for metastatic breast cancer is 4 mg/kg followed by a weekly trastuzumab maintenance dose of 2 mg/kg beginning 1 week after the loading dose. The first dose should be administered as a 90-minute IV infusion and the patient observed for at least 6 hours after the start. They should also be observed for 2 hours after the start of subsequent infusions for infusion-related symptoms of hypersensitivity. If the treatment is tolerated, subsequent infusions can be administered over 30 minutes.

(b) The licensed loading dose for early breast cancer is 8 mg/kg, followed 3 weeks later by 6 mg/kg, then repeated every 3 weeks. In practice, patients with metastatic breast cancer are also treated with this schedule. Three-weekly administrations are usually infused over 90 minutes.

Mrs DC will have to have another baseline cardiac assessment including an echocardiogram before restarting trastuzumab.

Is it appropriate to restart docetaxel? What dose should be prescribed?

A19 It is appropriate to restart docetaxel. The dose is 100 mg/m^2 for metastatic breast cancer.

The use of taxanes in the adjuvant setting is relatively new; however, there is evidence that re-treating patients with a taxane in the metastatic setting is effective. The choice of taxane could be either paclitaxel or docetaxel, according to local policy. Docetaxel is licensed in combination with trastuzumab in patients with HER2-positive metastatic breast cancer at a dose of 100 mg/m^2 administered over 1 hour as an IV infusion every 3 weeks. Usually up to a maximum of six cycles are administered.

Is it appropriate to continue pamidronate and trastuzumab treatment? How long should they be continued for?

A20 Yes, it is appropriate to continue pamidronate and trastuzumab. They should be continued until disease progression.

Pamidronate is continued until it is no longer effective in controlling Mrs DC's bone pain, or until the disease progresses.

Trastuzumab is usually continued until disease progression; however, there is some evidence that it remains effective if combined with other chemotherapy agents on disease progression. Therefore, some centres may have policies to continue trastuzumab through more than one chemotherapy treatment.

What monitoring is required?

A21 Mrs DC needs to have her cardiac function monitored every 3 months while on trastuzumab treatment. She needs to have her renal function and electrolytes monitored while she is on disodium pamidronate.

Mrs DC should have her baseline cardiac assessment and cardiac function tests prior to starting trastuzumab for metastatic breast cancer. These include an echocardiogram, ECG, or MRI, as per the recommendations for adjuvant treatment. Patients with symptomatic heart failure, a history of hypertension or coronary artery disease, or with a LVEF of 55% or less must be treated with caution. If the LVEF drops by 10% from baseline and to below 50%, trastuzumab treatment must be stopped, and a repeat LVEF assessment undertaken. If there is no improvement or further deterioration of LVEF, trastuzumab treatment should be discontinued. Cardiac assessments should be repeated every 3 months while on treatment.

Disodium pamidronate can cause hypophosphataemia, hypomagnesaemia, and hypocalcaemia, so these plasma electrolytes need to be monitored while she is on treatment. Her bone pain and side-effects to the treatment also need to be monitored.

How would you counsel Mrs DC on her dexamethasone treatment?

A22 Mrs DC must be informed that she needs to take the dexamethasone 8 mg (four 2 mg tablets) twice a day, that is, in the morning and early afternoon. She must also be informed of the possible side-effects.

Mrs DC must be informed that it is essential that she continue with the dexamethasone treatment for her brain metastases. The dexamethasone will reduce her headache by treating the inflammation and fluid retention in the brain caused by the radiotherapy treatment and the metastases. She must take the dexamethasone twice daily, which will be four 2 mg tablets each morning and at lunchtime/early afternoon. She will be given a steroid card, which she must carry with her at all times. She must not stop the steroids without a gradual reduction in dose, on the advice of her doctor, and must be advised that when she starts reducing the dose, if her headache returns it may necessitate the dose being increased again.

The possible longer-term side-effects of the dexamethasone must be discussed with Mrs DC. These include muscle weakness, bone fractures, dyspepsia and peptic ulceration, risk of thrush due to the immunosuppressive effect, and Cushing's syndrome (fat face). She must be advised not to take her second dose too late in the day, as it may keep her awake at night. She must be informed of the possible increase in appetite with dexamethasone, with a resultant weight gain, mood swings or mood changes, and the risk of the treatment inducing diabetes (rare).

What should happen about Mrs DC's pamidronate and trastuzumab treatment?

A23 Mrs DC's trastuzumab treatment should be stopped. Her pamidronate treatment can continue.

Lapatinib is an epidermal growth factor receptor (EGFR) and HER2 dual tyrosine kinase inhibitor which is indicated for patients who have received prior treatment with trastuzumab, taxanes and anthracyclines. As both lapatinib and trastuzumab target the HER2 receptor, trastuzumab treatment must be stopped before lapatinib commences. Clinical trials have shown that treating HER2-positive metastatic breast cancer patients who have progressed following treatment with previous chemotherapy regimens (including an anthracycline, a taxane and trastuzumab) with lapatinib and capecitabine delays the time to further cancer growth compared to the administration of capecitabine alone. Lapatinib is more effective than trastuzumab for brain metastases in metastatic breast cancer as it crosses the blood–brain barrier.

Mrs DC's disease has progressed in her brain, but not in her skeleton. Therefore, her disodium pamidronate treatment can continue.

What considerations need to be taken into account when prescribing oral chemotherapy?

A24 The considerations when prescribing oral chemotherapy are that the patient must be able to tolerate the oral route, they must be

educated on the recognition and management of side-effects, and must be counselled to ensure adherence to the regimen.

Patient information is key to successful oral chemotherapy. Patients are responsible for the administration of their drugs and need support so that they know what to do, for example if they vomit or miss a dose. Adherence to the regimen is essential, and there can be issues with patients forgetting their tablets when they are fatigued, or if there is morbidity causing short-term memory problems. Patients must also be informed of what to do if there are side-effects, such as abstaining from or delaying treatment.

Specific counselling points should include the name of the drug; its dose; what the capsule or tablet looks like; and when to take the drug in relation to food, drink and other prescribed drugs, such as antiemetic, etc. Patients and carers must be informed of the risks associated with handling cytotoxic drugs. They need to know where the drug should be stored, any precautions to be taken, and when to call the unit, doctor, nurse or pharmacist, and the contact details of who to call.

How should Mrs DC be counselled on her oral chemotherapy?

A25 **Mrs DC needs to be informed that her capecitabine chemotherapy is to be administered twice a day for 14 days, then she is to have a 1-week break before restarting treatment. Her lapatinib is to be taken at a dose of 1250 mg (five tablets) daily continuously.**

The dose of capecitabine for metastatic breast cancer in combination with lapatinib is 1000 mg/m^2 twice daily (total daily dose of 2000 mg/m^2). Mrs DC's dose of capecitabine would be 4000 mg/day, which should be administered as 2000 mg (four 500 mg tablets) twice daily for 14 days every 3 weeks. She must be advised to take the capecitabine with, or within 30 minutes after, food. Mrs DC needs to be aware of the cyclical nature of the capecitabine treatment, that is, 14 days on treatment, then 1 week off, which will be repeated every 3 weeks for up to six cycles of treatment, depending on her response. She must also be counselled on the possible side-effects and how to manage them (see **A26**). Mrs DC must be advised to moisturise her hands and feet two to three times a day to reduce the risk of them becoming sore. She must be counselled on her additional medication, which will include antiemetics and loperamide. Mrs DC must be advised to use regular mouthcare to keep her mouth clean. This will involve using a soft toothbrush and a saline or antiseptic mouthwash twice a day prophylactically.

It needs to be explained to Mrs DC that the lapatinib treatment is continuous. She must take 1250 mg (five 250 mg tablets) daily until her disease progresses. Lapatinib should be taken at least 1 hour before food, or at least 1 hour afterwards. It should be taken at the same time each day, for example always before breakfast. As lapatinib is mainly metabolised by CYP3A, and also inhibits CYP3A4 and CYP2C8 *in vitro,* it potentially interacts with a large range of drugs. The Summary of Product Characteristics (SPC) should be referred to for a comprehensive list of lapatinib's potential drug interactions. For example, CYP3A4 inhibitors (e.g. grapefruit juice, ritonavir, saquinavir, telithromycin, ketoconazole, itraconazole, voriconazole, posaconazole, nefazodone) increase lapatinib exposure and should be avoided. CYP3A4 inducers (e.g. rifampicin, rifabutin, carbamazepine, phenytoin, St John's wort) will reduce the exposure to lapatinib and must also be avoided.

Inhibitors and inducers of the transport proteins Pgp and BCRP can alter the exposure and distribution of lapatinib, as lapatinib is a substrate for these proteins (e.g. ketoconazole, itraconazole, quinidine, verapamil, ciclosporin, erythromycin (inhibitors); rifampicin, St John's wort (inducers)). As the solubility of lapatinib is pH dependent, concomitant treatment that increases gastric pH must be avoided, otherwise lapatinib absorption could be reduced. Drugs with a narrow therapeutic index that are substrates of CYP3A4 (e.g. cisapride, pimozide, quinidine) or CYP2C8 (e.g. repaglinide) must also be avoided with lapatinib. Mrs DC must be given a list of drugs that could interact with lapatinib and advised to inform her GP and pharmacist if they add any other treatments, to ensure that her new medicines do not interact with the lapatinib.

What side-effects should Mrs DC be warned about?

A26 There are a number of side-effects associated with both capecitabine and lapatinib that must be discussed with Mrs DC.

The main side-effects of capecitabine include diarrhoea, nausea, vomiting, stomatitis, abdominal pain, tiredness, loss of appetite, and hand–foot syndrome (palmar-plantar erythema) where the palms of the hands or soles of the feet can become numb, painful, red or swollen. Capecitabine has minimal risk of causing nausea and vomiting. Mrs DC must be advised that if she has an increased frequency of opening her bowels with diarrhoea four or more times a day compared to her normal bowel movements, or if she has diarrhoea overnight, she must contact the hospital for advice. She must be advised that if her hands and feet become sore and red, painful, swollen, or the skin starts peeling off, she must contact the hospital. It may necessitate the capecitabine being stopped for that cycle and subsequent doses being reduced. If her mouth becomes painful, red or swollen she must contact the doctor.

Mrs DC must be warned of the potential of neutropenic sepsis with chemotherapy. She must be informed that if she has a temperature of 38°C or above, or any sign of infection, she must contact the hospital immediately. She will need an urgent full blood count to check her neutrophil count, and may need to be admitted for IV antibiotics.

Capecitabine can cause cardiotoxicity, including myocardial infarction, angina, dysrhythmias, cardiogenic shock, sudden death and electrocardiographic changes. Mrs DC must be informed that if she has any chest pain, particularly in the centre of the chest and during exercise, she must contact the doctor.

The side-effects of lapatinib include diarrhoea, a reduction in LVEF, pulmonary toxicity, hepatotoxicity, rash, anorexia and fatigue. Mrs DC must be informed that her heart and liver function will be monitored during her treatment, and that she must inform the hospital if she has any breathlessness.

What supportive treatment should be prescribed concurrently?

A27 The supportive treatment that should be prescribed concurrently with capecitabine includes loperamide, aqueous cream, metoclopramide and saline or antiseptic mouthwash, benzydamine hydrochloride 0.15% mouthwash.

(a) Loperamide 2 mg after each loose stool up to a maximum of eight capsules in 24 hours should be prescribed to treat any diarrhoea due to capecitabine.
(b) Aqueous cream topically administered to the hands and feet as a moisturiser two to three times a day should be prescribed to prevent hand–foot syndrome. Aqueous cream should also be used instead of soap.
(c) Metoclopramide 10–20 mg three to four times daily when required should be prescribed in case of any nausea with capecitabine. An alternative antiemetic such as cyclizine, domperidone or prochlorperazine could be prescribed instead, according to local policy.
(d) Either saline or antiseptic mouthwash, for example chlorhexidine mouthwash, should be prescribed two to three times a day after meals, to keep the mouth clean and reduce the risk of stomatitis.
(e) Benzydamine hydrochloride 0.15% mouthwash 15 mL up to every 1.5 hours should be prescribed if required for a sore mouth. If Mrs DC has mouth ulcers she can also use Bonjela or Adcortyl in Orabase.

How long should lapatinib and capecitabine treatment be continued for?

A28 **Capecitabine should be continued for up to six to eight cycles, depending on response and local policy. Lapatinib is continued until disease progression.**

Acknowledgement

The author wishes to thank Dr Nicola Levitt, Consultant Medical Oncologist, Cancer and Haematology Centre, Oxford Radcliffe Hospitals NHS Trust, Oxford, for her advice on developing the case for this chapter.

Further reading

Allwood M, Stanley A, Wright P (eds). *The Cytotoxics Handbook,* 4th edn. Radcliffe Medical Press, Abingdon, 2002.

American Society of Clinical Oncology. *American Society of Clinical Oncology Guidelines for Antiemetics in Oncology: Update 2006*. American Society of Clinical Oncology.

Brighton D, Wood M (eds). *The Royal Marsden Hospital Handbook of Cancer Chemotherapy. A Guide for the Multidisciplinary Team*. Elsevier, Edinburgh, 2005.

Cassidy J, Bissett D, Spence RAJ (eds). *Oxford Handbook of Oncology.* Oxford University Press, Oxford, 2002.

Gabriel S, Daniels S. *Dosage Adjustment for Cytotoxics in Hepatic Impairment* [online] 2003. The North London Cancer Network.

Gabriel S, Daniels S. *Dosage Adjustment for Cytotoxics in Renal Impairment* [online] 2003. The North London Cancer Network.

Summerhayes M, Daniels S. *Practical Chemotherapy. A Multidisciplinary Guide.* Radcliffe Medical, Abingdon, 2003.

Ward C. *Chemotherapy Dose Adjustments for Renal and Hepatic Impairment* [online] 2007. Derby-Burton Cancer Network.

26

Symptom control in palliative care

Colin Hardman

Case study and questions

Day 1 Eighty-year-old Mrs PF was admitted to hospital after a home visit by her consultant surgeon. She had a 6-month history of weight loss, altered bowel habits, rectal bleeding and abdominal pain. Investigations had revealed a carcinoma in her colon, but she had declined treatment. She had therefore been referred to her general practitioner (GP) for palliative care and had initially been prescribed co-codamol 30/500 and temazepam.

She lived with her 85-year-old husband in their own house and they had no children. She did not smoke and drank only very rarely. She had no other medical problems and did not take any regular medication other than that provided by her GP. She rarely bought medicines and in general did not like taking them. She looked after her husband, who had had a myocardial infarction some years ago and now had angina pectoris that limited his activities.

Recently, her pain had become more frequent and more severe. She had experienced nausea and vomiting, and had little appetite. She had not slept well for some time. Her GP had given her metoclopramide 10 mg orally every 6 hours, with little effect, and tramadol 50 mg to be taken every 6 hours when needed for severe pain, but she has been reluctant to take them. She was now in constant pain, bed-bound, and experiencing frequent bouts of vomiting. She reluctantly agreed to let her consultant admit her to hospital for control of her symptoms.

On the ward she was noted to be drowsy, but responded appropriately when asked questions. She was dehydrated. White plaques were seen in her mouth, and areas of her tongue were red and sore. Masses were palpable in her abdomen. She described her pain as constant, but said it varied in intensity. The pain was largely confined to her abdomen. A rectal examination was not carried out because Mrs PF would not agree to it. The clinical impression was that Mrs PF had partial bowel obstruction from her tumour and constipation.

Her serum biochemical results were as follows:

- Glucose 4.1 mmol/L (reference range 3.3–11)
- Sodium 131 mmol/L (136–148)
- Potassium 3.0 mmol/L (3.6–5.0)
- Calcium (corrected for albumin) 2.31 mmol/L (2.1–2.6)
- Urea 10.1 mmol/L (2.5–10)
- Creatinine 125 micromol/L (55–120)

She was initially prescribed intravenous (IV) fluids and the following oral drugs:

- Morphine sulphate 10 mg (as solution) every 4 hours
- Prochlorperazine 12.5 mg every 6 hours by intramuscular injection
- Co-danthramer liquid 25/200 10 mL at night
- Temazepam 10 mg orally at night

Q1 Outline a pharmaceutical care plan for Mrs PF.
Q2 What factors are likely to be contributing to Mrs PF's drowsiness?
Q3 Why is Mrs PF vomiting so frequently?
Q4 Do you agree with the choice of antiemetic therapy?
Q5 What might be the cause of Mrs PF's oral problems, and what action would you recommend?
Q6 Was morphine sulphate solution the most appropriate analgesic for Mrs PF's initial pain control? Is the starting dose appropriate?
Q7 What should be considered when starting a patient on opiate therapy?
Q8 What might be the cause of Mrs PF's abdominal masses?
Q9 Was co-danthramer liquid the best choice of laxative?

Day 2 Mrs PF was still in pain, so her morphine dose was increased to 20 mg every 4 hours. She was less nauseated but still vomited once or twice a day. The consultant noted that she had a palpable liver edge.

Q10 What is the significance of Mrs PF's palpable liver?

Day 3 Mrs PF still complained of some abdominal pain. She added that it was different from her original pain, but difficult to describe. Dexamethasone 16 mg daily by mouth was prescribed and the dose of co-danthramer was increased to 10 mL twice daily.

Q11 Why has dexamethasone been prescribed for Mrs PF, and is the dose appropriate for this indication?
Q12 How should the dexamethasone therapy be monitored?
Q13 Should a proton pump inhibitor (PPI) be co-prescribed?
Q14 Would Mrs PF benefit from the addition of a non-steroidal anti-inflammatory drug (NSAID) to her therapy?
Q15 Is doubling the dose of co-danthramer the best way of managing Mrs PF's continuing constipation?

Day 4 Mrs PF passed some soft stools.

Day 6 Mrs PF reported that her pain was better. IV access had been removed and she was drinking, but not eating much. She still vomited, but rarely, and had little nausea.

Q16 Would you recommend any changes to Mrs PF's morphine therapy?
Q17 What other analgesics could be considered if Mrs PF develops pain unresponsive to her current therapy?

Day 12 Mrs PF was not sleeping well and complained of pain at night. Additional doses of morphine were given as required, with occasional benefit.

Q18 What other factors may affect Mrs PF's pain control, and how should they be addressed?

Day 14 Mrs PF was feeling better but a little drowsy. She complained of a headache and was given paracetamol, with good effect.

Q19 Why does paracetamol work in the presence of morphine?

Day 17 Transfer was arranged to a local hospice for continuing care. Her medication regimen at transfer was:

- Slow-release morphine 80 mg orally twice daily
- Haloperidol 0.5 mg orally at night
- Co-danthramer liquid 25/200 10 mL orally twice daily
- Temazepam 10 mg orally at night
- Diazepam 2 mg orally twice daily
- Morphine sulphate 10 mg/5 mL liquid for breakthrough pain

Q20 What factors may affect Mrs PF's adherence to this regimen?
Q21 If Mrs PF becomes unable to tolerate her therapy orally, what options could be considered?

Answers

Outline a pharmaceutical care plan for Mrs PF.

A1 **The pharmaceutical care plan for Mrs PF should include the following:**

(a) Ensure that all her symptoms are defined and managed optimally by considering all sources of the symptoms and choosing drugs appropriate to them.

(b) Define possible adverse drug reactions or interactions and plan a monitoring system.
(c) Ensure that Mrs PF can manage the regimen prescribed in her current state of health. Be certain that the dose forms are appropriate and that she can comply with the regimen both physically and mentally.
(d) Counsel Mrs PF (and/or her carer) on her regimen and be able to answer confidently and honestly any anxieties she may have about the drugs prescribed.
(e) Monitor any relevant laboratory tests that may be available.
(f) As her regimen evolves, ensure that the drugs prescribed are easily available in the community.
(g) Review her regimen regularly to ensure that all drugs and doses are relevant to her current problems.
(h) Recognise that many uses of medicines in palliative care are unlicensed, and consider who will need to be aware of such uses.

What factors are likely to be contributing to Mrs PF's drowsiness?

A2 **Several factors may be contributing. These include her advancing disease, divergence from normal sleep patterns as a result of pain and constipation, and her drug therapy. Prolonged nausea and vomiting prior to admission have probably also made her very tired. Uraemia and hypercalcaemia can also cause drowsiness, but these are not contributory factors in Mrs PF's case.**

It is important to consider all possible causes of symptoms in a patient such as Mrs PF who has terminal malignant disease, as each symptom may have a variety of causes, only some of which may be drug related. In Mrs PF's case there are possible iatrogenic causes of her drowsiness: the codeine in co-codamol and the tramadol are both opioids. She also has been taking temazepam, although her use of this at home may be variable. Older people are more prone to central nervous system side-effects from drugs, and this tendency could have been increased in Mrs PF's case by her underlying malignancy.

Why is Mrs PF vomiting so frequently?

A3 **Intestinal obstruction from her advancing disease, constipation, anxiety and her drug therapy are all possible contributory factors.**

Her original disease has not been actively treated and has continued to progress, and possibly to metastasise, and her bowel may be partially or completely obstructed. There is a well-recognised association between obstruction and nausea and vomiting. In addition to this, she is dehydrated, has been bed-bound for some time, and has been taking opiates, which are all contributory causes to constipation. Constipation in advanced cancer can cause nausea with or without vomiting. However, Mrs PF does not have significant hypokalaemia or hypercalcaemia, which are also possible contributory factors to the pathogenesis of vomiting.

Anxiety can create or exaggerate many symptoms, and if Mrs PF is concerned about her disease, her symptoms or her invalid husband, this could be a source of her increasing symptoms. In addition, she has not been sleeping well, and insomnia adds to the overall perception of many symptoms.

Furthermore, since her admission to hospital she has been prescribed oral morphine regularly in place of irregular doses of the previously prescribed opiates. The introduction of opiates, or a dose increase, is a common cause of vomiting and may lead to an increase in her symptoms if inadequately managed.

Do you agree with the choice of antiemetic therapy?

A4 **No. Oral haloperidol 1.5 mg at night, plus oral cyclizine 50 mg as required would be a better choice. The prescription should also allow each drug to be given by an appropriate alternative route if Mrs PF is vomiting.**

It is important to determine the source(s) of vomiting (see A3) because this facilitates selection of the most appropriate treatment.

Drug-induced vomiting, such as that associated with opiates, is mediated through the chemoreceptor trigger zone, which in turn is linked to the vomiting centre. Both sites lie in the floor of the fourth ventricle. Opiate-induced vomiting is not inevitable and is normally short-lived (remitting within a period of 3–4 days), but when it occurs, or has been known to occur in the past, then haloperidol is often effective at a starting dose of 1.5 mg at night. This dose could be increased if necessary, but with care because of Mrs PF's age (extrapyramidal side-effects should be monitored for).

Mrs PF's bowel obstruction is another probable cause of her vomiting, so an antiemetic such as cyclizine, which has a direct effect on the vomiting centre, should also be considered. As prokinetic antiemetics such as domperidone or metoclopramide may cause colic in patients with obstruction, these should be avoided.

Levomepromazine at a dose of 6–25 mg daily is an alternative if the above do not produce an adequate response. In some centres levomepromazine is the first-choice antiemetic rather than haloperidol. In the UK 6 mg tablets are available on a named-patient basis (see www.palliativedrugs.com for details).

If Mrs PF continues to vomit then the absorption of drugs from the gastrointestinal tract must be considered to be unreliable, and alternative routes should be used until such time as her vomiting is adequately controlled. For many patients with intestinal obstruction a realistic goal is to eliminate nausea, but to be prepared for the patient to vomit occasionally. It should also be remembered that many antiemetics can cause constipation, and this must be considered as a cause of prolonged nausea and vomiting.

Finally, if anxiety is an important component of Mrs PF's vomiting and cannot be resolved by non-drug means, then a low dose of a benzodiazepine such as diazepam might be effective. Although cumulative drowsiness caused by haloperidol, cyclizine and diazepam may be a problem, it can be controlled by dose adjustment. Regular review of laboratory tests that give an indication of renal and hepatic function can provide a guide to dosage and help to minimise the risk of adverse reactions.

What might be the cause of Mrs PF's problems, and what action would you recommend?

A5 **The most likely cause is a *Candida albicans* infection, which should be treated by fluconazole 50 mg daily (as syrup) plus regular mouthcare.**

Oropharyngeal and oesophageal candidiasis is a common consequence of chronic illness, which can be made worse by factors such as immunosuppressive drugs, a dry mouth caused by antimuscarinic drugs or dehydration, and poor oral hygiene. The soreness and discomfort produced by the infection may further reduce the intake of food and liquid, thereby compounding the patient's problems. Treatment with drugs such as nystatin, amphotericin or fluconazole will normally be effective: fluconazole syrup has the added advantage of providing a topical and systemic therapeutic effect.

Additional symptomatic support, such as artificial saliva solutions for a dry mouth, may be useful, and sucking small pieces of ice or pineapple can help to relieve discomfort by stimulating saliva production. Good oral hygiene will help to maintain improvement. Careful attention should also be paid to factors such as adequate cleaning of dentures, or they may become a source of continuing infection.

Was morphine sulphate solution the most appropriate choice for Mrs PF's initial pain control? Is the starting dose appropriate?

A6 **Yes. Her pain was not controlled by co-codamol 30/500 (an analgesic for mild to moderate pain), but it is at least partially opiate responsive. The starting dose is appropriate, but an 'as-required' dose of 10 mg for breakthrough pain could have been added.**

Three-quarters of patients with advanced cancer experience pain, and of those one-fifth have one pain, four-fifths have two or more pains, and one-third have four or more pains. It is important to establish the sources of a patient's pain in order to choose drugs with the greatest chance of achieving analgesia.

Not all pains are reliably relieved by opiates, nor do all pains require strong opiates immediately: it is often worth trying simple or intermediate analgesics before progressing to morphine. In this case oral morphine is appropriate, but it is important to choose an initial dose carefully. As Mrs PF has only used weak opioids regularly before admission, 10 mg morphine sulphate (as solution) every 4 hours is appropriate. Morphine and diamorphine have a duration of analgesia of 4 hours, and it is important to adhere to this regimen wherever possible. Morphine is available in a variety of presentations, which allows greater individualisation of drug regimens to improve adherence and so maintain analgesia. Diamorphine is usually reserved for injection, where its greater solubility allows a wide range of doses to be administered in small volumes. Diamorphine is particularly useful for continuous subcutaneous infusions.

When oral morphine is introduced it is important to increase the daily dose regularly until pain relief is obtained or side-effects are encountered. Morphine solution should be administered every 4 hours regularly and the same dose prescribed 'as required' for breakthrough pain. After 1 or 2 days the total daily dose of morphine needed to control the pain should be calculated, and from this the new 4-hourly dose and breakthrough dose can be created. If it becomes apparent that morphine is not treating the pain adequately then the prescription should be reviewed.

Continual review of a patient's response to analgesia is essential because pains may increase or diminish, and new or different pains may arise that require separate consideration. When monitoring pain control it is important always to remember that pain is what the patient says hurts.

What should be considered when starting a patient on opiate therapy?

A7 **(a) That predictable side-effects should be managed appropriately by prophylactic therapy.**

(b) Less predictable side-effects should be monitored for and action taken as appropriate.
(c) The opiate dose should be optimised according to response.
(d) Any concerns expressed by the patient or a carer about taking regular opiate therapy must be addressed.

The predictable side-effects associated with opiate therapy are drowsiness, nausea, vomiting and constipation, and have already been discussed. Appropriate advice and treatment should be provided and monitored. Although patients may become tolerant to the drowsiness, nausea and vomiting, they will not become tolerant to the constipation and regular laxative therapy will be essential.

The dose of morphine can be titrated according to response by increasing it by 25–50% overall in regular increments every 24 hours, with any extra doses that have been necessary on an 'as-required' basis during the previous 24-hour period being added into the next day's regimen. About two-thirds of patients never need more than 30 mg every 4 hours, although much higher doses are sometimes necessary.

Morphine does not cause respiratory depression in patients who have chronic pain, nor does dependence become a problem. Doses can be reduced if other analgesic procedures such as radiotherapy or nerve blocks prove effective, and can sometimes be stopped altogether and be replaced by simple analgesics. Alternative oral opiates include hydromorphone and oxycodone; fentanyl is available as a transdermal delivery system that is applied as a patch. This can be useful for patients who have difficulties in swallowing or managing their oral medicines; however, it should not be considered as an automatic choice but chosen in response to individual patient criteria. Fentanyl has an advantage that it is suitable for patients with renal impairment. Buprenorphine is also available in a patch formulation which may be suitable for some patients. These alternatives may be considered when side-effects from morphine become intolerable but morphine remains the oral opiate of choice. Each of these alternatives has its own range of adverse effects and the prescriber should be familiar with them before changing a prescription.

What might be the cause of Mrs PF's abdominal masses?

A8 The most likely causes are tumour or constipation.

Colonic tumours tend to spread locally, but unrelieved constipation should also be considered as this may also be a source of Mrs PF's symptoms on presentation.

Was co-danthramer liquid the best choice of laxative?

A9 **Mrs PF has a combination of constipation and partial obstruction, and co-danthramer may exacerbate some of her symptoms; however, overall, laxative therapy is necessary for her and a small dose of co-danthramer is probably the best choice under the circumstances.**

Mrs PF has constipation arising from a number of causes, which include dehydration (which is being corrected with IV fluid replacement), poor diet and drug therapy. Mrs PF may also have a history of constipation, and she should be asked what her normal bowel habits were prior to her current illness. She had taken co-codamol and tramadol before being admitted to hospital, and she is now taking regular morphine, which carries an almost inevitable risk of causing constipation. It is also important to appreciate that elderly patients are more prone to opioid side-effects. As Mrs PF has elected not to have her tumour treated and is being treated symptomatically, it is important that she be prescribed laxative therapy.

Laxatives can be broadly divided into bulk-forming agents, stool softeners, stimulants and osmotics. Where constipation is an established problem, bulk-forming agents may add to the stool mass and should be avoided. Where stools are capable of being moved, then simple measures such as glycerine suppositories may help, along with simple stimulants such as senna or bisacodyl, although if there is proven or suspected obstruction from tumour then stimulant drugs should ideally be avoided. Very often stools need softening before they will move, and drugs such as docusate alone (as a softening agent), co-danthramer or co-danthrusate (which contain both stool softeners and stimulants) are appropriate. The latter are particularly useful in opiate-induced constipation. Where stimulant laxatives cause pain and discomfort, lactulose may be preferable. Macrogols are also effective for some patients. The choice of laxatives should be considered in the same way that analgesics or antiemetics are selected. The level of severity, the effect on the patient, the possible causes of constipation and the capacity of the individual patient to take products will guide the final choice.

Mrs PF did not permit a rectal examination on admission so it was not possible to say whether or not her rectum was loaded with faeces. Had this been the case, or if it was suspected, then a glycerine suppository should have been used. In the event of continuing constipation not responding to changes of laxative or an increase in laxative dose, a phosphate enema could be suggested.

What is the significance of Mrs PF's palpable liver?

A10 **That she may have secondary disease in the liver. Colonic tumours tend to expand locally and to metastasise to the liver.**

Liver capsule pain is often opiate responsive, but dexamethasone therapy may also be helpful.

Why has the dexamethasone been prescribed for Mrs PF, and is the dose appropriate for this indication?

A11 **The dexamethasone has been prescribed primarily to relieve her probable bowel obstruction. The dose is appropriate for this indication.**

Dexamethasone is a corticosteroid which is seven times more potent than prednisolone, and this means that a dose of 16 mg dexamethasone is approximately equivalent to 112 mg prednisolone. Corticosteroids are powerful anti-inflammatory drugs and are prescribed to reduce inflammation and oedema around the site of the tumour, which in turn may reduce local pressure and hence pain.

Corticosteroids are also used for the symptomatic relief of a range of other problems, including nerve pains, spinal cord compression, dyspnoea, superior vena cava obstruction, liver capsule stretch and other symptoms with an inflammatory component. The use of dexamethasone as a co-analgesic may help to improve effective analgesia and in doing so reduce opiate requirements. In addition, steroid therapy may improve appetite and general wellbeing. Several studies have demonstrated a noticeable, if short-lived, improvement in appetite, which in turn may help to reduce nausea, pain perception and analgesic consumption. Patients report an improvement in quality of life during dexamethasone treatment, but the use of corticosteroids for prolonged periods must be balanced against the risk of side-effects.

The use of dexamethasone in bowel obstruction is controversial, and some authorities believe that its value in these circumstances is unproven. Doses of 16–24 mg/day for 5 days have been advocated, although other centres have used 4 mg twice daily for 5 days, with a maintenance dose of 5 mg daily if improvement is noted. High initial doses of dexamethasone are sometimes required in order to achieve a response. The dose is then gradually reduced to one that maintains symptom control. Dexamethasone is often given in divided doses, although some authorities prefer a single daily dose. Where divided doses are used, the last dose should be given no later than 6 pm to avoid insomnia.

How should the dexamethasone therapy be monitored?

A12 Dexamethasone therapy should be monitored both clinically and biochemically.

Regular monitoring of urine (for the presence of glucose), blood pressure (for signs of hypertension) and for signs of oedema is necessary.

Mrs PF should be asked regularly about her mouth, as corticosteroids may cause candidiasis. Mental disturbances may also occur. These include euphoria or more florid symptoms such as psychosis, and are especially associated with high doses or prolonged treatment. Signs and symptoms of Cushing's syndrome may occur with high doses, and corticosteroids have a weak association with peptic ulceration.

Should a proton pump inhibitor (PPI) be co-prescribed?

A13 Mrs PF does not need gastric protection at this stage.

The causes of gastrointestinal problems in a patient with terminal cancer can be very varied and range from features of the cancer itself to drugs and other unrelated causes. Mrs PF does not have a history of peptic ulceration and does not complain of symptoms such as heartburn. Although drug-induced causes of gastrointestinal symptoms are common in advanced cancer, where polypharmacy increases the number of potential causative agents, Mrs PF is not taking an NSAID as well as dexamethasone. She is thus in a low-risk category and prophylaxis is unnecessary.

Would Mrs PF benefit from the addition of a non-steroidal anti-inflammatory drug (NSAID) to her therapy?

A14 No, as she has no evidence of bone metastases.

NSAIDs are widely used for the relief of pain associated with bone metastases, and the effectiveness of this group of drugs is believed to derive from their action on blocking prostaglandin synthesis, although the evidence for their efficacy is limited. Any potential benefits must also be balanced against the potentially serious side-effects that they can produce. Mrs PF does not have signs or symptoms of metastatic bone pain and colonic cancers do not normally metastasise to bone. NSAID therapy is thus not justified.

Is doubling the dose of co-danthramer the best way of managing Mrs PF's constipation?

A15 Yes, as an initial step.

Mrs PF has not opened her bowels since her admission and her constipation is probably contributing significantly to her symptoms. It is essential to review the extent and causes of her constipation regularly, to ensure that therapy is as effective as possible.

Mrs PF is now taking oral opiates regularly and the need for protection against worsening constipation is very important. She has been taking dexamethasone for her presumed obstruction, and as she has not experienced colic with her previous dose of co-danthramer a cautious increase in dose is appropriate. If she eventually passes hard, dry stools, then consideration should be given to prescribing extra stool softeners, such as docusate.

Would you recommend any changes to Mrs PF's morphine therapy?

A16 A change to twice-daily slow-release morphine tablets is now appropriate.

Her pain control has reached a level that provides acceptable analgesia, so the opiate component may be changed to slow-release morphine as a more convenient but equally reliable method of opiate administration. To do this the total daily intake of morphine is calculated and converted to two equal doses of a slow-release preparation. A small extra increase in dose is often included. For patients with swallowing difficulties a suspension version (as sachets) is available, as is a capsule whose contents can be sprinkled on food. Similarly, a once-daily capsule is marketed that can be swallowed whole or the contents sprinkled on food.

Mrs PF has been taking 20 mg of oral morphine every 4 hours, which makes a total of 120 mg/day. She has also taken an extra 20 mg daily on an 'as-required' basis, to give a total daily dose of 140 mg. This can be rounded up to 160 mg to give a little extra analgesia and to give a convenient dose of 80 mg twice each day of slow-release morphine tablets. Mrs PF can be reassured that this change in treatment will not affect her pain control, and she can also be told that the dose can be increased when necessary. Modified-release dose forms of hydromorphone and oxycodone could be considered as alternatives.

What other analgesics could be considered if Mrs PF develops pain unresponsive to her current therapy?

A17 A number of agents have value as adjuvant treatments for a variety of pains.

When a patient continues to experience pain while taking opiates then the causes of pain should be reviewed again. There are some pains that are less responsive to opiates, and adjuvant treatment may help to bring such pains under control. A common example would be bone pain, which may respond to NSAIDs, although radiotherapy is often preferred.

Pains from nerve-related sources are frequently encountered, and patients will often describe them as shooting, stabbing or burning types of pain. Antidepressants, anticonvulsants and corticosteroids can be prescribed in these situations and have varying degrees of success. Gabapentin and pregabalin are licensed for the treatment of neuropathic pain. Methadone and ketamine are used for some neuropathic pains, and colic may be relieved by hyoscine.

What other factors may affect Mrs PF's pain control, and how should they be addressed?

A18 **Fear and anxiety or depression may be affecting her pain control.**

Factors such as fear, anxiety, uncertainty about the future and spiritual crises can all have a profound effect on an individual's perception of pain and their response to treatment. Mrs PF may be worried about her husband and what will happen to him if she dies. In this situation appropriate professionals simply listening to her anxieties may help to improve the situation; it may also be possible to suggest some practical solutions.

Where necessary, severe anxiety may be helped by low doses of an anxiolytic such as diazepam, and this may be appropriate for Mrs PF. Taking into account her age and concurrent therapy, a modest dose of diazepam (e.g. 2 mg twice daily) could be initiated. Alternatively, if depression is diagnosed then active treatment for that should be considered, with the choice of drug and dose being individualised as necessary.

Why does paracetamol work in the presence of morphine?

A19 **Simple analgesia often works for simple symptoms.**

Patients with advanced cancer are as likely to experience minor problems as the rest of the population, and symptoms from simple causes, such as an occasional headache, frequently respond to simple therapy.

What factors may affect Mrs PF's adherence to this regimen?

A20 **The main factors are the number of drugs that are frequently required for effective palliative care, together with the physical problems that accompany a terminal illness.**

Good palliative care regimens may eventually require a large number of drugs to treat all of the patient's symptoms. The potential complexity of the treatment may lead to problems in timing for the patient, and confusion about uses and doses. In addition, drug-induced symptoms such as a dry mouth or oral candidiasis can make swallowing solid dose forms difficult. The pharmacist can help by providing detailed counselling, and by helping to simplify and manipulate the regimen to provide the best symptom control. Liquid preparations may help to ease swallowing difficulties, and the use of appropriate compliance aids may help to resolve the organisation of drug administration. Mrs PF was reluctant to take medication before her admission, and counselling should focus on helping her to understand the importance of the regular use of her slow-release morphine to maintain her analgesia, and the purpose and value of the other components of her regimen.

If Mrs PF becomes unable to tolerate her therapy orally, what options could be considered?

A21 Her treatment may be provided rectally, transdermally, by the buccal route or via a syringe pump.

Some drugs are available for administration by a variety of routes. Although alternative routes may be suitable in some situations, there are also some potential disadvantages. For example, someone with a dry mouth may not be able to absorb a drug effectively by the buccal or sublingual route, and rectal administration may not be practical in someone with rectal disease or diarrhoea.

A continuous subcutaneous syringe driver is a convenient and practical method of administering a range of drugs, including analgesics and antiemetics. Diamorphine is the analgesic of choice for subcutaneous administration because of its greater solubility, and has been subjected to laboratory studies to define its stability in solution, both alone and with a variety of other drugs. When a patient is changed from oral morphine to subcutaneous diamorphine appropriate dosage adjustment is required: guidance on this can be found in the current edition of the *British National Formulary*.

Octreotide is a somatostatin analogue that has been used in palliative care for the relief of diarrhoea and large-volume vomiting. Intestinal obstruction has also been treated with octreotide, but its value for this indication is uncertain. It can be administered by subcutaneous infusion or as bolus subcutaneous injections. Octreotide should be used on the advice of a palliative care specialist.

Fentanyl transdermal patches are an alternative method of opiate administration, the patches being changed every 72 hours. The choice of starting dose depends on whether or not the patient has previously received opioids: when a change is made from oral morphine to fentanyl patches an appropriate dose can be calculated from information provided with the patches. Transdermal fentanyl should not be used for the treatment of acute pain because of the nature of its formulation, and if the patches are withdrawn for any reason the transfer to another form of analgesia must take into account the gradual fall in fentanyl serum concentration. Buprenorphine patches are also available.

Further reading

Dickman A, Littlewood C, Varga J. *The Syringe Driver – Continuous Subcutaneous Infusions in Palliative Care*. Oxford University Press, Oxford, 2002.

Doyle D, Hanks GWC, Macdonald N. *Oxford Textbook of Palliative Medicine*, 3rd edn. Oxford University Press, Oxford, 2003.

Twycross RG. *Introducing Palliative Care*, 4th edn. Radcliffe Medical Press, Oxford, 2002.

Twycross RG, Wilcock A. *Symptom Management in Advanced Cancer*, 3rd edn. Radcliffe Medical Press, Oxford, 2001.

Twycross RG, Wilcock A *et al*. *Palliative Care Formulary*, 3rd edn. palliative drugs.com 2007.

27

Eczema

Christine Clark

Case study and questions

Year 1 Mrs JR took her 5-year-old son Liam to the general practitioner (GP) because he had developed a patchy rash.

Mrs JR explained that Liam's rash had developed over the past week, but that his skin had been dry for a couple of weeks before then, during a beach holiday. Liam had now become very miserable, cried a lot and seemed to be uncomfortable: quite a change, as he was normally a happy child. He used to sleep through the night, but over the past week he had been waking and complaining that his skin hurt him. This behaviour disturbed the sleep of both his parents and his younger sister.

There had been no contact with infectious diseases and the family had no pets. On questioning Mrs JR remembered that Liam's father had had eczema as a child, and that Liam had suffered from 'dry skin' when he was a baby but that it had cleared up within a few months with regular emollient treatment.

On examination Liam had inflamed, red patches on the insides of his elbows and wrists, around the back of his neck and behind his knees. The affected areas looked sore and were excoriated in places. Liam repeatedly attempted to scratch the affected areas. The GP diagnosed atopic eczema.

Q1 How is the diagnosis of atopic eczema established?
Q2 What factors are thought to contribute to the development of atopic eczema?
Q3 What are typical trigger factors for atopic eczema?
Q4 A holistic approach to the management of atopic eczema is recommended. What does this involve in practice?

The GP prescribed Doublebase gel, Oilatum Junior bath oil and hydrocortisone 1% ointment and spoke to Mrs JR about 'stepped care'.

Q5 Outline a pharmaceutical care plan for Liam.
Q6 What is 'stepped care' for atopic eczema?
Q7 Why has Doublebase been prescribed, and how should it be used?
Q8 What is 'complete emollient therapy'?
Q9 Liam's itching makes it difficult for him (and the rest of the family) to sleep. How might the itching be controlled?
Q10 What is the role of bath emollients?
Q11 What can you recommend for washing Liam's hair?
Q12 Can you suggest any other (non-drug) measures to help to keep Liam's eczema under control?
Q13 What kind of advice/information should Liam and his parents be given to help them manage his eczema?

Year 2 Mrs JR and Liam attended the hospital outpatient department to see the dermatology specialist nurse because Liam was experiencing a flare-up of eczema, which seemed worse than usual. He had inflamed red patches on his inner forearms, around the back of his neck and behind his knees. The patches were weeping and crusted, and there were some pustules. Mrs JR said that it looked 'angrier' than usual and Liam was noticeably more distressed than usual. The dermatology specialist nurse diagnosed infected eczema.

Q14 What is the appropriate treatment for infected eczema?
Q15 What is the role of antiseptic-containing creams and bath products?

Year 3 Liam's eczema had flared up again on his face and arms. The skin around his eyes was red, inflamed and itchy, and his hands, forearms and legs were also affected. Mrs JR said that the family had recently acquired a dog and it had become Liam's constant companion. The dog was sleeping in Liam's bedroom.

The dermatology specialist nurse suggested wet-wrapping to improve the condition of the skin on Liam's arms and legs and prescribed Eumovate 0.05% and hydrocortisone 1% in addition to his regular emollients.

Q16 How should the topical corticosteroids be used?
Q17 How would you tackle 'steroid phobia'?
Q18 How might you suggest that Liam's exposure to dog dander be reduced?
Q19 What is wet-wrapping, and how can it be used safely?

Year 4 Liam's younger sister had caught head lice at school and Mrs JR feared that Liam might also have become infested because he had a flare-up of eczema affecting the skin at the back of his neck, and she had found a live louse when she examined his scalp.

Q20 How might head lice be linked to Liam's eczema flare-up?
Q21 What advice can you offer about suitable treatments for head lice for Liam?

At the dermatology clinic Mrs JR told the specialist nurse that Liam had complained to her that he hated the feel of Doublebase and did not want to use it any more.

Q22 How should a suitable replacement emollient be selected for Liam?

Year 9 Liam, now 14, returned to the dermatology clinic with his mother. He had now been using topical steroids intermittently for 8 years and had become good at looking after his skin; however, he had experienced more flare-ups recently which his mother had put down to the ups and downs of adolescence. At the clinic it was clear that Liam was becoming very conscious of his appearance and was anxious to find a way to control his eczema.

Q23 What is the role of topical calcineurin inhibitors (tacrolimus, pimecrolimus) in atopic eczema?

Answers

How is the diagnosis of atopic eczema established?

A1 **There is no test for atopic eczema. The diagnosis is based on a typical history.**

Atopic eczema is diagnosed when a child has an itchy skin condition plus three or more of the following:

(a) Visible dermatitis involving the skin creases (or visible dermatitis on the cheeks and/or extensor areas in children aged 18 months or under).
(b) A personal history of flexural dermatitis (or dermatitis on the cheeks and/or extensor areas in children aged 18 months or under).
(c) A personal history of dry skin in the last 12 months.
(d) A personal history of asthma or allergic rhinitis (or history of atopic disease in a first-degree relative of children aged under 4 years).
(e) The onset of signs and symptoms under the age of 2 years (this criterion only applies to children aged over 4 years).

What factors are thought to contribute to the development of atopic eczema?

A2 Atopic eczema is believed to be linked to genetic variations that lead to a breakdown of the skin barrier.

The skin barrier prevents the ingress of irritants, allergens and micro-organisms, and at the same time prevents the loss of excessive quantities of water. Critical elements of the skin barrier are tightly packed skin cells (corneocytes) in the horny layer (stratum corneum), which is the uppermost layer of the epidermis, and the lipid bilayers that surround them. This is sometimes described as being like a brick wall in which the cells are the bricks and the lipid bilayers the mortar. Natural moisturising factor is a complex mixture of substances, including urea and amino acids, which attracts moisture into the cells and keeps them swollen. The corneocytes are also linked to each other by corneodesmosomes. These links are cleaved by skin proteases when the time comes for the surface cells to be shed.

Factors that weaken the skin barrier allow irritants and allergens to enter and also allow more water loss from the skin. This can lead to dry and inflamed skin.

A number of genetic variations have been identified and it is likely that more will come to light in the future. For example, a genetic deficiency of the skin protein filaggrin is associated with atopic eczema. Filaggrin is formed in skin cells and is the starting material for natural moisturising factor and some components of the lipid bilayers. A genetic excess of skin proteases, causing premature skin shedding (desquamation), has also been linked to atopic eczema.

What are typical trigger factors for atopic eczema?

A3 Typical trigger factors for atopic eczema include physical and chemical irritants and allergens.

Skin irritants such as soaps and detergents (including shampoos, bubble baths, shower gels and washing-up liquids) remove skin lipids and dry the skin. Industrial chemicals such as solvents can also damage the skin and trigger bouts of eczema.

Inhaled allergens such as those arising from animal dander, grass or tree pollen, or from house dust mites often give rise to eczema flare-ups. Contact allergens such as perfumes or preservatives in cosmetics and toiletries can also play a role. Food allergy can be a cause of eczema in infants and young children

Simple physical irritants such as rough fabrics, tight clothing, low-humidity environments, sea water, heavily chlorinated swimming pool water and sweat can also trigger eczema in susceptible individuals. Stress is also known to play a role.

A holistic approach to the management of atopic eczema is recommended. What does this involve in practice?

A4 A holistic approach to the management of atopic eczema takes into account both the severity of the atopic eczema and how it affects the child and its family.

It should be remembered that there is not necessarily a direct relationship between the severity of the atopic eczema and its impact on quality of life. For example, a small patch of eczema in a visible area of skin can have a big impact.

Eczema can be graded using Table 27.1. The impact of eczema on quality of life and psychosocial wellbeing can be graded using Table 27.2.

Table 27.1 The grades of eczema

Grade	*Description*
Clear	Normal skin. No evidence of active eczema
Mild	▪ Areas of dry skin ▪ Infrequent itching (with or without small areas of redness)
Moderate	▪ Areas of dry skin ▪ Frequent itching ▪ Redness (with or without excoriation and localised skin thickening)
Severe	▪ Widespread areas of dry skin ▪ Incessant itching ▪ Redness (with or without excoriation, extensive skin thickening, bleeding, oozing, cracking and alteration of pigmentation)

Table 27.2 The impact of eczema on quality of life and psychosocial wellbeing

Grade	*Description*
None	No impact on everyday activities, sleep and psychosocial wellbeing
Mild	Little impact on everyday activities, sleep and psychosocial wellbeing
Moderate	Moderate impact on everyday activities and psychosocial wellbeing, frequently disturbed sleep
Severe	Severe limitation of everyday activities and psychosocial functioning, nightly loss of sleep

Outline a pharmaceutical care plan for Liam.

A5 **The goals of treatment are to keep the skin in good condition so as to minimise the frequency of flare-ups, and to control flare-ups as quickly as possible.**

Atopic eczema is a chronic inflammatory skin disease. Many children grow out of it, but others continue to experience problems as teenagers and adults.

A long-term pharmaceutical care plan would include:

(a) Ensuring that Liam and his carers understand what is known about eczema and its treatment.
(b) Ensuring that Liam and his carers are able to identify trigger factors for his eczema.
(c) Involving Liam in the choice of treatments as soon as he is old enough to express a view.
(d) Ensuring that Liam and his carers know how to use emollients and topical corticosteroids effectively.
(e) Ensuring that Liam and his carers are able to recognise flare-ups and signs of infection, and take appropriate action.
(f) Ensuring that Liam and his carers know how to obtain supplies of the treatments that will enable him to undertake effective self-care.

What is 'stepped care' for atopic eczema?

A6 **The basic principle of stepped care is that treatment increases or decreases in steps according to the severity of the eczema.**

Emollients are used all the time, and if the eczema flares up then treatment is 'stepped up' by adding a topical corticosteroid. If this is insufficient to control the eczema then the next step could involve increasing the potency of the topical corticosteroid, adding topical calcineurin inhibitors and/or wet-wrapping. There are two important aspects to stepped care: if a patient presents with a flare-up it is important to match the step of treatment to the severity of the eczema, and then step up or down as required.

When treating a flare-up, treatment should be continued for 48 hours after the symptoms have subsided and then be stepped down.

Why has Doublebase been prescribed, and how should it be used?

A7 **Doublebase has been selected because it is unperfumed, has a fairly high lipid content and is very 'spreadable'. It should be applied after bathing, showering or washing, and several times during the day.**

Emollients work by putting a film of lipid over the skin and in so doing help to restore the defective skin barrier. The efficacy of an emollient depends largely, but not entirely, on its lipid content. The effectiveness of emollient therapy in practice depends on finding products that the patient likes and which match their needs and preferences.

When selecting emollients for children with eczema there are several points to consider. The emollient should be unperfumed because perfume ingredients can be contact allergens that could make the eczema worse (it is possible to develop allergic contact eczema on top of atopic eczema). A secondary consideration is that patients may dislike the smell of the product. In general, the higher the lipid content, the more effective the emollient and the stickier or greasier it will feel. Creams and lotions (which are dilute creams) generally have a lower lipid content than ointments; however, there is a vast array of creams ranging from light, watery products to lipid-rich products. Creams are usually preferable for daytime use, whereas ointments are often better tolerated at night. Some emollient ingredients are quite stiff and difficult to spread (e.g. petrolatum), whereas others (e.g. isopropyl myristate, liquid paraffin) are very 'spreadable'. A more spreadable emollient is easier to apply and less likely to cause irritation during application.

Doublebase contains 15% isopropyl myristate and 15% liquid paraffin. It is unperfumed and easily spreadable. Alternative options could include Oilatum emollient, Unguentum Merck, Diprobase, E45 Cream, and Dermol Cream.

The emollient should be applied quickly and generously to all the skin, not just that which is visibly affected by eczema. It should be smoothed on and left to 'sink in' rather than be rubbed in, in order to avoid making the skin itch.

Aqueous cream is not recommended for children. A recent study showed that 50% of children prescribed it as a moisturiser developed stinging, itching, redness and burning. Aqueous cream was originally designed as a wash product rather than as a leave-on moisturiser.

What is 'complete emollient therapy'?

A8 'Complete emollient therapy' involves using leave-on emollients and emollient wash products regularly and avoiding the use of soap and detergents at all times.

Complete emollient therapy involves regular, frequent application of emollients after bathing, showering or washing, and several times during the day. In addition, it involves the use of emollient wash products. Soap and harsh detergents (including bubble-bath products) dry the skin and can undo the beneficial effects of emollient therapy, and so emollient wash products should be used instead. Most water-based emollients can be used for skin cleansing in this way. Aqueous cream is particularly suitable for this purpose, but purpose-formulated emollient wash products can also be used e.g. E45 Wash. Epaderm and emulsifying ointment are also suitable for washing: they mix easily with water and form an aqueous cream on the spot. Emollients do not lather in the same way as soap but they do emulsify dirt and grime, and can be rinsed away with water; however, there are considerable differences in their use which may govern usability and patient choice, for example how the skin feels after using the product. Also, emulsifying ointment can leave a lot of scum, which makes baths difficult to clean. In some situations a single product can be used both as a leave-on emollient and as a wash product. Dermol Lotion has been specifically formulated with this in mind. It is also helpful to use an emollient bath oil (see **A10**).

Liam's itching makes it difficult for him (and the rest of the family) to sleep. How might the itching be controlled?

A9 **A sedating antihistamine could be given. Promethazine 15–20 mg at night would be suitable.**

A sedating antihistamine can be used during acute flare-ups if sleep disturbance is a severe problem. Promethazine 15–20 mg at night would be suitable. In the first instance a trial of 7–14 days' treatment should be offered. If this is successful it can be repeated for subsequent flares.

Although routine use of oral antihistamines is not recommended for the management of atopic eczema in children, a 1-month trial of a non-sedating antihistamine may be considered in children with severe eczema, or children with mild or moderate eczema where there is severe itching or urticaria.

Other measures that could help include keeping Liam's bedroom cool and keeping the container of emollient in the fridge so that it has a cooling effect when it is applied.

What is the role of bath emollients?

A10 **Bath emollients serve as an additional way of applying emollients to the skin and also, in the case of emollient wash products, as soap-free skin cleansers.**

Bathing can remove some of the natural oils from the skin, and using a bath emollient is one way of mitigating this effect. Bath emollients also make the bath water feel soothing and pleasant and less likely to sting if the skin is sore and scratched. Suitable products include Oilatum Bath Oil, Doublebase Emollient Bath Additive and E45 Bath.

It is difficult to apply emollients to some young children because they dislike the sensation of having creams applied. For this group, bath emollients may be the only effective solution and are therefore of critical importance. Users of bath emollients should, however, be warned to take care when bathing as these products can make the bath extremely slippery during and after use.

What can you recommend for washing Liam's hair?

A11 A mild shampoo formulated for people with eczema.

Conventional shampoos can be too harsh for people with eczema. Appropriate products are usually described on the label as being suitable for people with eczema. Alternatively, a list of shampoos free of sodium lauryl sulphate (a particularly irritant surfactant) can be obtained from the National Eczema Society.

Can you suggest any other (non-drug) measures to help to keep Liam's eczema under control?

A12 Avoidance of trigger factors that are known to, or are likely to, irritate Liam's skin.

A number of items commonly irritate sensitive, eczema-prone skin. These include rough fabrics, contact irritants and allergens, and low-humidity environments. Liam should have soft cotton or silk (medical grade, sericin-free) underwear and sleepwear. Common allergens such as animal dander, grass pollen and house dust mites can all trigger eczema, and Liam should avoid these as far as possible if he is affected by them.

If possible, Liam should not be exposed to drying situations such as cold winds, excessive air-conditioning or over-heated rooms.

Other measures that might be considered could be avoidance of biological washing powders and the use of cotton mittens at night to prevent scratching during sleep.

What kind of advice/information should Liam and his parents be given to help them manage his eczema?

A13 Liam and his parents need information about how to keep his skin in good condition, how to recognise and treat flare-ups, and when to seek medical attention.

Liam and his parents should be given an explanation about atopic eczema and what the treatments are intended to achieve. They should have information about how much of the treatments to use and how often to apply them, and the concept of stepped care should be explained together with when and how to step treatment up or down.

It is essential they know how to recognise a flare-up. A flare-up is characterised by increased dryness, itching, redness, swelling and general irritability. It is also important for them to be able to recognise infected atopic eczema, which is often a cause of rapid deterioration of eczema.

Bacterial infection with *Staphylococcus* and/or *Streptococcus* is associated with weeping, pustules, crusts, atopic eczema failing to respond to therapy, rapidly worsening atopic eczema and, in severe cases, fever and malaise.

Eczema infected with herpes (eczema herpeticum) requires urgent medical attention. It is associated with areas of rapidly worsening, painful eczema along with fever, lethargy and distress. Clustered blisters similar to early-stage cold sores may be seen, and there may be small, punched-out erosions that coalesce.

What is the appropriate treatment for infected eczema?

A14 The most likely infecting organism is *Staphylococcus aureus*, for which the first-line treatment is oral flucloxacillin.

The skin of people with eczema is almost always colonised with *S. aureus*, but treatment is only required when there is evidence of infection. Streptococcal infections can also occur. Small, localised areas of infection can be treated with topical antibiotics, but larger areas should be treated with systemic antibiotics. Treatment should continue for 1–2 weeks. Flucloxacillin is the first-line treatment; erythromycin should be used in cases of resistant organisms or flucloxacillin allergy. Clarithromycin may be substituted in patients who are intolerant of erythromycin.

What is the role of antiseptic-containing creams and bath products?

A15 Antiseptic-containing creams and bath products can be used as adjunct therapy to reduce the bacterial load in cases of recurrent infected atopic eczema.

Antiseptic-containing creams and bath products, typically containing triclosan, chlorhexidine or benzalkonium chloride, are not suitable treatments for infected eczema but may be useful in reducing the overall bacterial load, and this could help to reduce the frequency of episodes of infection. Examples include Dermol 500 Lotion and Dermol 200 Shower Cream (which contain benzalkonium chloride 0.1%, chlorhexidine hydrochloride 0.1%), and Oilatum Plus (a bath additive which contains benzalkonium chloride 6.0% triclosan 2.0%).

How should the topical corticosteroids be used?

A16 The topical corticosteroids should be applied to the areas of eczema only. Moderate-potency steroid should be used for the limbs and mild-potency steroid for the face, and treatment should be continued until 48 hours after symptoms subside, then stepped down.

Topical corticosteroids reduce inflammation and itching. Long-term use of excessively potent topical corticosteroids can lead to skin thinning, telangiectasia (dilation of surface blood vessels causing permanent reddening of the skin) and striae (stretch marks). There is also a danger of systemic absorption and consequent suppression of the hypothalamopituitary–adrenal axis and growth retardation in children. Children, especially infants, are particularly susceptible to side-effects because their skin is thinner than adult skin and they have a large surface area relative to their mass.

In order to obtain the benefits and minimise the risks of topical steroid therapy the patient should use the lowest-potency steroid that is fully effective for the shortest possible period – hence the 'step-up, step-down' approach. Concern about the safety of topical corticosteroids in children should not result in under-treatment: inadequate treatment will perpetuate the condition. Thus, a short period of treatment with a moderate- or high-potency product is preferable to a long period of treatment with a mild product that does not control the disease.

The topical corticosteroids should be applied thinly, so that there is no excess cream or ointment left on the skin. One way to measure the dose is to use the fingertip unit: this is the amount that can be squeezed out from the last crease on the index finger to the tip of the finger, and amounts to about 0.5 g of cream or ointment. This quantity should be sufficient to cover the area covered by the flats of two hands (i.e. twice the area obtained when the flat hand is put down on a piece of paper and drawn round). To make use of this measure one needs to assess the area of eczema in terms of hand areas and divide the result by 2; this gives the number of fingertip units required. This may need to be carefully explained to patients.

Steroid creams should be applied to the areas of eczema even if the skin has been broken by scratching. This should be emphasised to patients (and/or parents or carers) because the package patient information leaflets often advise against application to broken skin, and this can be a reason for treatment failure. Topical corticosteroids should be applied once or twice a day at most. Treatment with emollients should continue, but the times of application of steroid and emollient should be separated by 20–30 minutes so that the corticosteroids are not diluted. Treatment with topical corticosteroids should be continued until 48 hours after symptoms subside, then stepped down to a lower-potency corticosteroid or to emollients alone.

How would you tackle 'steroid phobia'?

A17 **By explaining that the benefits of topical corticosteroids outweigh the risks when applied correctly.**

It is important to educate parents about the purpose and benefits of correctly applied topical corticosteroids. This includes explaining that treatment with topical corticosteroids combats inflammation and itching and prevents further deterioration of the skin condition. In order to do this a topical corticosteroid of suitable potency must be applied as soon as possible after a flare-up starts. If a suitable potency steroid is used, the flare can usually be brought under control in a few days and then treatment can be stepped down. It is also worth pointing out that using correct (large) amounts of emollient together with topical steroids is beneficial and results in the same effect but with a lower overall 'dose' of topical corticosteroid than would otherwise be required.

It should be emphasised that the alternative, of using a mild corticosteroid or avoiding topical corticosteroids altogether, can result in prolonged bouts of eczema and extensive skin damage.

How might you suggest that Liam's exposure to dog dander be reduced?

A18 **By reducing contact with the dog.**

It may not be possible or desirable to remove the dog from the home completely, but restricting it to the downstairs areas of the house would be one way of reducing Liam's exposure to dog dander.

What is wet-wrapping, and how can it be used safely?

A19 **Wet-wrapping describes the application of wet and dry bandages over topical corticosteroids and emollients. Wet-wrapping intensifies the effects of topical corticosteroids, but used incorrectly can make eczema worse.**

Traditional wet-wrapping involves the application of a topical corticosteroid followed by generous quantities of emollient. A cool, damp bandage (usually a tubular bandage or garment) is then applied, followed by a dry bandage on top.

The advantages of wet-wrapping are that it is occlusive, so that it intensifies the effects of the topical corticosteroid and holds the emollient in place. It is also pleasantly cooling as the water evaporates, and physically it prevents scratching.

Wet-wrapping with topical corticosteroids should only be used for 7–14 days to bring a flare under control and it should always be started by a healthcare professional who is trained in the technique. It should be noted that wet-wrapping can make infected eczema worse.

Dry-wrapping is also used occasionally as a means of holding very greasy emollients in place. It should be noted that bandages soaked in liquid paraffin are highly inflammable, and so people wearing dressings of this type must avoid naked flames at all costs.

How might head lice be linked to Liam's flare-up of eczema?

A20 The reaction to the head lice causes itching, which leads to a flare-up of eczema.

Itching occurs during infestations with head lice as a result of a delayed hypersensitivity reaction to louse saliva. The itching and consequent scratching can damage normal skin, but in eczema-prone skin it can precipitate a flare-up.

What advice can you offer about suitable treatments for head lice for Liam?

A21 Dimeticone lotion or wet-combing are the preferred methods of treatment for people with eczema.

An alcohol-free aqueous product should be used as alcohol-containing lotions can irritate the skin and precipitate a flare-up of eczema. Insecticide products are more often associated with skin irritation than is dimeticone. Two applications of dimeticone lotion or wet-combing, using the correct technique, are the preferred methods of treatment for people with eczema.

How should a suitable replacement emollient be selected for Liam?

A22 Liam should be given a choice of unperfumed emollient products to test so that he can select the product(s) that he likes.

Liam should be offered a selection of creams of differing degrees of stickiness, including a couple of humectant-containing emollients (one containing glycerine, e.g. Neutrogena Dermatological, and one containing urea, e.g. Eucerin). It might be useful to include at least one product that contains an anti-itch ingredient, such as lauromacrogols (Balneum Plus, E45 Itch) or colloidal oatmeal (Aveeno).

Liam should be encouraged to take tester products away to try them at home for several days. He should be reminded that he might need more than one product: he might need different emollients for limbs and face, and for day- and night-time use.

Aqueous cream should be avoided as it does not contain sufficient lipid to be an effective leave-on emollient.

What is the role of topical calcineurin inhibitors (tacrolimus, pimecrolimus) in atopic eczema?

A23 **Topical tacrolimus and pimecrolimus have a role in eczema that is not controlled by topical corticosteroids and in situations where there is a risk of important adverse effects from topical corticosteroid treatment.**

Topical tacrolimus or pimecrolimus are not indicated for the treatment of mild eczema and do not have a place in the first-line management of eczema; however, if atopic eczema is not controlled by topical corticosteroids, or if there is a risk of serious adverse effects from long-term or frequent topical corticosteroid treatment, then their use can be considered. Tacrolimus can be used for moderate to severe atopic eczema in children aged 2 years and over. Pimecrolimus can be used for moderate atopic eczema on the face and neck in children aged 2–16 years.

Topical calcineurin inhibitors should only be applied to areas of active atopic eczema, including areas of broken skin. They should not be used under occlusion, such as a dry bandage.

At present it is recommended that the prescribing of topical calcineurin inhibitors should be restricted to physicians with a specialist interest and experience in dermatology.

Liam has now been using topical corticosteroids intermittently for 8 years. If regular application of hydrocortisone is not controlling the eczema affecting his face, then treatment with a topical calcineurin inhibitor should now be considered. The options for treatment are tacrolimus for moderate to severe atopic eczema or pimecrolimus for moderate atopic eczema on his face and neck.

Further reading

Atopic eczema in primary care. *MeRec Bull* 2003; **14**: No 1.

Barnetson R StC, Rogers M. Childhood atopic eczema. *Br Med J* 2002; **324**; 1376–1379.

Bath emollients for atopic eczema: why use them? *Drug Ther Bull* 2004; **10**: 73–75.

Burgess IF, Brown CM, Lee PN. Treatment of head louse infestation with 4% dimeticone lotion: randomised controlled equivalence trial. *Br Med J* 2005; **330**: 1423.

Carr A, Patel R, Jones M *et al.* A pilot study of a community pharmacist intervention to promote the effective use of emollients in childhood eczema. *Pharm J* 2007; **278**: 319–22.

Charman CR, Morris AD, Williams HC. Topical corticosteroid phobia in patients with atopic eczema. *Br J Dermatol* 2000; **142**: 931–936.

Conroy S. New products for eczema. *Arch Dis Child Educ Pract Ed* 2004; **89**: ep23–ep26.

Cork MJ, Robinson DA, Vasilopoulos Y *et al.* New perspectives on epidermal barrier dysfunction in atopic dermatitis: Gene–environment interactions. *J Allergy Clin Immunol* 2006; **118**: 3–21.

Cork MJ, Britton J, Butler L *et al.* Comparison of parent knowledge, therapy utilization and severity of atopic eczema before and after explanation and demonstration of topical therapies by a specialist dermatology nurse. *Br J Dermatol* 2003; **149**: 582–589.

Cork MJ, Timmins J, Holden C *et al.* An audit of adverse drug reactions to aqueous cream in children with atopic eczema. *Pharm J* 2003; **271**: 747–748.

Hoare C, Li Wan Po A, Williams H. Systematic review of treatments for atopic eczema. *Health Technol Assess* 2000; **4**: 1–191.

Long CC, Finlay AY. The finger-tip unit – a new practical measure. *Clin Exp Dermatol* 1991; **16**: 444–447.

National Institute for Health and Clinical Excellence. CG57. *Atopic Eczema in Children: Management of Atopic Eczema in Children from Birth up to the Age of 12 Years*. NICE, London, 2007.

National Institute for Health and Clinical Excellence. TA82. *Pimecrolimus and Tacrolimus for Atopic Dermatitis (Eczema)*. NICE, London, 2004.

National Institute for Health and Clinical Excellence. TA81. *Frequency of Application of Topical Corticosteriods for Eczema*. NICE, London, 2004.

National Patient Safety Agency. Rapid Response Report Number 4. *Fire Hazard with Paraffin Based Skin Products on Dressings and Clothing*. NPSA, London, 2007.

Palmer CN, Irvine AD, Terron-Kwiatkowski A *et al.* Common loss-of-function variants of the epidermal barrier protein filaggrin are a major predisposing factor for atopic dermatitis. *Nature Genetics* 2006; **38**: 441–446.

Staab D, Diepgen TL, Fartasch M *et al.* Age related, structured educational programmes for the management of atopic dermatitis in children and adolescents: multicentre, randomised controlled trial. *Br Med J* 2006; **332**: 933–938.

Williams H. New treatments for atopic dermatitis. *Br Med J* 2002; **324**; 1533–1534.

28

Psoriasis

Christine Clark

Case study and questions

Year 1 Miss JG, a 17-year-old schoolgirl, had developed thickened, red patches on her elbows, knees and shins. The patches had clear red edges and were covered in silvery-white scales that came off easily. The lesions were only mildly itchy but Miss JG was distressed by their appearance and the fact that they tended to crack and bleed as she flexed her knees and elbows. She suspected that they were caused by psoriasis because her mother, aunt and one cousin all suffered from psoriasis. Miss JG smoked 10 cigarettes a day.

Her general practitioner (GP) confirmed the diagnosis of plaque psoriasis and prescribed calcipotriol cream twice daily and Oilatum emollient.

Q1 What changes occur in the skin in people with psoriasis?
Q2 Outline a pharmaceutical care plan for Miss JG.
Q3 How do vitamin D analogues such as calcipotriol act in psoriasis?
Q4 What is the role of emollients in the management of psoriasis?
Q5 What is the role of cigarette smoking in psoriasis?
Q6 What information/advice can you give to Miss JG to help her to use the calcipotriol safely and effectively?

Month 6 Miss JG had been working for exams and was experiencing a flare-up of psoriasis. In addition to the patches on her elbows, knees and shins she also had numerous patches on her trunk, both back and front, and some on her hands. Once again the patches were thickened, red and scaly, with clear edges.

In view of Miss JG's distress and the extent of the disease she was referred to a specialist for treatment. After discussion of the various options the specialist prescribed a course of UVB treatment.

Q7 How is psoriasis measured and monitored?

Q8 What is UVB treatment for psoriasis?
Q9 What is PUVA treatment for psoriasis?
Q10 What advice can you give Miss JG about sunbathing and the use of sunbeds with respect to managing her psoriasis?

Year 2 Miss JG's skin had been clear for several months but over the past 2 weeks she had experienced a minor flare-up of psoriasis. She had a few clearly demarcated patches affecting her knees, elbows and lower back.

She discussed the treatment options with her GP and they decided that a combination product containing calcipotriol and betamethasone (Dovobet) was the most suitable option.

Q11 Would dithranol or coal-tar products be helpful to Miss JG?
Q12 What are the benefits of using a combination of calcipotriol and betamethasone?
Q13 What information/advice can you give to Miss JG to help her to use the calcipotriol/betamethasone combination product safely and effectively?

Year 3 The psoriasis affecting Miss JG's trunk and limbs was well controlled using the combination product. She had been able to treat flare-ups quickly and was happy with the way she has been able to manage her skin condition. However, recently she had begun to have intermittent problems with scalp psoriasis. This had taken the form of patches of psoriasis on her scalp with some diseased skin affecting the edges of her face. The skin around her hairline was noticeably reddened and scaly. She had also developed some sore patches in her armpits.

Miss JG was very anxious about the deterioration in her skin. She was going to be married in 2 months' time and wanted to look her best for the occasion. At the very least she wanted to get her scalp and face clear.

She discussed her problems with a GP with a special interest (GPwSI) in dermatology. The GPwSI was sympathetic and diagnosed scalp psoriasis and flexural psoriasis. She assured Miss JG that these were common aspects of plaque psoriasis and that there were effective ways of treating them. She prescribed Cocois ointment, Ceanel shampoo, calcipotriol scalp application and hydrocortisone 1% cream.

Q14 What information/advice can you give to Miss JG to help her to use the scalp treatments effectively?
Q15 What is the role of topical steroids in facial and flexural psoriasis?

Year 6 Miss JG returned to the specialist clinic with extensive severe psoriasis affecting her trunk and limbs. She said that she could not face any more topical treatments because they were too messy and took too long to apply and to work. She begged for 'tablets' that she had heard about from other members of her family.

Ciclosporin was initiated at a dose of 3 mg/kg/day.

Q16 Is there a role for systemic corticosteroids in the management of extensive, severe psoriasis?

Q17 What are the roles of ciclosporin, methotrexate and etretinate in the management of psoriasis?

Q18 What monitoring needs to be undertaken before ciclosporin treatment is started?

Eight weeks later Miss JG returned to the clinic. Her skin had improved dramatically, but a blood test showed that her creatinine level had risen from 80 micromol/L to 110 micromol/L, suggesting some impairment of renal function. The ciclosporin was discontinued immediately. Miss JG was very upset. She said that she could not go back to topical treatments and wanted to know what other options there were.

Q19 What are the advantages and disadvantages of infliximab, adalimumab, efalizumab and etanercept in the treatment of psoriasis?

Answers

What changes occur in the skin of people with psoriasis?

A1 **In patches of psoriasis there is proliferation of keratinocytes which means that the epidermis becomes much thicker than usual. The skin cells do not differentiate in the normal way and are shed in large, visible flakes. There is also development of new blood vessels in the plaque, which contributes to their thickened and reddened appearance.**

These changes involve activation of inflammatory processes in which T lymphocytes play a central role. The exact sequence of events is not yet fully understood. It is postulated that in response to an unknown trigger T lymphocytes are activated and then release cytokines and other inflammatory mediators that drive the proliferative and inflammatory responses seen in the skin. This also results in further T-cell activation and the disease process is continued. It is not known why patches appear in different places at different times, although some sites are more common. It is known that minor skin trauma can start a patch, as can a surgical incision, piercing or tattoo, but these stimuli do not account for most patches that appear.

Outline a pharmaceutical care plan for Miss JG.

A2 **The goals of treatment in psoriasis are to identify and avoid known trigger factors and to control flare-ups as quickly as possible.**

Psoriasis is a chronic inflammatory skin disease for which there is no cure. The frequency of flare-ups varies greatly, and the psychological burden imposed by the threat of flare-ups can be considerable.

A long-term pharmaceutical care plan would include:

(a) Ensuring that Miss JG understands what is known about psoriasis and its treatment. This should include:

  (i) Reassurance that psoriasis is not infectious and cannot be spread to other parts of the body by application of topical treatments.
  (ii) Reassurance that psoriasis is not a type of skin cancer.

(b) Ensuring that Miss JG is able to identify factors that make her psoriasis better or worse.
(c) Involving Miss JG in the choice of treatments.
(d) Ensuring that Miss JG knows how to use emollients and topical treatments effectively.
(e) Ensuring that Miss JG is able to recognise flare-ups and take appropriate action.
(f) Ensuring that Miss JG knows how to obtain supplies of the treatments that will enable her to undertake effective self-care.

How do vitamin D analogues such as calcipotriol act in psoriasis?

A3 **Vitamin D analogues such as calcipotriol (Dovonex), tacalcitol (Curatoderm) and calcitriol (Silkis) reduce keratinocyte proliferation, normalise differentiation and reduce immune activation in psoriatic plaques.**

These agents have weak effects on calcium metabolism. Unlike tar and dithranol products they do not smell unpleasant or stain the skin, nor do they carry the risk of skin atrophy seen with topical corticosteroids. The main effects of the vitamin D analogues are to reduce the rapid proliferation of skin cells and to restore the normal pattern of differentiation. In psoriasis plaques more skin cells than normal are in the growth phase, and this accounts for much of the skin thickening. In addition, the skin cells do not mature in the normal way as they progress upwards from the basal layer to the horny (surface) layer. Many of the surface cells are still nucleated and still linked to each other, so that they are shed in visible flakes rather than as single cells.

The maximum weekly doses of the vitamin D analogues are limited to avoid the risk of systemic absorption and the development of hypercalcaemia (calcipotriol 100 g of the 50 microgram/g preparations; calcitriol 210 g of the 3 microgram/g prepartion; tacalcitol 70 g of the 4 microgram/g preparations).

Treatment with a vitamin D derivative is as effective as topical corticosteroids for psoriasis and superior to dithranol. Furthermore, combined therapy using calcipotriol and a potent corticosteroid is more effective than calcipotriol alone.

What is the role of emollients in the management of psoriasis?

A4 Emollients restore pliability to the skin and reduce the shedding of scales.

Miss JG should be encouraged to use an emollient regularly. Emollients have several beneficial effects in psoriasis: they restore pliability to the skin and help to prevent painful cracking and bleeding; they also reduce the shedding of scales and can help to reduce itching.

Miss JG should be encouraged to experiment with emollients until she finds ones that suit her, bearing in mind that different products may be needed for different areas of skin.

In order to combat the cracking and scaling it may be helpful to recommend that Miss JG try products containing humectants such as urea or glycerin. Suitable products would be Eucerin, Calmurid and Neutrogena Dermatological. An emollient bath additive may also be helpful.

What is the role of cigarette smoking in psoriasis?

A5 Cigarette smoking increases the risk of developing psoriasis and is believed to make existing psoriasis worse.

The risk of psoriasis is almost twice as high in smokers and ex-smokers as in non-smokers. Heavy (more than 20 per day) and long-term smoking are associated with severe disease in women.

Miss JG should be advised to give up smoking.

What information/advice can you give to Miss JG to help her to use the calcipotriol safely and effectively?

A6 Miss JG should be advised to apply the product generously but to avoid sensitive areas such as the face and flexures.

Successful treatment with vitamin D analogues depends on using adequate quantities of cream or ointment. Patients should be advised that, in contrast to topical corticosteroids, calcipotriol should be applied fairly thickly. One fingertip unit (0.5 g) is sufficient for an area of 100 cm^2 (approximately the area of a medium-sized adult palm). In one study about two-thirds of apparent 'non-responders' to calcipotriol obtained marked improvements when optimal amounts were applied.

Transient skin irritation, resulting in increased redness, dryness and stinging or burning, can be a problem, and for this reason calcipotriol should not be used on the face or flexures. Miss JG should be warned about this because sometimes the irritation makes people feel that the disease is getting worse and they are tempted to stop treatment.

Calcitriol is significantly less irritant and is suitable for use on the face and flexures. The use of a combination product containing calcipotriol and betamethasone dipropionate also overcomes the problem of transient skin irritation.

How is psoriasis measured and monitored?

A7 **Psoriasis can be measured using the psoriasis area and severity index (PASI) and/or by asking the patient how the bad the disease is and how bothersome it is on a scale of 1–10.**

Numerous measures have been devised for estimating psoriasis severity, covering both the disease and its impact on the patient's quality of life. The PASI has been used in many trials. It relies on the clinician scoring each area of the body (arms, legs, trunk and head) for redness, thickening and scaling, and estimating the proportion of the skin surface in each area affected. Scores range from zero to 72. In practice this is too cumbersome to use on a regular basis. It is also insensitive. For example, it would give a low score to a patch of psoriasis on the face, which a patient may find very disabling. For day-to-day use, such as assessing the effectiveness of a new treatment, it is more practical to ask the patient how bad their disease is and how bothersome it is to them on a scale of 1–10.

Specific quality of life scores have also been developed, e.g. the Psoriasis Disability Index and the Psoriasis Life Stress Inventory.

What is UVB treatment for psoriasis?

A8 **UVB treatment is irradiation with ultraviolet B light at wavelengths between 290 and 320 nm.**

UVB is ultraviolet light of wavelengths 290–320 nm. It is the part of the absorption spectrum that is responsible for sunburn. In the past UVB was used in combination with coal tar for the treatment of psoriasis, but now it is usually used alone. UVB treatment is particularly suitable for extensive psoriasis with numerous small plaques that would be difficult to treat with topical agents. The main disadvantage is the time required to attend the clinic.

Because UVB can burn skin the dose has to be adjusted to match the patient's skin type. This is done by determining the 'minimal erythemogenic dose' (MED) of UVB. This is the dose that causes faint skin pinkness 24 hours after irradiation. A series of test patches are irradiated, typically for 10, 20, 30 and 40 seconds, and examined 24 hours later. Once the MED has been established, a reduced dose, usually 80% of the MED, is calculated. This is given three times a week until the psoriasis clears, which usually takes 4–6 weeks. Each treatment takes only a few minutes.

Antipsoriatic activity appears to be associated with the wavelengths 300–313 nm and so most experts now use 'narrowband' UVB, using lamps that produce mainly 311 nm ± 2 nm wavelengths. The removal of the shorter wavelengths reduces the risk of burning. Some areas of skin are very sensitive to the effects of UVB: male patients receiving UVB treatment have an increased risk of developing tumours in the genital skin, and for this reason the genitals should be covered during treatment. UVB therapy is contraindicated in patients who are taking photosensitising medicines such as thiazide diuretics or tetracyclines, and in patients with underlying photosensitive diseases such as systemic lupus erythematosus or polymorphous light eruption. The risks of developing non-melanoma skin cancer with UVB are as yet unknown.

Recently, a number of studies have been conducted using UVB light from an excimer ('excited dimer') laser. Excimer lasers are characterised by short wavelengths, high intensities and short pulse durations. Unlike conventional lasers they do not generate heat, which could damage surrounding tissue. Treatment times are shorter than with traditional UVB and the light can be directed at the affected areas. Excimer laser treatment may, in the future, be an option for faster treatment of isolated lesions, but it is not yet widely available.

What is PUVA treatment for psoriasis?

A9 PUVA treatment comprises the use of psoralen (a photosensitiser) with ultraviolet A (UVA) light.

UVA is light of wavelengths 320–400 nm. It penetrates deeper into the skin than UVB but has little action on its own. When given together with a psoralen photosensitiser the effects of UVA are greatly enhanced. The UVA induces a phototoxic reaction that causes the psoralen to form cross-links between complementary strands of DNA. The resulting effects are slowing of keratinocyte proliferation and suppression of the immune reaction in skin. There is melanogenesis (tanning) and effects on fibroblasts and endothelial cells.

The most commonly used sensitiser is 8-methoxypsoralen (8-MOP), which is available as tablets, lotion, paint or as a bath solution. It is important to ensure that the psoralen is present in the skin at the time that the UVA is given. Oral 8-MOP is given 1–2 hours before irradiation, and topical psoralens are applied immediately before irradiation.

The UVA dose can be determined either by an assessment of the skin type or by individual testing to determine the minimal phototoxic dose (MPD). Skin type assessment involves deciding which of the following six skin groups best matches the patient's skin:

I Always burns, never tans
II Always burns, but sometimes tans
III Sometimes burns, but always tans
IV Never burns, always tans
V Moderately pigmented people (Chinese, Indian)
VI Black people (West Indies, Africans)

Patients who have taken psoralens remain photosensitive until the psoralen has cleared from the body (12–24 hours). During this time they are vulnerable to the effects of natural sunlight and need to protect their skin with sunscreens. In order to minimise the risk of cataract formation they are also advised to wear dark glasses during this time. Some patients experience nausea with the oral psoralen. PUVA treatment is given twice a week until the psoriasis clears.

Prolonged exposure to PUVA is associated with an increased risk of non-melanoma skin cancer and photo-ageing of the skin. As with natural sunlight, fair-skinned individuals are more susceptible to these effects. The British Photodermatology Group has recommended that the maximum lifetime exposure to UVA should be $<1000\ J/cm^2$ or 250 treatments, but unless careful records are kept it is easy for this limit to be exceeded.

PUVA treatment is particularly suitable for extensive psoriasis with numerous small plaques that would be difficult to treat with topical agents. The main disadvantages are the time required to attend the clinic and the fact that it is more complicated to organise, as it is crucial that the patient accesses the photosensitiser at the correct time and protects their skin until the psoralen has cleared from the body. For these reasons, and because of the known long-term risks associated with PUVA, narrowband UVB is often the UV treatment of choice, provided the patient is not so pale that they burn easily.

What advice can you give Miss JG about sunbathing and the use of sunbeds with respect to managing her psoriasis?

A10 Miss JG can be advised that sunbathing may be helpful but that sunbeds will not be.

Sunbeds use UVA radiation, and this would not have much effect on psoriasis without the use of a photosensitiser. Alternatively, if she has taken a photosensitiser and still has some in the body, she could be badly burned by using a sunbed. It is rarely possible to measure the exact doses of radiation delivered from tanning sunbeds in the same way as in a PUVA clinic.

Natural sunlight is often beneficial for people with psoriasis, although many avoid public sunbathing because of embarrassment about the appearance of their skin.

Would dithranol or coal-tar products be helpful to Miss JG?

A11 Neither dithranol nor coal tar products would be as pleasant, convenient or effective to use as Dovobet.

Dithranol (anthralin) has been used for the treatment of psoriasis for decades. It is a yellow powder that is profoundly irritant to normal skin, causing inflammation and severe blistering. It causes a purple-brown residual (temporary) staining of skin and also stains clothing and bathroom fittings permanently.

Dithranol is traditionally incorporated into Lassar's paste (zinc and salicylic acid paste BP) so that it can be applied to the psoriasis plaques and kept away from uninvolved skin. This can be made in concentrations from 0.1% up to 3%, and the concentration used is gradually increased according to the patient's response. It is believed to have a direct anti-proliferative effect on epidermal keratinocytes. Dithranol has been used in two main ways. Traditionally, inpatient treatment involves application of the paste for 12–24 hours, after which the paste is removed and the patient has a tar bath and UVB irradiation. This is known as the Ingram regimen. Short-contact dithranol treatment (SCDT) is now more commonly used. This involves the application of dithranol in concentrations of up to 8% for 15–30 minutes, with or without UVB irradiation. Some patients can undertake SCDT by themselves at home.

Micanol is a temperature-sensitive dithranol formulation that releases the drug at skin temperature. It must be washed off with lukewarm water (no soap) to avoid further release of the drug.

A response to dithranol treatment can be expected within 20 days. Great care must be taken to avoid contact with normal skin and facial skin. Dithranol treatment is impractical if there are multiple small plaques, and it is not suitable for the treatment of psoriasis affecting the flexures or facial skin because of its irritant nature.

Coal tar has been used in the treatment of psoriasis for decades. Its mode of action is not fully understood and the active component (among the thousands in crude coal tar) is unknown. Coal tar is believed to have keratolytic, anti-inflammatory and anti-proliferative effects. In addition to proprietary preparations such as Clinitar and Psoriderm, crude coal tar, 1–5% in white or yellow soft paraffin or emulsifying ointment, has been used. Crude coal tar stains clothing and smells unpleasant to many people. It has been combined with UVB phototherapy (Goeckerman regimen).

Crude coal tar contains a number of carcinogens and percutaneous absorption of mutagens is known to occur; however, there is no evidence that topical coal tar treatment increases the risk of skin or other cancers.

What are the advantages and disadvantages of using a combination of calcipotriol and betamethasone?

A12 **Advantages include the fact that the combination product works better than either of the ingredients separately, and that it only needs to be applied once a day. Disadvantages include the risks associated with topical steroids plus the risk of adverse effects on withdrawal.**

The potential disadvantages of a combination product containing calcipotriol and betamethasone are that if she forgets that it contains a potent corticosteroid and uses it continuously for long periods (many months) without a break she could be at risk of side-effects, such as skin thinning and stretch marks, and even of systemic effects if she exceeds the recommended doses. In addition, when treating psoriasis with topical corticosteroids there may be a risk of generalised pustular psoriasis or of rebound effects when treatment is discontinued. This can be very distressing, and is the reason why medical supervision needs to be continued during withdrawal from long-term or high-dose corticosteroid treatment. 'Accidental withdrawal' can occur if the patient does not realise that the product contains a potent topical corticosteroid.

Combination products such as Dovobet would not have been a good option for Miss JG earlier in the course of her disease when she had lots of small lesions: it is better (easier to apply) when they are reasonably large patches. Also it is not recommended for use in patients under 18.

What information/advice can you give to Miss JG to help her to use the calcipotriol/betamethasone combination product safely and effectively?

A13 Miss JG should be advised to start treatment when her psoriasis flares up and continue until the plaques have flattened.

Miss JG should keep a supply of the combination product available so that as soon as her skin flares up she can start treatment. She should apply the product to the plaques once a day, and treatment should continue until the plaques flatten – that is, they no longer feel thickened or bumpy. At this stage the areas may still be reddened, but she should discontinue active treatment. The discoloration could take several weeks to subside.

What information/advice can you give to Miss JG to help her to use the scalp treatments effectively?

A14 The Cocois ointment should be applied and left overnight to soften and lift the thickened scale. When the scale has been removed, the calcipotriol scalp application can be applied.

Miss JG has been prescribed treatment to soften and lift the thickened scale on her scalp, and also some antipsoriatic treatment (calcipotriol scalp application) to reduce the underlying inflammation. The antipsoriatic treatment will be more effective once the layer of scale has been removed. This requires patience and persistence: simply pulling or scratching the scale off would be painful and could cause more inflammation.

The Cocois ointment should be applied quite thickly, parting the hair in several places so as to cover the whole scalp. It should be left in place for at least an hour, but ideally overnight. A plastic shower cap can be worn over the hair, and pillows need to be protected with an old towel. In the morning, before shampooing the hair to wash out the ointment, she should comb very gently to remove the loosened scales. A blob of the Ceanel shampoo should be gently worked into the hair near the scalp before water is added, as this removes the ointment more effectively.

Most people find scalp treatment easier if someone else can help with the application and the combing-out processes.

Miss JG should be warned that several applications might be required to get the scalp and hair back into a satisfactory condition. The softening and shampooing routine may need to be repeated daily for a few days. The second step, active treatment with calcipotriol scalp application, can then be performed. Again, careful, thorough application is needed, gently parting the hair and working across the whole scalp. She should take care not to allow the lotion to trickle over her face.

What is the role of topical steroids in facial and flexural psoriasis?

A15 **Short-term mild topical corticosteroids offer an effective way of controlling psoriasis in sensitive areas such as the flexures and the face.**

Topical corticosteroids do not smell, stain or cause irritation, and are often effective at bringing a flare-up under control. These advantages have to be balanced against the risks of local side-effects such as skin atrophy, striae, telangiectasias, and the risk of rebound and worsening of psoriasis after discontinuation. An additional problem is tachyphylaxis (the need for increasing amounts to achieve the same effect as treatment progresses).

Mild topical corticosteroids are used for psoriasis affecting the face, flexures or genitalia, and potent corticosteroids are used for recalcitrant lesions on the trunk or limbs. One fingertip unit of a corticosteroid cream or ointment is sufficient to treat an area equivalent to the flats of two adult hands. (The flat is the area you get if you put your hand down on a piece of paper and draw round it – fingers and thumb included.)

The use of topical corticosteroids to treat psoriasis requires careful supervision, and the British Association of Dermatologists (BAD) has formulated guidelines for their safe use (see Box 28.1).

Box 28.1 BAD guidelines for the management of psoriasis: topical corticosteroids

No topical steroid should be used regularly for more than 4 weeks without critical review

Potent corticosteroids should not be used regularly for more than 7 days

No unsupervised repeat prescriptions should be made: patients should be reviewed every 3 months

No more than 100 g of a moderately potent or higher potency preparation should be applied per month

Attempts should be made to rotate topical corticosteroids with alternative non-corticosteroid preparations

Use of potent or very potent preparations should be under dermatological supervision

The fingertip unit is a measure that helps patients to know how much ointment or cream to apply

Steroid phobia prevents some patients from using topical corticosteroids effectively, and this needs to be addressed with clear explanations. Another issue is confusion between concentration and potency. People with psoriasis often receive several different topical corticosteroids and, on occasions, have assumed that lower concentrations equate to lower potencies: an analogy with artificial sweeteners is a useful way to explain the difference.

The moderate potency steroid clobetasone butyrate 0.05% may not be sold for the treatment of psoriasis.

Is there a role for systemic corticosteroid therapy in the management of extensive, severe psoriasis?

A16 No. Systemic corticosteroids are rarely used in the management of psoriasis.

Treatment of psoriasis with systemic corticosteroids is associated with severe side-effects and rebound pustular psoriasis. For this reason systemic corticosteroids are held as a treatment of last resort and should always be closely supervised by an experienced dermatologist. If systemic corticosteroids are used at all then they must be withdrawn very slowly to minimise the risk of rebound disease. Some sources, for example the *Merck Manual*, recommend that systemic corticosteroids should never be used for any form of psoriasis, whereas the British National Formulary says 'Systemic or potent topical corticosteroids should be avoided or given only under specialist supervision in *psoriasis* because, although they may suppress the psoriasis in the short term, relapse or vigorous rebound occurs on withdrawal (sometimes precipitating severe pustular psoriasis).'

What are the roles of ciclosporin, methotrexate and acitretin in the management of psoriasis?

A17 Systemic therapy for psoriasis using methotrexate, ciclosporin or etretinate is reserved for severe disease that is unresponsive to topical treatments and/or phototherapy.

Methotrexate is a dihydrofolate reductase inhibitor that interferes with DNA synthesis by preventing the formation of tetrahydrofolate. It has been used for many years in the treatment of malignant disease, but is also used, in much lower doses, in the management of psoriasis. Its action was presumed to be immunosuppressive, and recent studies have shown that methotrexate inhibits other enzymes, causing adenosine, a T-cell toxin, to accumulate. This may account for its immunosuppressive activity.

For psoriasis treatment methotrexate is given in a single weekly dose of 12.5–20 mg. It is used both for clearance of disease (it can clear psoriasis in 8 weeks) and for maintenance treatment.

Methotrexate should not be given to people with active infections or during pregnancy or lactation. It also inhibits spermatogenesis and should not be given to men who wish to father children. The azoospermia is reversible, but a washout period is required.

A test dose is normally given before regular treatment is started to check that the patient is not unusually sensitive to the immunosuppressive effects. Regular monitoring for signs of bone marrow suppression and the development of liver fibrosis is essential during methotrexate treatment.

Patients must be advised to look out for signs of infection, such as a sore throat, which could be the result of bone marrow suppression. Avoidance of alcohol is recommended to minimise the risks of liver damage. Nausea is the most common side-effect. It usually starts within 12 hours of taking the dose and can persist for up to 3 days. Folic acid, at a dose of 5 mg daily, can be more helpful than conventional antiemetics. Other side-effects of methotrexate include mucosal ulceration, stomatitis, macrocytic anaemia and pneumonitis.

Accidental overdose can be a serious risk for people taking weekly doses of methotrexate. The National Patient Safety Agency has published a patient safety alert setting out the steps that need to be taken by healthcare professionals to ensure that methotrexate is used safely.

Methotrexate is cleared by the kidneys, so drugs such as some penicillins, salicylates, non-steroidal anti-inflammatory drugs and probenecid can reduce clearance and increase toxicity.

Ciclosporin has for many years been used as an immunosuppressant in organ transplantation. In psoriasis it blocks the intracellular components of T cell activation through a series of interactions resulting in the inhibition of calcineurin phosphatase, which in turn inhibits nuclear factor of activated T-cells (NFAT). NFAT regulates transcription of T-cell cytokines. Ciclosporin in doses of 2.5–5.0 mg/kg can clear psoriasis in 6–8 weeks.

Ciclosporin is sometimes used for maintenance treatment, but many clinicians feel that the risks of side-effects outweigh the benefits. Ciclosporin is contraindicated in pregnancy and breastfeeding and should not be given to people who are immunosuppressed. The most common side-effects are mild nausea and indigestion. The most serious are nephrotoxicity and hypertension. Both are dose dependent and have gradual onset. Regular monitoring of renal function using serum creatinine levels is essential. If the level rises more than 30% above baseline (even if this is still within the normal range) then the ciclosporin dose should be reduced or treatment discontinued. Moderate hypertension can be treated with nifedipine. Other side-effects include hypertrichosis and neurological events such as dysaesthesiae (abnormal sensations of the skin – typically pins and needles), tremors and headaches. In spite of its immunosuppressive activity, the use of ciclosporin in dermatology does not appear to cause internal malignancies or increased susceptibility to infection. Ciclosporin is metabolised via CYP3A (cytochrome P450 3A) and excreted mainly in the bile. Numerous drugs interact with ciclosporin to raise or lower blood levels, and put the patient at risk of increased toxicity or reduced effect. One commonly seen interaction is when erythromycin is prescribed, causing ciclosporin levels to rise, often with beneficial effect on the psoriasis and causing the patient to assume that erythromycin is good for psoriasis.

Retinoids are vitamin A analogues. They bind to nuclear receptors that regulate gene transcription. In psoriasis they induce keratinocyte differentiation, thereby normalising maturation of keratinocytes and reducing epidermal hyperplasia. The major limitation to the use of acitretin is its teratogenicity. In women of childbearing age the possibility of pregnancy must be excluded before treatment and pregnancy avoided during treatment and for a period of 2 years afterwards. Because of the difficulty of meeting these provisions in practice, many dermatologists prefer not to use acitretin in women of childbearing age. Acitretin is sometimes used in combination with PUVA (known as re-PUVA: retinoid plus PUVA). The maximum effect is seen after 4–6 weeks. The most common side-effects involve skin and mucous membranes, such as dry and cracking lips, dry skin and mucosal surfaces. Other side-effects include hair thinning, paronychia, and soft and sticky palms and soles. Liver function and blood lipids should be monitored.

What monitoring needs to be undertaken before ciclosporin treatment is started?

A18 **Miss JG's blood pressure and serum creatinine level should be checked. A check for pre-existing malignancies (including skin and cervix) should also be carried out.**

What are the advantages and disadvantages of adalimumab, infliximab, efalizumab and etanercept in the treatment of psoriasis?

A19 **The major advantage of biologics is that the treatment is given by injection and, in general, the side-effects appear to be less wide-ranging than with the conventional systemic agents. The**

main disadvantage is that patients need to learn to self-inject, or be prepared to spend time in hospital at regular intervals for intravenous (IV) infusions, and that the long-term effects of these agents are as yet unknown.

The biologics act by blocking components of the immune response that play a part in psoriasis. Adalimumab, etanercept and infliximab block tumour necrosis factor (TNF)-α; efalizumab blocks the activation of T cells. Ustekinumab blocks the activation of T cells by inhibiting the actions of interleukin (IL)-12 and IL-23.

At the time of writing NICE has made recommendations on the use of infliximab, etanercept, efalizumab and adalimumab, stating that they should only be used when the following two criteria are met:

(a) The disease is very severe, as defined by a total Psoriasis Area Severity Index (PASI) of 20 or more and a Dermatology Life Quality Index (DLQI) of more than 18.
(b) The psoriasis has failed to respond to standard systemic therapies such as ciclosporin, methotrexate or PUVA, or the person is intolerant of or has a contraindication to these treatments.

Since this decision efalizumab has been voluntarily withdrawn by its manufacturer from the market due to an increased risk of progressive multifocal leukoencephalopathy. Ustekinumab has a marketing authorization but has not yet been reviewed by NICE. One recent study showed that adalimumab and infliximab were the most cost-effective agents.

Before starting treatment with a biologic, checks should be made for latent tuberculosis and hepatitis B, which can both be reactivated by treatment with biologics that influence the immune system.

Treatment of psoriasis with biologics should only be undertaken by specialist physicians experienced in the diagnosis and treatment of psoriasis.

Table 28.1 overleaf summarises the dosing and features of the biologics available at the time of writing.

When therapy for psoriasis using biologics was first introduced intermittent treatment was recommended; however, in practice patients who respond to biologic therapy often receive more or less continuous treatment because this is the only way that their disease can be adequately controlled. Results so far suggest that continuous treatment is generally safe and well tolerated, with adverse effects being no more common than in short-term studies. Re-treatment with infliximab after a gap of 20 weeks is associated with antibody formation, reduced efficacy and increased risk of allergic responses. For this reason, infliximab is sometimes given together with methotrexate.

Table 28.1 The dosing and features of the biologics available at the time of writing

Drug name	*Dose and frequency*	*Features*
Adalimumab (Humira)	40 mg by subcutaneous injection at week 1, week 2 and then every 2 weeks	Fully human monoclonal antibody Preloaded pen injector system
Etanercept (Enbrel)	25 mg by subcutaneous injection twice weekly or 50 mg once weekly	Fusion protein 50 mg preloaded syringe available
Infliximab (Remicade)	5 mg/kg by IV infusion over 2 hours at week 1, then at 2 and 6 weeks after the first infusion, then every 8 weeks	Chimeric human–mouse monoclonal antibody
Ustekinumab (Stelara)	45mg (or 90 mg if >100 kg) by subcutaneous injection at week 0, week 4 and then every 12 weeks	Fully human IgG1κ monoclonal antibody

Further reading

Ashcroft DM, Li Wan Po A, Williams HC, Griffiths CEM. Systematic review of comparative efficacy and tolerability of calcipotriol in treating chronic plaque psoriasis. *Br Med J* 2000; **320**: 963–967.

Boudreau R, Blackhouse G, Goeree R, Mierzwinski-Urban M. *Adalimumab, Alefacept, Efalizumab, Etanercept and Infliximab for Severe Psoriasis Vulgaris in Adults: Budget Impact Analysis and Review of Comparative Clinical and Cost-Effectiveness.* Ottawa: Canadian Agency for Drugs and Technologies in Health (CADTH) 2007: 48.

British Association of Dermatologists & Primary Care Dermatology Society. Recommendations for the initial management of psoriasis. 2003. www.pcds.org.uk

Camarasa JM, Ortonne J-P, Dubertret L. Cacitriol shows greater persistence of treatment effect than betamethasone dipropionate in topical psoriasis therapy. *J Dermatol Treat* 2003; **14**: 8–13.

DermNet NZ. New Zealand Dermatological Society Incorporated. UVA photo(chemo)therapy. http://dermnetnz.org.

Mason J, Mason AR, Cork MJ. Topical preparations for the treatment of psoriasis: a systematic review. *Br J Dermatol* 2002; **146**: 351–364.

Medonca CO, Burden AD. Current concepts in psoriasis and its treatment. *Pharmacol Ther* 2003; **99**: 133–147.

National Patient Safety Agency: Patient Safety Alert NPSA/2006/13. *Improving Compliance with Oral Methotrexate Guidelines*. NPSA, London, 2005.

Nelson AA, Pearce DJ, Fleischer AB Jr *et al*. Cost-effectiveness of biologic treatments for psoriasis based on subjective and objective efficacy measures assessed over a 12-week treatment period. *J Am Acad Dermatol* 2008; **58**: 125–135.

National Institute for Health and Clinical Excellence. TA134. *Infliximab for the Treatment of Adults with Psoriasis*. NICE, London, 2008.

National Institute for Health and Clinical Excellence. TA103. *Etanercept and Efalizumab for the Treatment of Adults with Psoriasis*. NICE, London, 2006.

National Institute for Health and Clinical Excellence. TA146. *Adalimumab for the Treatment of Adults with Psoriasis*. NICE, London, 2008.

Ortonne J-P, Humbert P, Nicolas JF *et al*. Intra-individual comparison of cutaneous safety and efficacy of calcitriol 3 $\mu g\ g^{-1}$ ointment and calcipotriol 50 $\mu g\ g^{-1}$ ointment on chronic plaque psoriasis localized in facial, hairline, retroauricular or flexural areas. *Br J Dermatol* 2003; **148**: 1–8.

Osborne JE, Hutchinson PE. The importance of accurate dosage of topical agents: a method for estimating dosage and its application to apparent calcipotriol treatment failures in psoriasis. *Br J Dermatol* 2000; **143**: 63–64.

Rott S, Mrowietz U. Recent developments in the use of biologics in psoriasis and autoimmune disorders. The role of autoantibodies. *Br Med J* 2005; **330**: 716–720.

Walsh SRA, Shear NH. Psoriasis and the new biologic agents: interrupting a T-AP dance. *Can Med Assoc J* 2004; **170**: 1933–1941.

29

Anticoagulant therapy

Christopher Acomb and Peter A Taylor

Case study and questions

Day 1 Mr WS, a 52-year-old 65 kg overlooker in the local wool mill, was referred to hospital by his general practitioner (GP) with a red, swollen left leg. He said that he had not knocked his leg but that 'it had just come up during the night'. He had taken some painkillers before going to his GP, who had referred him.

Mr WS's past medical history revealed that he had been started on co-amilozide 5/50 tablets (amiloride hydrochloride 5 mg, hydrochlorothiazide 50 mg) 6 months earlier for mild breathlessness on exertion. He had been treated for epilepsy in the past, but had not had any fits for over 5 years and was not currently taking any medication for this. He had been thinking of going back to his GP because he had recently become more breathless, particularly at night.

On examination Mr WS was found to be short of breath, with a regular pulse and a raised jugular venous pressure. His left calf was inflamed and painful to the touch. When measured, his calf circumferences were: left leg 39.5 cm, right leg 38 cm. His left thigh was also swollen. Chest X-ray showed some fluid retention but no apparent pulmonary emboli, and he was haemodynamically stable.

He was diagnosed as having a left deep-vein thrombosis (DVT) and mild left ventricular failure. Although seemingly a spontaneous DVT it was considered that this could have been linked to his worsening heart failure. Because of his clinical history a confirmatory test for pulmonary embolism (PE) was not felt necessary, as initial treatment would be similar. If his clinical picture changed and a PE was suspected then a CTPA (pulmonary angiogram) was to be carried out to confirm the diagnosis.

Mr WS was admitted and prescribed:

- Furosemide 40 mg orally each morning
- Amiloride 5 mg orally each morning

- Warfarin, loading dose to be given over 3 days
- Tinzaparin 14 000 units subcutaneously once a day

Q1 Why does Mr WS need both low-molecular-weight heparin (LMWH) and warfarin therapy?
Q2 What laboratory indexes would you check before starting oral anticoagulant therapy?
Q3 Was the dose of LMWH prescribed for Mr WS appropriate?
Q4 How is the LMWH treatment monitored in the laboratory?
Q5 Is there a place for intravenous (IV) unfractionated heparin?
Q6 What loading dose of warfarin would you recommend for Mr WS? What factors did you take into account when making this recommendation?
Q7 How is warfarin treatment monitored in the laboratory?
Q8 Why is it important that a complete drug history is taken from Mr WS?
Q9 Outline the key elements of a pharmaceutical care plan for Mr WS.

Day 2 Mr WS was slightly less breathless, although his leg was still swollen and painful. He was prescribed ibuprofen for the pain.

Q10 What changes in drug therapy would you recommend?

Day 4 Mr WS was still a little breathless and had now developed a cough with green sputum. He was diagnosed as having a chest infection and prescribed erythromycin 500 mg orally three times a day.

His prothrombin time (reported as an international normalised ratio – INR) was 3.5 (target range 2–3) after a loading dose of 7 mg arfarin daily for 3 days.

His LMWH was continued at a dose of 11 000 units subcutaneously once a day and a maintenance dose of warfarin was prescribed.

Q11 How long should Mr WS's LMWH therapy be continued?
Q12 What maintenance dose of warfarin would you recommend? How should his therapy be monitored after the maintenance dose is initiated?
Q13 How long should Mr WS's warfarin therapy be continued?

Day 5 Mr WS's chest infection appeared to be improving and his leg was much better.

Day 6 Mr WS continued to do well. His LMWH was discontinued; however, his INR was reported as 5.4 (2–3). Adjustment to his treatment for left ventricular failure was also undertaken by reducing his diuretics and adding the angiotensin-converting enzyme (ACE) inhibitor ramipril. His blood pressure was carefully monitored during this change.

Q14 What are the possible causes of Mr WS's high INR?

Q15 How should Mr WS's high INR be managed?

Day 8 Mr WS was doing very well, with both his chest and leg much improved. His INR was 2.9 (2–3) and it was decided to discharge him.

His discharge medication comprised:

- Erythromycin 500 mg orally three times a day for 1 day, then stop
- Furosemide 20 mg orally daily
- Ramipril 1.25 mg orally daily
- Warfarin 1.5 mg orally daily

His GP was asked to increase the dose of ramipril as necessary, in accordance with the *British National Formulary* (BNF), and to monitor urea and electrolytes.

Q16 What points would you cover when giving medication advice to Mr WS about his warfarin therapy?

Day 12 On his visit to the outpatient clinic, Mr WS's INR was found to be 2.6 (2–3) and his warfarin dose was continued at 1.5 mg orally daily for a further week.

Day 19 At Mr WS's outpatient attendance his INR was found to have fallen to 1.8 (2–3).

Q17 What are the possible causes of Mr WS's low INR?

Mr WS was prescribed warfarin 2.5 mg daily.

Day 33 Mr WS was admitted with epistaxis and haematuria. The only change in treatment was a prescription for azapropazone from his GP 2 days before admission. This had been prescribed for acute gout.

Q18 What are the probable causes of Mr WS's problems? What action would you recommend?

Q19 What other drugs should be avoided or prescribed with caution and careful monitoring while Mr WS continues to take warfarin?

Answers

Why does Mr WS need both low-molecular-weight heparin (LMWH) and warfarin therapy?

A1 **Mr WS requires anticoagulant therapy to prevent the extension of the clot that has formed in his leg. LMWH therapy provides an immediate anticoagulant effect until the slower-acting oral warfarin therapy exerts its full anticoagulant activity.**

A LMWH is now often used alone while awaiting a definitive diagnosis by Doppler ultrasound scan. Clinical symptoms and history, along with a positive or equivocal result from D-dimer testing, will reduce the likelihood of an incorrect diagnosis, enabling early intervention with an LMWH and the prevention of a hospital admission. A confirmatory diagnosis can then be made following a planned Doppler ultrasound scan, at which time warfarin can be introduced and the LMWH stopped once warfarin has achieved therapeutic control. This form of treatment can be easily organised in the community.

Heparin and LMWH form a complex with antithrombin III which, in therapeutic doses, inhibits the action of thrombin and activated factor X. Warfarin is a vitamin K analogue and prevents the formation of vitamin K-dependent clotting factors II, VII, IX and X.

LMWHs act rapidly but must be given parenterally. They have the advantage over unfractionated heparin because (for the treatment of thromboembolism) they can be given as a once-daily subcutaneous injection, whereas unfractionated heparin needs to be given as a continuous IV infusion. This simpler administration has led in many areas to the development of home/outpatient treatment of DVT and PE.

The LMWH will need to be continued for at least 6 days and until the warfarin is exerting a full therapeutic effect. Mr WS will be at risk of further thrombosis for a number of weeks after this first incident.

In contrast to heparin, warfarin takes 3–4 days to exert its full anticoagulant effect and is therefore not effective in limiting the extension of the thrombosis in the early phase; however, being orally active, it is very useful for long-term anticoagulant treatment.

Newer oral anticoagulants are being introduced based on small molecule inhibitors of specific coagulation enzymes. At the time of writing two such products, rivaroxaban (inhibitor of factor Xa) and dabigatran etexilate (a direct thrombin inhibitor), have been licensed but only for prophylaxis of venous thromboembolism. These newer medicines do not so far have a requirement for monitoring, and so if licensed for the treatment of DVT may be more acceptable to patients and clinicians for longer-term treatment.

What laboratory indexes would you check before starting oral anticoagulant therapy?

A2 **A pre-treatment clotting screen should be carried out. Although other indexes (such as haemoglobin level, platelet adhesiveness and liver function tests (LFTs)) are indicated in some patients, Mr WS's history does not suggest that these are warranted in his case.**

A pre-treatment clotting screen is essential to ensure that a patient has not already been anticoagulated and that organic changes, such as liver disease, have not disrupted his clotting mechanism. Either of these conditions would mean an excessive response to the initial warfarin dose, but not necessarily the heparin dose.

There are other laboratory indexes that will help make anticoagulation safer, but they are not necessary for every patient and should only be carried out if there is evidence, either from a previous or a current medical history, that they may be grossly abnormal. They include the following:

(a) **A haemoglobin level**. A patient with anaemia may have occult bleeding which would be exacerbated by anticoagulation. A baseline haemoglobin level would also be useful to detect bleeding in the future.
(b) **A platelet level**. Platelets are involved in the clotting process and thrombocytopenia would make the patient very prone to bleeding; however, platelet counts can be deceptive, as it is the ability to adhere to one another and not just the number of platelets that determines their activity. This adhesiveness is seldom checked routinely, but such a measurement would detect the antiplatelet activity of non-steroidal anti-inflammatory drugs (NSAIDs).
(c) **LFTs.** The liver is involved in both the production of clotting factors and the metabolism of warfarin. Its normal function is therefore essential for safe anticoagulation.

Mr WS only requires his international normalised ratio (INR) to be measured at this point. Although he may have a history of taking NSAIDs ('painkillers') and there is thus a slight chance he may have had a gastrointestinal bleed, he has given no history of dyspepsia and has no obvious signs of anaemia. His heart failure may have caused some changes to his LFTs but it is unlikely that they are significant enough to influence his loading dose, although they may influence his maintenance dose and frequent INR monitoring will be required until a safe maintenance dose is established. Any future changes in his heart failure or its treatment will also affect the warfarin maintenance dose and should be monitored for. In our own practice many patients will have slightly deranged LFTs because of other pathologies, but this does not seem to affect warfarin loading decisions and so LFTs are not done routinely, but instead only when there are other clinical reasons for doing so.

Was the dose of LMWH prescribed for Mr WS appropriate?

A3 The dose was rather large and should be adjusted.

The LMWHs used to treat thromboembolism are dosed according to body weight. Renal function should also be considered, as poor function may increase the risk of bleeding during anticoagulation. Tinzaparin is dosed at 175 units/kg and so the correct dose for Mr WS is 11 375 units. A dose of 11 000 units (0.55 mL from a 2 mL multidose vial) would be appropriate, being a reasonable volume to be measured. At the time of writing all the LMWHs used for the treatment of thromboembolism come as prefilled syringes or as multidose vials. There are some small differences between the different brands, so the Summary of Product Characteristics should be consulted for specific details on dosing.

How is the LMWH treatment monitored in the laboratory?

A4 Patients receiving therapy for more than 5 days should have a platelet count and their potassium level measured.

The LMWHs differ from unfractionated heparin in that they do not require therapeutic monitoring. They have little effect on the activated partial thromboplastin time (APTT), which is the measure used to monitor unfractionated heparin. Anti-factor Xa has been used in research studies to monitor the effect of LMWHs, but this is not necessary for routine use. The LMWHs are associated with a small incidence of thrombocytopenia, and so patients who remain on them for longer than 5 days should have a platelet count carried out as part of a full blood count.

Patients may also require their potassium level to be monitored if LMWHs are used for this extended time, as heparins have been associated with reduced aldosterone levels, and although most patients will respond with an increase in renin production, some may not be able to, resulting in an increased potassium level.

Is there a place for intravenous (IV) unfractionated heparin?

A5 **Dalteparin, enoxaparin and tinzaparin all have an evidence base to support their use in thromboembolism and are all licensed for DVT and PE, so there is little place for IV unfractionated heparin at the start of thromboembolism treatment.**

The LMWHs are easier to dose and more consistent in the degree of anticoagulation produced. The main advantage to using IV unfractionated heparin is that it is controllable. The relatively short half-life of unfractionated heparin means that stopping an IV infusion quickly results in a return to normal clotting status. Furthermore, the effect of unfractionated heparin can be reversed by using protamine. This is in contrast to the LMWHs which, once given subcutaneously, have an effect for 24 hours and are not fully reversible by protamine. Therefore, when it is necessary to control carefully or to stop anticoagulation rapidly, unfractionated heparins still may be used. For example, IV unfractionated heparin can be used when therapeutic anticoagulation is required prior to surgery, with the infusion being switched off 6–8 hours prior to the procedure.

What loading dose of warfarin would you recommend for Mr WS? What factors did you take into account when making this recommendation?

A6 **Warfarin 7 mg daily for 3 days. This loading dose takes into account the fact that Mr WS has left ventricular failure.**

Warfarin is highly protein bound and has a long half-life. The administration of a loading dose therefore reduces the time taken for the drug to achieve steady state.

The standard warfarin loading dose is 10 mg daily for 3 days. This should be reduced in the presence of conditions that might potentiate the action of warfarin. The following factors should be considered:

(a) **Age**. In general, elderly patients are more sensitive to warfarin. It is recommended that a reduced loading dose is given to patients over 60 years of age, although in practice we find that, with a healthier older population, in many of these patients a significant age effect may not be seen until much later, in some cases nearer 80 years.
(b) **Body weight**. Given that the volume of distribution is at least partially linked to body weight, a reduced loading dose should be given to patients weighing <60 kg.
(c) **Plasma protein-binding capacity**. This will be reduced in patients with low plasma protein levels or in those already taking drugs that are highly protein bound. Albumin is the principal plasma protein fraction that binds warfarin.

(d) **Concurrent pathology**. Some diseases, such as congestive cardiac failure, reduce the liver's ability to produce clotting factors and to metabolise warfarin effectively.

(e) **Other drugs**. Although already mentioned under plasma protein-binding capacity, concurrent drug therapy can also interfere with warfarin activity in many other ways, and nearly all types of drug interaction have been reported.

Taking the above factors into consideration will ensure a safer loading dose for most patients; however a small number of patients will still respond in an unpredictable way. This may be due to genetic differences between patients. Cytochrome P450 isoform 2C9 (CYP2C9) and vitamin K epoxide reductase complex 1 (VKORC1) contribute significantly to the way in which warfarin acts and is metabolised. Genetic polymorphisms in CYP2C9 and VKORC1 occur in the population and may explain some of the interpatient variation seen. Technologies to screen for these polymorphisms are developing, but at the time of writing are not used routinely.

In Mr WS's case his loading dose should be reduced to 7 mg daily for 3 days on the basis that his left ventricular failure may enhance the activity of warfarin. If he had had two or more of the above factors, then his loading dose should have been reduced further to 5 mg daily for 3 days.

It should be noted that prescribers sometimes reduce the loading dose by giving 10 mg, 5 mg and then 5 mg over the 3 days. The first dose (10 mg) will often produce an exaggerated response on day 4, which makes calculation of the maintenance dose difficult and can lead to doses being omitted because of the seemingly high INR.

There are a number of nomograms and methods available to initiate warfarin therapy. Certainly we favour lower loading doses, particularly for those managed on an outpatient basis. Provided patients continue to receive adequate anticoagulation with LMWH, it is better to be slow and cautious when initiating oral anticoagulation.

How is warfarin treatment monitored in the laboratory?

A7 **Warfarin activity is monitored in the laboratory by measuring the prothrombin time.**

The citrate in the blood sample is neutralised with excess calcium ions and thromboplastin added. The time taken for the sample to clot is then known as the prothrombin time. Comparing this with a sample containing no anticoagulant will give a prothrombin time ratio.

The thromboplastin used in this test has been standardised so as to allow a patient to be controlled by any laboratory. This standardisation has resulted in the test being named the international normalised ratio: INR.

INR values in the range of 2.0–4.5 are accepted as being therapeutic, although target INRs within this range are used to cover the various indications for warfarin anticoagulation. In Mr WS's case a target range of 2.0–3.0 would be appropriate to prevent an extension of his DVT.

Why is it important that a complete drug history is taken from Mr WS?

A8 A drug history is essential prior to starting oral anticoagulant therapy with warfarin or other coumarin derivatives because many drugs can interact with warfarin to a clinically significant extent.

Two important facts were elicited from Mr WS's medication history. First, it was noted that Mr WS has a history of epilepsy. On questioning, he indicated that he had been taking phenytoin some 3 months earlier. Phenytoin and other drugs that induce warfarin metabolism may exert their effect for up to 6 weeks after stopping therapy. This demonstrates that not only current medication, but also any other medication taken over the previous 6 weeks, should be considered in an effort to reduce potential complications of warfarin treatment.

Second, Mr WS had referred to 'painkillers' he had taken at home. When questioned further, he said that he usually took Aspro Clear tablets, but as he had run out he had taken some of his wife's Anadin Extra. Both of these over-the-counter products contain aspirin ('Anadin' has become a brand name associated with a range of analgesic products, only some of which now contain aspirin). This means that he should be counselled regarding their future use, as he will need to avoid aspirin and aspirin-containing products while he is taking warfarin. In addition, attention should be given to the possibility that his recent ingestion of aspirin may cause aspirin-induced low platelet activity, which may lead to bruising or other minor bleeding despite normal INRs, or that drug-induced gastrointestinal erosions may cause major bleeding complications.

Outline the key elements of a pharmaceutical care plan for Mr WS.

A9 This is high-risk treatment and a care plan to ensure adequate anticoagulant control is essential.

All patients starting anticoagulant therapy should have a clear pharmaceutical care plan which ensures, wherever possible, that the patient is protected from the potential risks of the treatment.

Warfarin activity monitoring should be planned, with the first significant laboratory result being reported on day 4 after introducing the drug. Thereafter, INRs should be done regularly and with a gradually increasing interval between tests, as stability is achieved.

The care plan should include discharge arrangements and should allow time for providing medication advice to ensure he has a good understanding of the treatment and its implications, before discharge.

Mr WS will need to be followed up at the anticoagulant clinic after leaving hospital, and these arrangements (e.g. when and where) along with communications with the clinic should be included in the care plan. In our own hospital these clinics are run by our pharmacists, making the organisation much simpler. We also use Intermediate Care Centres (or peripheral clinics) to provide a more local service for patients.

The plan should also consider how to communicate with both the patient's GP and, if possible, their community pharmacist. Good communication is essential in order to reduce the risks to the patient.

What changes in drug therapy would you recommend?

A10 Consider changing ibuprofen to paracetamol, co-codamol or co-dydramol.

Ibuprofen does not usually affect warfarin activity (it does not normally increase INRs), but should probably be stopped because of the small risk of gastrointestinal bleeding associated with NSAIDs. A gastrointestinal bleed while on warfarin can have disastrous consequences. Furthermore, ibuprofen and other NSAIDs could exacerbate Mr WS's heart failure. Paracetamol, co-codamol and co-dydramol should not affect his warfarin activity.

Although the use of paracetamol products for acute episodes of pain do not usually influence the anticoagulant effect of warfarin, we have seen a small number of patients (particularly elderly patients) on regular full doses of paracetamol who have developed significantly raised INRs. Clinical staff monitoring patients should be made aware of this possibility, as it is not well documented.

How long should Mr WS's LMWH therapy be continued?

A11 LMWH therapy should continue until the desired effect of warfarin has been achieved.

The INR value on day 4 is the first indication of warfarin activity and is the level from which the maintenance dose of warfarin can be calculated. Mr WS's INR was already in the therapeutic range by day 4; however, we would usually recommend continuing the LMWH until day 6, as some patients can have high INRs but still have coagulation problems because of an imbalance in the clotting process. This may be seen as a worsening of the DVT. It is usually desirable to overlap the LMWH with warfarin at therapeutic INRs for at least 24 hours.

What maintenance dose of warfarin would you recommend? How should his therapy be monitored after the maintenance dose is initiated?

A12 **Warfarin 2.5 mg daily. INR monitoring should take place after 2–3 days; thereafter, depending on the results, it may be carried out at increased intervals.**

This dose is calculated using the method of Dobrzanski, which relates the maintenance dose to the cumulative loading dose over 3 days (in this case 21 mg, rounded down to 20 mg) and the INR achieved on the fourth day. This relationship is shown in Table 29.1.

Table 29.1 Warfarin dose calculation using the method of Dobrzanski

	Cumulative warfarin dose (mg)						
INR	15	20	25	30	35*	40*	45*
2.0	3.5	4	5	5.5	6	7	7.5
2.2	3.5	4	4.5	5	5.5	6	6.5
2.5	3	3.5	4	4	4.5	5	5.5
3.0	2.5	3	3.5	3.5	4	4	4
3.5	–	2.5	3	3	3.5	–	–
4.0	–	–	3	3	3	–	–
4.5	–	–	2.5	3	3	–	–
5.0	–	–	2.5	2.5	3	–	–

* Values of cumulative doses exceeding 30 mg may be found when the INR has not been measured at the correct time. Such values should not normally be used.

Although many factors can affect this relationship, in general it gives a good conservative estimate of the maintenance dose required.

To use the table, the cumulative loading dose given prior to the time of INR measurement should be calculated. The horizontal line corresponding to the measured INR should then be followed to the point where it intersects with the vertical column headed by the cumulative loading dose. The value at the point of intersection represents the recommended maintenance dose.

Further monitoring should be carried out after 2–3 days and then, depending on the results obtained, the interval can be increased, initially to once a week and then to every 2, 4 and even 6 weeks. If a graph is drawn of INR against time, the slope will indicate the need for more frequent monitoring, e.g. a sharp change in the slope of the graph would indicate the need for more frequent monitoring or intervention to prevent values going outside the agreed limits.

Changes in treatment, or in a patient's pathology, also necessitate more frequent monitoring. The overall aim must always be to ensure that sufficient monitoring is undertaken to enable adverse changes to be detected without inconveniencing the patient excessively.

How long should Mr WS's warfarin therapy be continued?

A13 For 6 months, provided there is no recurrence of his DVT.

A first DVT with no complications is normally treated with warfarin for a period of 3 months, although some authorities feel that patients who have suffered a thrombotic episode may be predisposed to this condition for much longer. In the case of Mr WS, his mild heart failure could have been a contributing factor: until this is controlled he will continue to be at risk (it was judged to be a spontaneous DVT). We would recommend at least 6 months' anticoagulant therapy, and if the DVT should recur, then continuous treatment.

What are the possible causes of Mr WS's high INR?

A14 There are a number of possible causes of the high INR, including changes in Mr WS's fluid balance (as a result of furosemide therapy), worsening of his heart failure (no clinical signs), drug interactions and failure to take the correct dose. However, the most likely explanation is an interaction between erythromycin and warfarin.

Warfarin is available as a racemic mixture of *S* and *R* isomers. Erythromycin is known to inhibit isoenzymes CYP3A4 and CYP1A2 involved in *R*-warfarin metabolism (as do clarithromycin, ciprofloxacin and norfloxacin) and is best avoided in patients anticoagulated with warfarin. If erythromycin therapy is necessary, a reduction of 50% in the dose of warfarin is required before the antibiotic is started. Weekly monitoring should also be recommended until the effect of the erythromycin is no longer seen, which may be 2 or 3 weeks after antibiotic therapy is stopped.

How should Mr WS's high INR be managed?

A15 Omit one dose, then recommence treatment with 1.5 mg warfarin orally daily.

The BNF gives good guidance on the management of excessive anticoagulation. Mr WS has a high INR but no apparent bleeding, and the probable cause of the increase in INR is known. He should therefore have one dose of warfarin withheld to quickly reduce the risk of a bleed, and he should then continue treatment with a lower dose. Reducing the dose to approximately 50% of that previously suggested would be appropriate. His INR should be monitored after a further 2 days and the dose readjusted if necessary.

When the erythromycin therapy is stopped, Mr WS's hepatic enzyme systems will return to normal; however, this return will not be as sudden as the inhibition, and monitoring should therefore continue at least weekly and his dose of warfarin should be adjusted until he returns to his pre-erythromycin dose.

What points would you cover when giving medication advice to Mr WS about his warfarin therapy?

A16 **It is essential to give medication advice to patients who have been prescribed warfarin for the first time. There is a large amount of information to be conveyed and it requires a high level of skill and a substantial amount of time. We take the view that it is unethical for a patient on warfarin to be discharged from hospital without being given medication advice. The National Patient Safety Agency (NPSA) information pack for patients should be supplied along with an individual discussion with the patient to ensure a sound understanding of the treatment and its risks.**

The major points to be covered with Mr WS include the following:

(a) What warfarin is and what it does.
(b) Why Mr WS is taking warfarin, and how its action can help.
(c) How much to take and how the dose can be described (i.e. the colour or strength of the tablet, and how dose changes may involve different combinations of the four strengths of tablet available).
(d) When to take the dose, what happens if a dose is missed, and the importance of regular dosing.
(e) Factors that affect the action of warfarin. These include food (diets high in vitamin K in particular), social activities (smoking, drinking, travel, exercise), and other medicines, including over-the-counter products and alternative medicines.
(f) Who Mr WS should tell that he is on anticoagulant therapy (GP, dentist, pharmacist).
(g) What symptoms to look for which may indicate too much anticoagulant activity (e.g. gum bleeding, bruising, blood in urine), what the significance of each might be, and what to do about it.
(h) Who to contact if there are problems or doubts about treatment.
(i) What to do about diseases that might occur during treatment (for instance influenza).

(j) When to come to clinic and why monitoring is important.
(k) What the treatment goals are (to help Mr WS visualise his therapy and thereby assist his adherence and cooperation).

The advice and information sessions will also be an opportunity to develop a clinical relationship between Mr WS and the pharmacist which will continue after discharge.

What are the possible causes of Mr WS's low INR?

A17 His warfarin dose was not increased when his erythromycin therapy was stopped.

This is the most likely cause of Mr WS's low INR. Non-adherence is a possibility, but assuming it at this stage would be inappropriate. The effect of hepatic enzyme inhibition may take a week or two to be fully reversed, so monitoring and small dose increases (in this case 0.5 mg aliquots) will be required during this time and until the original activity is resumed. It should be noted that if a patient has very low INRs early on in treatment and is at risk of further thromboembolism it may be necessary to restart therapeutic doses of LMWH for a few days until therapeutic INRs are achieved again.

What are the probable causes of Mr WS's problems? What action would you recommend?

A18 Azapropazone therapy is the most likely cause of his problems. It should be withdrawn and replaced by alternative therapy if needed.

On admission Mr WS was found to have a very high INR (>7.0), which was most probably caused by the addition of azapropazone to his warfarin therapy.

Most NSAIDs have some antiplatelet activity and, as such, can enhance bleeding, although this does not affect the INR. Similarly, although many NSAIDs are protein bound, the warfarin that is displaced by their competitive binding is rapidly eliminated by the liver so that, at most, only a small transient rise in INR (usually for no longer that a day or two) may be seen. However, as with the classic reaction between phenylbutazone and warfarin, azapropazone is not only capable of displacing a significant amount of warfarin from its protein-binding sites, but can also inhibit hepatic enzyme activity very rapidly. This produces a very profound increase in free warfarin levels and, as a consequence, in anticoagulant activity.

The use of azapropazone must be avoided wherever possible in patients already taking warfarin.

NSAIDs also affect the gastrointestinal mucosa, causing damage and some blood loss, and this will be enhanced in the presence of warfarin.

Mr WS's acute symptoms of gout may require an NSAID, but diclofenac would have been a more appropriate choice, being potent enough to treat the pain while having no effect on warfarin metabolism and only a small effect on the protein binding of warfarin. The Committee on Safety of Medicines (CSM) has restricted azapropazone to use in rheumatoid arthritis, ankylosing spondylitis and acute gout **only when other NSAIDs have been tried and failed.**

In our experience we have seen problems with high INRs following the use of colchicine for gout. Whether this is a result of an interaction between colchicine and warfarin or a physiological effect of gout on warfarin therapy is unknown.

The use of allopurinol for long-term prophylaxis of gout may also be considered, provided that increased monitoring of Mr WS's warfarin therapy is undertaken while allopurinol therapy is being introduced, as this drug is also reported to have an effect on anticoagulant therapy. An increase in warfarin activity is likely, although the size of the response varies from patient to patient.

Finally, the diuretics taken by Mr WS should be reviewed to see whether improvements in control or choice could be made, as they are the likely cause of his acute episode of gout.

Whichever method is used to control Mr WS's gout, more frequent monitoring of his anticoagulant treatment must be initiated.

What other drugs should be avoided or prescribed with caution and careful monitoring while Mr WS continues to take warfarin?

A19 **Warfarin and related compounds interact with many different drugs. A comprehensive - but not exhaustive – list of compounds involved can be found in the BNF and further explanation of these interactions in *Martindale: The Complete Drug Reference.***

Warfarin is present as a racemic mixture of *R* and *S* isomers, of which the *S* isomer is the more potent form. Isoenzyme CYP2C9 affects the *S* isomer and can be inhibited by drugs such as fluconazole and amiodarone. Polymorphism in CYP2C9 makes predicting the outcome of a drug interaction difficult. Isoenzymes CYP3A4 and CYP1A2 are involved in *R*-warfarin metabolism, and inhibition of these isoenzymes has already been discussed in **A14**.

Patients can vary quite markedly in their response to interactions, sometimes making it difficult to predict the outcome. For this reason it is important to:

(a) Recognise known drug interactions before the interacting medicine is given and initiate treatment changes that will avoid marked disruption of anticoagulant control.
(b) Ensure that the patient (and their GP and community pharmacist) is aware of the problem of drug interactions and that the clinic is informed before any new medication, including complementary and over-the-counter medicines, is started. As more medicines transfer from prescription only to over-the-counter status, e.g. cimetidine, fluconazole, the involvement of the community pharmacist becomes essential. Also, regular reminders should be given to the patient that many health store products taken in large doses can also have a marked effect on anticoagulant control. Ubidecarenone (Coenzyme Q10), vitamin E and fish oils have all been implicated, the latter two probably affecting platelet activity rather than the INR. Patients often do not equate health store products with medical products.
(c) Remember that changes in the doses of concurrent medication may influence the anticoagulant effect.
(d) Use the smaller range of medicines known to be safe in the presence of anticoagulants.
(e) Monitor patients carefully when medication is being changed.

It is very easy to recognise a drug interaction after a marked change in anticoagulant control has occurred. It is more beneficial to the patient if that change is anticipated and prevented.

The NPSA's Patient Safety Alert 18 highlighted the need to be extremely cautious and vigilant when using anticoagulants. A comprehensive package of information and self-audit tools has been produced which help clinical staff reduce the harm caused to patients by anticoagulants. The pack also contains a large number of references to support the use of anticoagulants. Reducing the risks associated with anticoagulation is also the focus of the Safer Patient Initiative run by the Health Foundation in conjunction with the Institute for Healthcare Improvement.

Further reading

Baglin TP, Keeling DM, Watson HG. Guidelines on oral anticoagulation (warfarin): third edition – 2005 update. *Br J Haematol* 2005; **132**: 277–285.

Baglin TP, Cousins D, Keeling DM, Watson HG. Recommendations from the British Committee for Standards in Haematology and National Patient Safety Agency. *Br J Haematol* 2007; **136**: 26–29.

Bates SM, Weitz JI. New anticoagulants; beyond heparin, low molecular weight heparin and warfarin. *Br J Clin Pharmacol* 2005; **144**: 1017–1028.

Clemerson J, Payne K. Pharmacogenetics – background and future potential. *Hosp Pharm* 2008; **15**: 159–164.

Clemerson J, Payne K. Pharmacogenetics – current applications. *Hosp Pharm* 2008; **15**: 167–173.

Dobrzanski S. Predicting warfarin dosage. *J Clin Hosp Pharm* 1983; **8**: 247–250.

Qaseem A, Snow V, Barry P *et al.* Current diagnosis of venous thromboembolism in primary care: a clinical practice guideline from the American Academy of Family Physicians and the American College of Physicians. *Ann Fam Med* 2007; **5**: 57–62.

Schraibman IG, Milne AA, Royle EM. *Home Versus In-patient Treatment for Deep Vein Thrombosis* (Cochrane Review). In: Cochrane Library 2. Update Software, Oxford, 2003.

Stockley IH. *Drug Interactions*, 8th edn. Pharmaceutical Press, London, 2007.

30

Colorectal surgery

Stan Dobrzanski

Case study and questions

Day 1 Mrs DH, a 71-year-old woman taking warfarin and atenolol for atrial fibrillation (AF) who had recently started oral hypoglycaemic medication for type 2 diabetes mellitus, attended the anticoagulant clinic. She told the clinic pharmacist that she had experienced a change in bowel habit during the past 2 months and had been buying senna tablets. She had been passing blood rectally when going to the toilet.

The pharmacist advised an immediate visit to her general practitioner (GP), who referred her to hospital where a malignant mid-rectal growth was identified that would require an anterior resection. As it would not be possible to carry out the surgery laparoscopically because of previous complicated gynaecological surgery, the approach would have to be through an abdominal incision. The cancerous section of the rectum would be excised and an end-to-end anastomosis formed between the sigmoid colon and the rectal remnant. Additionally, to protect the easily damaged anastomosis, a temporary loop ileostomy would be created that could later be reversed.

Day 16 At the preadmission clinic her drug history was:

- Furosemide 20 mg daily
- Atenolol 50 mg daily
- Warfarin 4 mg each evening
- Gliclazide 80 mg twice a day
- Metformin 500 mg twice a day
- Simvastatin 20 mg at night

She had once developed a rash when taking penicillin. Her biochemistry results were normal apart from a creatinine of 110 micromol/L and a potassium level of 3.5 mmol/L. She weighed 78 kg and her random blood glucose reading at the preadmission clinic was 7.6 mmol/L, with a glycosylated haemoglobin (HbA_{1c}) of 8.3%.

Mrs DH said that she was worried about contracting meticillin-resistant *Staphylococcus aureus* (MRSA) and asked whether having surgery meant that she needed to stop warfarin.

Q1 What steps can be taken at the preadmission clinic to minimise the incidence of postoperative MRSA?
Q2 When should warfarin be stopped before elective surgery, and what are the risks involved?

Day 20 (preoperatively) The junior doctor admitting Mrs DH asked the pharmacist whether there were risks associated with prescribing low-molecular-weight heparin (LMWH) in patients who might require epidural analgesics postoperatively. He also asked if this patient would require sliding-scale insulin. In the evening Mrs DH was given a Fleet Enema to clean the bowel.

Q3 What is the risk of venous thromboembolism (VTE) occurring in this patient?
Q4 What are the risks of using LMWHs in patients who are to have an epidural infusion?
Q5 How should the hypoglycaemic drugs be managed perioperatively?

Day 21 (operation day) Because there was a NIL ORALLY notice placed over her bed, Mrs DH was not given any of her tablets that morning.

Q6 Does a NIL ORALLY instruction mean that medication cannot be taken by mouth?

Before going to theatre Mrs DH was given another Fleet Enema. The anaesthetist in theatre was about to prescribe intravenous (IV) cefuroxime 1.5 g and metronidazole 500 mg when he noticed that she was allergic to penicillin.

Q7 Would the use of a cephalosporin be safe? When should the antibiotics be administered? Should antibiotic use continue postoperatively?

The anaesthetist used propofol to induce sleep and sevoflurane for general anaesthesia, remifentanil for analgesia and rocuronium as a muscle relaxant. An epidural line was inserted and an infusion of morphine 5 mg in 100 mL bupivacaine 0.125% commenced at a rate of 6 mL/h. She was also catheterised. As surgery finished the anaesthetist injected glycopyrronium and neostigmine.

Q8 Why is the anaesthetist using a muscle relaxant, and why was an injection of glycopyrronium and neostigmine given at the end of the procedure?

Mrs DH continued to be 'NIL ORALLY' immediately after the operation. The junior doctor was unsure which IV fluids to prescribe in addition to the sliding-scale regimen.

Q9 What IV fluids might be prescribed?

Day 22 (first postoperative day) Mrs DH was now allowed 15 mL sips of water. She was complaining of some discomfort despite the morphine and bupivacaine infusion. The doctor had written up morphine 10 mg injections 'when required' and wondered if he could add diclofenac to supplement the analgesia.

Q10 Would morphine and diclofenac be suitable analgesics for this patient?

One of the nurses attaching a new epidural syringe said that she was sometimes worried about connecting the syringe to the wrong line.

Q11 How might the administration of epidural injections be made safer?

During the evening ward round it was pointed out that Mrs DH was now exhibiting slight pyrexia of 37.5°C.

Q12 Should the pyrexia be treated with a continued course of antibiotics?

As her blood pressure was also low and as she was now hypokalaemic, the furosemide 20 mg tablets were stopped. The surgeon said that diuretics were risky in patients with an ileostomy.

Q13 What are the risks of diuretics in ileostomy patients?

Day 23 Mrs DH was now taking 30 mL sips of fluid and was now able to take her usual tablets, with the exception of her oral diabetes medication. On the ward round the pharmacist was asked to recommend a suitable dose with which to restart warfarin.

Q14 What dose of warfarin should be given? When should Mrs DH visit the anticoagulant clinic? When should the use of enoxaparin stop?

Day 24 Mrs DH was offered 60 mL sips of fluid and later on in the day, free fluids, and was told that normal food intake could resume.

Day 25 The pain management team recommended that her epidural line could be removed. Oral codeine was prescribed to thicken her ileostomy output. That evening her insulin sliding-scale regimen was stopped and gliclazide and metformin were restarted. Unfortunately, in the night Mrs DH developed a raised temperature again, this time of 38.5°C.

Q15 What are the most likely causes of high postoperative pyrexia?

Day 29 (8 days after surgery) The pharmacist carrying out discharge planning was concerned to learn that Mrs DH had a supply of senna at home.

Q16 Why are laxatives not recommended in patients with an ileostomy?

Day 30 Mrs DH went home with a supply of her usual medication except for the furosemide, which had been stopped. A month later, she was re-admitted following a fall. Her blood pressure was low again and she was hypokalaemic. It emerged that her GP had restarted her prescription for furosemide.

Q17 Why had the furosemide been represcribed?

Answers

What steps can be taken at the preadmission clinic to minimise the incidence of postoperative MRSA?

A1 **Preadmission clinics commonly screen patients for MRSA and, where appropriate, provide a preoperative eradication regimen.**

The Department of Health has suggested universal screening for MRSA, and new polymerase chain reaction techniques enable identification of MRSA within hours of testing. If Mrs DH tested positive for MRSA, or even if she had previously been positive, then she would be supplied with an eradication regimen. This would comprise:

(a) Chlorhexidine 4% solution for use in the shower daily, starting 5 days before surgery and paying particular attention to the groin, axillae and behind the ears.

(b) Mupirocin Nasal Ointment to be applied three times a day for 5 days.

In addition she would be offered appropriate MRSA antibiotic prophylaxis at the time of surgery.

When should warfarin be stopped before elective surgery, and what are the risks involved?

A2 **Warfarin should stop 4 days before surgery. It can restart as soon as oral intake is possible.**

White (1995) carried out a study showing that if warfarin stops 4 days before surgery then in most cases the International Normalised Ratio (INR) will be <1.5 on the day of the operation. Most surgeons would be prepared to operate with an INR below this level without fear of excessive bleeding.

Kearon and Hirsh (1997) produced the first definitive guidelines relating to the risks of stopping warfarin perioperatively and concluded that in patients with AF, such as Mrs DH, the risks were low. More recently there has been a debate about the need for 'bridging therapy', which entails replacing warfarin with a 'therapeutic' dose of LMWH (or intravenous (IV) heparin) before an operation. Postoperatively, bearing in mind the possibility of haemorrhage, lower 'prophylactic' doses would be used. This may be appropriate for high-risk patients such as those with old mechanical mitral valve replacements; however; at present there is no general consensus about the value of implementing such a strategy.

Postoperatively warfarin should restart once oral intake is possible.

What is the risk of venous thromboembolism (VTE) occurring in this patient?

A3 **Each patient should be individually assessed to determine the risk of thromboembolism and appropriate thromboprophylaxis prescribed.**

The NICE Clinical Guideline Number 46 recommends that each patient should be individually assessed to identify their risk factors for the development of VTE prior to surgery. The guideline lists the various risk factors, but in general the risk of thromboembolism increases with age, increasing infirmity, and as the nature of the surgery becomes more radical. An elderly patient with cancer, such as Mrs DH, represents a high level of risk.

To ensure that thromboprophylaxis is prescribed, some hospital inpatient treatment charts incorporate a special section making it mandatory for doctors either to prescribe thromboprophylaxis or to specify why it is not appropriate.

What are the risks of using LMWHs in patients who are to have an epidural infusion?

A4 When an epidural infusion is planned LMWHs are usually given on the evening before surgery rather than immediately beforehand, in order to minimise the possibility of a spinal bleed.

There have been reports in America of bleeding leading to spinal cord compression following the administration of LMWHs shortly before spinal injections or the placement of epidural lines. Paralysis resulting from spinal cord compression is very insidious, as in its early stages it is difficult to distinguish from the effects of the local anaesthetic. As a result, anaesthetists prefer that products such as enoxaparin be administered the evening before any surgery that involves spinal/epidural drug administration.

There have been reports of vertebral canal haematoma in patients taking clopidogrel, and this drug may need to be stopped 7 days before surgery, provided the risks of having no antiplatelet therapy are judged acceptable. It is generally thought that aspirin is safe.

Where patients are admitted on the day of surgery, LMWHs may be administered postoperatively provided this is carried out at least an hour after any spinal/epidural drug administration.

Removal of epidural catheters should be delayed until at least 12 hours after injection of LMWH.

How should the hypoglycaemic drugs be managed perioperatively?

A5 The oral hypoglycaemic drugs should be stopped and a sliding-scale insulin regimen introduced.

The decision as to whether to start perioperative insulin in maturity-onset diabetes depends on the patient's existing blood glucose control and the nature of the surgery. The stress of surgery may cause hyperglycaemia, and not being able to eat will cause hypoglycaemia. All this makes perioperative blood glucose levels difficult to control.

In the case of Mrs DH the gliclazide should be omitted the evening before surgery when she starts her bowel-cleansing regimen. At that point she would also stop taking solid food to ensure that her bowel will be clean the next day, and an insulin sliding-scale regimen such as the one set out below should start:

(a) IV 10% dextrose with 20 mmol/L potassium: infuse at 50 mL/h.
(b) IV 50 units insulin (Human Actrapid) in 50 mL sodium chloride 0.9% infused as on the sliding-scale regimen below (Table 30.1).

Table 30.1 Insulin sliding-scale regimens

Blood sugar (mmol/L)	*Units of insulin/ hour Gentle*	*Units of insulin/ hour Standard*	*Units of insulin/ hour Aggressive*
<4.0 or signs of hypoglycaemia: give 25 mL IV glucose 50% and call medical staff for review			
<4.0	0.2	0.5	1
4.0–9	0.5	1	2
9.1–11	1	2	4
11.1–17	2	3	8
17.1–28	4	4	10
>28	6 (call doctor to review regimen)	6 (call doctor to review regimen)	12 (call doctor to review regimen and/or call diabetic team)

A typical starting rate might be 1 unit of insulin per hour, as shown in the 'Standard' scale. Initially, blood glucose is monitored every hour for 6 hours and then every 2 hours if the blood glucose levels are stable. If the standard scale does not provide adequate control (the target range being between 5 and 10 mmol/L) a switch to the 'Aggressive' or 'Gentle' scale as appropriate can be considered. Postoperatively, hourly monitoring of blood glucose will again be required until stable control is assured.

When the patient is able to resume their usual pattern of food intake postoperatively, oral treatment should start again at a meal time when the patient would normally take their gliclazide. At that point the insulin infusion should be stopped and the dose of gliclazide administered.

With metformin there may be an increased risk of lactic acidosis in procedures linked with hypoxia, such as cardiac or vascular surgery, or where there is renal failure that reduces metformin excretion. Therefore, it is often the custom for metformin to be stopped for 2 days before surgery; however, no recent studies support this practice. When renal function is normal, metformin has a half-life of <5 hours and so it is often accepted that it need only be omitted on the morning of surgery. Metformin should then resume when food intake and hydration become normal.

Does a NIL ORALLY instruction mean that medication cannot be taken by mouth?

A6 Oral medication taken with 30 mL of water can normally be continued up until 30 minutes before surgery.

Pharmacists should work with preadmission clinics to draw up guidelines governing which drugs to stop and which to continue before surgery. These guidelines should be supplemented by a formal 'nil orally' policy that defines the precise meaning of this term.

Most medicines need not be omitted before surgery, and beta-blockers *currently* being taken by the patient, such as atenolol, **must not** be omitted perioperatively. Until very recently, the available evidence even pointed to deliberately starting beta-blockers at the time of surgery to reduce the risk of myocardial infarction; however, the recent POISE trial showed that high perioperative doses of metoprolol also increased the risk of stroke. The use of beta-blocker 'prophylaxis' to prevent heart attacks at the time of surgery remains controversial.

Would the use of a cephalosporin be safe? When should the antibiotics be administered? Should antibiotic use continue postoperatively?

A7 Cephalosporin use would be safe in the absence of an immediate (type 1) penicillin allergy. The antibiotics should be administered before 'knife to skin'.

In a recent review Pichichero described the widely quoted cross-allergy risk of 10% between penicillins and cephalosporins as a myth. The chemical side chain of cefuroxime is very different from that of penicillin and this makes cross-allergy unlikely. Where there is a history of an immediate (type 1) penicillin allergy, then gentamicin would offer an alternative.

Clean surgery, such as a breast biopsy, does not normally require antibiotic prophylaxis, which is reserved for contaminated or dirty surgery, such as that encountered when operating on the bowel, where antibiotic prophylaxis given at the time of surgery prevents postoperative infection. IV cefuroxime and metronidazole are commonly used to provide broad-spectrum plus anaerobic antibacterial cover. For maximum prophylactic effect the timing of the antibiotic injection is important, and the usual aim is to have completed antibiotic administration just before 'knife to skin'. If administration is delayed for only a few hours after surgery then the 'golden period' during which prophylaxis is effective passes and the possibility of postoperative wound infection increases. One dose given at the right time is more effective than many doses given later on.

Why is the anaesthetist using a muscle relaxant, and why was an injection of glycopyrronium and neostigmine given at the end of the procedure?

A8 **Muscle relaxants are used to prevent spasms when abdominal muscles are cut, and facilitate ventilation.**

Rocuronium relaxes abdominal muscle tone, which in turn makes it possible for the surgeon to retract the abdominal musculature and prevent diaphragmatic movement following incision. Muscle relaxants also allow easier insertion of an endotracheal tube, which is used for the mechanical ventilation that is required because of the respiratory depression produced by high-potency opiates such as remifentanil. The muscle relaxants themselves paralyse muscular control of breathing, but this does in turn facilitate mechanical ventilation.

Neostigmine is a cholinesterase inhibitor and reverses the action of a competitive neuromuscular blocker at the nicotinic receptor; however, as the cholinesterase inhibitor also stimulates acetylcholine effects at muscarinic receptors, this might cause salivation, bradycardia and increased gastrointestinal tract activity. Glycopyrronium is an atropine-like muscarinic receptor blocker and prevents these undesirable side-effects.

What IV fluids might be prescribed?

A9 **The patient's fluid requirements should be met by combining sodium chloride 0.9% with the infusion of dextrose 10% with 20 mmol/L of potassium.**

In patients *without* the complication of diabetes mellitus, the aims of postoperative prescribing of IV fluids are broadly to maintain a urine output of between 1 and 2 L/day and to assume the need to replace further 'insensible' fluid losses of approximately 1.5 L/day lost through perspiration through the skin and water vapour via the lungs. As an example, an 'average' patient might in 24 hours require 1 L sodium chloride 0.9% plus 20 mmol potassium over 8 hours, and then 2 L dextrose 5%, each with 20 mmol potassium over the next 16 hours, by IV infusion.

The sodium chloride provides 154 mmol of sodium and maintains extracellular fluid volume. The dextrose 5% provides free water which distributes both intra- and extracellularly (adding 50 g dextrose to 1 L water makes it nearly isotonic and capable of being given IV). For a 70 kg patient the above regimen is very loosely based on giving fluid 40 mL/kg; sodium 2 mmol/kg; potassium 1 mmol/kg each day.

Other losses from nasogastric aspirate or losses from drains are normally replaced with sodium chloride 0.9%, which is given in addition to the regimen above. Maintenance of accurate fluid balance records and monitoring of electrolyte levels is pivotal to the rational prescribing of fluids postoperatively.

Mrs DH, a type 2 diabetic, already has a dextrose 10% plus potassium 20 mmol/L infusion running continuously. At 50 mL/h this provides her with 1200 mL of water, 451 kcal and 24 mmol of potassium per day. Any additional fluid requirements would have to be met by the use of sodium chloride 0.9%, with potassium added if necessary. It is important to monitor potassium levels in a diabetic patient, as insulin causes increased uptake of potassium into cells and a consequent fall in plasma potassium levels. As Mrs DH's oral intake increases, the sodium chloride 0.9% would need to be reduced; however, the sliding-scale insulin together with the glucose 10% with potassium 20 mmol/L would need to be continued until normal food intake can be established.

Would morphine and diclofenac be suitable analgesics for this patient?

A10 Diclofenac should ideally be avoided because of the risks of kidney damage. Additional doses of morphine could lead to respiratory depression. IV paracetamol would be a more suitable option.

Non-steroidal anti-inflammatory drugs (NSAIDs) such as diclofenac can cause kidney damage. Because Mrs DH is a diabetic with already poor renal function (creatinine clearance 50 mL/min), the use of NSAIDs should ideally be avoided.

Duplicating opiates by prescribing 'as-required' morphine injections on top of a morphine (or fentanyl)-containing epidural infusion would carry the risk of respiratory depression. Initially, the safest option would be pre-emptively to use regularly administered IV paracetamol on top of the epidural. The World Health Organization has developed the concept of an analgesic ladder, whereby analgesia is given regularly and 'stepped up' from non-opioids to mild opioids and then strong opioids as pain worsens. With surgery, pain is most severe directly after an operation, but then pain scores gradually start to decline as the patient recovers. The monitoring and adjustment of ongoing postoperative pain control would be based on 'stepping down' an analgesic ladder as the patient recovers.

How might the administration of epidural injections be made safer?

A11 The recent National Patient Safety Agency (NPSA) Patient Safety Alert Number 21 offers guidance related to safer practices with epidural injections and infusions.

There is a danger of cardiac arrhythmias and death if epidural bupivacaine is administered IV by mistake. A 'spaghetti-like tangle' of central and peripheral lines as well as epidural lines is therefore worrying, and the NPSA has recommended that all epidural bags and syringes be labelled 'For Epidural Use Only', and has endorsed the use of colour and design to differentiate between epidural and other lines. An example includes using yellow-tinted lines specifically for epidurals. Other recommendations include relying on the use of pharmacy-/commercially prepared infusions, separating the storage of such infusions from products that are given IV and training all staff in the dangers of IV administration of local anaesthetics. Initiatives are under way to look at making physical connections between epidural devices and IV lines incompatible.

'Lipid rescue' regimens are available that neutralise the cardiotoxic effects of accidental IV administration of bupivacaine.

Should the pyrexia be treated with a continued course of antibiotics?

A12 **Transient mild postoperative pyrexia <38°C is common following elective surgery and may be due to the stress, trauma and inflammation resulting from the surgery itself. It is not caused by infection, and is not a reason for prolonging antibiotic use.**

What are the risks of diuretics in ileostomy patients?

A13 **Patients with ileostomies are particularly vulnerable to diuretic-induced dehydration and electrolyte imbalance.**

The colon is a major organ of water absorption. This is evidenced by the severe dehydration or even death caused by diarrhoeal conditions where the function of the colon is impaired. Therefore, in the absence of a functioning colon diuretics can have a disproportionately significant effect, as is the case in ileostomy patients. Although the use of diuretics in ileostomy patients is not contraindicated, they should be prescribed with caution.

What dose of warfarin should be given? When should Mrs DH visit the anticoagulant clinic? When should the use of enoxaparin stop?

A14 **Normally the postoperative dose of warfarin is the same as before admission to hospital.**

If the patient makes a full recovery then their maintenance dose of warfarin will usually be the same as it was before the operation. A reloading dose regimen can be used to produce a rapid rise of the INR into the patient's usual therapeutic range and may reassure the worried patient about being 'subtherapeutic' for any length of time. The reloading dose depends on the patient's usual maintenance dose as follows:

> If the usual maintenance dose is 3 mg or below, then add 3 mg warfarin to this dose for 2 days and then continue with the normal dose after that.

or

> If the usual maintenance dose is above 3 mg, then add 5 mg warfarin to this dose for 2 days and then continue with the normal dose after that.

The thromboprophylactic dose of enoxaparin should continue until the fifth day postoperatively, but could then be stopped provided her INR has reached 2. For patients requiring a shorter hospital stay, enoxaparin would only be required until discharge and/or the return of normal mobility.

At the time of discharge, and provided her INR is near the desired level, an appointment should be made for Mrs DH to attend the anticoagulant clinic in about 10 days. Some very frail patients may not cope well at home following very major surgery, and if, for instance, they do not regain their normal appetite, then their vitamin K intake will fall and there is the danger of a steep rise in INR.

What are the most likely causes of high postoperative pyrexia?

A15 Following abdominal surgery the surgeon would suspect chest infection, urinary tract infection or wound infection.

Pyrexia, a raised white blood cell count and a C-reactive protein very much greater than 10 mg/L are all signs of postoperative infection. The surgeon might suspect a chest infection caused by atelectasis. This occurs when postoperative pain or discomfort causes the patient to lapse into shallow breathing, which in turn causes air to stagnate in the lungs leading to the collapse of alveoli and infection. The surgeon would also examine the wound for pus, pain and inflammation. In the case of Mrs DH a urinary tract infection caused by catheterisation could also be a possibility. This proved to be the case, and trimethoprim was prescribed.

Why are laxatives not recommended in patients with an ileostomy?

A16 Patients with ileostomies are never constipated, and the effect of laxatives might lead to dehydration.

Ileostomy output is very liquid. If it is not being produced then the most likely cause is intestinal obstruction. The patient should seek medical help and not rely on laxatives. In addition, laxatives may cause dehydration by increasing the volume of ileostomy output.

Why had the furosemide been re-prescribed?

A17 The discharge letter written by the pharmacist had only stated what drugs had been prescribed and not what had been stopped. The GP may have thought that the furosemide was missing because of a medication history error in hospital.

Prescribing in surgical patients is essentially procedure based. Usually drugs that are taken for long-standing medical conditions such as hypertension will not be affected by surgery. It is possible that the GP issuing the repeat prescription may have assumed that the furosemide had been left off the discharge letter through an oversight, and by re-prescribing the diuretic had caused a hospital readmission.

It is therefore vital that the hospital discharge letter informs the GP and the patient about drugs that have been stopped because of side-effects. One simple way of ensuring that this happens is to design the discharge letter so that it becomes mandatory for the prescriber either to indicate whether there have been any changes to regular medication or to sign confirming that there have been no changes.

Further reading

Cusson GJ. Medications affecting ostomy function. In: Colwell J, Goldberg M, Carmel J (eds). *Fecal & Urinary Diversions,* Mosby, St Louis 2004 pp. 339–350.

Department of Health. *Screening for Meticillin-Resistant* Staphylococcus Aureus *(MRSA) Colonisation. A Strategy for NHS Trusts: A Summary of Best Practice.* DOH, London, 2007.

Duncan AI, Koch CG, Xu M *et al.* Recent metformin ingestion does not increase in-hospital morbidity or mortality after cardiac surgery. *Anesth Analg* 2007; **104:** 42–50.

Fleischer LA, Poldermans D. Perioperative beta blockage: where do we go to from here? *Lancet* 2008; **371**: 1813–1814.

Kearon C, Hirsh J. Management of anticoagulation before and after elective surgery. *N Engl J Med* 1997; **336**: 1506–1511.

National Institute for Health and Clinical Excellence. CG46. *Venous Thromboembolism: Reducing the Risk of Thromboembolism (Deep Vein Thrombosis and Pulmonary Embolism) in Inpatients Undergoing Surgery.* NICE, London, 2007.

National Patient Safety Agency Safety Alert 21. *Safer Practice with Epidural Injections and Infusions*. NPSA, London, 2007.

Pichichero ME. Cephalosporins can be prescribed safely for penicillin-allergic patients. *J Fam Pract* 2006; **55**: 106–112.

Rahman MH, Beattie J. Managing post-operative pain through giving patients control. *Pharm J* 2005; **275:** 207–210.

Rowlingson JC. Lipid rescue: A step forward in patient safety? Likely so! *Anesth Analg* 2008; **106**: 1333–1336.

Turner DAB. Fluid, electrolyte and acid–base balance. In: Aitkenhead AR, Smith G, Rowbotham D, eds. *A Textbook of Anaesthesia,* 5th edn. Churchill Livingstone, London, 2007, pp. 416–430.

White RH, McKittrick T, Hutchinson R *et al.* Temporary discontinuation of warfarin therapy: changes in the international normalised ratio. *Ann Intern Med* 1995; **122**: 40–42.

31

Cholecystectomy

Sharron Millen and Anne Cole

Case study and questions

Day 1 Fifty-six-year-old Mrs FS was admitted at 7am on the day of surgery for an elective laparoscopic cholecystectomy. She had been seen 2 weeks previously at the pre-assessment clinic, having presented to her general practitioner (GP) 3 months earlier complaining of pain in the right upper quadrant of her abdomen after eating. The pain radiated to her back and usually lasted for about 4 hours, and was associated with nausea. Her GP made a diagnosis of biliary colic and prescribed diclofenac, co-codamol 30/500 and metoclopramide; however, the episodes of biliary colic had not resolved and Mrs FS had been referred for an ultrasound scan, which had revealed a 1.5 cm gallstone in the gallbladder.

Her drug history at pre admission clinic as documented by the pharmacist and reconciled with the GP record was:

- Diclofenac 50 mg orally, up to three times daily, when required
- Co-codamol 30/500, two tablets every 4–6 hours when required, up to a maximum of eight tablets in 24 hours
- Metoclopramide 10 mg orally, up to three times daily when required
- Bendroflumethiazide 5 mg every morning
- Simvastatin 40 mg every evening
- Estraderm TTS patches 50 micrograms/24 h twice a week

Q1 What advice should the pharmacist have given Mrs FS about her medication at the pre admission clinic?
Q2 Is diclofenac an appropriate choice of analgesic for biliary colic?

Mrs FS had no known allergies. She smoked 20 cigarettes a day and drank occasionally. Her weight at the pre admission clinic was 93 kg. She was taking bendroflumethiazide for hypertension, simvastatin for hypercholesterolaemia, and using Estraderm TTS patches 50 micrograms/24 h as hormone replacement therapy (HRT) (she had undergone a hysterectomy 3 years previously). Mrs FS had a family history of gallstones. She herself had no other previous medical history of note.

On examination her pulse was 82 beats per minute (bpm) and regular. Her blood pressure was 150/86 mmHg. A pressure sore assessment risk by the nursing staff gave a score of 5, which indicated that Mrs FS was not at risk of pressure sores. A nutritional assessment by the nursing staff triggered a referral to the dietitian. Mrs FS mentioned to the nursing staff that she would like to try and give up smoking.

Q3 How should Mrs FS's smoking cessation be managed?
Q4 How should Mrs FS's estradiol patches be managed preoperatively?
Q5 Is thromboembolic prophylaxis important in this case?
Q6 Are combination paracetamol products appropriate?
Q7 Are the nutritional and pressure sore risk assessments important for Mrs FS?
Q8 Outline a pharmaceutical care plan for Mrs FS.

The surgical trainee outlined the procedure to Mrs FS and the associated risks were described. Mrs FS agreed that she understood what she had been told and signed a consent form. She was prescribed enoxaparin 40 mg subcutaneously once daily for prophylaxis against deep-vein thrombosis (DVT) and pulmonary embolism (PE), with the first dose to be given 4 hours postoperatively. The nursing staff measured and fitted Mrs FS with thigh-length graduated compression/antiembolism stockings as recommended by NICE, and the importance of her continuing to wear these until discharge was emphasised, along with maintaining as much mobility as possible and drinking plenty of fluids.

The clinical pharmacist spoke to Mrs FS about her medication and reconciled the medicines prescribed with her GP's record of her current medication, the pre admission clinic record and the medicines that she had brought into hospital with her. Mrs FS asked the pharmacist why she had to have the injections to prevent blood clots, and wondered whether there was a tablet that she could take instead.

Q9 How should the pharmacist respond?

The anaesthetist visited to review the elective cases. The anaesthetist spoke to Mrs FS about the drugs she would receive perioperatively and how she would feel during the various stages of the procedure. Epidural and patient-controlled analgesia (PCA) were discussed as possible methods of controlling her postoperative pain, and the risk factors were explained. Mrs FS consented to have an epidural. The anaesthetist documented on the drug chart that enoxaparin could be administered postoperatively, 4 hours after the insertion of the epidural cannula, as long as haemostasis had been secured.

Q10 What combinations of drugs are used in epidurals?
Q11 How do these agents work?
Q12 What are the side-effects of epidurals, and how can they be managed?
Q13 What other methods of opioid analgesic administration could have been used for Mrs FS?
Q14 What is meant by 'patient-controlled analgesia' (PCA)?
Q15 When is PCA not a suitable choice of analgesia?
Q16 What counselling points would have needed to be covered if Mrs FS had chosen PCA for postoperative analgesia?
Q17 Is there an advantage to using an epidural over PCA for Mrs FS?

The following premedication was administered at 10 am:

- Temazepam 20 mg orally
- Cyclizine 50 mg intramuscularly

Q18 What is the purpose of 'premedication'?
Q19 Do you agree with the choice of Mrs FS's premedication?

Mrs FS was drowsy within 30 minutes and was taken down to theatre at 11 am. On induction she received:

- Cefuroxime 750 mg intravenously (IV)
- Metronidazole 500 mg IV
- Morphine 2 mg IV

An intermittent compression device was set up on Mrs FS's calves and used for the duration of the procedure. The anaesthetist used physiological responses to pain throughout the operation to manage Mrs FS's analgesia. Small bolus doses of morphine were administered as needed.

Q20 Why was Mrs FS given antibiotics and morphine at induction?

In theatre the surgeon found an inflamed gallbladder containing many large gallstones. A laparoscopic procedure was not possible, so the surgeon performed an open cholecystectomy. A nasogastric tube was inserted and a bile sample was sent for culture and sensitivities.

In recovery an epidural infusion of bupivacaine 0.15% with fentanyl 2 micrograms/mL was started at 8 mL/h. This was to run via a dedicated, coloured antisiphon epidural line and the dose titrated accordingly.

Q21 How should epidurals be prescribed, supplied, stored, administered and monitored?
Q22 What methods of thromboembolic prophylaxis are being used for Mrs FS?

Mrs FS was returned to the ward, where she continued to receive the following medication:

- Cefuroxime 750 mg IV three times daily
- Metronidazole 500 mg IV three times daily
- Enoxaparin 40mg subcutaneously once daily (first dose 4 hours postoperatively)
- Bupivacaine 0.15% with fentanyl 2 micrograms/mL, 8 mL/h via epidural cannula
- Estraderm TTS patches 50 micrograms/24 h twice a week

The 'when required' medication was as follows:

- Cyclizine 50 mg intramuscularly up to three times daily
- Diclofenac 50 mg suppositories rectally or 50 mg orally three times daily
- Paracetamol 1 g orally, rectally or by IV infusion every 4–6 hours when required, up to a maximum of 4g in 24 hours

Day 2 The epidural was controlling Mrs FS's pain well. She was comfortable and apyrexial. During the immediate 24-hour postoperative period she had received sodium chloride 0.9% with 3 g potassium chloride IV at 125 mL/h. This was sufficient to replace her losses from the drain at the wound site, losses via the nasogastric tube, urine output, faecal and insensible losses.

Q23 What is meant by 'insensible losses'?
Q24 Is there a rationale for co-prescribing non-steroidal anti-inflammatory drugs (NSAIDs) and paracetamol with opioids postoperatively?
Q25 Should gastrointestinal prophylaxis have been co-prescribed with the NSAID?

Day 3 Her serum biochemistry and haematology results were:

- Sodium 142 mmol/L (reference range 135–145)
- Potassium 4.0 mmol/L (3.5–5.0)
- Urea 3.6 mmol/L (3.0–6.5)
- Creatinine 72 micromol/L (60–125)
- Albumin 28 g/L (32–50)
- White blood cells (WBC) 9.8×10^9/L ($4.0–10.0 \times 10^9$)
- C-reactive protein (CRP) normal

Bowel sounds had returned and the nasogastric tube and wound drains were removed. Mrs FS was started on 30 mL sips of water every hour, to increase to 60 mL/h during the afternoon. The epidural was stopped. The bile culture and sensitivity results came back negative. Mrs FS was apyrexial and her pulse was 50 bpm. The IV fluid replacement regimen was stopped. Mrs FS's medication was now as follows:

- Cefuroxime 750 mg IV three times daily
- Metronidazole 500 mg IV three times daily
- Enoxaparin 40 mg subcutaneously once daily
- Estraderm TTS patches 50 micrograms/24 h twice a week

The 'when required' medication was as follows:

- Paracetamol 1 g orally or rectally every 4–6 hours when required, up to a maximum of 4 g in 24 hours
- Diclofenac 50 mg tablets orally up to three times daily
- Dihydrocodeine 30 mg every 4 hours up to a maximum of 240 mg in 24 hours
- Morphine oral solution 10 mg orally every 4 hours

The pharmacist requested that the surgical house officer discontinue the antibiotics.

Q26 Was the pharmacist right to request this?
Q27 Do you agree with the choice of oral analgesia for Mrs FS?
Q28 Should the first dose of morphine be given as the epidural stops?
Q29 How long should her thromboembolic prophylaxis continue?

Day 4 Mrs FS was eating a light diet. The dietitian visited her and provided her with some nutritional advice with an aim to achieve a weight loss of no more than 2 kg per week.

Day 5 Mrs FS was discharged from hospital, with an outpatient appointment in 6 weeks. Her discharge medication was as follows:

- Paracetamol 1 g every 4–6 hours when required, up to a maximum of 4 g in 24 hours
- Ibuprofen 400 mg three times daily when required
- Bendroflumethiazide 5 mg every morning
- Simvastatin 40 mg every evening
- Estraderm TTS patches 50 micrograms/24 h twice a week

The pharmacist performed a clinical check on the discharge prescription and the medicines management technician issued prelabelled discharge packs of paracetamol and ibuprofen from the ward stock, and returned Mrs SF's own medicines that were to continue. Mrs FS was counselled about how to take her medication and her consent was obtained to send the medication that she had brought into hospital on admission that was no longer prescribed, for destruction.

Q30 What advice should Mrs FS be given about her medication prior to discharge?

Answers

What advice should the pharmacist have given Mrs FS about her medication at pre-admission clinic?

A1 To continue all her regular medications up until admission.

Mrs FS should have been advised to continue with her hormone replacement therapy (HRT) to prevent the return of any undesirable menopausal symptoms. She should continue her simvastatin and metoclopramide. A decision on whether to continue the diuretics perioperatively would depend on the individual centre. There is no direct evidence as to whether these should be continued or stopped preoperatively; however, owing to the risks of dehydration intraoperatively many centres advise omitting diuretics such as bendroflumethiazide on the day of surgery.

Is diclofenac an appropriate choice of analgesic for biliary colic?

A2 Yes. However, diclofenac is contraindicated in some situations.

Diclofenac is a non-steroidal anti-inflammatory drug (NSAID) that may induce or worsen peptic ulcer disease (PUD). If the differential diagnosis of Mrs FS's disease had included any possibility of active PUD, dyspepsia or pyloric stenosis, then an NSAID would not have been an appropriate choice. NSAIDs must also be avoided in patients with a history of an allergic reaction to NSAIDs. They should be used with caution in patients with asthma, hypertension, cardiac failure, ischaemic heart disease, peripheral arterial disease, cerebrovascular disease, renal or hepatic disease, or a history of PUD: combination therapy with protective agents such as misoprostol or a proton pump inhibitor should be considered for such patients.

Recent clinical trials have highlighted the cardiovascular (CV) safety concerns about NSAIDs and cyclo-oxygenase-2 (COX-2) selective inhibitors. Current evidence suggests that diclofenac (especially at a dose of 150 mg/day) is associated with a similar prothrombotic risk as COX-2 selective inhibitors. Naproxen (1000 mg/day) and low-dose ibuprofen (e.g. ≤1200 mg/day) are associated with a lower prothrombotic risk and are a more appropriate choice for patients who require a NSAID when CV risk is of concern.

Mrs FS is receiving bendroflumethiazide to control her hypertension. NSAIDs can worsen hypertension as a result of their effects on renal function and sodium and water retention. It is therefore important that Mrs FS receives NSAIDs for as short a time as possible. This will also minimise the risk of other side-effects such as PUD or thrombosis. The total daily dose of NSAID can be reduced by co-prescribing additional analgesia. In this case Mrs FS was prescribed co-codamol 30/500, a combination product of paracetamol 500 mg and codeine 30 mg per tablet. If additional analgesia is required then morphine is the opioid of choice. Historically pethidine was used in biliary disease because it was reported to cause less spasm of the sphincter of Oddi (the sphincter at the base of the gallbladder) than other opioids, but this is now disputed. All opioids can affect smooth muscle tone.

How should Mrs FS's smoking cessation be managed?

A3 **Unless patients are suffering from severe nicotine withdrawal, it is not appropriate to initiate nicotine replacement therapy perioperatively while they are away from their normal environment and usual support network. However, if Mrs FS shows signs of withdrawal, or there are concerns about anxiety because she is abstaining from smoking, then patches should be prescribed at an appropriate dosage. Prior to discharge Mrs FS should be provided with encouragement, information, support groups and products available to aid smoking cessation.**

A good starting point is for Mrs FS to make a list of reasons for giving up smoking and to keep referring back to the list to ensure she maintains her commitment to stopping. Nicotine replacement therapy has been found to increase the chance of smoking cessation about 1.5–2 fold. Both individual counselling and group therapy increase the chance of quitting by up to four times. Most hospitals have nicotine replacement patches, but these are not the only type of smoking cessation aid available. Nicotine replacement is also available in the form of chewing gum, nasal spray, inhaler, sublingual tablets and lozenges. Bupropion (mode of action for enhancing the ability of patients to abstain from smoking currently unknown) and varenicline (a selective partial nicotine receptor agonist) are also available. There is little direct evidence that one nicotine replacement product is more effective than another. The decision about which to use should be guided by individual preferences, and Mrs FS should be advised to consult her GP or community pharmacist after she has returned home with a view to attending a specialist smoking clinic. NICE has issued public health programme guidance on smoking cessation services (2008) and technology appraisals on the place of bupropion and nicotine replacement therapy (2002, updated 2006) and varenicline (2007).

How should Mrs FS's estradiol patches be managed preoperatively?

A4 It is recommended that HRT be continued during elective surgical admissions in order to prevent the return of postmenopausal symptoms. HRT is an additional minor risk factor for deep-vein thrombosis/pulmonary embolism (DVT/PE) in patients undergoing surgery; however, the decision to continue HRT prior to admission should be made on the basis of weighing up additional risk factors for thromboembolism against the risk of patient distress due to stopping the drug.

Postmenopausal women (both hysterectomised and non-hysterectomised) using oestrogen therapy have an increased risk of biliary tract disease.

Is thromboembolic prophylaxis important in this case?

A5 Yes. In the UK PE following hospital-acquired DVT causes between 25 000 and 32 000 deaths each year. Mrs FS is undergoing abdominal surgery that will last for more than 30 minutes. This carries a significant risk factor for the development of postoperative DVT or PE which may be fatal.

Mrs FS also has other risk factors for the development of postoperative DVT/PE. She is obese and admits to smoking 20 cigarettes per day. She is also on HRT. Using the NICE and American College of Chest Physicians (ACCP) guidance, these factors put her at high risk of developing a postoperative DVT/PE, and for this reason it is essential that she receives thromboembolic prophylaxis.

The risk assessment must be documented in the patient's notes so that staff are clear about her risk factors and which prophylaxis is indicated.

Are combination paracetamol products appropriate?

A6 No. Combination paracetamol products prevent patients being able to titrate their individual analgesic requirements to their needs, and may thus lead to unnecessary side-effects.

Products such as co-codamol 30/500 with high concentrations of weak opioid mean that patients take 60 mg codeine per dose. Doses of 60 mg provide little more analgesia than the 30 mg dose, but a higher incidence of constipation and sedation.

Are the nutritional and pressure sore risk assessments important for Mrs FS?

A7 Yes. Ideally all patients admitted to hospital should have a nutritional and pressure sore risk assessment.

The reason for performing these assessments when patients are admitted to hospital and during their stay is to identify those who have deficits in their nutritional status. These patients may require dietary advice or may be at risk of developing pressure sores. The results of these assessments trigger positive action by the nursing staff, which is important from both a quality of care and a risk management perspective. In the past, the nutritional and tissue breakdown risk of patients was underestimated. There is now a wealth of evidence demonstrating that where nutrition and pressure sore risk assessments take place, the incidence of post-operative complications and hospital-acquired pressure sores reduces significantly. Regular mattress audits should also be undertaken to ensure worn mattresses are removed from use. During her admission, Mrs FS's skin should be examined daily for any sign of tissue breakdown.

Outline a pharmaceutical care plan for this patient.

A8 **The pharmaceutical care plan for Mrs FS should consist of a problem list, aims of pharmaceutical treatment, interventions or monitoring required, and an evaluation section. The pharmaceutical aspects of Mrs FS's care that need to be included in the care plan are:**

(a) Risk assessment of medicines contributing to biliary disease.
(b) Choice of antiemetic.
(c) Choice and method of administration of analgesia.
(d) Choice and duration of prophylactic antibiotics.
(e) Methods and duration of thromboembolic prophylaxis.
(f) Medicines reconciliation, discharge medication planning and patient counselling.
(g) Smoking cessation.

How should the pharmacist respond?

A9 **The pharmacist needs to explain to Mrs FS that the reason for the injections is to reduce the risk of her developing a blood clot.**

All drugs currently licensed in the UK for thromboembolic prophylaxis following general surgery are administered via injection. Warfarin therapy would not be appropriate owing to the difficulty of achieving and maintaining a stable therapeutic level for the short period of time thromboprophylaxis is required.

At the time of writing two new oral thromboembolic prophylaxis agents have been launched. Dabigatran and rivaroxaban have been licensed for elective total hip or knee replacement, but not for general surgery at present. However, oral absorption of agents after general surgery would be unpredictable, and in many cases unlikely, due to gut stasis.

What combinations of drugs are used in epidurals?

A10 **Epidurals are usually a mixture of a local anaesthetic agent and an opioid.**

Occasionally local anaesthetic agents are used alone. The most commonly prescribed solution is bupivacaine with fentanyl. The concentrations used in these solutions vary: a Patient Safety Alert issued by the National Patient Safety Agency (NPSA) aims to address this (see **A21**). A review of the literature suggests that bupivacaine 0.125–0.15% with fentanyl 2 micrograms/mL results in effective pain relief without increasing the side-effect profile.

The effectiveness of the analgesia depends on many factors, including:

(a) The drugs chosen.
(b) The site of the epidural.
(c) The volume and concentration of the local anaesthetic.

These all contribute to the degree of sensory and motor block achieved.

How do these agents work?

A11 **Opioids selectively block pain transmission by their action on opioid receptors, whereas local anaesthetics inhibit nerve transmission. In combination they act synergistically, which reduces the dose of each agent required to produce adequate analgesia. This reduces the incidence of side-effects.**

(a) **Fentanyl.** Opioids diffuse across the dura mater into the cerebrospinal fluid. Here they bind with the opioid receptors in the dorsal horn of the spinal column and modify transmission of pain impulses to the brain. The remainder of the drug is absorbed into the epidural veins and passes into the systemic circulation, which may produce a small degree of systemic analgesia.
(b) **Bupivacaine.** Local anaesthetic agents block sodium channels along the nerve fibre, which results in a local block of pain transmission in the spinal cord. The degree of blockade depends on the total amount of drug instilled, which in turn depends on the solution concentration and the rate of infusion. Small unmyelinated fibres are affected first, large myelinated fibres last. Loss of nerve function occurs in the following order: pain, temperature, touch, deep pressure, skeletal muscle power and finally autonomic blockade.

What are the side-effects of epidurals, and how can they be managed?

A12 **Side-effects may include urinary retention, hypotension, sensory loss, and (rarely) pruritus, respiratory depression and nausea.**

Side-effects can be minimised by close monitoring of the patient, adhering to a standardised system and the use of colour-coded, dedicated epidural lines (see A21). Serious adverse incidents result from the accidental intravenous (IV) administration of epidurals. There is also a small risk of paralysis during the insertion of the epidural cannula.

As a result of media attention patients are often concerned about having an epidural inserted. These concerns need to be discussed and informed consent obtained. Patients also need to understand that as a result of epidural administration they may become unaware of the need to urinate, as sensory awareness of the bladder can be lost. Depending on local practice, patients will either be routinely catheterised on initiation of therapy or monitored for this adverse event and catheterised if needed.

Specific side-effects are as follows:

(a) **Epidural fentanyl.** Side-effects as any opioid.

- (i) Pruritus is caused by histamine release, although it is not that common with fentanyl. If it occurs it is likely to be on the face, chest and abdomen, and within the first few hours of epidural initiation.
- (ii) Respiratory depression is uncommon with low-dose infusions because the high lipid solubility of fentanyl confines its effect mainly to the spinal cord. If it is going to occur it is most likely within the first hour of the infusion. It can be reversed with naloxone.
- (iii) Nausea is rare with low-dose epidural infusions but is a result of systemic action.
- (iv) Urinary retention is a result of the inhibition of the micturition reflex and is not readily reversed.
- (v) Slowing of gastrointestinal motility is less likely than with parenteral administration.

(b) **Epidural bupivacaine.**

- (i) Hypotension is the most commonly occurring cardiovascular side-effect, especially if the patient is hypovolaemic. It can result in reduced heart rate and blood pressure. If not a symptom of hypovolaemia it can be treated with ephedrine, a potent vasoconstrictor (α and β agonist), by administering 3–6 mg by slow IV injection, repeated every 3–4 minutes to a maximum dose of 30 mg.
- (ii) Sensory loss may include numbness of the legs and tongue and shivering.

(iii) Urinary retention. As a result of the sacral level block there is a reduced ability for the urinary sphincter to relax.

(iv) Neurotoxicity. This is generally only in the case of overdose or accidental systemic administration, and includes light-headedness, dizziness, and visual/auditory disturbances, e.g. tinnitus and inability to focus. In severe cases twitching, tremors and convulsions may occur.

What other methods of opioid analgesic administration could have been used for Mrs FS?

A13 **The other major methods of administering postoperative opioid analgesia are via fixed regular or 'when required' doses of intramuscular injections, or a patient-controlled analgesia (PCA) system.**

Administering opioid analgesia via fixed regular or 'when required' doses of intramuscular injections is fraught with problems, such as the difficulty of assessing how much opioid will be required and how frequently it should be given for each individual patient. Numerous factors influence the amount and frequency of analgesia required. These include the patient's age, weight, height, gender, and the type of operation. Many factors also influence the kinetics of an intramuscular dose in a patient after surgery, such as temperature and circulating blood volume. Therefore, a patient who returns to the ward hypothermic after a lengthy procedure, and hypovolaemic because of inadequate fluid replacement, will have poor perfusion of skeletal muscle with resultant poor absorption of any opioid analgesia administered. If an increased amount of opioid analgesic is prescribed to overcome this situation and provide an adequate level of pain relief, there is a serious risk that as the contributing factors to the poor skeletal muscle perfusion are corrected the patient will become 'overdosed' with opioid, which may increase the risk of respiratory depression and sedation. Sometimes patients also feel reticent about asking for an injection, either because they do not want to 'bother the nursing staff' or they wish to avoid an injection. This results in inadequate levels of analgesia. Infusion devices, epidurals or PCA provide much better analgesia and therefore aid recovery.

What is meant by 'patient-controlled analgesia' (PCA)?

A14 **PCA is a method of pain control whereby patients self-administer small doses of an IV opioid analgesic at set intervals using a specially designed pump.**

This method of opioid administration is generally accepted as safe and effective. In contrast to conventional intramuscular opioid analgesia,

PCA is associated with fewer adverse effects, better pulmonary recovery after abdominal surgery, reduced nursing time for drug administration, improved individualisation of drug dosages, improved analgesia and reduced length of hospital stay. It also allows patients to take control of their own pain relief.

Many devices are available to administer opioid analgesia via PCA. The electronic infusion pumps used consist of a microprocessor programmed to deliver a set volume of analgesic with a lockout period during which the patient can receive no further doses. Some PCA pumps include the facility to print a report detailing everything that has occurred to the device since it was set up, e.g. the number of times the patient has pressed the demand button, the number of doses received and the volume of analgesic remaining. The disposable devices used to administer PCA are simpler, with a fixed lockout period and fixed volume delivered by each press of the demand button outside the lockout period.

A needle-free transdermal fentanyl PCA is also available for use in hospital that is licensed for acute postoperative pain. It allows patients complete freedom of mobility compared to other mechanical PCAs; however, morphine remains the first choice of PCA in the UK.

The devices used to administer PCA differ enormously and there should be careful multidisciplinary evaluation of the products available before any choice to purchase is made.

When is PCA not a suitable choice of analgesia?

A15 Exclusion criteria for the use of PCA would include:

(a) Major, complex procedures.
(b) Any known allergies to the opioid used for PCA.
(c) Pregnancy.
(d) Breastfeeding.
(e) History of drug abuse.
(f) Patients with rheumatoid arthritis or any other finger disabilities that prevent them from operating the device.
(g) Patients with pre-existing neurological disease.
(h) Patients who are unable to understand how to use the device (literature is available for some PCA devices in a number of different languages, and many UK hospitals have translators available which can help address this).
(i) Those who do not wish to use PCA.
(j) Emergency surgical procedures, when there is insufficient time preoperatively to explain about PCA and how to use the device, or when the patient is too unwell to understand.

What counselling points would have needed to be covered if Mrs FS had chosen PCA for postoperative analgesia?

A16 **If patients are deemed suitable for PCA it is essential that they be counselled on its use prior to surgery and are given the opportunity to refuse to use it if they do not wish to take control of their analgesia.**

The nurse, doctor or pharmacist counselling Mrs FS prior to surgery would need to explain how PCA works, how to obtain a dose, how hard to press the demand button, the lockout period, what this means, and what to do if she remained in pain. They would also need to offer reassurance about the safety of the device with regard to overdosing, and address any concerns about 'addiction'. A demonstration PCA kit would have been available so that Mrs FS could handle the device and practise pressing the demand button before going to theatre. A patient information booklet about PCA would also have been provided for Mrs FS to read, and she would have been encouraged to ask any questions she had about the PCA. There are also videos available to help with patient counselling. Mrs FS would have been made aware that the nursing staff had been assessing her pain score every hour and told how the pain scoring method works. The nursing staff would have regularly monitored the PCA device during use.

Is there an advantage to using an epidural over PCA for Mrs FS?

A17 **Yes. Epidurals manage pain more effectively than PCA.**

Laparoscopic cholecystectomy requires several small incisions in the abdomen to allow the insertion of operating ports, small cylindrical tubes approximately 5–10 mm in diameter, through which surgical instruments and a video camera are placed into the abdominal cavity. The surgeon watches a monitor and performs the operation by manipulating the surgical instruments through the operating ports.

Significant pain will occur postoperatively and although PCA could be used, an epidural is likely to provide better analgesia. The degree of postoperative pain following open cholecystectomy is expected to be even higher as the incision is larger and the abdominal muscles are cut.

What is the purpose of 'premedication'?

A18 **The purpose of premedication is to allow patients to go through the preoperative period free of apprehension and sedated enough to be comfortable, but still rousable and able to cooperate fully in their care.**

Prior to anaesthesia the anaesthetist will explain to Mrs FS what is to happen, where she will wake up and how she will feel on waking. Premedication is best administered 1 hour before surgery.

Do you agree with the choice of Mrs FS's premedication?

A19 **Yes. Oral premedication with a short-acting benzodiazepine such as temazepam is common practice, as benzodiazepines meet the criteria outlined in A18.**

Antiemetics are not routinely administered during premedication, but on induction Mrs FS will receive an IV dose of morphine. As antiemetics are best administered 30 minutes prior to emetic stimuli, it is sensible to administer an antiemetic with the premedication. Also, Mrs FS had been suffering with nausea preoperatively, therefore it is sensible to treat this prior to induction.

Why was Mrs FS given antibiotics and morphine at induction?

A20 **The antibiotics were administered prophylactically and the morphine was given to supplement the analgesic effects of the anaesthetics.**

Antibiotic prophylaxis is defined as 'administration of an antimicrobial drug in the absence of known infection in order to decrease the likelihood of subsequent infection at a surgical site'. Prophylactic antibiotics are most effective if they are administered during the 2-hour period before the surgical incision. This is because high levels of antibiotics are needed in the bloodstream and tissues in the minutes after the incision to prevent bacterial seeding of the operative wound.

As Mrs FS is to undergo surgery on her biliary tract, the most likely organisms to be encountered are Enterococci and Enterobacteriacae 'coliforms'. The need for metronidazole in this situation is debatable because anaerobes are not usually present in the biliary tract, and cefuroxime should provide adequate prophylactic cover for the organisms most likely to be present.

Morphine is administered intraoperatively to supplement the analgesic effects of anaesthetics which, if used alone, may not provide adequate analgesia for a patient undergoing major surgery. The administration of opioid analgesics such as morphine with anaesthetic agents also reduces the total amount of anaesthetic required.

How should epidurals be prescribed, supplied, stored, administered and monitored?

A21 **In 2007 the NPSA issued a Patient Safety Alert which identified a number of actions that can make administering epidural injections and infusions safer.**

Epidural infusions and injections need to be prescribed according to hospital policy. In most cases this will be on the main drug chart. Epidurals should be supplied to the ward in a premixed solution to prevent calculation errors in mixing, and be clearly labelled 'For Epidural Use Only' in a large font with judicious use of colour and design to clearly differentiate them from products for administration by IV and other routes. The range of epidural infusions and injections should be rationalised and procedures introduced for preparing and administering these products.

As epidurals can be plain local anaesthetic agents or a mixture of local anaesthetic with opioid, their storage requirements differ. All controlled drug (CD) epidurals must be stored in a locked cupboard with no IV or other types of infusion or injection. Plain local anaesthetic epidurals should be stored in separate cupboards or refrigerators from those holding IV or other types of infusion or injection, to minimise the risk of selection error.

Epidurals need to be administered using clearly labelled epidural administration sets and cannulae with dedicated pumps or syringe drivers that distinguish them from those used for IV infusions or injection. The devices used to administer CD mixtures need to be lockable.

All staff involved in epidural therapy must receive adequate training and have the necessary work competencies to undertake their duties safely. An annual audit should be carried out to ensure that epidural practices adhere to the agreed range of products and procedures.

The detailed monitoring of an epidural will depend on hospital policy. Generally patients with epidurals have blood pressure, heart rate, respiratory rate and level of block monitored every hour. The total amount of drug remaining in the syringe and the total amount infused are also checked hourly to prevent the chance of mechanical error.

The level of block is checked using ethyl chloride spray (because it is cold). This is sprayed over the patient's torso and the patient identifies where they can feel it. If the analgesia is felt to be insufficient then the nurses can increase the epidural rate gradually until the maximum prescribed rate is reached. If the epidural is still not providing adequate relief then an alternative analgesic strategy must be used or the epidural resited.

What methods of thromboembolic prophylaxis are being used for Mrs FS?

A22 Mrs FS will receive prophylactic subcutaneous enoxaparin injections postoperatively. She has also been fitted with thigh-length graduated compression/antiembolism stockings, and intermittent compression devices were used on her calves during surgery.

A larger reduction in the incidence of postoperative DVT and/or PE is achieved when these three different methods of thromboembolic prophylaxis are used together, rather than in isolation. Enoxaparin is used because it is a once-daily injection and currently costs less than unfractionated heparin. At the time of writing there is no evidence demonstrating that any of the low-molecular weight heparins (LMWHs) available are superior to unfractionated heparin in reducing the incidence of DVT/PE following general surgery. In this case Mrs FS received the first dose of enoxaparin postoperatively owing to the difficulties of ensuring that preoperative doses of LMWH are administered at least 12 hours before, or at least 4 hours after, insertion of the epidural cannula to reduce the risk of haematoma.

Thrombi start to form during surgery, therefore mechanical thromboprophylaxis in the form of intermittent calf compression devices were used to promote blood flow by rhythmically altering the pressure in an envelope around the calves. These may be continued postoperatively for as long as they are tolerated, or until Mrs FS is fully mobile. Properly fitted graduated compression/antiembolism stockings were used in addition to enoxaparin postoperatively to increase the velocity of venous return. Early postoperative ambulation may also help to reduce the incidence of DVT, but this is not proven. It has been recommended that individual clinicians, units and hospitals in the UK should develop written policies for prophylaxis, and the use of prophylaxis should be included in clinical audit and care pathways.

What is meant by 'insensible losses'?

A23 **The term 'insensible fluid loss' refers to water loss from the body via evaporation from the skin and water vapour expired from the lungs. It can be estimated at 0.5 mL/kg/h at 37°C.**

Is there a rationale for co-prescribing non-steroidal anti-inflammatory drugs (NSAIDs) and paracetamol with opioids postoperatively?

A24 **Yes. Opioid analgesics, paracetamol and NSAIDs have different modes of action and are complementary in their analgesic effects.**

It has been demonstrated that by administering opioids with paracetamol or diclofenac during the postoperative period, opioid requirements can be reduced by one-third. However, NSAIDs should be reserved for patients for whom analgesia cannot be provided by opioids and simple analgesics alone. This is because NSAIDs can have serious side-effects (see **A2**). Also, there is a risk that using NSAIDs for postoperative analgesia may lead to wound haematoma, especially if the patient is receiving enoxaparin.

Paracetamol is now available as an IV formulation. This allows administration to a range of patients not previously able to receive it. However, because of the increased risks associated with the IV formulation and the high bioavailability via the IV route, its use should be restricted to appropriate patients and for short durations. The high bioavailability of paracetamol by the IV route may make it necessary to consider reducing the dose to 8-hourly if long-term use is necessary.

Should gastrointestinal prophylaxis have been co-prescribed with the NSAID?

A25 This will depend on local policy or guidelines.

Mrs FS has some risk factors for perioperative acute gastrointestinal haemorrhage: she is a smoker, and is receiving thromboprophylaxis and NSAIDs. However, she has no history of gastrointestinal haemorrhage, is expected to have a short hospital admission, and is unlikely to be nil by mouth for very long. Mrs FS should be counselled to take her oral diclofenac after food, but to stop it immediately if she experiences any symptoms of indigestion

Was the pharmacist right to request this?

A26 Yes. The current local antibiotic prophylaxis guidelines for biliary surgery are for one dose of IV cefuroxime and metronidazole on induction and two doses at 8-hourly intervals postoperatively. Additional prophylactic doses should be given if surgery continues for more than 4 hours, or the patient loses more than 1.5 L blood or suffers haemodilution over 15 mL/kg. These recommendations differ from those of the Scottish Intercollegiate Guidelines Network (SIGN), which considers antibiotic prophylaxis for open cholecystectomy but does not support prophylaxis for a routine laparoscopic cholecystectomy.

The answer to this question therefore depends on the surgical antibiotic prophylaxis guidelines in place in the hospital. Prophylactic antibiotics should not be continued for more than 24 hours, although most of the evidence is for three doses in total, with single doses appropriate for several procedures. The *British National Formulary* now recommends single doses for gastrointestinal procedures, with additional doses only if the procedure is prolonged (2–4 hours) or the patient has blood loss >1.5 L.

If spillage of bowel contents occurs during surgery or there is some other form of wound contamination, the surgeon may request that antibiotics be continued for 3–5 days. This would then be classed as treatment and should be documented as such in the patient's case notes, switching administration to the oral route as soon as the patient is able to take sips and can tolerate oral therapy.

Ensuring the narrowest spectrum of antimicrobials possible for the shortest period of time prevents the development of bacterial resistance.

Do you agree with the choice of oral analgesia for Mrs FS?

A27 **Yes. Once the immediate postoperative requirement for opioid analgesia has passed a combination of paracetamol with a weak opioid plus an NSAID, if needed, usually provides good analgesia for general surgical patients, provided there are no contraindications. Combined preparations are no better than individual agents, and it is more difficult to titrate the dose to achieve the required level of analgesia while minimising side-effects (see A6).**

The nursing staff should be educated that these different forms of analgesia are additive in their effects when given in combination, and should be encouraged to use them together.

Should the first dose of oral morphine be given as the epidural stops?

A28 **This again would depend on individual hospital guidelines. There is no clinical reason why the first dose of opioid cannot be given immediately the epidural stops, but most hospitals have policies that stipulate a gap of about 4 hours between stopping the epidural and giving the first dose of opioid.**

How long should her thromboembolic prophylaxis continue?

A29 **Following most general surgical procedures, thromboembolic prophylaxis should continue at least until discharge, rather than for any predetermined time.**

Mrs FS is obese, smokes, and is on HRT. She has undergone major abdominal surgery. These factors put her into a high-risk category for the development of DVT/PE (see **A5**). Prophylaxis with enoxaparin should continue until discharge. Thromboembolism can occur up to 6 weeks postoperatively, and patients should be encouraged to remain mobile following their return home and maintain hydration by drinking plenty of water. If Mrs FS was found to have abdominal cancer during the procedure this would further increase her thromboembolic risk, and it would then be recommended that she should receive extended thromboprophylaxis for 28 days postoperatively (if curative surgery is performed or there are residual tumors *in situ*).

Mrs FS must not have her epidural cannula removed until at least 12 hours after a dose of enoxaparin to prevent the risk of an epidural haematoma.

What advice should Mrs FS be given about her medication prior to discharge?

A30 **There are several important medication counselling points that Mrs FS should receive prior to discharge.**

The medication counselling should include the importance of taking the tablets to remain pain free, rather than trying just to tolerate the pain. Ibuprofen has fewer gastrointestinal side-effects than diclofenac but is also less potent; however, in combination with regular paracetamol this should be adequate. Mrs FS should be advised to consult her GP if the analgesia is ineffective. In this situation diclofenac could be substituted for ibuprofen, and codeine phosphate 30 mg every 4 hours when required prescribed in addition to paracetamol.

The importance of taking her ibuprofen after food must be stressed to Mrs FS, and she should be advised to stop taking it if she has any signs of dyspepsia and to consult her GP immediately. She should be advised of the maximum dose of paracetamol (4 g in 24 hours, or eight 500 mg tablets) and reminded to avoid any over-the-counter preparations containing paracetamol or NSAIDs that may inadvertently take her over the maximum doses.

Mrs FS should be reminded to restart her bendroflumethiazide and simvastatin tablets on discharge and to continue using her HRT patches.

Following Mrs FS's expressed interest in giving up smoking she should be provided with encouragement and information and advised to consult her GP, community pharmacist or free NHS smoking helpline after she has returned home, with a view to attending a specialist smoking cessation clinic (see **A3**).

Further reading

Chan KL, Hung LCT, Suen BY *et al*. Celecoxib versus diclofenac and omeprazole in reducing the risk of recurrent ulcer bleeding in patients with arthritis. *N Engl J Med* 2002; **347**: 2104–2110.

Cirillo DJ, Wallace RB, Rodabough RJ *et al*. Effect of estrogen therapy on gallbladder disease. *J Am Med Assoc* 2005; **293:** 330–339.

Gedney JA, Liu EH. Side-effects of epidural infusions of opioid bupivacaine mixtures. *Anaesthiology* 1998; 53: 1148–1155.

Hirsch J, Guyatt G, Albers G *et al*. Executive Summary of American College of Chest Physicians: Evidence-Based Clinical Practice Guidance (8th Edition). *Chest* 2008; **133**: 71–109.

Lancaster T, Stead L, Silagy C *et al*. Effectiveness of interventions to help people stop smoking: findings from the Cochrane Library. *Br Med J* 2000; **321**: 355–358.

McQuay HJ, Moore RA. *An Evidence-based Resource for Pain Relief.* Oxford University Press, Oxford, 1998.

Millen S, Warwick D. Implementing standards for prophylaxis against venous thromboembolism. *Hosp Pharm* 2008: **15**: 375–376.

National Institute for Health and Clinical Excellence. TA39. *Guidance on the Use of Nicotine Replacement Therapy (NRT) and Bupropion.* NICE, London, 2002.

National Institute for Health and Clinical Excellence. CG46. *Venous Thromboembolism (Surgical).* NICE, London, 2007.

National Patient Safety Agency. *Safer Practice with Epidural Injections and Infusions.* NPSA, London, 2007.

National Prescribing Centre. Update on the prescribing of NSAIDs. *MeReC Monthly* May 2008.

Ozalp G, Guner F, Kuru N *et al.* Postoperative patient controlled epidural analgesia with opioid bupivacaine mixtures. *Can J Anaesth* 1998; 45: 938–942.

Rahman MH, Beattie J. Managing post-operative pain. *Pharm J* 2005; **275**: 145–148.

Rahman MH, Beattie J. Managing post-operative pain through giving patients control. *Pharm J* 2005; **275**: 207–210.

Scottish Intercollegiate Guidelines Network. *Guidance on Antibiotic Prophylaxis in surgery.* SIGN, Edinburgh, 2008.

32

Medicines management

Kym Lowder

Case study and questions

Day 1 Mrs KW was visited in her home by a primary care visitor (PCV). A PCV is a qualified healthcare assistant (HCA) who has been given additional training in how to assess clients for falls risks and carry out a general basic medical assessment, and also how to help individuals access social benefits. Basic training in commonly prescribed medicines and their side-effects, compliance issues, and other medicines-related issues to be aware of is provided to all PCVs by a Primary Care Trust (PCT) prescribing adviser. All visits take the same format. The service is targeted at those over 75 who live alone and are not in regular contact with any medical or social care agencies.

The resulting medication report (see Table 32.1) and general health report (see p. 621) was sent to the PCT prescribing adviser for comment:

- Date of birth: 4.12.30
- Resting blood pressure (BP) 176/92 mmHg
- Standing BP 180/92 mmHg
- Lying BP 175/90 mmHg
- Urine: nothing abnormal detected
- Falls in past 12 months: 1
- Dizziness: occasional

Q1 Is Mrs KW's BP a cause for concern?
Q2 Comment on the dose of aspirin.
Q3 Which medicines could be contributing to her dizziness?
Q4 Comment on the possible problems associated with purchasing ibuprofen over the counter (OTC).
Q5 What could explain the varying quantities of Mrs KW's medication?
Q6 What additional information might be provided through a pharmacist domiciliary visit?

Week 2 Based on the information received, the prescribing adviser decided that a domiciliary visit was indicated. Further details of Mrs KW's

Table 32.1

Medication	*Dose*	*Quantity in home*
Glyceryl trinitrate (GTN) sublingual tablets	as required	2 × 50 plus 20
Aspirin dispersible	75 mg twice daily	30
Isosorbide mononitrate	20 mg twice daily	84 (takes am and 6 pm)
Atenolol	100 mg daily	112
Fluoxetine	20 mg daily	65 (takes at night)
Co-codamol 30/500	two tablets four times daily as required	160
Lactulose	10 mL as required twice daily	400 mL
Senna tablets	two at night when required	98
Ferrous sulphate tablets	200 mg daily	30
Nitrazepam tablets	5 mg at night	44
Oxybutynin tablets	2.5 mg twice daily	140
PLUS: purchased ibuprofen tablets taken as required.		

medical condition had been obtained from the medical notes at her surgery. These showed that Mrs KW's main medical problems were stable angina and osteoarthritis of the knees (awaiting replacement). She was also being treated for moderate depression and nocturnal urinary frequency.

Q7 Outline the key elements of a pharmaceutical care plan for Mrs KW.
Q8 How would you recommend her medication regimen be rationalised?
Q9 Outline how you could change or withdraw Mrs KW's nitrazepam.
Q10 What additional drug therapy may be indicated for Mrs KW?

During the pharmacist's visit, Mrs KW began to talk more openly about the way she managed her medication. She lived alone and had occasional visits from her son, who was particularly vocal about how she should take her pills. It became apparent that she was quite confused over why she was on *so* many tablets, as they did not make her feel better – in fact, she often felt worse. In a low voice she confessed that constipation in particular bothered her. She felt particularly sluggish and drowsy in the mornings, which in turn meant that she was often late taking her tablets, if she managed to remember at all. She was only taking her fluoxetine intermittently, as she thought they were for when she was a little 'down in the dumps' and they didn't help her sleep anyway! However, her angina appeared to be well controlled as she rarely had to take the little white tablets that 'you have to put under your tongue'. The bottle of GTN looked somewhat aged and had no date of opening visible.

The pharmacist used the opportunity to explain the reasons for taking the medication she had been prescribed, and to discuss the possible significant side-effects. She suggested that Mrs KW take her fluoxetine in the morning, as it was then less likely to disturb her sleep. The need to take it regularly for it to work properly was emphasised. The pharmacist suggested that if she still felt 'down' after 3–4 weeks then she should see her general practitioner (GP) again.

Q11 Why do you think Mrs KW is not taking her medication as directed?
Q12 What are the medicines management options to help Mrs KW remain independent and in her own home?
Q13 Which option would you recommend for Mrs KW?

Week 3 After discussions between the prescribing adviser and GP, Mrs KW's regular repeat medicines were amended in line with the advice from the prescribing adviser.

To give Mrs KW a fresh start with her medication all old medicines were removed from the house and a fresh prescription written so that all the medicines would finish at the same time, thereby allowing rational ordering. The surgery would then also notice any subsequent abnormal ordering patterns. Although this might appear an expensive option in the form of wasted medication, the benefits in terms of keeping Mrs KW safely in her own home significantly outweighed this cost. Items that were no longer taken by Mrs KW were removed from the repeat slip to ensure that she could not order them in error.

The prescribing adviser visited the community pharmacist and discussed Mrs KW's problems and her identified pharmaceutical needs.

Q14 What role can the community pharmacist play in caring for patients like Mrs KW?

The prescribing adviser arranged a follow-up visit to explain the changes to Mrs KW's therapy and to answer any questions that had subsequently occurred to her.

Week 6 A follow-up appointment for Mrs KW showed that her BP was well controlled at 148/85 mmHg. The results of her serum lipid test showed that a statin was indicated (>30% risk over 10 years), but Mrs KW declined and 'informed dissent' was marked in her notes. Her osteoarthritis still troubled her at times, but she felt more in control of her pain and was much happier as she no longer relied on laxatives. She was still considering what to do about her nitrazepam, as she had been on it for 15 years since her husband died. The ferrous sulphate therapy was discontinued as her haemoglobin level was 11.8 g/dL.

Her final list of medication was as follows:

- GTN spray sublingually when required for chest pain
- Aspirin 75 mg orally each morning after breakfast
- Monomax XL 60 mg orally each morning
- Atenolol 100 mg orally each morning
- Fluoxetine 20 mg orally each morning
- Paracetamol 1 g orally four times daily when required for pain
- Codeine phosphate 30 mg one orally when required for severe pain, up to four times daily
- Ibuprofen 5% topical gel
- Senna two orally at night when required for constipation
- Nitrazepam 5 mg orally at night when required to aid sleep
- Oxybutynin SR 5 mg orally each morning

Answers

Is Mrs KW's BP a cause for concern?

A1 Yes. Her BP should be controlled to the level recommended by the NICE hypertension guideline (CG034) for patients with existing coronary heart disease (CHD).

Mrs KW's BP was taken while she was sitting, standing and lying. This was to exclude the possibility of postural hypotension, which can be a cause of dizziness in some patients.

Both her diastolic and systolic BP were considerably higher than the British Hypertension Society, NSF and NICE guidelines; however, abnormal BP readings should be repeated two or three times over a period of a few days to rule out the possibility of anxiety-induced hypertension brought on by the PCV equivalent of 'white coat' syndrome. The target blood pressure for Mrs KW, who is not diabetic but who suffers from ischaemic heart disease (IHD), should be <140/90 mmHg. Patients who are hypertensive and with no other risk factors should only be considered for treatment if their BP is consistently above 160/100 mmHg. The

Quality and Outcomes Framework Audit standard for BP for patients with CHD is <150/90 mmHg.

High systolic BP is an independent risk factor for stroke, and hypertension in general is a major risk factor for worsening CHD and myocardial infarction. Mrs KW is already on a beta-locker for her angina, so suitable choices for additional therapy for someone of her age and ethnicity would be a dihydropyridine calcium-channel blocker (CCB) or a thiazide diuretic. Beta-blockers are no longer recommended as first-line agents for the treatment of hypertension, as they appear to be less effective at reducing the risk of stroke. Angiotensin-converting enzyme inhibitors (ACEIs) are thought not to add significantly to the hypotensive effects of beta-blockers, and also are less effective in older people owing to their less sensitive renin–angiotensin systems, so should not be considered as a first-line addition for Mrs KW. CCBs are well known for their adverse side-effect profile (e.g. headache and angioedema), which can lead to a 20% drop-out rate, so a trial of 2.5 mg bendroflumethiazide would probably be the best initial option. However, if Mrs KW's angina had been poorly controlled a CCB might have been a good option.

Comment on the dose of aspirin.

A2 The dose of aspirin is higher than routinely recommended for CHD prophylaxis.

Aspirin is one of the mainstays of cardiovascular event prophylaxis in patients with IHD; however, it comes with a risk of gastrointestinal side-effects that can be minor, in the form of dyspepsia, or fatal, in the form of a major gastrointestinal bleed in susceptible individuals. The risk in the older person is significantly higher, and IHD is also an independent risk factor for an increased risk of bleeding. In addition, Mrs KW is prescribed a selective serotonin reuptake inhibitor (SSRI), which is another risk factor for gastrointestinal bleeding.

Aspirin-induced gastrointestinal bleeds are known to be dose related, and reducing Mrs KW's dose of aspirin to 75 mg will reduce her risk of bleeding by 40%. Various doses have been studied to try to establish the optimum level required to protect from a cardiovascular event. A meta-analysis of these studies has shown that 75 mg is an effective dose, and therefore considering the risks involved it would be prudent to reduce her dose to 75 mg. The aspirin should be taken once daily, in water and after breakfast, to minimise gastrointestinal irritation and dyspepsia. The use of buffered or enteric-coated formulations has not been shown to be of clinical benefit in reducing gastrointestinal adverse events.

Which medicines could be contributing to her dizziness?

A3 **Co-codamol 30/500, nitrazepam and oxybutynin.**

Dizziness can be caused by a variety of factors, both physiological and pharmacological. As older people are already at increased risk of falling owing to muscle weakness and poor balance, it would be logical to ensure that all avoidable risks are either eliminated or minimised. Postural hypotension can be a problem, but is not so in this case, according to the PCV's report. The cumulative effects of the following three drugs could, however, be contributing to Mrs KW's problems.

(a) **Co-codamol 30/500**. The high dose of codeine prescribed will accumulate in the older person's body due to failing liver function and can cause significant daytime drowsiness, poor coordination and lethargy.

(b) **Nitrazepam**. The role of long-acting benzodiazepines in causing falls and accidents is well documented. This effect is particularly pronounced in the older person owing to the drug's extended half-life and poor elimination. An alternative option would be to try to withdraw Mrs KW's hypnotic gradually or to substitute a shorter-acting drug such as oxazepam, which may not cause the same 'hangover' effects.

(c) **Oxybutynin**. This drug is known to cause cognitive impairment. There are several alternatives to oxybutynin, and trospium is known not to cross the blood–brain barrier; however, switching would not generally be considered a first-line option in Mrs KW's case, unless a direct link had been made between her fall and the initiation of therapy.

Comment on the possible problems associated with purchasing ibuprofen over the counter (OTC).

A4 **Self-medication is of concern in patients with other medical problems, especially when there may be no clinical input if purchasing occurs in outlets such as supermarkets and garages.**

Medicines bought OTC will not generally appear on patients' medication records at the surgery or pharmacy unless it has been previously prescribed by the general practitioner (GP). This can lead to problems of over-medication, interactions, and side-effects that are not attributed to the OTC product.

Ibuprofen, albeit the non-steroidal anti-inflammatory drug (NSAID) with the lowest risk of gastrointestinal side-effects at standard doses, could cause a fatal bleed in a susceptible patient, particularly if taken regularly at high doses. In Mrs KW's case the prescribed aspirin and fluoxetine will also increase her risk of a gastrointestinal bleed. Mrs KW should initially be prescribed simple analgesia such as paracetamol 1000 mg, taken regularly. Further analgesic effect may be achieved by the addition of a topical NSAID which has been shown to be beneficial, particularly for knee and hand osteoarthritis. If Mrs KW's pain cannot be controlled by these options an NSAID may be the answer; however, it should be prescribed under the supervision of her GP, who will need to bear in mind the increased risk of cardiac events associated with the use of diclofenac and cyclo-oxygenase-2 agents. A proton pump inhibitor should also be prescribed to provide cover against gastrointestinal side-effects.

What could explain the varying quantities of Mrs KW's medication?

A5 Erratic ordering, unmatched quantities and non-adherence.

A common explanation is that Mrs KW is ordering unmatched quantities via her repeat prescription slip. Ticking all drugs for reorder, whether or not they are required, is common. An immense amount of work is going on in many surgeries to rationalise repeat prescribing through improved processes and patient education. Unintentional non-adherence can arise from the inability to obtain medicines, or through the patient not managing to take them as instructed owing to difficulties with memory or the packaging. Adherence may also be poor in patients who have not had a discussion with the prescriber about the purpose, benefits and risks of their therapy. Readers may wish to refer to the NICE Clinical Guideline on medicines adherence (CG76, January 2009) for further information and advice around the complexities associated with medicines adherence.

What additional information might be provided through a pharmacist domiciliary visit?

A6 Insight into the patient's attitudes to medication, evidence of hoarding and social issues.

A domiciliary visit has the immediate advantage of assessing the patient in surroundings where they feel more comfortable and at ease. Time is not as limited as in the clinical setting, and patients are generally more open about how they feel and cope with their medication. It is also an opportunity to ask to see where medicines are kept to check storage conditions and to review the quantities being held. Previously unmentioned OTC medicines and herbal/vitamin supplements that may be of clinical significance can also come to light. Social problems may become apparent which can then be passed on to the appropriate agencies for further action.

Outline the key elements of a pharmaceutical care plan for Mrs KW.

A7 **The pharmaceutical care plan should address each of Mrs KW's problems to ensure that positive, patient-centred outcomes are obtained for all of her medical conditions. Key issues include:**

(a) Optimise her medication regimen with respect to frequency of dosing, timing of dosing and continued therapeutic need for each medication.
(b) Ensure that Mrs KW is fully informed about her medication, its basic mode of action and the reason for its prescription.
(c) Review medication that may be causing Mrs KW's problems due to side-effects.
(d) Try to ascertain the cause of her fall and dizziness.
(e) Ensure that medication, where applicable, is producing the desired effect, e.g. pain relief.
(f) Monitor her therapy appropriately.
(g) Question Mrs KW as to her own personal feelings and beliefs about her therapy and counsel her accordingly, in order to help ensure she will be adherent with her therapy.
(h) Identify ways in which she can be supported with her medication taking, so that she can remain independent.
(i) Ensure her medication record is up to date.

In order to support Mrs KW's care should she need to be seen in another care setting, her current medication record should be accurate and up to date. This will ensure that her medicines can be reconciled speedily should she be admitted to hospital. Medicines reconciliation can be summarised as 'a complete list of medicines accurately communicated' and was the topic of the first Technical Patient Safety Solution issued jointly by NICE and the National Patient Safety Agency. The aim of the guidance is to reduce the number of medication-related adverse events and errors that occur when patients move between care settings.

How would you recommend her medication regimen be rationalised?

A8 **The aim will be to simplify the drug regimen to one best suited to Mrs KW and her daily routine.**

Clinically unnecessary medication should be stopped, and dose frequencies that Mrs KW has trouble remembering should be reviewed.

(a) **GTN tablets.** These could be changed to a GTN spray, which will ensure that Mrs KW does not get muddled with more tablets. She will also always have an effective rescue therapy, which is not out of date, in the event of breakthrough chest pain.

(b) **Aspirin**. Reduce the dose to 75 mg daily as discussed in A2.

(c) **Isosorbide mononitrate 20 mg**. An extended-release formulation of once-daily isosorbide mononitrate 60 mg may suit Mrs KW better and ensure that she has a nitrate-free period to avoid nitrate tolerance. Branded prescribing is now recommended in many primary care organisations for sustained-release products, and will ensure that Mrs KW will receive consistent therapy each month from the community pharmacy at an economic cost.

(d) **Atenolol 100 mg**. This dose is correct for the treatment of angina.

(e) **Fluoxetine**. This and other selective SSRIs are known to cause sleep disturbance and therefore should not be taken at night. Mrs KW should be advised to take her medication regularly and in the morning.

(f) **Co-codamol 30/500**. Paracetamol is the recommended treatment for relief of pain due to osteoarthritis, so regular four times daily dosing is the best option. It is generally accepted that multiple dosing for pain relief is not a problem in the majority of patients, as it enables them to manage their pain relief on an individual basis. Removal of regular, and high-dose, codeine from the regimen will significantly help Mrs KW's constipation and would also improve her daytime alertness and wellbeing (see also **A3**).

(g) **Lactulose and senna**. Lactulose is not a first-line treatment for constipation unless the condition is chronic. Adequate fluids, exercise and dietary fibre are the first approach to treating and preventing constipation, with senna used when required for acute episodes.

(h) **Ferrous sulphate**. Iron salts are also known to cause constipation, and at the dose prescribed are unlikely to be of therapeutic value. Withdrawal could be discussed with the GP.

(i) **Nitrazepam**. The use of nitrazepam for Mrs KW's 'insomnia' is of particular concern. Its implication in falls has already been mentioned (see **A3**). It also appears that Mrs KW is getting up in the night for the toilet, so the risk of falling is significantly increased.

(j) **Oxybutynin**. The twice-daily dose could be changed to the once-daily sustained-release formulation.

Outline how you could switch or withdraw Mrs KW's nitrazepam.

A9 **Switching or withdrawal of hypnotics can be successfully achieved, but only with the close collaboration and commitment of the patient.**

Patient education is vital when trying to reduce benzodiazepine use. Mrs KW should be made aware of all the problems associated with benzodiazepine and the benefits of therapy withdrawal. Benefits have been shown to include improved memory (which may improve adherence to her other medicines), better coping skills and increased dexterity. Mrs KW can be reassured that there is no evidence to show a relationship between reduced hypnotic usage and worsened sleep. Education regarding good sleep hygiene, which involves the use of relaxation strategies, hot baths, milky drinks etc., can be provided.

There are two main options: either withdrawal of the nitrazepam in a managed way or by switching to a shorter-acting drug such as oxazepam (equivalent doses are found in the *British National Formulary*), and then withdrawal. The newer 'z' drugs such as zopiclone should not be considered as there is little evidence to show any superiority over traditional benzodiazepines, and they are generally more expensive. As nitrazepam has such a long half-life, a managed gradual reduction in dose over a period of several weeks may be the most suitable option. Mrs KW would need to be fully committed to the reduction plan and regular support from a healthcare professional will be required. This service can be offered by GPs, nurses or community pharmacists, and should if possible be backed up by counselling services.

What additional drug therapy may be indicated for Mrs KW?

A10 A cholesterol-lowering agent and the ACEI ramipril.

Mrs KW's medical records should be checked for results of recent serum lipid tests; however, current guidelines promote the use of lipid-lowering agents for secondary prevention irrespective of serum cholesterol levels. Simvastatin 40 mg should be offered to Mrs KW as an addition to her drug therapy. She could also be advised to try a cardioprotective diet which includes five portions of fruit and vegetables a day, and two portions of oily fish a week.

Following the HOPE trial, ramipril was licensed for the prevention of coronary events in patients over the age of 55 following myocardial infarction or with IHD and one other risk factor (e.g. smoking, hypertension, diabetes). Again, Mrs KW should be fully informed as to the therapeutic options open to her. Ramipril therapy may also help to reduce her BP to target levels; however, if her BP remains high then an additional antihypertensive, as previously discussed, would also be indicated.

Why do you think Mrs KW is not taking her medication as directed?

A11 The reasons are probably multifactorial.

Mrs KW appears to show key signs of non-adherence with her prescribed therapy. She would not be unusual in this, as it is estimated that at least 50% of patients do not take their medication as the prescriber intended, figures for adherence to arthritis and hypertension therapies being 25% and 40%, respectively.

Achieving concordance on what therapies will be taken demands that there is a discussion and perhaps negotiation between the practitioner and the patient that results in agreement about how the patient's condition should be managed. Practitioners must accept that this agreement may not reflect what they consider to be optimal therapy for the individual.

The following factors can affect an individual's adherence:

(a) Satisfaction with the consultation.
(b) Personality and credibility of the practitioner.
(c) Severity of the condition (perceived and actual).
(d) Complexity of regimen.
(e) Effectiveness.
(f) Patient's expectations.
(g) External influences (people).
(h) 'Who cares anyway?'

The first two points reflect the relationship the patient has with the practitioner – in this case her GP – and her previous experiences within the health service. A series of rushed and impersonal appointments at the surgery will not usually give a patient the confidence that she has been treated as an individual, or that her needs have been listened to and understood. These factors will influence the importance Mrs KW places on her treatment and hence the likelihood of her adhering to prescribed medication.

The beliefs of the practitioner are equally important, in that a GP who does not appear to believe in the course of action being prescribed will not engender confidence in the patient that they are doing the right thing.

'Silent' illnesses such as hypertension and hypercholesterolaemia generally lead to lower levels of adherence because the treatments do not result in day-to-day observable benefit, whereas the pain brought on by the angina and osteoarthritis are regular reminders to patients of the consequences of not taking their medication. In such cases a clear explanation about the nature of the problem and its possible long- and short-term consequences is extremely important, as is quantifying any risks in terms that the patient can relate to real life. In addition, the effectiveness of the therapy should be regularly demonstrated to the patient through the sharing of test results and other clinical markers, so that the patient can 'see' progress being made. Results that are not as expected could indicate poor adherence, which could be discussed; or ensure that therapy is regularly reviewed and adjusted by the doctor.

The patient should have realistic expectations about what their therapy is likely to achieve for them. In some cases this will be a total cure, in others a control of symptoms, and in some cases the patient will not physically feel any different at all or may even feel worse as a result of side-effects.

A patient's personal health beliefs and previous successes or failures will also play a role in whether therapy will be adhered to or even accepted.

Influences from external sources, which can include friends, family, the media and the internet, should never be underestimated. Negative comments are much more likely to jeopardise the way a patient feels about their condition or therapy than are positive or corroborative ones.

The patient's self-esteem and the place they hold in society will also affect adherence. A patient who feels that they are not valued, are a burden or a nuisance will have no interest in ensuring their therapy is effective.

It has never been established that levels of adherence can be related to race, gender, intelligence, occupation, income, or cultural background. The relationship between age and adherence is also complex and, contrary to popular belief, some studies have shown that younger people are less adherent than their older counterparts.

The PCV's and pharmacist's conversations with Mrs KW suggested that there had been little communication with her about her condition and treatment options, or if there had been, it had been forgotten or not understood.

What are the medicines management options to help Mrs KW remain independent and in her own home?

A12 **Possible options include a domiciliary carer, help from neighbours/relatives, monitored dose systems and a medication review.**

Using the domiciliary situation as a memory aid should not be underestimated. Tick-box charts on the fridge, tablets next to the kettle or by the toothbrush are useful methods of aiding memory and hence adherence. Help from other people such as neighbours or relatives, or someone supplied by a care agency or social services, could also support Mrs KW and give her the confidence to maintain her independence. Monitored dose systems (e.g. Nomad, Medidose) of various types and quality are available. Supplies of tablets or capsules are dispensed into cells for each specific dose period, or blister-packed into individual dose units. However, it should be remembered that some older people find these foil and blister packs very difficult to manage owing to their reduced manual dexterity and finger strength. All of these systems can help those who get easily muddled with several different types of tablet, but they will not solve problems due to failing memory, also known as poor (mental) capacity.

The value of a medication review has already been discussed.

Which option would you recommend for Mrs KW?

A13 **An easy 'domestic' memory aide that was individually tailored to Mrs KW.**

Following a discussion of the various options with Mrs KW, she considered that a tick-box chart system on her fridge door would help her to remember her medication; it would also ensure that she did not double-dose. Her son would check, weekly, that the system was working.

The idea of using a monitored-dose system (MDS) was ultimately rejected because, once her medication had been rationalised, Mrs KW felt that her own personal systems were less confusing and easier to use.

What role can the community pharmacist play in caring for patients like Mrs KW?

A14 **The community pharmacist is ideally placed to advise on and monitor any problems Mrs KW may have with prescribed medication as well as advise on items she may wish to purchase over the counter. In addition, her regular community pharmacist will be able to carry out a medicines use review (MUR) annually, or more often if a specific problem arises, to confirm that Mrs KW is still managing her medicines appropriately.**

As a result of the above initiatives Mrs KW felt a lot more confident about managing her medication and said that, in future, she would not hesitate to ask her local pharmacist if she had any queries.

All of the information gained and the interventions carried out require the intervening pharmacist, whether from primary or secondary care, to share the relevant information with Mrs KW's usual community pharmacist. Otherwise, there is a significant risk that the new care plans will not be continued as intended.

When the prescribing adviser talked to Mrs KW's local pharmacist she asked if it was possible for Mrs KW's medication to be dispensed in readily distinguishable packaging. For example, a mixture of large and small bottles, cartons, and bold writing for analgesics. They both thought it would be a good idea if Mrs KW was offered an MUR in around 3 or 4 months' time.

Other patients will of course require different solutions to their problems, and the community pharmacist is ideally placed to make a significant contribution. A number of local schemes are already running that have been immensely successful in keeping older people in their own homes and out of costly care homes. One such scheme is the provision of MDSs to suitable clients, paid for by the PCT. Access to this service is through referral from a variety of sources: secondary care, primary care, social services and community pharmacists. The client is visited in their own home by a member of the medicines management team who assesses their pharmaceutical needs according to a standard form. Where appropriate, arrangements are made for an MDS to be supplied by the client's local pharmacy, which is then paid a fee for providing the service. In over 50% of cases referred it has been found that an MDS is either not necessary or unsuitable. Other problems that arise from this visit are dealt with by direct liaison with the GP or community pharmacist. It has been found that direct contact with the prescriber is essential to ensure appropriate action is taken.

PCTs are also using community pharmacists to refer medication issues back to surgeries in a variety of schemes that include recommending aspirin for cardiovascular patients, reporting regimen problems, following up patients on antidepressants by telephone, and managing hypnotic withdrawal.

Further reading

Anon. Medicines management services – why are they so important? *MeReC Bull* 2002; **12**(6).

Clyne W, Blenkinsopp A, Seal R. *A Guide to Medication Review*. National Prescribing Centre, Liverpool, 2008.

Department of Health. *National Service Framework for Coronary Heart Disease*. Department of Health, London, 2000.

Department of Health. *National Service Framework for Older People*. Department of Health, London, 2001.

Ogden J. *Health Psychology: A Textbook*. Open University Press, Buckingham, 1996.

National Pharmaceutical Association. *NSF for Older People: A Guide for Community Pharmacists*. NPA, St Albans, 2002.

National Institute for Health and Clinical Excellence: Clinical Guidelines CG067, CG034, CG059. NICE, London.

National Institute for Health and Clinical Excellence. CG76. *Medicines Adherence. Involving Patients in Decisions about Prescribed Medicines and Supporting Adherence*. NICE, London, 2009.

National Institute for Health and Clinical Excellence: Technical Patient Safety Solution PSG001. *Medicines Reconciliation*. NICE, London, 2007.

National Prescribing Centre. Moving towards personalised medicines management. Improving outcomes for people through the safe and effective use of medicines. Liverpool, 2008. www.npc.co.uk.

Royal Pharmaceutical Society of Great Britain. *RPS ePIC References. Brown Bag and Medication Reviews*. Royal Pharmaceutical Society of Great Britain, London, 2002.

Taylor K, Harding G. *Pharmacy Practice*. Taylor & Francis, London, 2001.

33

Managing medicine risk

Gillian F Cavell

Case study and questions

Day 1 Seventy-four-year-old Mrs MR was admitted to hospital after being referred with frank haematuria by her general practitioner (GP). She had presented to her GP 3 days earlier complaining of increasing confusion and urinary incontinence. A urinary tract infection was suspected for which the GP had prescribed ciprofloxacin 250 mg twice daily. Her past medical history included atrial fibrillation, type 2 diabetes mellitus and osteoporosis. The medication history, documented on the handwritten GP referral letter, included digoxin 0.625 mg daily, warfarin, furosemide 20 mg daily, gliclazide 80 mg twice daily, Tylex two tablets when required for pain, alendronate and Adcal-D3 plus ciprofloxacin 250 mg twice daily. An allergy to penicillin was also noted by the GP.

On examination Mrs MR appeared dehydrated. Her blood pressure was 110/70 mmHg and her pulse was normal at 80 beats per minute (bpm). Her temperature was elevated at 38.5°C. She was noted to be confused and unable to answer questions put to her by the junior doctor. Her serum biochemistry was as follows:

- Sodium 141 mmol/L (reference range 135–145)
- Potassium 3.6 mmol/L (3.5–5)
- Creatinine 128 micromol/L (60–120)
- Random blood glucose 16.5 mmol/L (3.5–10)
- Red blood cells (RBC) 5×10^9/L ($4.5–6.5 \times 10^9$)
- White blood cells (WBC) 15×10^9/L ($4–11 \times 10^9$)
- Haemoglobin 11.8 g/dL (13–18)
- International normalised ratio (INR) 7

An intravenous IV sliding-scale insulin regimen was commenced to reduce her blood glucose level. The furosemide was discontinued. IV fluids were written up as follows: 40 mmol potassium in 1000 mL sodium chloride 0.9% infusion, followed by 1000 mL sodium chloride 0.9% infusion.

Day 2 The pharmacist identified Mrs MR as a newly admitted patient on a medical ward. The following drugs were prescribed on her inpatient prescription chart:

Regular:

- Digoxin 625 micrograms at 0800
- Gliclazide 80 mg at 0800 and 1800, with the instruction to withhold while on sliding-scale insulin
- Alendronate 70 mg at 0800
- Adcal D3 at 1800
- Ciprofloxacin 250 mg 0800 and 2200
- Warfarin with the instruction to withhold

As required:

- Tylex two tablets every 8 hours for pain relief
- Paracetamol two tablets every 6 hours for pain relief

'Once only' doses:

- Vitamin K 1 mg IV stat

The penicillin allergy was appropriately documented on the chart.

Q1 How should the medication history be confirmed?
Q2 Which drugs in Mrs MR's medication history might make her susceptible to pharmaceutical problems?
Q3 Outline a pharmaceutical care plan for Mrs MR.
Q4 Which of the drugs prescribed on the inpatient chart indicates that the patient has an elevated INR?
Q5 What was the most likely cause of Mrs MR's elevated INR?

The patient's prescription was corrected as recommended. Trimethoprim 200 mg twice daily was added to treat her urinary tract infection.

Q6 Comment on the digoxin dose.
Q7 What other changes would you make to Mrs MR's prescription?

When reviewing the IV therapy the pharmacist noted that the potassium infusion had been prepared on the ward by the addition of 40 mmol of potassium chloride to a 1 L infusion of sodium chloride 0.9%.

Q8 What hazards are associated with IV potassium replacement therapy?
Q9 How are the risks associated with the preparation of injectable medicines assessed?
Q10 What risk factors apply to the preparation of an infusion of 40 mmol potassium chloride in sodium chloride 0.9% solution?
Q11 Should concentrated potassium solutions be held in clinical areas?

The pharmacist noted that the alendronate prescription had been signed as given on 2 consecutive days before the prescription had been changed. The patient had been given two doses of 70 mg from her own supply of medicines.

Q12 What are the likely causes of this error?
Q13 Suggest ways in which this type of error might be avoided in future.

Day 3 Mrs MR remained confused and was now refusing to take anything orally. A nasogastric tube was passed to facilitate the administration of oral fluids and medicines.

Q14 What risks are associated with drug administration through enteral feeding lines, and how can they be managed?
Q15 What advice would you give the nurses to facilitate administration of the tablets through the nasogastric tube?

Day 5 Mrs MR was much improved. Her temperature had reduced to 37.2°C and she was much less confused and able to talk to her daughter who came to visit. Her INR had returned to within the target range for thromboprophylaxis in atrial fibrillation (2–3) and warfarin was re-prescribed at her usual maintenance dose.

Q16 How should information about Mrs MR's medication be communicated to her GP?

Answers

How should the medication history be confirmed?

A1 **The medication history should be confirmed by using at least two sources to ensure the information is accurate.**

Although this medication list has been taken directly from a GP letter the information in the letter may not be complete or accurate, and may not reflect what the patient is actually taking. For example, the GP may have written it while in the patient's home, without access to the full medical and prescription notes, or there may have been recent adjustments to the medication regimen that the person writing the letter may not be aware of. The patient may also not be taking the medications as prescribed.

In December 2007 the UK National Patient Safety Agency (NPSA) and NICE issued joint guidance to ensure accurate medicines reconciliation when patients are admitted to hospital in order to avoid unintentional changes to their regular medication. This involves documenting an accurate list of all medications being taken at the time of admission, and should be carried out for every adult admitted to hospital either electively or as an emergency.

A medication history can be confirmed in several ways: interview the patient; identify a list of prescribed medicines from the patient's repeat prescription form; identify a list of prescribed medication from a handwritten or printed card or list the patient may carry; identify the patient's current medication from the patient's own supply if it is available; contact the patient's GP to discuss the current medication regimen and doses. If patients are admitted from a nursing home the home may be contacted to request a faxed copy of the medication administration record or a list of current medication. If the patient has a regular pharmacist this may also provide useful information, as may contacting any clinics the patient attends regularly (e.g. anticoagulant, renal unit etc.).

When patients (or carers) are interviewed about their medicines it is important to make sure that this is done systematically, ideally following a checklist, and that appropriate questions are asked. Many patients consider only oral preparations as medicines, and may not volunteer information about injections, eye drops, creams and ointments, inhalers etc. unless specifically asked. As Mrs MR is confused it would not be appropriate to obtain a medication history from her directly. She (or a relative or carer) may, however, have a copy of a repeat prescription or a list of her current medications. The most appropriate way of confirming the medication history would be to ask Mrs MR's husband to bring in all her medicines and, as she is on warfarin, her yellow anticoagulant booklet. Any outstanding queries can then be clarified by speaking directly to her GP.

Other important information that should be noted from the medication history includes medicines recently discontinued and those recently prescribed. It is also important to determine whether the patient is taking any over-the-counter or herbal medicines that might have relevance to the admission or to future management. If any problems in medicines management are identified during the medicines reconciliation process at admission, for example the need for specific adherence support, these can be noted and addressed in good time before the patient's discharge.

Which drugs in Mrs MR's medication history might make her susceptible to pharmaceutical problems?

A2 Mrs MR is prescribed two drugs which may put her at particular risk of pharmaceutical problems: warfarin and digoxin.

Mrs MR presented with haematuria which, in a patient taking anticoagulants, suggests over-anticoagulation. This is confirmed by her elevated

INR. She is also prescribed digoxin, another drug with a narrow therapeutic index.

Outline a pharmaceutical care plan for Mrs MR.

A3 The pharmaceutical care plan for Mrs MR should include the following:

(a) Ensure that Mrs MR's medication history is accurate and complete.
(b) Ensure all prescriptions are accurate, complete and unambiguous.
(c) Ensure all medicines are prescribed according to the *British National Formulary* prescribing guidelines.
(d) Ensure that allergy documentation is complete.
(e) Monitor the prescription for drug interactions and therapeutic duplication.
(f) Advise medical staff on the appropriate choice of antibiotic.
(g) Provide advice to nursing staff on the safe administration of medicines.
(h) Advise nursing staff of the availability of ready-made potassium-containing infusions.
(i) Provide medication-related information appropriate to the needs of Mrs MR and/or her carers after discharge.

Which of the drugs prescribed on the inpatient chart indicates that the patient has an elevated INR?

A4 Vitamin K therapy is an indicator of over-anticoagulation in patients prescribed warfarin.

Vitamin K is prescribed to adults for coagulopathies associated with hepatic dysfunction and to reverse over-anticoagulation with warfarin. It is therefore a good indicator of either liver disease or problems with warfarin therapy.

Mrs MR had an INR of 7 on admission and has haematuria, possibly as a consequence of the high INR. Warfarin doses have been correctly withheld and 1 mg of vitamin K has been administered to partially reverse the effects of warfarin.

Small doses of vitamin K are used to reduce the risk of haemorrhage without rendering the patient resistant to warfarin. Larger doses of vitamin K (e.g. 10 mg) are often prescribed to treat high INRs due to reduced hepatic synthetic function of clotting factors in liver disease, and may reduce the response to warfarin therapy for a week or more after warfarin is resumed, thereby increasing the risk of subsequent thrombosis.

What was the most likely cause of Mrs MR's elevated INR?

A5 **The elevated INR was most likely to have been caused by an interaction between ciprofloxacin and warfarin. Ciprofloxacin enhances the effects of warfarin, leading to over-anticoagulation.**

This event can be described as a clinically significant prescribing error. A prescribing error has been defined in the UK literature as follows: 'a clinically meaningful prescribing error occurs when, as a result of a prescribing decision or prescription writing process, there is an unintentional significant reduction in the probability of treatment being timely and effective or an increase in the risk of harm when compared with generally accepted practice'.

Prescribing errors often occur as a result of lack of knowledge about the drug or about the patient. Errors can also occur where there is a lack of understanding of how the patient's clinical condition may alter the way the drug is handled by the body, e.g. renally excreted drugs in a patient with renal impairment.

In this instance an incorrect prescribing decision has been made as a result of lack of knowledge of the interaction between warfarin and ciprofloxacin, or the GP and the pharmacist who dispensed the prescription not knowing that the patient was taking warfarin.

Anticoagulants are a therapeutic group of drugs that have been identified by the NPSA as being associated with adverse drug events which have resulted in severe harm or death. Effective communication and appropriate monitoring are essential for the safe use of anticoagulants.

The prescriber should be contacted to advise him of the interaction between ciprofloxacin and warfarin, which may affect the patient's INR when warfarin is restarted. There is also increasing evidence of a link between the use of quinolone antibiotics and the emergence of *Clostridium difficile* infections in patients taking these antibiotics.

A suitable alternative antibiotic according to local microbiology guidelines should be recommended.

Comment on the digoxin dose.

A6 **The digoxin dose is unlikely to be correct, possibly owing to a decimal point error.**

The digoxin dose is written on the GP referral letter as 0.625 mg, which is equivalent to 625 micrograms, which is what the junior doctor has written up. This dose is unlikely to be correct. It is more likely to be a transcription error with a misplaced decimal point.

Tenfold errors with oral drugs in adults are often difficult to make, as it would mean giving the patient five or 10 tablets or capsules, which should appear unusual to a nurse administering a medicine; however, with digoxin it is relatively easy to give this dose without realising an error by using two 250 micrograms tablets and one 125 micrograms tablet.

The error must be corrected immediately, ideally before the patient is given the incorrect dose.

What other changes would you make to Mrs MR's prescription?

A7 The following changes to the prescription should be recommended:

(a) The alendronate dosage frequency should be changed from daily to weekly.

A dose of 70 mg has been prescribed to be administered at 8 am. This should only be given once a week and not within 30 minutes of any other drug. The prescription should be suitably endorsed to ensure the dose is not given every day. It should also be endorsed to ensure it is given at the correct time with respect to food and other prescribed drugs.

(b) The timing of the Adcal-D3 dose should be changed from 8 am to 6 pm.

Adcal D3, used as a calcium and vitamin D supplement, should not be administered at the same time of day as alendronate. Ideally, the calcium supplement should be administered in the evening.

(c) The 'as-required' Tylex should be discontinued and the need for the regular codeine-containing analgesic reviewed.

Tylex is a combination analgesic containing 30 mg codeine phosphate and 500 mg paracetamol (co-codamol 30/500). The indication for regular use is unclear and is likely to be contributing to confusion and constipation in Mrs MR. Mrs MR is also prescribed as-required doses of paracetamol up to the maximum daily dose (4 g). The use of Tylex and paracetamol may result in paracetamol overdosage, especially if the nurses are unaware that Tylex contains paracetamol.

In view of Mrs MR's confusion it would be appropriate to omit the opiates from the analgesic regimen, continuing instead with 1 g paracetamol four times a day. Her pain relief and analgesic requirements should be reassessed in 24–48 hours.

What hazards are associated with IV potassium replacement therapy?

A8 High concentrations of IV potassium administered rapidly can cause fatal cardiac arrhythmias. Such situations can arise as a result of accidental administration of concentrated potassium

solutions, or when concentrated potassium solutions are added to large infusions without adequate mixing during preparation.

Potassium chloride is one of the cocktail of drugs used to carry out the death sentence of convicted criminals in certain parts of the world. There have been reports in the literature of deaths associated with inadvertent use of potassium chloride in hospitals, where ampoules of concentrated potassium solutions have been mistaken for ampoules of sodium chloride 0.9%, Water for Injection or furosemide.

IV administration of concentrated potassium chloride solutions is one of eight 'Never Events' described by the NPSA. Never Events are serious and potentially avoidable patient safety incidents. All hospitals should have effective systems in place to minimise or eliminate the risk of Never Events. In the future, NHS trusts may be liable to pay severe financial penalties if 'Never Events' occur.

How are the risks associated with the preparation of injectable medicines assessed?

A9 **Risks with the preparation of injectable medicines can be assessed using standardised assessment tools which take into account the number and complexity of steps in the preparation of the final product.**

The NPSA uses the following criteria when assessing risks with injectables:

(a) **Therapeutic risk**: where there is a high risk of patient harm if the medicine is not used as intended.
(b) **Use of a concentrate**: if further dilution is required before administration.
(c) **Complex calculation**: for example a double dilution or a complex rate of administration needs to be calculated.
(d) **Complex method**: for example more than five manipulations, or syringe-to-syringe transfer.
(e) **Reconstitution of a powder.**
(f) **Use of multiple or parts of vials or ampoules.**
(g) **Use of a pump with an associated calculation.**
(h) **Use of a non-standard giving set.**

Final products with risk scores >6 are considered to be 'high risk' and steps should be put in place to reduce those risks. Products with risk scores between 3 and 5 are considered to be 'moderate risk' and risk reduction strategies are recommended for these drugs. If the risk score is <3 risk reduction could be considered, but efforts should be focused on products with higher risk scores.

The risk assessment is useful but does not take into account risks associated with incorrect product selection due to look-alike packaging, which should be considered alongside this risk assessment process.

What risk factors apply to the preparation of an infusion of 40 mmol potassium chloride in sodium chloride 0.9% solution?

A10 **The following four risk factors apply to the preparation of solutions containing 40 mmol potassium chloride in sodium chloride 0.9%:**

(a) Therapeutic risk. There is a high risk of patient harm if the medicine is not used as intended.
(b) Use of a concentrate. Dilution of the potassium concentrate available in ampoules is required before its administration.
(c) Use of multiple parts of vials or ampoules.
(d) Use of a pump with an associated calculation.

This gives a risk score of 4, and parenteral potassium administration is therefore classed as 'moderate risk'.

Risk reduction strategies that have been proposed to prevent errors with IV potassium chloride administration include the use of ready-made infusions wherever possible, and standardisation of the prescription of potassium chloride infusions to enable the administration of ready-made infusions.

Should concentrated potassium solutions be held in clinical areas?

A11 **If ready-made infusions containing potassium chloride are available in clinical areas the need for concentrated potassium chloride solutions will be minimised.**

Policies should be available and staff trained to recognise the risks associated with potassium infusions. Clinicians should be trained to prescribe and administer ready-made infusions whenever possible.

What are the likely causes of this error?

A12 **Daily and weekly doses have been confused, possibly as a result of lack of flexibility of the inpatient prescription chart and lack of knowledge of the different formulations of alendronate.**

There are a number of causes of this error. Typically hospital medication administration records do not facilitate the prescribing of intermittent doses. Even if a weekly prescription is intended, there is scope for daily administration of drugs unless the days on which doses should not be given are crossed through on the drug chart to indicate that no dose is due. If the nursing staff are unfamiliar with the usual doses of the medicine or the availability of different formulations of a medicine, the risk of administration of doses each day is compounded. Mrs MR's drug chart had not been reviewed by a pharmacist until after the second dose had been given, and so no endorsement highlighting the need for a weekly dosing regimen had been made.

Mrs MR received the inappropriate dose of alendronate because the product was available on the ward, having been dispensed for another patient. Medicines dispensed by hospital pharmacy departments and stored in medicine trolleys tend to be treated as 'stock' drugs and may be used for more than one patient. The increasing trend towards reuse of patients' own drugs in hospitals and bedside storage of medicines is likely to reduce this tendency to 'share' non-stock drugs between patients.

Fortunately, Mrs MR is unlikely to experience any permanent harm from the overdose, although her serum calcium and phosphate levels should be monitored because of the risk of hypocalcaemia and hypophosphataemia. However, the risks from similar errors with other medicines may be more significant. Confusion between daily and weekly doses of methotrexate and vindesine have resulted in serious patient harm.

Suggest ways in which this type of error might be avoided in future.

A13 **Reporting and then collating error reports in order to develop an understanding of how and why they occur is a way of reducing the incidence of errors. Where errors are known to occur, risks can be identified and solutions put in place.**

This is an example of an error which has resulted from multiple system failures rather than the action of any individual.

In the past, error reporting has tended to focus on the actions of individuals and has been associated with blame and punishment. It is now recognised that errors occur as a result of *active failures* and *latent conditions*. Active failures are unsafe practices of people working within a system. Latent conditions are organisational issues, such as resource allocation, management, environment and processes which, either alone or in combination with an active failure, can result in error. Blaming individuals discourages error reporting, making it difficult for organisations to identify trends in the types of error that occur and hence to understand their risks. By understanding the conditions that may predispose to error, safe systems of work can be developed to reduce future risks. In *An Organisation with a Memory*, the Department of Health highlights the need for the NHS to learn from its mistakes; the NPSA was set up to collect, assimilate and analyse adverse incidents, and to propose solutions to prevent their recurrence.

Although this error is unlikely to result in permanent harm it is an example of an error that should be reported as an adverse incident through the Trust's incident-reporting scheme to the NPSA.

The use of electronic prescribing systems could eliminate this type of error by preventing the daily prescription of a product designed to be prescribed and administered weekly. In the future, electronic prescribing combined with barcode technology, in which the product to be administered is identified by scanning a barcoded prescription and the product's barcode, may be a means of confirming that the product selected is the correct one for the prescription.

Pharmacists have an increasing role in teaching both undergraduate medical students and newly qualified junior doctors so that they understand the risks associated with prescribing, how errors can occur and, most importantly, how they should prescribe to minimise the risks.

What risks are associated with drug administration through enteral feeding lines, and how can they be managed?

A14 **In order to administer drugs safely through enteral feeding lines issues such as formulation, interactions with the feed and method of dose preparation need to be considered.**

Not all formulations intended for oral administration are suitable for crushing for administration via an enteral feeding line. In addition, where patients also have IV access, there is a risk of inadvertent IV administration of oral medicines if an IV syringe is used to prepare the dose.

For oral medicines to be administered through a nasogastric tube they need to be either formulated as a liquid medicine or prepared by crushing and suspending the oral solid dosage forms. Not all solid oral dose forms can be crushed without altering their pharmacokinetic profile. Modified and controlled-release tablets and enteric-coated formulations should not be crushed for administration in this way.

When tablets are suitable for crushing they should be suspended in plenty of water and the tube flushed after administration to prevent it blocking.

Some medicines interact with the feed, possibly reducing drug absorption. Depending on the drug being administered, the feed will need to be discontinued for a while before and after medicines administration.

In hospitals IV syringes have been traditionally used to administer doses of oral medicines to patients via enteral (nasogastric, gastrostomy or jejunostomy) lines, and also to administer doses of liquid medicines which cannot easily be measured in a graduated measuring pot. When oral medicines are drawn up in IV syringes there is a risk of wrong-route errors, that is, inadvertent administration of an oral medicine via the IV route, especially if the patient has an IV access line in place. There have been reports of fatalities as a result of the administration of oral medicines via the IV route.

Increasingly the additive ports on the enteral giving sets are being designed without the Luer connectors that meant that IV syringes had to be used to access the line. Instead, ports incompatible with Luer-tipped IV syringes are being incorporated into enteral giving sets to avert the potentially disastrous consequences of wrong-route errors.

What advice would you give the nurses to facilitate administration of the tablets through the nasogastric tube?

A15 Wherever possible, liquid formulations or soluble tablets of the prescribed medicines should be administered, ideally by using a suitably sized oral syringe. For some drugs differences in the bioavailability between the liquid and the solid dosage forms will need to be considered when the formulation is switched.

For Mrs MR, the digoxin and trimethoprim should be dispensed as the liquid preparations and the prescription endorsed to show that these formulations have been made available. Although digoxin elixir is more bioavailable than the tablets (80% for the liquid, compared to 70% for the tablets) a dosage adjustment is unlikely to be needed unless the patient has significant renal impairment.

A soluble formulation of calcium and vitamin D, such as Adcal D3 effervescent, Cacit D3 effervescent granules or Calfovit D3 sachets, may be substituted for the Adcal D3.

Alendronate tablets cannot be crushed for administration in this way, so alendronate should be withheld until Mrs ME can swallow the tablets whole.

Depending on the outcome of the analgesic review a soluble paracetamol-containing analgesic could be supplied.

The feed should be discontinued before the medicines are administered and the line flushed with 20–30 mL of water using a large – ideally 50 mL – oral syringe. The medicines should be administered one at a time using an oral syringe, with flushing between each one. The line should be finally flushed through prior to restarting the feed.

How should information about Mrs MR's medication be communicated to her GP?

A16 Accurate, complete and timely information about a patient's medication should be transferred to the patient's GP as soon as possible after her discharge. Ideally this should be done electronically.

Medication errors can occur when patients move from one healthcare setting to another. Effective communication is especially important at these stages. On discharge, the patient's new drug regimen and treatment plan need to be communicated in a timely and reliable way to ensure safe and seamless transfer of care back to the primary care team.

When patients move between healthcare settings communication is often slow and incomplete. Delays in communicating information about the discharge medication mean that the information may not be available to the GP when he or she next prescribes for that patient. The patient may then be inadvertently prescribed medicines that are no longer indicated, duplicate drugs, drugs that interact, or even drugs that are contraindicated. This can lead to readmission to hospital with a preventable, drug-related problem.

When Mrs MR is discharged from hospital it is important that changes in her medication are communicated with her GP so that she does not continue to receive the medicines she was prescribed prior to her admission. There is also evidence that communicating with the community pharmacist helps to reduce the incidence of discrepancies between the discharge medication and medication subsequently prescribed by the GP. Ideally this information should be transferred electronically to reduce delays, reduce the risk of transcription errors and help ensure seamless care at the interface.

As Mrs MR is taking warfarin it is essential that arrangements for monitoring her INR are set up before she is discharged, and that she is aware of both her warfarin dose and the arrangements for future blood tests.

Further reading

Cambridgeshire Health Authority. *Methotrexate Toxicity. An Inquiry into the Death of a Cambridgeshire Patient in April 2000*. Cambridgeshire Health Authority, Cambridge, 2000.

Dean B, Barber N, Schachter M. What is a prescribing error? *Qual Health Care* 2000; **9**: 232–237.

Department of Health. *An Organisation with a Memory*. Department of Health, London, 2000.

National Institute for Health and Clinical Excellence. *Technical Patient Safety Solutions for Medicines Reconciliation on Admission of Adults to Hospital*. NICE, London, 2007.

National Patient Safety Agency. Patient Safety Alert 19. *Promoting Safer Measurement and Administration of Liquid Medicine via Oral and other Enteral Routes*. March 2007. Available at: www.npsa.org.uk.

National Patient Safety Agency. *Safety in Doses*. NPSA, London 2007. www.npsa.nhs.uk.

National Patient Safety Agency. *Never Events*. NPSA, London, 2008. www.npsa.nhs.uk.

National Patient Safety Agency. *Patient Safety Alert (PSA01)*. NPSA, London, 2002. www.npsa.nhs.uk.

Phillips J, Beam S, Brinker A *et al*. Retrospective analysis of mortalities associated with medication errors. *Am J Health Syst Pharm* 2001; **58**: 1835–1841.

Index